# Principles and Practice of Surgery

[Books.] other Surgery books.

    (a) BROWSE. — ✓

    (b) Hamilton Bailey.

    (c) Hobbsley.

# Principles and Practice of Surgery

A Surgical Supplement to
*DAVIDSON'S PRINCIPLES AND PRACTICE OF MEDICINE*

## A. P. M. Forrest
MD ChM FRCS(Ed., Eng. & Glas.) HonDSc (University of Wales) HonFACS FRSE
Regius Professor of Clinical Surgery, University of Edinburgh

## D. C. Carter
MD FRCS(Ed. & Glas.)
St Mungo Professor of Surgery, University of Glasgow

## I. B. Macleod
BSc MB ChB FRCS(Ed.)
Consultant Surgeon, Royal Infirmary of Edinburgh

CHURCHILL LIVINGSTONE
EDINBURGH LONDON MELBOURNE AND NEW YORK 1985

CHURCHILL LIVINGSTONE
Medical Division of Longman Group UK Limited

Distributed in the United States of America by
Churchill Livingstone Inc., 1560 Broadway, New York, N.Y.
10036, and by associated companies, branches and representatives throughout the world.

First published 1985
  Reprinted 1985
  Reprinted 1986

0-443-01565-1

British Library Cataloguing in Publication Data

Principles and practice of surgery.
  1. Surgery
  I. Forrest, A. P. M.      II. Carter, D. C.
  III. Macleod, I. B.
  617      RD31

Library of Congress Cataloguing in Publication Data

Main entry under title:
Principles and practice of surgery.
  Companion v. to: Davidson's Principles and practice
of medicine.
  Includes index.
  1. Surgery.   2. Surgery, Operative.   I. Forrest,
A. P. M.   II. Carter, David C.   III. Macleod, I. B.
(Ian Buchanan)   IV. Davidson, Leybourne Stanley
Patrick, Sir, 1894–    . Principles and practice
of medicine.   [DNLM: 1. Surgery.   2. Surgery,
Operative.   WO 100 P9565]
RD31.P85   1984              617              84-9619

Typeset by H Charlesworth & Co Ltd, Huddersfield
Printed in Great Britain by
Clark Constable, Edinburgh and London

# Preface

The need for a 'surgical companion' to *Davidson's Principles and Practices of Medicine* was suggested by Dr John Macleod some years ago. His concept was logical in that the teaching of surgery as an undergraduate discipline should complement that of medicine and requires a strong foundation of medical knowledge. In the event we have compiled a surgical text which although still a companion to Davidson, is complete in itself and will allow the undergraduate to appreciate the medical as well as the surgical implications of the diseases he will encounter in surgical wards.

These are the days of shorter and shorter textbooks of surgery for undergraduates. We make no apology for not attempting to follow the trend. In addition to providing the undergraduate with a reasoned and readable textbook, we hope also to have provided a text which will prove useful to postgraduates studying for the proposed new Part I examination in Surgery in General for the Fellowship of the Royal College of Surgeons of Edinburgh.

Most of this book has been written, cross-checked and rewritten by the three of us. We have been assisted in the chapter on gall bladder and liver by Mr T. V. Taylor, in the chapter on the large intestine by Mr J. Guest and the vascular chapter by Mr M. G. Walker. Chapters on specialist subjects have been contributed by Professor D. J. Wheatley (Surgery of Cardiac Disease and Chest and Mediastinum), Professor E. R. Hitchcock (Principles of Neurosurgery), Professor G. D. Chisholm (Urological Surgery), Dr J. D. Cash (Blood Transfusion) and Mr D. J. Stewart (Thyroid and Parathyroid) who, with Mr. I. M. C. Macintyre, prepared the Appendices. We are grateful to them for allowing us to edit their work stringently so that it conforms to the style of the rest of the book.

Mr Alastair Ritchie and Mr Robert Steele have made a major contribution in helping to plan the illustrations which have been drawn by Mrs Anne McNeill, our medical artist. We have relied greatly on Mrs Janet Wake and Mrs Ann Dunsire (secretarial staff) and wish to acknowledge our indebtedness to them for their patience and forbearance.

1985

A.P.M.F.
D.C.C.
I.B.M.

# Contributors

**J. D. Cash** PhD MB ChB FRCP MRCPath
National Medical Director,
Scottish National Blood Transfusion Service

**G. D. Chisholm** ChM FRCS(Ed., Eng.)
Professor of Surgery,
University of Edinburgh

**J. Guest** MD MB ChB FRCS(Glas.)
Senior Registrar,
Royal Postgraduate Medical School, London

**E. R. Hitchcock** ChM FRCS(Ed., Eng.)
Professor of Neurosurgery,
University of Birmingham

**I. M. C. Macintyre** MB ChB FRCS(Ed.)
Consultant Surgeon,
Leith Hospital, Edinburgh

**D. J. Stewart** ChM MB ChB FRCS(Ed.)
Consultant Surgeon,
Preston Royal Infirmary

**T. V. Taylor** MD ChM FRCS(Ed., Eng.)
Consultant Gastrointestinal Surgeon,
Manchester Royal Infirmary

**M. G. Walker** ChM FRCS(Ed.)
Senior Lecturer in Clinical Surgery,
Ninewells Hospital and Medical School,
Dundee

**D. J. Wheatley** MD ChM FRCS(Ed.)
Professor of Cardiac Surgery,
University of Glasgow

# Contents

# 1. Investigation and Diagnosis of Surgical Problems

The general approach to a patient with a 'surgical condition' differs little from that used in other branches of medicine. However, there are matters of detail and sometimes of timing which are influenced by the particular nature of a surgical disease. Establishment of a clear diagnosis and assessment of the severity and extent of disease are the foundations for rational therapy, which need not necessarily include operation.

The approach may have to be modified if the rate of progress of disease does not allow time to confirm the suspected diagnosis before treatment becomes mandatory. The surgeon must then use his experience and judgement to dictate the course to be followed. For example, approximately 20% of appendices removed on a clinical diagnosis of 'appendicitis' are normal. This figure can be reduced if patients are observed until diagnosis is 'certain', but only at the expense of an increased incidence of perforated appendicitis, peritonitis and even death.

Fundamental to the selection of investigative procedures is a clear definition of the patient's problems based on a detailed history and meticulous clinical examination. Neglect of this principle leads to unnecessary and indiscriminate investigation with inherent risks, discomfort and expense.

Investigations are required not only to confirm the diagnosis but also to monitor the course of the disease and response to therapy. For example, radiology and endoscopy are used to monitor the response of a gastric ulcer to treatment, while serial liver function tests monitor the progress of a patient with obstructive jaundice.

## EXAMINATION OF THE URINE

### ROUTINE ANALYSIS

Analysis of the urine is mandatory on admission to hospital. Recognition that a patient is diabetic is particularly important as metabolic acidosis may develop and seriously influence cardiac performance during anaesthesia. Microscopic examination of the urine may help define the cause of acute abdominal pain e.g. pyelonephritis (pus cells), renal colic (red cells, abnormal crystals) and appendicitis (usually, but not always, clear).

Microscopic examination of the urine may also be used to monitor progress. For example, the number of red cells reflects progress after renal injury while counts of casts can be used to monitor rejection of a kidney transplant.

### SPECIFIC GRAVITY (OSMOLALITY)

Measurement of urine specific gravity is all too often neglected. In the shocked patient who develops oliguria, it will help differentiate acute renal tubular failure from inadequate renal perfusion due to hypovolaemia. The treatment of these two situations is quite different. Measurement of urinary specific gravity can be made on one drop of urine using a portable 'refractometer', which measures total solids.

Measurements of urine osmolality by freezing-point depression is a more sophisticated technique for estimating the total concentration of

1

solids in the urine in patients with complicated fluid and electrolyte problems.

## 24-HOUR COLLECTION

In some instances, 24-hour urine collections are required to determine the excretion of substances including:

1. *Creatinine* to determine creatinine clearance as a test of renal function;

2. *11-hydroxycorticosteroids* and *17-oxosteroids* and *oestrogens* in the diagnosis of adrenocortical hyperactivity;

3. *3-methoxy 4-hydroxy-mandelic acid (VMA)* in the diagnosis of phaeochromocytoma;

4. *5-hydroxyindole acetic acid (5-HIAA)* in the diagnosis and monitoring of the carcinoid syndrome;

5. *Calcium* in suspected hyperparathyroidism or to monitor the progress of metastatic disease of bone;

6. *Porphyrins* so that porphyria may be excluded as a cause of abdominal pain;

7. *Amylase* to estimate amylase clearance relative to that of creatinine in the diagnosis of acute pancreatitis;

8. *Electrolytes* (Na, K, Cl) when complicated problems of fluid balance require estimation of losses from all sources;

9. *Hydroxyproline* (OHP) to monitor progress of metastatic disease in bone.

## EXAMINATION OF THE BLOOD

When a patient comes to hospital for investigation or treatment of a surgical condition, samples of venous blood should be taken *as a routine* for measurement of haematological parameters (haemoglobin concentration, packed cell volume, white cell count), blood urea and serum electrolyte concentration (sodium, potassium and bicarbonate). Routine determination of the ESR is not necessary unless chronic inflammatory, malignant or collagen disease is suspected.

The indications for specific haematological investigation are discussed elsewhere with reference to individual clinical situations. The following general principles should be remembered:

1. The haemoglobin level does not reflect the magnitude of acute haemorrhage as compensatory haemodilution may not be complete for 48 hours. A low haemoglobin in a patient admitted with acute haemorrhage usually signifies chronic blood loss.

2. Patients undergoing routine surgical operations should generally have a haemoglobin level of at least 10 g/100 ml.

Depending on urgency, patients with lower levels should either be transfused or have their anaemia treated before operation.

3. Patients undergoing all but minor surgery should have blood taken for grouping and cross-matching before operation.

4. Patients being treated by intravenous infusion and nasogastric aspiration should have daily determination of plasma urea, sodium, potassium and bicarbonate levels.

5. Patients with chronic or acute respiratory disease who require operation should have respiratory function estimated (FEV1,FVC) arterial blood taken to determine $H^+$ ion concentration and blood gas pressures ($Pa_{O_2}$ $Pa_{CO_2}$), and standard bicarbonate. These investigations should also be performed in patients about to undergo intrathoracic procedures.

6. All patients with a history of jaundice should have serological testing for hepatitis B-associated antigen.

7. Bio-assays employing bacteria (e.g. determination of serum cyanocobalamin [$B_{12}$] and folate) are affected by antibiotics, and should *not* be performed while a patient is receiving antibiotic therapy.

## EXAMINATION OF THE STOOL

Examination of the abdomen is incomplete without digital examination of the rectum (Fig. 1.1). Rectal examination is in turn incomplete without inspection of any faeces on the examining finger and testing for the presence of faecal occult blood. Every rectal tray should carry the appropriate reagents (e.g. Haemoccult test cards).

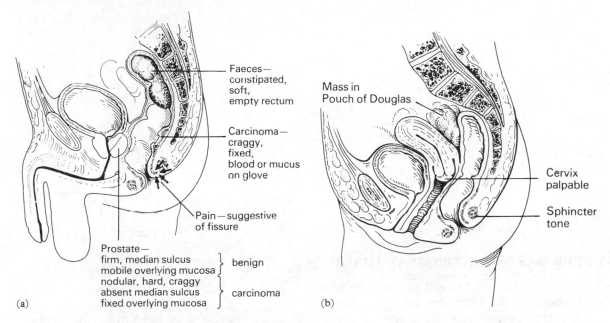

**Fig. 1.1** Possible findings on digital examination of the rectum. (a) Male. (b) Female.

Simple inspection of the stool is helpful in patients with diarrhoea. Slime and obvious blood may point to an inflammatory process, clay-coloured stools to obstructive jaundice; bulky or frothy stools to malabsorption.

Microscopic examination of a fresh specimen of faeces is indicated in patients with diarrhoea. Pus cells, trophozoites, cysts of *Entamoeba histolytica*, and parasites such as *Giardia lamblia* may be found. The presence of undigested meat fibres points to malabsorption. A preponderance of coccal organisms is noted in certain superinfections of the intestine. Bacteriological culture of the stool is essential in the investigation of patients with diarrhoea and in some hospitals is used to select antibiotics for pre-operative colon preparation.

## BACTERIOLOGICAL INVESTIGATIONS

Bacteriological investigations are important in surgical practice.

1. Direct smears and culture of body fluids, tissues, exudates and excreta provide evidence of infection.

2. Assessment of the sensitivity of an infecting organism is necessary for rational antibiotic therapy. Ideally, the administration of antibiotics should be delayed until sensitivities are known. If delay is dangerous, the bacteriologist and clinician select 'blind' therapy to deal with those organisms believed most likely to be causing the infection.

3. From time to time, surgical wards develop a 'run' of infection in operated patients. The bacteriologist can define precisely the type of organism and its sensitivity to antibiotics, and may then trace the source by bacteriological examination of nursing and medical staff, and the ward and theatre environment. The source may prove to be an asymptomatic carrier, a faulty steriliser or a patient with sepsis.

4. Bacteraemia should always be considered as a possible cause of unexplained shock in a surgical patient. Serial blood samples are taken for culture. The optimal timing of these samples relative to temperature elevations is debated. A good rule is to take 3 or 4 samples at one hour intervals. The infecting organism is often a Gram-negative bacillus, and arises most frequently from the urinary tract, biliary tract or large bowel. In a patient with persistent pyrexia following an operation, infection due to the surgical procedure must first be ruled out.

## ENDOSCOPY

Endoscopy is defined as the viewing of the interior of hollow viscera and body cavities by instruments introduced through natural or created orifices. The development of flexible fibreoptic viewing and lighting systems in which the light image is transmitted through thousands of tiny glass fibres, each coated with an opaque medium, has extended the scope, range and diagnostic accuracy of endoscopy. Most endoscopes have facilities for irrigation and suction, tissue biopsy and photography.

### UPPER GASTRO-INTESTINAL TRACT

The first oesophagoscopes and gastroscopes were rigid instruments. Their passage was uncomfortable and general anaesthesia was preferred. Perforation of the oesophagus in the neck or at the entrance to the stomach was a risk. This has been reduced by the introduction of fibreoptic endoscopes. These modern instruments are flexible, have controllable tips and can be swallowed relatively easily under mild sedation and local anaesthesia. However, rigid endoscopes are still used for sigmoidoscopy and cystoscopy, and in some clinics for bronchoscopy and oesophagoscopy.

The following flexible instruments are available:

*Oesophagoscope.* This is end-viewing and rather shorter and thicker than the gastroscope.

*Gastroscope.* This is available in end-viewing or side-viewing forms. The end-viewing instrument is better for all-purpose use, whereas the side-viewing gastroscope allows better inspection of the lesser curvature, particularly in its upper part.

*Gastroduodenoscope.* This is a longer version of the gastroscope which can be negotiated through the pylorus to inspect the duodenum. Using a side-viewing gastroduodenoscope the ampulla of Vater may be cannulated and radio-opaque contrast injected to visualise the common bile duct and pancreatic duct (ERCP: endoscopic retrograde choledocho-pancreatography). (Fig. 1.2). This investigation may be used to define the lower part of the bile duct in patients with

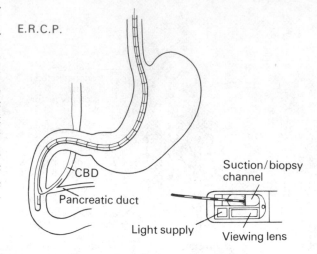

Fig. 1.2 Endoscopic retrograde cholangio-pancreatography (ERCP)

jaundice and is of great value in the investigation of patients with suspected pancreatic disorders. Cytological examination of pancreatic secretions may help in the diagnosis of pancreatic disorders.

*The choledochoscope* may be used to inspect the interior of the bile ducts during operation and to detect residual calculi. Modern instruments have a wider channel which permits the passage of a 'stone catcher' for the removal of retained stones. This may be inserted postoperatively along the drainage track following choledochotomy.

### LOWER GASTRO-INTESTINAL TRACT

*The proctoscope* is a short instrument (10 cm) introduced *per anum* to inspect the anal canal and lower rectum (Fig. 1.3). Haemorrhoids and other lesions of the anal canal, e.g. fissure and carcinoma, can be detected. Haemorrhoids can be injected and tumours biopsied. Proctoscopy is normally undertaken with the patient lying in the left lateral position, with his knees drawn up to his chest. It is always preceded by careful inspection of the perianal area and digital rectal examination. The instrument is well lubricated (KY jelly) and introduced gently so that it passes upwards and forwards in the direction of the anal canal. Painful conditions such as acute fissure-in-ano are associated with marked anal spasm and proctoscopy is usually impossible. In these

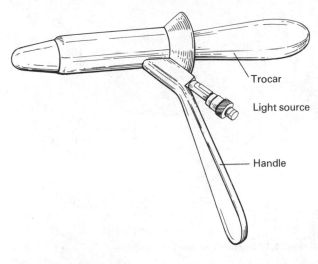

Trocar

Light source

Handle

**Fig. 1.3** Proctoscope

circumstances the examination should be abandoned, and the patient examined subsequently under general anaesthesia. If the patient adopts the knee-elbow position, up to 10 cm of rectum may be visualised through the protoscope. However this position is embarrassing for the patient and seldom used.

*The standard sigmoidoscope* is a rigid steel or plastic instrument, 25–30 cm in length, which is used to inspect the interior of the rectum and lower sigmoid colon. In modern instruments the lighting system is fibreoptic. During inspection of the rectum, the bowel is *gently* distended with air to allow better visualisation of the mucosa.

Sigmoidoscopy is best carried out with the patient in the left lateral position and without special preparation.

Digital rectal examination precedes introduction of the instrument. This relaxes the anal sphincter and determines if the rectum is empty. If the rectum is full of faeces, examination is deferred pending bowel preparation.

The lubricated instrument, with its obturator in place, is passed gently through the sphincter, following the direction of the anal canal for a few centimetres.

It is then directed more posteriorly and the obturator is removed. The eyepiece and insufflator are attached and the instrument is now passed upwards under vision for its full length or until further progress is prevented by a pathological process or an anatomical feature. Negotiation of the pelvic-rectal junction (12–15 cm from the anal verge) can be difficult if there is an acute bend in the bowel and may give rise to excessive patient discomfort. One should not persist if this is the case.

The bowel wall is carefully inspected during slow withdrawal of the instrument, and specially designed forceps can be used to take punch biopsies from a lesion or from the rectal mucosa.

Two sizes of rigid sigmoidoscope are available and flexible fibreoptic sigmoidoscopes are now also in use. If a biopsy has been taken during sigmoidoscopy, the patient must not have any form of enema *including barium examination* for five days. Otherwise there is a definite risk that the forcible distension of the rectum by the enema will perforate the bowel at the biopsy site or result in air or barium embolisation. In some radiological departments barium enemas are not performed for a week after any sigmoidoscopy even when no biopsy has been taken.

The following are noted during examination:

1. general appearance of the mucosa: colour, consistency, signs of inflammation;

2. presence of contact bleeding: in contrast to normal mucosa, inflamed mucosa bleeds if stroked lightly with forceps, a swab, or the edge of the sigmoidoscope;

3. presence of abnormalities such as ulcerating neoplasia;

4. nature of the bowel content: abnormal faeces, the presence of mucus, fresh or altered blood, or pus. These findings may signify pathology beyond the reach of the instrument. If faeces are encountered, a specimen is tested for occult blood;

5. biopsies are taken of obvious abnormalities or, in some instances, of apparently normal mucosa.

Some lesions such as small polyps may be removed completely at sigmoidoscopy. Larger polyps are normally removed under anaesthesia using an *operating sigmoidoscope*. This is a shorter and broader variety of the instrument. Diathermy can be used to fulgurate small mucosal lesions.

The *colonoscope* is a fibreoptic instrument which can be used to inspect the whole of the interior of the large bowel. It is particularly useful in investigation of patients with colonic polyps as these tend to be multiple and are frequently difficult to demonstrate radiologically. Abnormal features may be biopsied, and polyps can be removed for histological examination using a diathermy snare. The procedure requires considerable patience on the part of both the operator and the patient, and meticulous bowel preparation is essential.

## THE PERITONEAL CAVITY

The interior of the peritoneal cavity may be inspected through a *laparoscope*. General anaesthesia is preferred so that the abdominal wall can be relaxed for induction of a pneumoperitoneum. A needle is inserted through the abdominal wall just below the umbilicus and carbon dioxide is delivered through a water seal which acts as a safety-valve to prevent excessive intra-abdominal pressure. The laparoscope is inserted through a small sub-umbilical incision and, by appropriate elevation of the head or foot of the operating table, different parts of the peritoneal cavity are inspected. Structures lying posteriorly cannot be visualised. The examination is particularly useful for:

1. examination of pelvic organs in the female and sterilisation by tubal diathermy;

2. inspection of the liver in jaundiced patients; the detection of multiple hepatic metastases may obviate the need for laparotomy;

3. biopsy of organs under direct vision. This is particularly useful for liver biopsy as the biopsy needle can be directed to areas of obvious pathology (Fig. 1.4).

The procedure is well tolerated, even by frail patients, and is followed by little discomfort. Considerable care is needed in patients who have previously undergone laparotomy. Adhesions limit the view and bowel adherent to the anterior abdominal wall may be perforated during introduction of the instrument.

## THE RESPIRATORY SYSTEM

*The laryngoscope* is a short, curved or straight instrument used to inspect the pharynx and vocal cords. It is used regularly by anaesthetists for passing an endotracheal tube under direct vision.

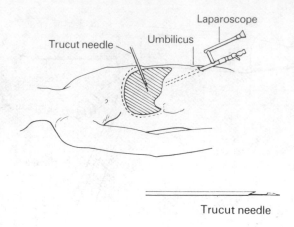

**Fig. 1.4** Laparoscopy and liver biopsy

*The bronchoscope* is used to inspect the trachea and main bronchi either under local or general anaesthesia. A rigid instrument is still preferred by some. Large biopsies can be taken through this instrument and pus can be aspirated from the bronchial tree in patients with post-operative pulmonary collapse or severe chest infection. Flexible fibreoptic bronchoscopes are now available which are smaller than the rigid instruments and allow inspection of smaller bronchi. They may detect more peripheral lesions, but substantial biopsies cannot be obtained (Fig. 1.5).

*The mediastinoscope* is a rigid instrument which is introduced into the mediastinum through a short transverse incision in the suprasternal notch. Mediastinal tissues can be biopsied. The finding of involved mediastinal nodes in a patient with bronchogenic carcinoma may prevent fruitless operation.

*The thoracoscope* is an instrument similar to the laparoscope which is used to visualise the pleural space. Pleural or peripheral lung lesions may be biopsied without recourse to formal thoracotomy.

## THE URINARY SYSTEM

The interior of the bladder may be inspected through a *cystoscope*, a rigid instrument introduced via the urethra (Fig. 1.6). The bladder is subsequently distended with distilled water so

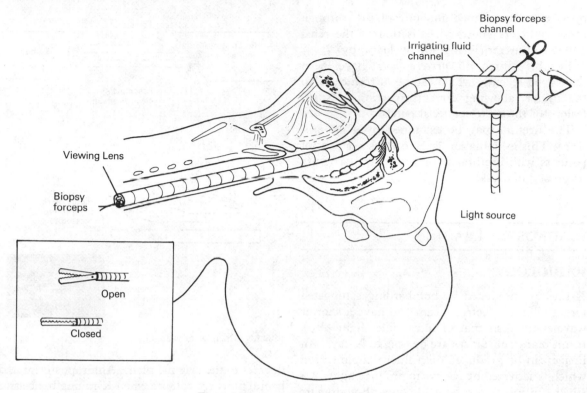

**Fig. 1.5** Fibreoptic bronchoscopic biopsy

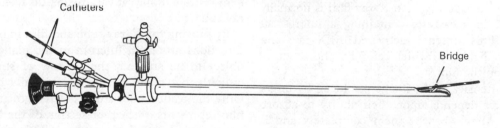

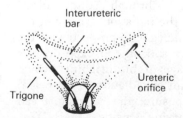

**Fig. 1.6** Cystoscope and ureteric catheterisation

that its entire interior is viewed clearly. Modern cystoscopes have fibreoptic lighting systems which allow excellent illumination without heat. Forceps or diathermy leads can be introduced through the instrument to allow a biopsy or fulguration.

The ureteric orifices are visible at cystoscopy and can be cannulated by fine catheters. Radio-opaque contrast medium introduced through these catheters allows visualisation of the renal pelvis and ureter (retrograde pyelography).

Flexible fibreoptic *ureteroscopes* have been developed recently which can be introduced into the ureter, allowing direct inspection of small lesions of the ureter or renal pelvis.

The urethra may be examined by a *urethroscope*. This examination is used in assessment of patients with urethral trauma, urethral stricture or prostatic disease.

# DIAGNOSTIC IMAGING

## RADIOLOGY

X-rays are produced by bombarding a tungsten target with an electron beam and have a shorter wavelength than that of ultra-violet light. As a result many substances are opaque to X-rays. An image can be produced on a fluoroscopic screen which is activated by X-rays to produce light, or a silver precipitate can be made on a photographic plate or film coated with an emulsion sensitive to both light and X-rays. An X-ray film is normally enclosed in a cassette containing a fluorescent screen. This screen is activated by X-rays and produces light rays which reinforce the action of X-rays on the film.

The intensity of the image produced by target substances depends upon their ability to absorb X-rays. Metal absorbs them completely and is absolutely radiopaque; fat or air are non-absorbent and are therefore completely radiolucent.

Passage of X-rays through solid objects depends not only on the radiation density of the object, but on electromagnetic properties of the X-rays, their quantity and time of exposure. By varying the kilovoltage of his machine (which determines the amount of radiation in the beam) and the time of exposure, the radiologist can visualise tissues of varying densities (Fig.1.7).

### Dimensions

An X-ray plate gives a two-dimensional reproduction of a three-dimensional target so that radiologists frequently take additional films at 90

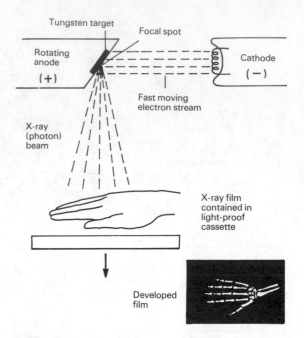

**Fig. 1.7** Principles of radiology

degrees to the original plane. Anteroposterior and lateral films are routine when X-raying bones and chest. Various obliquities of projection help to demonstrate tissues at varying depths from the X-ray tube.

By moving the X-ray tube and film in opposite directions around a fulcrum in the plane of the object to be studied, the shadow of structures outwith that plane can be intentionally blurred. Only the plane under study is left in focus. Each film represents a 'slice' or section of the body or tissue and is called a *tomogram*. This technique has been brought to its ultimate sophistication by computerised transverse axial tomography (see below).

Stereoscopic techniques are also used in radiology. Two pictures are taken by shifting the position of the X-ray tube by a distance equal to that between our eyes. When viewed through a stereoscopic projector, a three-dimensional image is seen. This technique has most commonly been used to detect small linear fractures of the skull but now is being applied to the examination of soft tissues.

Sequential changes to demonstrate moving organs or to study the flow of contrast material can be studied by serial radiographs on rapid

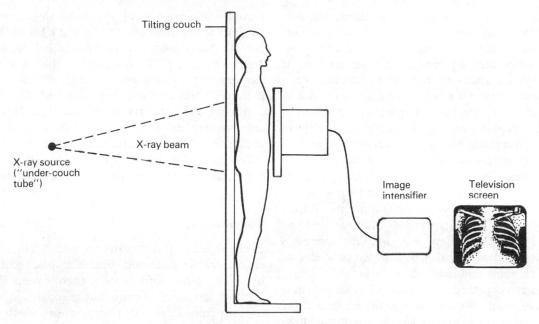

**Fig. 1.8** Modern television screening

change cassettes or by continuous viewing of the image on a fluorescent screen or by television (Fig.1.8). These techniques have proved of particular value in such dynamic investigations as coronary angiography or the study of deglutition.

Radiological investigations expose the patient, radiologist and radiographer to potentially harmful irradiation. Radiation received by staff is monitored constantly by a small badge containing an X-ray film. Protective lead clothing is worn whenever staff are in an exposed situation. The hands of the radiologists are particularly vulnerable and lead gloves are worn when appropriate. The first sign of excessive radiation is vertical ridging and brittleness of the nails, followed by atrophy of the skin, excess keratinisation and fissures.

Protection of the patient is also the responsibility of the radiological staff. They must know which levels of irradiation are safe and the amount of radiation involved in routine investigations. In addition, it is now recommended that elective radiological investigations in women of child-bearing age should be carried out only in the 10 days following menstruation so that irradiation of an unsuspected recently conceived fetus is avoided. This is the 'ten day rule'.

Because of the radiation risk requests for unnecessary radiological investigations must be avoided.

## SPECIAL CONTRAST TECHNIQUES

In plain films the different densities of the body tissues, liquids and contained air provide contrasts between adjoining structures and produce shades of greyness on photographic film. Natural contrasts can be augmented by introduction of air, barium sulphate and media containing iodine into body cavities and hollow viscera, and the oral or parenteral administration of radio-opaque materials which are secreted or excreted in body fluids.

An emulsion of barium is used to examine the alimentary tract and may be swallowed to study the oesophagus, stomach and small intestine or introduced by enema to outline the rectum and colon. Relatively small amounts of barium are used. Accuracy is improved if air is insufflated to distend the organ and spread barium thinly on the mucosa. These 'air contrast' or 'double contrast' examinations allow detection of fine mucosal abnormalities. At some sites distension is possible only if a relaxing agent is administered. For example, air distension of the duodenum requires injection of an anticholinergic agent such as propanthalene (Buscopan) and may reveal abnormalities not shown by routine barium studies. If there is clinical evidence of obstruction or a perforated bowel is suspected barium must not be used. It may initiate complete obstruction or cause dense adhesions in the peritoneal cavity. In these circumstances the water-soluble iodine-containing 'Gastrografin' is preferred.

A variety of other iodine-containing organic chemicals are available for contrast radiology of hollow viscera, ducts and other conduits. Water-soluble compounds specifically filtered and excreted by the kidneys are used for excretion urography, but can also be injected to delineate arteries, veins, sinus tracts or ducts.

Other compounds are prepared in an oily base and are used to visualise lymphatics and those sinus tracts in which only a more viscous medium will remain for sufficient time to be radiographed. Oily media are particularly suitable for lymphangiography as they are trapped by phagocytes in lymph nodes and allow serial X-rays over a period of months. Iodine-containing fluids of varying solubility are available which mix freely with particular body fluids, e.g. joints (arthrography), spinal canal (myelography) or ventricles of the brain (ventriculography).

Compounds containing iodine have been developed which are excreted by the liver. Some are fat-soluble and used to visualise the gall bladder. Other media such as biligrafin are water-soluble and following intravenous injection are excreted directly by the liver and outline the bile ducts (intravenous cholangiography).

## Xero-radiography

Xero-radiography uses a plate consisting of an aluminium sheet coated with a thin layer of positively charged selenium. The charge is retained until the plate is exposed to light or to X-rays, when it leaks out from the exposed areas. The pattern of the charge which remains is determined by the amount of X-radiation which has passed through the part examined and therefore by the radiation-absorbing properties of the tissues. This pattern of the remaining charged particles is made visible by blowing a blue plastic powder containing negatively-charged particles onto the plate. This adheres to the positively charged ions to produce an image which is impressed on plastic-coated paper by heat (Fig. 1.9).

A particular property of the technique is 'edge enhancement' due to heaping-up of powder at lines of differing electrical charge. This makes it particularly suitable for the study of soft tissues, e.g. the breast, and for the detection of foreign bodies.

## Thermography

Every object at a temperature above absolute zero emits infra-red radiation which a may be recorded by an infra-red camera as a thermogram (Fig. 1.10). Thermograms must not be confused with conventional infra-red photographs which are taken with an ordinary camera equipped with filters to remove visible light, and use film sensitive to long-wave light. In infra-red photography the object must be illuminated by an external source whereas a thermogram may be taken in total darkness. An infra-red camera for thermography contains mirrors which focus the infra-red radiation onto a detector. Differences in temperature induce electrical activity which can be displayed on an oscilloscope and photographed. Areas of increased metabolic activity or vascularity are 'warmer' than surrounding areas.

Thermography is non-invasive and records natural body emissions. It has the drawback that the patient must be cooled in a constant ambient temperature for 15 minutes. It has been used for a variety of purposes including detection of breast tumours, determination of tissue viability following trauma or burns, definition of inflammatory lesions and recognition of incompetent communicating veins in patients with varicose veins.

## Computerised axial tomography (CT scanning)

Computerised axial tomography utilizes a slit beam of X-rays which are directed at points on the circumference of a narrow section of the body in the transverse axis. These rays fall sequentially

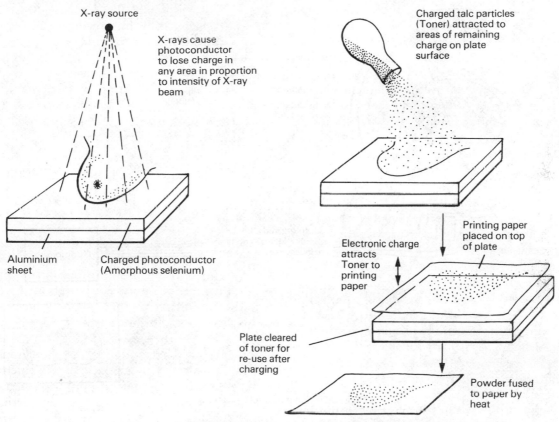

**Fig. 1.9** Principles of xero-radiography

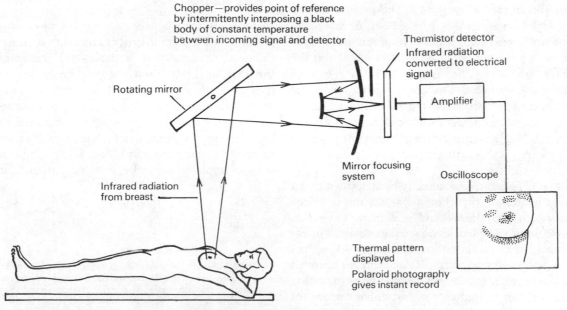

**Fig. 1.10** Principles of thermography

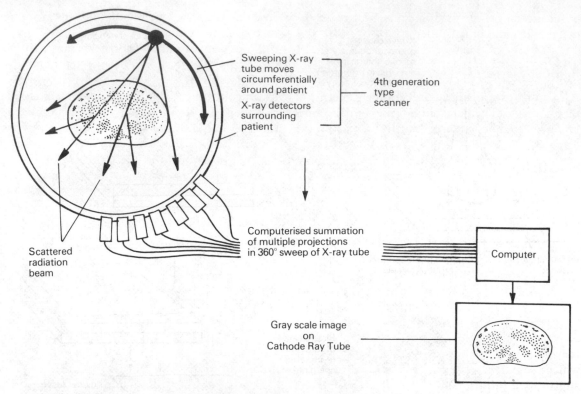

**Fig. 1.11** Principles of CT-scanning

on multiple scintillation crystal detectors with photomultipliers, each of which feeds impulses into a computer to build up a picture of the section being examined (Fig. 1.11). The picture can be displayed on a console, printed out, or stored on tape or disc. The patient is gradually moved through a ring of tubes and detectors so that the whole body can be examined in a series of transverse sections. The dose of radiation to the skin is similar to that received in routine radiology.

CT scans can detect minor differences in tissue density. Resolution is extremely fine, one point on the matrix representing an area of tissue of 0.75 mm × 0.75 mm.

The CT scanner has already been applied to the investigation of intracranial disease, and to examination of the thorax and abdomen. Owing to respiratory and cardiac movement, detail of intrathoracic or intra-abdominal structures is less than of intracranial structures. Resolution is improved by the simultaneous injection of iodine-containing media which produce 'contrast enhancement' of abnormal tissues.

# RADIOACTIVE ISOTOPES AND SCINTISCANS

## Trace studies

Isotopes emitting beta or gamma rays may be used as 'trace' substances in order to measure their non-radioactive counterparts in the body. For example, the size of body fluid compartments may be measured by injecting small amounts of radioactive substances, allowing time for equilibration, counting the isotope concentration and then calculating the total volume in which they are dissolved by the 'dilution principle' (Fig. 1.12). The turnover of radio-isotopically labelled proteins and

$$Q = [S] \ V$$

or

$$V = \frac{Q}{[S]}$$

**Fig. 1.12** The dilution principle. Qs the amount of a substance dissolved in a volume V equals the product of the concentration of the substance [S] and the volume. Q and [S] are known variables. This assumes that the substance is equally distributed and not excreted or metabolised

other substances can give valuable information on metabolism and organ function.

## Scintiscans

As gamma rays penetrate several centimetres of tissue, they can be detected by an external counting device. The counter usually consists of a detector which emits scintillations of light when exposed to gamma radiation. These scintillations are magnified by photo-multiplier circuits and counted or displayed visually. A mobile detector can be used to scan the patient (as in a rectilinear scanner) or multiple detectors can be used in a fixed device (as in the gamma camera). The pattern of isotopic emissions can be printed out on paper or displayed on an oscilloscope screen (Fig. 1.13).

Scintiscans can be used to study the circulation by estimating the flow of an isotopically-labelled substance through an organ or part. However, they are used most widely to visualise organs which selectively concentrate specific isotopes after oral or intravenous administration. The organ is scanned or photographed by the gamma camera and its position and size assessed. Areas of abnormally high or low uptake may point to contained disease. Scintiscanning does not disturb patients unduly.

To prevent radiation damage, isotopes suitable for scintiscanning should be excreted rapidly and have a short life. Thorium (Thorotrast) which was used at one time to outline the cerebral circulation had a half life of millions of years, accumulated in the liver and induced cancer formation.

*Liver scans.* The liver can be visualised by injecting dyes such as [131]I-labelled Rose Bengal which are concentrated by parenchymal cells (hepatocytes), or by injecting colloidal particles such as [99m]Tc-sulphur colloid which are removed by reticulo-endothelial (Kupffer) cells. In normal liver these isotopes are distributed uniformly. Lesions within the liver appear as areas of diminished uptake but must be at least 2 cm in size to be demonstrated. Liver scintiscans have a false-negative rate of 25%.

Simultaneous liver and lung scans may be used to demonstrate a subphrenic abscess by revealing a gap between the upper margin of liver and lower margin of lung.

*Pancreatic scans.* Methionine labelled with [75]Se is taken up by acinar cells and has been used for pancreatic scintiscanning. Accuracy is too low to justify its use.

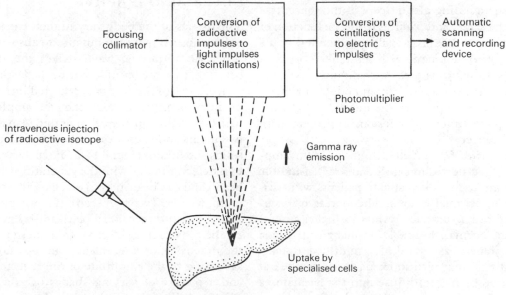

**Fig. 1.13** Principles of scintiscans

*Lung scans.* Two types of lung scan are used. In 'perfusion scans', micro-aggregates of serum albumin labelled with $^{131}$I or $^{99m}$Tc (technetium 99m) are injected intravenously to outline the pulmonary circulation. In 'ventilation scans' radioactive $^{133}$Xe is inhaled to outline the bronchi and alveoli. An area of diminished uptake on the perfusion scan may indicate pulmonary embolus. Post-operative atelectasis diminishes both perfusion and ventilation and produces an abnormality on both scans. A ventilation scan should be performed whenever interpretation of a perfusion scan is in doubt.

*Thyroid scans.* Radioactive isotopes of iodine ($^{131}$I and $^{125}$I) are trapped selectively by thyroid acinar cells. The determination of uptake by the gland related to its concentration in the blood and excretion in the urine was once the basis of thyroid function tests. This approach has been replaced by biochemical estimation of circulating thyroid hormone levels in peripheral blood.

Thyroid scanning is still used to detect localised increased or decreased uptake in patients with palpable thyroid nodules. However, radio-iodine has now been superseded by $^{99m}$Tc-sodium pertechnicate which is also taken up by the iodine-trapping mechanism but is easier to prepare, and exposes the patient to a lower dose of irradiation. The nodules are described as 'hot' if the isotopes are taken up to a greater degree than in the surrounding gland, 'cool' if the concentration is the same, and 'cold' if less. The function of a palpable nodule is a valuable pointer to its pathology. A hot nodule is most likely to be a benign adenoma, whereas a cold nodule is likely to be a cyst, degenerate benign nodule or cancer.

Total body scans after the injection of $^{131}$I are used to detect metastatic lesions in patients with thyroid cancer.

*Brain scans.* $^{131}$I-labelled human serum albumin, $^{99m}$Tc-pertechnicate and $^{113m}$In-indium chelate are used to investigate patients with suspected intracranial lesions. The increased vascularity of brain tumours results in higher uptake than in normal brain. Non-malignant cystic lesions appear as areas of diminished uptake. Haematomas may also show increased uptake but as the isotope has to diffuse into the haematoma and activity appears more slowly than in tumours.

Serial scans may differentiate between the two. Brain scintiscans have now been superseded by CT scans (see page 291).

*Skeletal scintiscans.* Increased turnover of bone minerals in areas of osteoblastic activity can be demonstrated by scintiscans following intravenous injection of bone-seeking isotopes. $^{18}$Fluorine, $^{85}$strontium and $^{47}$calcium were initially used but technetium $^{99m}$Tc-labelled diphosphonates and polyphosphates are now preferred.

Bone scanning is used mainly to detect bone metastases. The osteoblastic activity surrounding these metastases may be detected several months before radiological change. Areas of increased uptake may also be seen in Paget's disease, in arthritis and other degenerative conditions and at fracture sites.

*Venous thrombosis.* The early detection of deep venous thrombosis is facilitated by scintiscanning of the legs after intravenous injection of $^{125}$I-labelled fibrinogen. This is administered before operation and the legs are scanned daily for 7–10 days. As venous thrombosis forms it incorporates labelled fibrinogen and produces a localised hot spot. Prevention of deep venous thrombosis is more important than early detection and this technique has proved useful in assessing the value of prophylactic regimes.

## ULTRASONOGRAPHY

The tissues of the body vary in their capacity not only to absorb radiation but also to absorb sound. When an ultrasonic wave strikes the interface between two media of differing acoustic impedance, some of the energy is reflected into the first medium as an ultrasonic echo, the amplitude of which depends on the relative impedance of the two media and is greatest at the interface between solids and liquids (Fig. 1.14). The echo is recorded by a detector in line with the generating ultrasonic beam, and can be displayed on an oscilloscope as a unidimensional wave (A scan). If a sweeping beam is used a two-dimensional black and white picture can be constructed (B scan). In modern machines the intensity of the image can be modulated according to the amplitude of the reflected wave, and a picture of varying shades of grey can be produced. This is called *grey-scale ultrasound.*

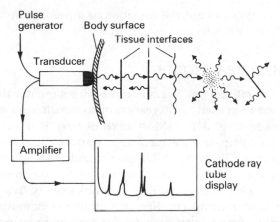

**Fig. 1.14** Principles of ultrasonography

Multiple generators and detectors in different planes can be used to construct an ultrasonic tomogram. In some sites, e.g. the pancreas, the image rivals the quality of CT scanning.

Ultrasound is non-invasive, carries no radiation risk, and has high resolution. In surgical practice, it has been used most commonly to determine whether a mass is solid or cystic. The progress of pancreatic cysts, deep-seated abscesses or an aortic aneurysm can be followed by serial examinations. Ultrasonography is also used to detect displacement of the falx cerebri by space-occupying intracranial lesions. Other uses include scanning the liver for metastases, monitoring the fetus *in utero* and defining intracardiac anatomy.

Ultrasonic flow meters have been developed which function on the Doppler principle. Movement of the red cells causes a shift in the frequency of the reflected signal from their interface with fluid blood. Transcutaneous flow meters are available which consist of an ultrasonic transmitter, a receiver, an audio-amplifier and loudspeakers (Fig. 1.15). When the transducer (which contains transmitter and receiver) is placed over a vein, venous flow is audible. In obstruction there is silence. In the normal limb, squeezing the leg distal to the transducer augments the venous flow and causes a roar from the loud-speaker, indicating patency of the vein. A similar system is used to study flow in peripheral arteries.

A sophisticated form of ultrasonography is used in echocardiography to obtain a time-based tracing of movements within the heart. The reflection of the moving valves and chamber walls

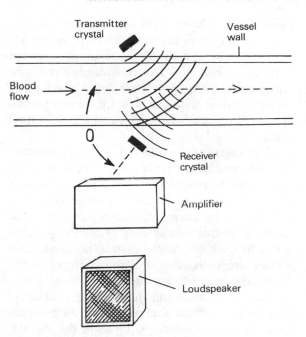

**Fig. 1.15** The Doppler principle applied to measurement of flow

can be printed out in grey-scale fashion, and intracardiac lesions can be defined.

## BIOPSIES

In many situations a sample of tissue must be obtained for histopathological or biochemical examination before a definitive diagnosis can be made. This is particularly important in the differentiation between benign and malignant disease, and in the liver or kidney where diseases of different aetiology can produce similar alterations in form or function.

### CYTOLOGY

Cytology refers to the examination of architecture of cells while histopathology denotes examination of the architecture of tissue and its cellular components.

Two main methods are used to obtain cells for examination:

*Exfoliative cytology.* Cells shed by epithelial linings of hollow viscera or ducts can be separated from secretions or excretions and examined for abnormalities. As the cells are suspended individually or in clumps the recognition of abnormalities rests on examining cellular as opposed to tissue morphology and considerable skill and experience is required. Exfoliative cytology is readily applied to disease of the upper gastrointestinal, respiratory, urinary and female genital tracts.

*Needle-aspiration cytology.* Cytological examination of a needle aspirate can aid diagnosis. A 1.5 mm needle is attached to a syringe and inserted into the tissue to be sampled. Suction is applied and the needle advanced several times through the tissue so that a small drop of cellular material is drawn into the needle shaft. The needle and syringe are withdrawn and the contents of the needle are smeared on a slide (Fig. 1.16).

Apart from obtaining material for cytological examination, needle aspiration can differentiate cystic from solid swellings. Cysts of the thyroid, breast and kidney can be readily distinguished from solid tumours and operation avoided. Radiological screening with X-rays or ultrasonic scanning can aid the direction of a needle into a deep-seated lesion.

## HISTOPATHOLOGY

*Needle biopsy.* Various types of hollow needle have been used for 50 years to obtain small cores of tissue (Fig. 1.17). Most needles have a trocar, cutting tip and mechanism to retrieve the tissue sample. The Vim-Silverman needle, Menghini needle and Travenol Tru-cut needle are good examples and are used to obtain biopsies of liver, kidney and muscle. Specially designed cannulas with cutting edges are used for bone and marrow biopsies.

*Drill biopsy.* Modern drill biopsy apparatus consists of a small sharp cannula attached to a high-speed compressed air drill which rotates at 15–20 000 rpm. The technique is cumbersome and noisy.

*Punch biopsy.* Punch biopsy forceps are available for removing pieces of tissue from skin tumours and from lesions within the mouth or

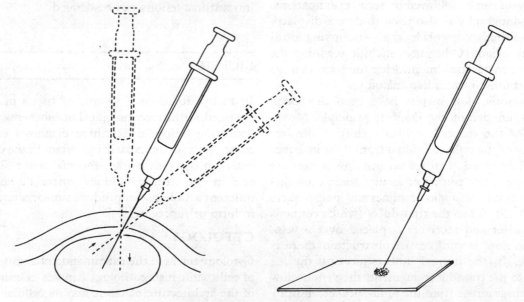

Fig. 1.16 Needle aspiration cytology

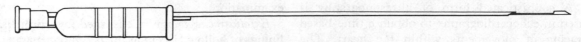

Fig. 1.17 Trucut biopsy needle

nose. Small punch biopsy forceps can be passed through endoscopes and have been used to obtain tissue samples from the gastro-intestinal tract, the urinary system and the bronchi. Forceps have been miniaturised to allow use through fibreoptic endoscopes and biopsies can now be obtained from any part of the gastro-intestinal tract, from within the bile ducts and from the lungs (Fig. 1.5). As these biopsies are small, multiple samples should always be taken, otherwise the true nature of a lesion may be missed.

*Crosby capsule biopsy*. This instrument is used to biopsy small bowel mucosa and is particularly valuable in the investigation of malabsorption. The Crosby capsule is a small metal cylinder containing a biopsy channel and a guillotine. It is attached to fine tubing through which suction can be applied (Fig. 1.18). It is swallowed by the patient and its position monitored radiologically. When the capsule is in the desired position suction is applied to the tube. This draws a portion of mucosa into the capsule which is snipped off and retained by the guillotine. The capsule is withdrawn slowly by traction on the suction tube. Alternatively, the tubing is cut and the capsule recovered from the faeces.

Modifications of this capsule allow biopsy specimens to be sucked up the tube so that multiple biopsies from different sites can be obtained.

*Open biopsy*. Open operation may be necessary if the site is otherwise inaccessible, if closed methods are thought dangerous, or if a large piece of tumour is required. The biopsy may be obtained by incision (cutting into the tissue to obtain a sample) or excision (removing the whole of the abnormal tissue). Immediate histological examination by frozen section technique is used when diagnosis is required urgently.

## SURGICAL EXPLORATION

In some patients it is necessary to resort to formal exploratory operation to establish the presence, extent and nature of disease. This is not an admission of diagnostic failure, and when used appropriately may save the patient numerous expensive and painful investigations. Further, the operative findings and immediate histological diagnosis may allow the conversion of an exploratory procedure into a therapeutic one. A special example is the *staging laparotomy* carried out in patients with lymphoma to establish the extent of the disease and allow more appropriate treatment.

## POPULATION SCREENING

The screening of normal populations of men and women for early disease has been used in this country to detect malignant disease of uterine cervix, lung and breast. In Japan, cancer of the stomach is common and the screening of normal persons by radiology and endoscopy has achieved early detection of this cancer and may have reduced mortality.

Screening methods should be inexpensive, fully acceptable to the patient and preferably non-invasive. They should detect over 90% of established lesions, and false-positive rates must be low. Screening is only applicable when the disease is sufficiently common to justify the expenditure of money and manpower, a requirement which may be met if 'high risk' groups are defined. Before screening is applied widely, there should be proof that earlier detection improves the prog-

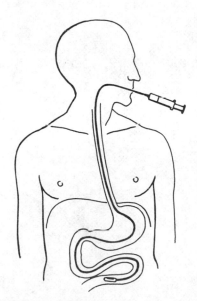

**Fig. 1.18** Crosby capsule

nosis of the disease in question. Large controlled randomised studies of population screening are usually required.

## TESTS OF FUNCTION

The techniques described are mainly concerned with the detection of anatomical abnormalities. Many disease processes do not produce anatomical change, but result in aberrations of function.

These can be detected by tests of organ and tissue function.

Simplest are the range of biochemical tests commonly used in the initial investigation of a patient — 'the biochemical profile'. Estimates of plasma urea and creatinine reflect renal function; of albumin, bilirubin and liver enzymes hepatic function; of electrolytes general metabolic functions. Some tests reflect the function of several tissues. For example, a raised alkaline phosphatase may be caused by disease of liver, bone or intestinal tract.

Such tests are based on the synthetic, secretory, absorptive or excretory functions of organs which in special circumstances can now be studied by a wide range of complex biochemical investigations.

Many organs and tissues have other than biochemical functions. For example the gastro-intestinal tract displays motor activity; a nerve conducts impulse; a muscle contracts. Intraluminal pressure measurements; the recording of electrical impulses, and the study of the effect of stimuli are all used to study disease processes. Many of these sophisticated techniques have originated in the physiological and clinical research laboratory, and should be applied clinically only when proven to be safe and to give valid information.

Details of the use of these and other investigative procedures in specific disease are given elsewhere.

# 2. Pre-Operative Assessment

Pre-operative assessment and preparation is an essential part of a surgical procedure. Elective operations should be carried out under optimal conditions with full physical and psychological preparation of the patient, who should be adequately informed of the reason for the operation, its nature and its implications. In emergency situations this may not be possible and an operation may have to be performed in less than ideal circumstances (see p.43).

## OUTPATIENT VISIT

Assessment and preparation begin at the first outpatient consultation. A good referral letter from the general practitioner is invaluable, providing an assessment based on a long professional relationship between family doctor and patient.

The first responsibility of the consulting surgeon is to reach a likely diagnosis, obtained by careful history, detailed physical examination and the results of investigations. Many of these can be carried out as an outpatient; but some require admission to hospital.

A decision to recommend operation is made once the cause of the patient's problem has been diagnosed and it is known to be amenable to surgical treatment. The patient must be fully informed of the nature of his illness, the reason for operation and its implications. The surgeon should indicate the likely duration of stay in hospital, the period of convalescence and the time of absence from work or household duties. The likelihood of residual deformity and disability e.g.

from an amputation or artificial stoma should be discussed frankly from the outset.

By the end of his outpatient visits the patient should be fully aware of what lies ahead. He will appreciate an estimate of the date of admission so that he can make appropriate arrangements.

The surgeon should write to the general practitioner after every outpatient visit to keep him informed of progress.

## FITNESS FOR OPERATION

### The pre-admission clinic

In most hospitals the house surgeon is primarily responsible for recording a full history and clinical findings in the patient's case notes. This serves as a data base and defines secondary problems which merit consideration. In addition, fitness for anaesthesia and operation must be carefully assessed. These duties are ideally performed in a 'pre-admission' outpatient clinic held some days before the admission date. The patient can then be admitted to the ward on the night before operation with all necessary investigations completed.

The following enquiries are routine:

*Fitness for anaesthesia.* Disease which increases the risk of anaesthesia and surgery should come to light during systematic enquiry. The patient must be questioned specifically about the use of drugs, notably steroids, insulin, thyroid medication, digitalis, diuretics, antihypertensive drugs, anticoagulants, bronchodilators, antibiotics and psychotropic agents. Women of child-bearing age should be asked whether they are taking the contraceptive pill. Particular attention is paid to a history of past cardiovascular, respiratory or renal disorders. Postoperative myocardial infarcts are more common in those with a history of previous infarcts, respiratory or renal problems in those known to have chronic respiratory or renal disease.

*Allergies and hypersensitivity.* Sensitivity to elastoplast and penicillin are common and must be recorded. Knowledge of sensitivity to iodine-containing compounds is essential as radiological investigations using contrast media may be performed and, in sensitive patients, can have fatal consequences.

*Previous operative and anaesthetic experience.* A specific enquiry must be made about previous operations and any complications, particularly chest, cardiac or renal, venous thrombosis, jaundice or infections. A history of unexplained jaundice or renal damage following halogenated hydrocarbons (e.g. halothane) or apnoea following muscle relaxants may influence the choice of anaesthetic agents. The case notes from previous admissions must be read in their entirety.

*Alcohol and drug abuse.* Possible abuse of alcohol and psychotropic drugs must be recorded. These can affect the tolerance to anaesthetic agents and lead to difficulty in inducing and maintaining anaesthesia. If chronic intake of these agents has led to drug dependence, withdrawal symptoms can be anticipated in the postoperative period.

## Smoking

Cigarette smoking is associated with a major increase in postoperative chest complications. All patients should be encouraged to stop smoking once the decision to operate has been made. The longer the interval between stopping smoking and operation, the lower the risk of postoperative problems.

## PHYSICAL ASSESSMENT

*General metabolic status.* The patient's weight is recorded. Ideally, height should also be recorded; the dose of some drugs is determined by surface area rather than weight. Emaciated malnourished patients withstand surgery poorly: the serum albumin and total protein levels are measured. If necessary, nutritional status can be improved by pre-operative dietary supplements, nasogastric tube feeding, parenteral nutrition (see ch. 4).

The obese patient presents many problems. Venepuncture and intravenous infusions are more difficult; landmarks are obscured; surgical exposure is tedious; postoperative respiratory problems are common; and the risks of thrombo-embolism, wound infection and wound dehiscence are increased. Unless operation is urgent, it should be postponed pending substantial weight reduction.

Fluid and electrolyte disturbances are more common in emergency situations but all patients undergoing elective surgery should be assessed for evidence of dehydration or overhydration (ankle or sacral oedema, pulmonary crepitations) including determination of blood urea and electrolyte levels.

*Haematology.* Routine operations should generally not be carried out if the haemoglobin concentration is less than 10 g per 100 ml. Such patients should either be transfused prior to surgery or the operation postponed until anaemia has been corrected. Patients having major operations should have their blood group determined and a minimum of two units of blood cross-matched in readiness for transfusion during the operation. Some procedures, e.g. open-heart surgery, will require more. A coagulation screen is performed if:

1. there is a history of previous bleeding disorder or of undue bleeding at a previous operation;
2. the patient has received cytotoxic chemotherapy or drugs affecting coagulation;
3. there is acute or chronic liver disease;
4. there is evidence of purpura or spontaneous bruising.

*Cardiovascular system.* Pulse rate and blood pressure must be recorded. Arrhythmias and hypertension usually require control as general anaesthesia may induce dangerous vasomotor responses. A catecholamine-secreting tumour (phaeochromocytoma) can be associated with fatal collapse which may occur during anaesthesia and surgery. The young hypertensive patient must be fully investigated.

Heart size and sounds are assessed clinically

and a pre-operative chest X-ray is examined for abnormalities of the size and shape of the heart. Auscultation of the lungs, examination of the neck veins, determination of liver size and examination of the ankles and sacrum for oedema are routine to detect incipient cardiac failure.

All patients over the age of 55 years should have an ECG performed. Postoperative myocardial infarcts are more common in those whose pre-operative ECG shows ischaemic changes. Changes in a postoperative ECG cannot be taken to indicate a recent myocardial infarction unless a pre-operative ECG is also seen.

*Respiratory system.* A postero-anterior radiograph of the chest is routine. Additional lateral views and tomograms may be required if it is abnormal. If there is a productive cough, a specimen of sputum is sent for bacteriological examination. Copious purulent sputum in chronic bronchitis or other forms of respiratory disease require full preoperative assessment and treatment (see p.50).

*Hepatic function.* All jaundiced patients and those with a previous history of liver disease, hepatomegaly, splenomegaly or high alcohol intake require tests of liver function, testing for circulating hepatitis B-associated antigen and a coagulation screen (including prothrombin time).

*Urinary system.* Postoperative urinary retention can be anticipated in male patients with prostatic hyperplasia. In all elderly males prostatic size is checked on rectal examination and bladder distension excluded by abdominal palpation and percussion. Suspected chronic retention of urine (i.e. incomplete emptying of the bladder) should be investigated pre-operatively.

Plasma urea and creatinine concentrations are a useful but insensitive screening test of renal function. Suspicion of renal disease demands more sensitive tests e.g. creatinine clearance. A sample of urine must always be tested by 'dipstick' before operation for sugar, ketones, bilirubin, urobilinogen and blood. Urine microscopy and culture are indicated if there is any suspicion of urinary tract infection or haematuria.

# ADMISSION TO HOSPITAL

Many hospitals now have admission departments where basic information such as the patient's name, address, date of birth, religion, occupation, next of kin, the general practitioner's name and address are documented in the patient's case folder. The patient should have received a booklet explaining hospital procedure. Once the documentation is complete he or she is admitted to the ward.

On arrival, the house surgeon checks that the patient's notes are complete, and that the results of pre-operative investigations have been received. He should explain again to the patient the nature of the operation and the risks and problems involved, and see that the consent form is completed. Arrangements are made to inform the relatives about the diagnosis, the operation to be performed and its likely outcome. This is mandatory in all serious diseases.

Finally the house surgeon ensures that all is ready for the final check in the pre-operative procedure: the pre-operative ward round. In some wards a pre-operative check list is used (Fig.2.1).

# THE PREOPERATIVE WARD ROUND

On the day before surgery the surgeon, his medical staff, and a member of the ward nursing staff visit the patient.

*Final examination of the patient.* The surgeon re-examines the patient, to confirm previous findings and to ensure that the proposed operative procedure is correct. In the case of unilateral conditions, e.g. hernia, breast lumps, or varicose veins, the operation side is marked with an indelible marker. The patient's records are checked to make certain that all essential investigations have been completed and that blood is available for transfusion during or after operation.

*Instructions to the medical staff.* The need for pre-operative intravenous infusion is discussed. In many cases, an infusion is not established until the patient arrives in theatre. Urethral catheteri-

PRE-OPERATIVE CHECK LIST

To be completed on pre-operative day

Name _____

Diagnosis _____

Operation scheduled _____

CVS _____

RS _____

BP _____ mmHg

|  | normal | abnormal |
|---|---|---|
| Urinalysis | ☐ | _____ |

| Chest X-ray (tick if taken) ☐ | ECG (tick if taken) ☐ | Hb (g%) ☐ |

...........................................................................

Units blood crossmatched    none ☐    number ☐

Consent form completed ☐

Other instructions _____

_____ Signed _____

**Fig. 2.1** Pre-operative check list

sation may be required, e.g. in pelvic operations. If possible this should be delayed until the patient has been anaesthetised.

When per-operative radiology is required (e.g. operative cholangiography during gall bladder surgery), the radiology department should be informed so that facilities are available at the desired time. If an immediate pathological report on a specimen is likely to be required, the requisite pathology form should be completed and the pathologist informed.

*Discussion of procedures.* At the pre-operative round the surgeon will discuss the plan of the operation and particular points in the postoperative care of the patient. Particular requirements during operation are communicated to the theatre staff.

*Instructions to the nursing staff.* The nursing staff are responsible for several standard pre-operative procedures. For example, they remove dentures, rings and other jewellery, administer the premedication and fix a plastic wrist band around the patients wrist indicating name, religion, dose and time of administering premedication. An orderly is usually responsible for washing and shaving the operation site if required. These duties may require modification in the light of particular problems brought to light at the pre-operative round.

To prevent risk of aspiration of vomitus during

induction of anaesthesia, patients undergoing general anaesthesia should take no food from 6.00 pm and no fluids from 9.00 pm on the day before surgery. If operation is scheduled for late afternoon (after 3.00 pm) a cup of tea is permitted on the morning of operation.

Many surgeons recommend the routine passage of a nasogastric tube in patients undergoing gastro-intestinal surgery. This is passed two hours before operation unless there is a history of gastric retention when it should be inserted for a few days before operation.

If the operation involves the large bowel, the surgeon will enquire about the success of the preparation.

The patient's drug chart is checked and essential medication prescribed. Problems such as diabetes and impaired coagulation require special attention (see ch. 5).

A fluid balance chart is commenced before all major operations and in all patients with abnormalities of fluid and electrolyte balance.

When all preparations have been checked, the surgeon has a final word with the patient, to reassure and allay anxieties. He makes certain that the operation consent form has been correctly completed, that relatives have been informed and arrangements have been made for him or a member of his staff to meet them postoperatively.

*The anaesthetist* will assess the patient's fitness for anaesthesia and prescribe premedication. These measures should have been taken *before* the pre-operative round, so that any problems can be discussed. Its purpose is to ensure that the patient arrives in theatre sedated but still conscious and able to co-operate. Effective premedication also facilitates the course of general anaesthesia and reduces the amount of anaesthetic required. A sedative hypnotic, usually a barbiturate or nitrazepam, is prescribed on the evening before operation to ensure a good night's rest. Forty-five minutes before surgery, a narcotic (e.g. morphine 10–15 mg subcutaneously) is given to sedate the patient. This is usually combined with atropine (0.6 mg subcutaneously) to reduce respiratory tract secretions and counter any tendency to bradycardia during induction of anaesthesia. Some anaesthetists prefer to give atropine intravenously immediately before induction.

# 3. The Operation

## GENERAL ANAESTHESIA

The aim of a *general* anaesthetic is to abolish pain and reaction to it by reversible loss of consciousness, and blockade of motor and autonomic functions.

A graded depression of all levels of activity in the nervous system can be produced by inhalation or intravenous anaesthetic agents. Loss of consciousness is attributed to depression of the ascending reticular activating system of the brain stem and midbrain, with consequent reduction in cortical activity. The other effects of anaesthesia, e.g. analgesia, are apparently independent of this reticular activating system, though the mechanism is not fully understood.

## AGENTS USED IN ANAESTHESIA

### Intravenous agents

*Ultra-short-acting barbiturates.* An intravenous injection of thiopentone (Pentothal) or thiamylal (Surital) will rapidly induce anaesthesia of relatively short duration. Weak (2.5%) solutions are used so that extravasation or arterial injection can be recognised before harm is done.

*Ketamine* (Ketalar), also given by intramuscular injection, produces a state of 'dissociative anaesthesia'. An intravenous injection of 1–3 mg/kg will produce analgesia, amnesia and a lack of response to verbal stimuli within 30 seconds. This effect lasts for some 5–10 minutes unless supplementary doses are administered. Spontaneous muscular movements may occur, but protective reflexes and respiration are not affected. Patients must recover in a quiet setting; otherwise

unpleasant hallucinations and violent reactions may occur. Ketamine is useful for minor procedures and burn dressings, but has little place in major operations. Its use now is largely limited to children.

### Inhalation agents

At room temperature these are stored as gases or volatile liquids under pressure. The following agents are commonly used.

*Nitrous oxide* is the least potent of the anaesthetic gases, and is seldom used alone for surgical anaesthesia. It must be given with at least 20% oxygen, and is frequently used in mixture with oxygen, nitrous oxide and halothane. It is non-explosive, non-toxic and does not produce respiratory depression. Nitrous oxide is a good analgesic for use in childbirth.

*Cyclopropane* is an inflammable gas. For economy and safety it is administered only in a closed rebreathing system. Low concentrations produce analgesia; higher concentrations surgical anaesthesia. Induction is quick and the patient passes rapidly into deep anaesthesia with respiratory depression. An unusual property of cyclopropane is that blood pressure is well maintained. Although now superseded by halothane (which is non-explosive) it is still useful in shocked patients.

*Halothane* is a volatile liquid which is potent and non-explosive. Induction is smooth but relatively slow, and it is most often given with nitrous oxide and oxygen. Progressive respiratory depression occurs as the concentration increases. Unlike cyclopropane, halothane produces hypotension. As the myocardium is sensitised to circulating catecholamines arrhythmias may occur and adrenaline should not be used at operation. Halothane causes some muscle relaxation but this is not sufficient for abdominal surgery, and additional relaxant drugs are required. It is hepatotoxic, and should not be given to patients with liver damage nor should it be given repeatedly within a 3-month period. It is expensive and administered in a closed system.

*Ether* (diethyl ether) is an irritant, volatile and explosive liquid. Induction is prolonged and unpleasant. All depths of surgical anaesthesia can be produced. Because of its irritant properties, respiration is maintained and even stimulated until the deeper stages of anaesthesia are reached. Ether has no toxic effects and has good muscle-relaxing properties. However, the prolonged induction period, stimulation of copious respiratory tract secretions and troublesome recovery with nausea and vomiting make it generally unsuitable.

## NEUROMUSCULAR BLOCKING AGENTS

Neuromuscular blocking agents are quaternary amines. They induce muscle relaxation and facilitate surgical manipulation without deep anaesthesia. As the respiratory muscles are paralysed, ventilatory support is essential. Blocking agents are given by intravenous injection. Two types of agents are used (Fig. 3.1):

*Non-depolarising compounds* [d-tubocurarine, gallamine (Flaxedil) and dimethyl tubocurarine] are competitive inhibitors and prevent combination of acetylcholine with muscle end-plate receptors. This effect can be reversed by cholinesterase inhibitors e.g. neostigmine, edrophonium.

*Depolarising agents* [succinylcholine (Scoline)] do not block the receptors but produce prolonged depolarisation of the end-plate which becomes refractory to stimulation by acetylcholine. A brisk contraction of the muscle therefore precedes relaxation. Cholinesterase inhibitors intensify their action. The action of succinylcholine is short-lived (2–4 minutes). It is the preferred agent and can be given at intervals when relaxation is required. In occasional patients prolonged apnoea follows the administration of succinylcholine '*Scoline-apnoea*'. This may be due to an atypical plasma pseudocholinesterase which is unable to hydrolyse succinylcholine. Assisted ventilation must be continued until spontaneous breathing returns, sometimes after many hours.

## ADMINISTRATION OF ANAESTHETICS

*Induction.* Anaesthesia can be induced by inhalation anaesthetics but an intravenous agent is preferable. The ultra-short-acting barbiturates are normally used and an IV injection of 2.5% solution of thiopentone (Pentothal) is effective within seconds. Great care is taken to ensure that the injection is intravenous. Intra-arterial injection can cause arterial occlusion, and extravasation causes sloughing of tissues at the injection site. As induction produces relaxation of the jaw and airways obstruction, the head is maintained in extension and the jaw elevated. An oropharyngeal airway may be inserted.

In major operations, the anaesthetist inserts an endotracheal tube to allow direct control of ventilation. This has an inflatable cuff which occludes the trachea and prevents aspiration of gastric contents into the respiratory tree. The endotracheal tube is inserted immediately after induction and following the injection of a short-acting muscle relaxant (succinylcholine).

General anaesthesia is induced only when an adequate airway can be guaranteed. Exceptionally, an anaesthetist may require the surgeon to perform tracheostomy under local anaesthesia before inducing general anaesthesia.

During induction, aspiration of secretions and gastric contents must be prevented. Except in emergencies an anaesthetic is only given to fasted patients or those in whom the stomach has been emptied by a naso-gastric tube.

*Maintenance of anaesthesia.* Anaesthesia is normally maintained by inhalation agents administered, along with oxygen, in either an 'open' or 'closed' system (Fig.3.2). In the former, expired gases are not recirculated. If allowed to accumulate in the theatre atmosphere these may be of risk to theatre staff (particularly if pregnant) and exhaust systems are now incorporated in all anaesthetic machines.

During administration of anaesthetics regular assessment of the patient's vital signs, his re-

(a) The myoneural junction

A Ch-Acetylcholine

AChE-Acetylcholinesterase

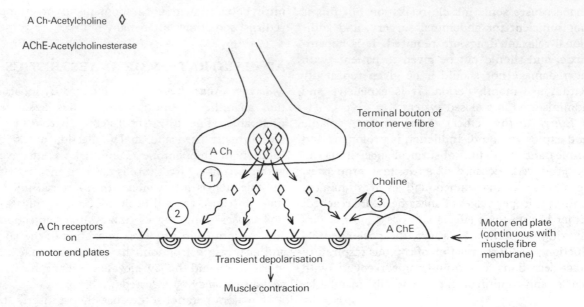

(b) Non-depolarising blockers (tubocurarine, gallamine, pancuronium)

A Ch

Blocking agent

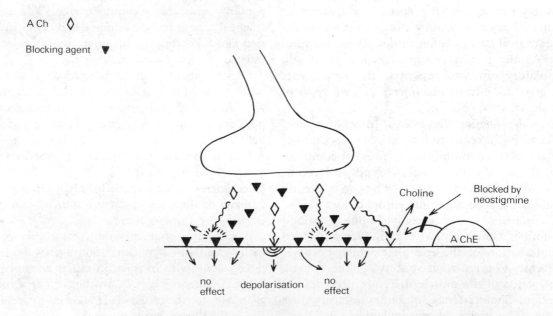

**Fig. 3.1** Neuromuscular blockade. (a) The myoneural junction. Sequence of events: 1. Nerve impulse releases quanta of ACh into synaptic gap. 2. ACh interacts with receptor to create a motor end plate potential. These potentials are summed to produce muscle contraction. 3. ACh is rapidly destroyed by AChE, and the resultant choline is taken back into the nerve fibre for ACh synthesis. (b) Non-depolarising blockers. These agents compete with ACh for receptors but do not cause depolarisation. Increasing the concentration of ACh by blocking AChE will reverse the effects of such compounds. (c) Depolarising blockers. These agents depolarise, but are not as rapidly inactivated as ACh. This results in prolonged depolarisation which prevents neuromuscular transmission, and is not reversed by inhibition of AChE.

(c) Depolarising blockers (suxamethonium)

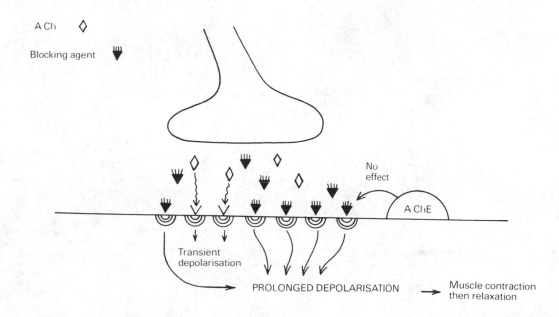

A Ch    ◇

Blocking agent    ♨

No effect

A ChE

Transient depolarisation

PROLONGED DEPOLARISATION

Muscle contraction then relaxation

sponse to surgical stimuli and the appearance of the operating field allow the anaesthetist to decide whether the anaesthetic is too light, adequate or too deep. The choice of anaesthetic agent and its rate of administration can then be adjusted to provide optimal conditions for the particular operation in progress.

For operations in the abdomen or chest, a dose of muscle relaxant is normally given at the completion of the procedure to facilitate closure.

## LOCAL ANAESTHESIA

A local 'anaesthetic' blocks transmission of impulses along nerve fibres by altering membrane permeability. Used to block sensory nerves, it prevents appreciation of painful stimuli so that operative procedures can be carried out within the area subserved by the blocked nerve. The anaesthetic agent may be injected into the operation site or injected proximally around the main trunks of the appropriate nerves.

Local anaesthesia is also of value in control of postoperative pain. For clinical use a local anaesthetic must be non-irritating, rapid in action, completely reversible and readily sterilized. If absorbed systemically, there is stimulation of the central nervous system and depression of the myocardium. Lignocaine is the local anaesthetic used most frequently and the total dose should not exceed 200 mg (see below).

## TOPICAL ANAESTHESIA

As anaesthetic agents are absorbed through the surface of mucous membranes, solutions and creams containing 0.5–4.0% lignocaine are used to anaesthetise the conjunctiva, mucosa of the mouth, nasopharynx and larynx, the urethra and the urinary bladder. They are applied as sprays, gargles, soaked pledgets of cotton wool, or gels. Anaesthesia develops rapidly and lasts for 30–60 minutes.

## LOCAL INFILTRATION

Solutions of lignocaine are available for local infiltration through a fine needle inserted into or

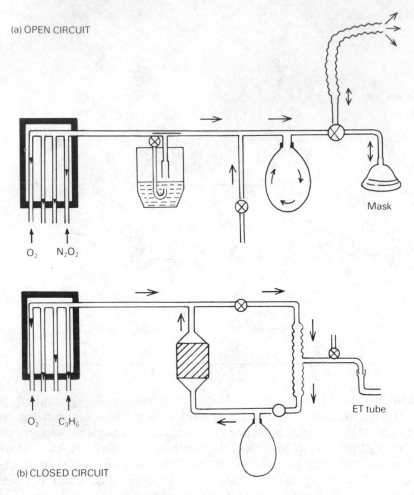

(a) OPEN CIRCUIT

Mask

$O_2$  $N_2O_2$

(b) CLOSED CIRCUIT

$O_2$  $C_3H_6$

ET tube

**Fig. 3.2** Open and closed systems of anaesthesia.

through the skin. The part to be operated on is infiltrated slowly with dilute (0.5%) solutions. Stronger solutions (1% and 2%) are available but these are normally reserved for nerve blocks. The maximum recommended dose of lignocaine is 200 mg.

Because of the dangers of rapid absorption, local anaesthetics must not be injected into inflamed tissues. The altered pH of the tissues also affects the action of the anaesthetic agent.

Larger doses (up to 500 mg) can be given if a vasoconstrictor, e.g. 1:200 000 adrenaline, is combined with the local anaesthetic. Patients with cardiac disease or thyrotoxicosis should *not* be given local anaesthetic agents containing adrenaline.

For dental anaesthesia, 2% lignocaine or 2% lignocaine with 1:800 000 adrenaline are used.

## NERVE BLOCK

Nerve block is performed by injecting small amounts of local aneasthetic around a main nerve trunk. 1% or 2% solutions of lignocaine are used either in plain solution or with adrenaline 1:200 000. The anaesthetist or surgeon carrying out the injection must be aware of the anatomical course of the nerve, its surface relationships and the type of surrounding tissues. As with all injections, aspiration must precede injection so that intravascular injection is avoided. Common sites for nerve block are the brachial plexus in the axilla or root of neck; ulnar nerve at the elbow; anterior or posterior tibial nerve at the ankle; digital nerve at the roots of the fingers or toes; intercostal nerve below the ribs. Solutions containing adrenaline

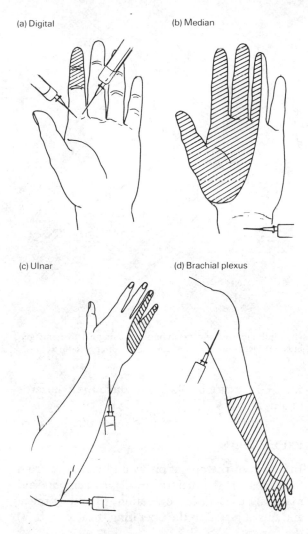

(a) Digital    (b) Median

(c) Ulnar    (d) Brachial plexus

**Fig. 3.3** Some common sites for nerve blocks.

must not be used in fingers or toes or other sites without good collateral circulation (Fig.3.3).

When there are multiple sensory nerves supplying a part e.g. the groin or scalp, a 'field block' can be carried out in which a series of injections block all the nerves.

## REGIONAL INTRAVENOUS ANAESTHESIA

The reduction of closed fractures and other simple surgical procedures on extremities can be performed under regional anaesthesia induced by the injection of a dilute solution of a local anaes-

thetic into a vein while the limb is kept ischaemic by a tourniquet.

A blood pressure cuff is first applied to upper arm or thigh and a plastic cannula inserted into a distal vein; the limb is elevated and an elastic bandage applied to empty it of blood. The cuff is then inflated to above systolic pressure (usually to 250 mm Hg) and 30–50 ml 0.5% lignocaine or pilocaine (but *not* marcaine) injected.

Anaesthesia lasts 30–60 minutes but the pressure of the cuff becomes intolerable at 30 minutes. The cuff must *not* be released before 15 minutes has elapsed or there is a danger of release of the agent into the general circulation with the induction of cardiac arrythmia (Fig.3.4).

## SPINAL AND EPIDURAL ANAESTHESIA

Injection of local anaesthetic agents into the subarachnoid or epidural spaces can be used to block spinal nerve roots as they course from the spinal cord to intervertebral foramina. Spinal anaesthesia is performed by injecting the agent through a lumbar puncture needle inserted between L3 and L4 (Fig.3.5). Solutions of lignocaine (5%) or dibucaine (0.05%) which are respectively lighter or heavier than cerebrospinal fluid (CSF) are used. These either float or sink according to position of the body. A 'high spinal' blocks nerves arising in the thoracic region; a 'low spinal', those in the lumbosacral. Leakage of CSF may cause headache and the patient should lie flat in bed for 12 hours after a spinal anaesthetic.

An epidural anaesthetic is administered by inserting a needle into the epidural space which lies between the ligamentum flavum and arachnoid membrane (Fig.3.6) A fine catheter is inserted through this needle and repeated injections of local anaesthetic will maintain anaesthesia for hours if need be. As the subarachnoid space is not punctured, headache due to leakage of CSF is not a problem. Epidural anaesthesia is of value in control of postoperative pain. It is most commonly used in the lower lumbar region to anaesthetise the perineum.

The sympathetic outflow along anterior nerve roots is also blocked by spinal and epidural anaes-

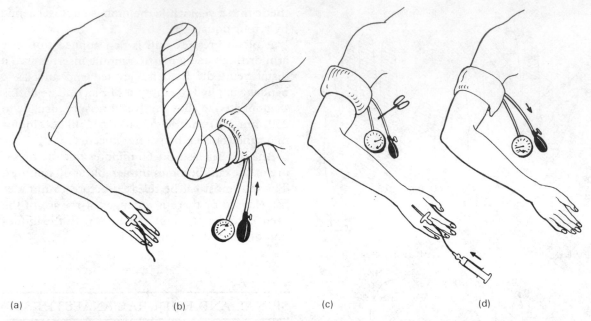

(a)                    (b)                    (c)                    (d)

**Fig. 3.4** Regional intravenous anaesthesia. (a) Cannula inserted. (b) Limb elevated and exsanguinated using elastic bandage, followed by inflation of cuff. (c) Injection of local anaesthetic. (d) Deflation of cuff at the end of the procedure.

thetics. Vasomotor paralysis can cause hypotension and bradycardia (slowing of the heart). These effects are particularly dangerous in the hypertensive arteriosclerotic patient.

## COMPLICATIONS

The main complication of local anaesthesia is overdose. Excitement, apprehension, muscle irritability and convulsions result from stimulation of the nervous system. This is followed by depression and a shock-like state. Cardiovascular and respiratory depression occur and death from hypoxia may follow. The most important steps in treatment are to oxygenate and if necessary ventilate the patient. Control of convulsions by barbiturates or muscle relaxants is occasionally necessary.

## THE OPERATION

During a surgical operation the patient is exposed to three main risks: infection, the effects of trauma, and postoperative thrombo-embolic dis-

ease. Great care is taken to reduce these hazards to a minimum.

## INFECTION

Infection of the operation wound can arise from four sites: (1) the theatre air; (2) instruments and materials used in the operation; (3) the surgical and nursing staff in the operating theatre; and (4) the patient.

### Theatre air

The ventilation systems of modern theatres ensure that there are frequent changes of atmosphere so that the density of organisms is kept low. The theatre atmosphere cannot be completely sterilised and there is always a 'fall-out' of organisms onto the operation site, the drapes used to surround the wound, and the floor. Laminar flow systems which blow a current of filtered air over the operating table will reduce, but not abolish this fall out (Fig.3.7).

As an operation 'list' proceeds, the bacterial count in the atmosphere increases and infection is more common in patients at the end of a list. If

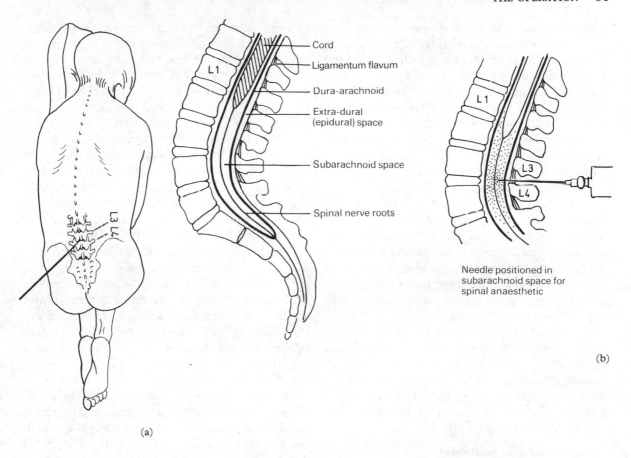

Cord
Ligamentum flavum
Dura-arachnoid
Extra-dural (epidural) space
Subarachnoid space
Spinal nerve roots

Needle positioned in subarachnoid space for spinal anaesthetic

(a)

(b)

**Fig. 3.5** Spinal anaesthesia. (a) Position of patient. (b) Position of needle within spinal canal.

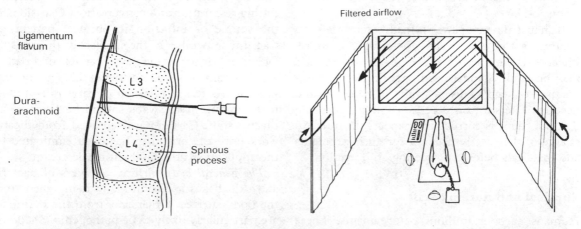

Ligamentum flavum

Dura-arachnoid

Spinous process

**Fig. 3.6** Epidural anaesthesia.

Filtered airflow

**Fig. 3.7** Laminar flow system in an operating theatre.

more than four major operations are to be performed in the same theatre, ideally there should be a break of an hour after the fourth case to allow the bacterial count to fall.

Infection rates increase when 'clean' and 'infected' cases are operated on in the same theatre. Ideally, infected cases should undergo surgery in a separate theatre. If this is not possible, they should be treated at the end of the list after all 'clean' cases have been dealt with.

Occasionally, a patient undergoing a 'clean' operation is found unexpectedly to have an abscess or other infective condition. After completion of the operation, the list should be suspended for one hour while the theatre is cleaned.

The longer an operation, the greater the risk of infection. Longer procedures inevitably involve greater tissue manipulation and damage and longer exposure to the atmosphere.

Currents of air may be caused by movements of staff in theatre. These may carry organisms from the floor or from crevices in the furniture to contaminate wounds or instruments. Movements of theatre staff should be orderly. Excess numbers of staff should not be allowed 'on the floor'.

## Instruments and materials

In well-run theatres, the risk of infection from instruments and other materials is slight. Routine checks of sterilisation procedures (autoclaves etc.) are the responsibility of a bacteriologist. At the end of each operation, all contaminated materials are removed from the theatre for re-sterilisation or disposal.

If an instrument or swab is inadvertently left in a wound at the end of an operative procedure, infection is the rule. This is frequently serious and may be fatal. Standardised counting procedures are used to keep a tally of swabs, instruments and needles. The surgeon is responsible for ensuring that the count is correct and expects the nurse in charge of the case to account for all instruments and materials before completing an operation.

## Surgical and nursing staff

Humans harbour millions of organisms. These are concentrated in hands, perineum, upper res-

piratory tract and usually are not pathogenic. However, infective organisms can be carried particularly when there is a pimple or boil or other septic focus. Staff with such infections are banned from theatre until the lesion has healed fully.

*The hands.* The 'scrub up' technique is designed to remove surface organisms from hands and forearms. It cannot remove organisms from sweat glands and hair follicles. After routine cleansing the skin surface is recolonized in approximately 20 minutes. Excess scrubbing should be avoided and many scrub-up rooms are equipped with a stop-clock (Fig.3.8).

This problem is overcome in two ways: (a) the use of sterile rubber gloves and gowns worn over a fresh laundered 'scrubsuit'; and (b) modern washing agents which combine a detergent with an antiseptic and remain active on the skin surface for a long time. Organisms arriving at the skin surface are killed for up to two hours after a 'scrub up' with povidone iodine (Betadine) or chlorhexidine (Hibitane).

Gloves are frequently punctured during operations. After a 3-hour operation, 70% of gloves contain puncture holes. If a puncture is recognised, gloves should be changed. The gown should be changed if the sleeve or other part of the gown becomes wet, as a channel is created for the transfer of organisms.

*The upper respiratory tract.* A mask to cover nose and mouth is worn routinely in theatre. This reduces the number of bacteria and bacteria-laden droplets expelled from the mouth and nose during respiration and conversation. Occasionally the source of infection in surgical patients is traced to a member of the surgical or theatre staff who is an unsuspecting nasal 'carrier' of a pathogenic organism. This occurs in 10% of normal persons. As the recognition of carriers is important, routine nasal swabs should be taken in all theatre staff. Carriers are removed from theatre work until the organism has been eliminated by the application of a nasal antibiotic cream.

*The general body surface.* Showers of bacteria and skin flakes are continually being shed from the body surface. Organisms from the perineum are particularly likely to be pathogenic. Shedding of flakes and bacteria increases for a period of

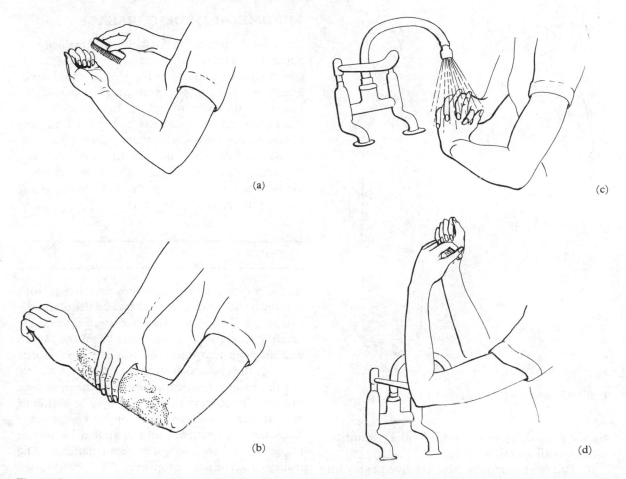

(a)

(c)

(b)

(d)

**Fig. 3.8** Scrub-up technique. (a) Fingernails scrubbed. (b) Forearms washed. (c) Hands rinsed. (d) Water allowed to run off in a proximal direction.

about two hours after a shower, which should not be taken immediately before an operation. Shedding is reduced by wearing a 'theatre cap' to cover the hair, and trousers gathered in at the ankle which prevent dispersion from the perineum (Fig.3.9).

## The patient

The most potent source of organisms causing wound infection is the patient. Such 'endogenous' infections are common and may occur in four ways:

1. The patient may be an asymptomatic 'carrier' of pathogens. This is more likely if he has been exposed to the hospital environment for some time. Some surgeons insist that in such patients nose, throat and perineal swabs are taken pre-operatively and appropriate antibiotic treatment given.

2. The patient may have intercurrent infection unrelated to his surgical problem. This consists of an infected skin lesion, a bad tooth or infection of the respiratory or urinary tract. This should be treated before elective surgery. If operation cannot be postponed, the intercurrent infection should be treated with appropriate antibiotics during and after surgery.

3. The disorder for which the patient is undergoing operation may have produced local sepsis e.g. an appendix abscess. When it is not possible to avoid entering the 'contaminated' area, steps must be taken to protect the wound from infec-

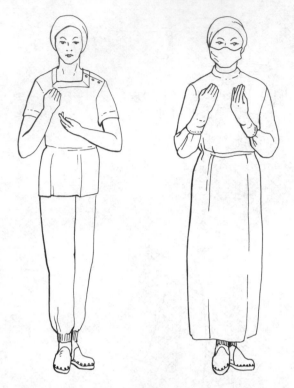

**Fig. 3.9** Protection of theatre personnel.

tion, e.g. by delay in its suture, or the administration of antibiotics (see p.63).

4. The operation may have involved entry into a contaminated viscus e.g. the small or large intestine. In elective procedures this hazard is reduced by preparation of the intestinal tract (see p.422).

## TRAUMA

Tissue damage is inevitable with any operation. Its degree affects:

1. The *metabolic demands* on the patient.

2. The risk of *infection* (dead or injured tissue is more liable to colonisation by bacteria.

3. The extent of postoperative *oedema* (the sequestration of circulating fluid causes a fall in effective circulating blood volume which, if severe, may lead to circulatory shock).

4. The amount of operative *blood loss*.

A good surgeon handles tissues and instruments gently and protects those tissues which lie outside the immediate operative field.

## THROMBO-EMBOLIC DISEASE

It is now recognised that in the majority of patients in whom deep venous thrombosis develops, the process starts during the operation itself. Measures taken in the postoperative period are therefore unlikely to affect the incidence of thrombosis and emphasis is now placed on prophylactic measures before and during surgery. These include low-dose subcutaneous heparin, the wearing of supportive stockings and the prevention of pressure on the calf veins while muscles are relaxed. (See p.41).

## RECOVERY

At the end of the operation the anaesthetist stops administering anaesthetic agents and ventilates the patient until spontaneous respiration occurs. He carefully sucks out all secretions from the mouth and pharynx and once the cough reflex returns removes the endotracheal tube. In modern hospitals the patient then proceeds from the operating theatre to a recovery room. This may be within or outside the 'clean' area, is adminstered by the anaesthetic department and is staffed by nurses trained in the care of unconscious patients. The trolleys must allow adoption of the head-down position; oxygen, suction and monitoring equipment should be available and all the facilities for immediate resuscitation should be at hand.

Patients remain in this recovery area until they are fully conscious, spontaneously breathing and have a stable circulation. It is the anaesthetist's responsibility to decide when they are fit to return to the ward. If there is any doubt, the patient remains under close supervision in the recovery room or may be transferred to an intensive care unit.

## INTENSIVE CARE

Intensive care may take several different forms and many larger hospitals support separate units for the care of those with specific problems such as myocardial ischaemia (coronary care unit), acute renal failure (renal unit), and respiratory failure (ventilatory unit); in addition, beds are generally available for general intensive nursing care combined with constant medical attention backed up by systems for continuous monitoring and treatment. Patients having major procedures e.g. cardiac surgery will proceed from theatre direct to an ICU.

In general the most effective method of arranging continuous patient monitoring is also the most simple. An ECG cardiac monitor is relatively cheap and easy to manage and allows continuous monitoring of the pulse rate. Blood pressure is measured readily by sphygmomanometry, and central venous pressure by a simple saline manometer through a central venous line. Urinary output is measured by a calibrated reservoir and catheter, electrolytes and blood gases by automated laboratory equipment.

Sophisticated methods of monitoring are required in some cases, but the equipment is expensive and techniques are often invasive. Continuous monitoring of arterial blood pressure requires an arterial line; monitoring of pulmonary wedge pressure requires an indwelling Swann-Ganz catheter which also allows the estimation of pulmonary venous blood gas concentration or cardiac output. Some sophisticated measurements can be made without invasive techniques, e.g. deep body or core temperatures can be measured by sensitive surface thermometers and aortic blood flow by an ultrasonic flow meter placed over the chest. Equipment apart, the main value of an intensive care unit is to facilitate continuous care of a patient by trained personnel. Changes in colour, in the level of consciousness, in the quality of the pulse and peripheral circulation are still important guides to progress (Fig.3.10). Recognition of 'pattern changes' is still of the greatest significance and good nursing care is the basis of intensive therapy.

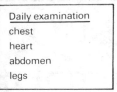

Daily examination
chest
heart
abdomen
legs

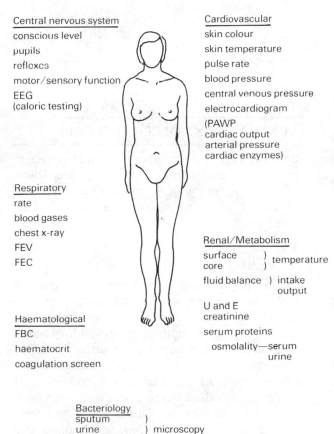

Central nervous system
conscious level
pupils
reflexes
motor/sensory function
EEG
(caloric testing)

Respiratory
rate
blood gases
chest x-ray
FEV
FEC

Haematological
FBC
haematocrit
coagulation screen

Cardiovascular
skin colour
skin temperature
pulse rate
blood pressure
central venous pressure
electrocardiogram
(PAWP
cardiac output
arterial pressure
cardiac enzymes)

Renal/Metabolism
surface    )
core       ) temperature
fluid balance ) intake
                output
U and E
creatinine
serum proteins
    osmolality—serum
                urine

Bacteriology
sputum      )
urine       ) microscopy
blood       ) and
wound swabs ) culture — aerobes
drain fluid )          anaerobes

Fig. 3.10 Monitoring of patient following serious operation.

# 4. Post-Operative Care and Complications

## GENERAL POST-OPERATIVE CARE

Following an operation there are three phases to the care of the patient. These are 1. immediate (recovery room care); 2. care on return to the surgical ward; 3. rehabilitation and convalescent care.

### Immediate (recovery room area)

During the first phase the patient must be kept under close observation until he is awake, breathing satisfactorily with a stable circulation and relieved of pain. Complications, should they occur, require immediate and skilled attention. This phase of recovery is generally regarded as the responsibility of the anaesthetist and in most modern hospitals, a *recovery area* is situated close to the operating theatre. This is staffed by nurses trained in care of the unconscious patient and is equipped with monitoring and resuscitation apparatus, and beds and trolleys which can be tilted to the head-down position.

### Care on return to the surgical ward

Once responsive with a clear airway, the patient is returned to the care of the surgical team in the general ward where regular observation by medical and nursing staff continues. Complications during this phase other than haemorrhage or cardio-pulmonary catastrophe rarely pose an immediate threat to life and are usually specifically related to the operation performed. After a major operation, this period of care generally lasts for a week.

### Rehabilitation and convalescent care

Although by now the patient is well on his way to full recovery, he may still require a period of professional care before he is able to return home and resume domestic and other duties. This is provided in a convalescent hospital or, if there is need for a programme of graded activity, in a rehabilitation centre.

The first two of these three periods of care are considered in detail below.

## IMMEDIATE CARE

### Cerebral state

Unconscious or drowsy patients are kept semi-prone with the thighs flexed and the head and neck supported in a slightly flexed position. The mouth must be free from obstructing bedclothes and the jaw is allowed to fall forwards. Inhalation of secretions, blood or vomitus is a major threat in all unconscious patients while their cough reflex is depressed. It is imperative to prevent such material pooling in the mouth and pharynx. Quiet surroundings and lack of restraint are desirable but some patients may become excited or disorientated with recovery of consciousness. Sedation is then necessary and should be ordered by the anaesthetist to ensure compatibility with the anaesthetic agents used.

### Circulatory stability

The patient should be haemodynamically stable at the end of the operation. Regular recordings of pulse rate and blood pressure ensure that circulatory stability is maintained. The skin should be warm and pink and when blanched by digital pressure the capillaries should rapidly refill. The veins also should be well-filled.

ECG monitoring is indicated if there is a history of cardiac disease or any concern about the state of the heart during anaesthesia.

Haemorrhage is a major cause of circulatory instability. It is important to observe and measure drainage from wound drains or gastro-intestinal tubes and to alert the surgeon if excessive blood loss be suspected.

## Myocardial ischaemia

Post-operative cardiac failure is most likely to occur in the immediate recovery period. While in most cases there is a history of preceding cardiac disease, myocardial ischaemia or cardiac arrest can occur in an otherwise fit patient. Patients with myocardial ischaemia may complain of gripping chest pain, but this is not invariable and hypotension may be the only sign. If ischaemia is suspected, an ECG is performed urgently and arrangements made for cardiac monitoring. A sample of blood is withdrawn for estimation of concentrations of cardiac enzymes.

*Cardiac arrest* results in an absent pulse in an unconscious and apnoeic patient. Closed cardiac massage is started immediately, a cuffed endocardial tube is inserted and the patient is ventilated. 150 mmol sodium bicarbonate is administered intravenously during the first 10 minutes to combat acidosis and is repeated as long as the circulation remains inadequate. An ECG is performed. If asystole is present, the heart can be stimulated by an electrical pacemaker. If ventricular fibrillation is present, it can be corrected by electrical defibrillation. The extent of recovery depends upon the degree of cerebral damage and is related to the duration of arrest. Persistent fixed dilatation of the pupils denotes irreversible cerebral damage.

## Respiratory care

Respiratory failure is defined as an inability to maintain normal partial pressure of oxygen and carbon dioxide ($Pa_{O_2}$ and $Pa_{CO_2}$) in the arterial blood. Blood gas estimations are essential for its early recognition and should be monitored in patients with previous respiratory problems. The normal $Pa_{O_2}$ is over 13 kPa at the age of 20 years, falling to around 11.6 kPa at 60. For practical purposes respiratory failure is denoted by a $Pa_{O_2}$ of less than 6.7 kPa. Severe hypoxaemia may result in visible central cyanosis.

The patient's airway must be kept clear at all times. *Airway obstruction* causes great distress with confusion, choking, croaking and audible rhonchi. The chest is often held hyperinflated so that cardiac dullness is absent.

A finger is hooked through the mouth and pharynx to ensure that there is no obstruction by the tongue, by false teeth or by a foreign body. The jaw is elevated and using a laryngoscope, the pharynx is inspected and sucked out and the larynx examined. If there is evidence of laryngeal obstruction, a cuffed endotracheal tube is inserted and artificial ventilation is commenced with an Ambu bag or other manual inflator while mechanical ventilation is arranged.

If the airway is clear, *hypoxia* is likely to be due to under-ventilation of areas of the lungs with discrepancies between ventilation and perfusion. Blood gases are measured and oxygen administered by a mask such as the MC or Hudson mask which delivers about 60% oxygen when the flow rate is 4–6 l/min. Mechanical ventilation with insertion of a cuffed endotracheal tube may still be required if an adequate $Pa_{O_2}$ cannot be maintained.

## Special problems

More complex methods of monitoring are required for certain groups of patients. For example, patients undergoing adrenalectomy require steroid replacement therapy; patients having neck surgery must be observed for accumulation of blood in the wound which can cause rapid asphyxia; and patients having open heart surgery require intensive cardiovascular monitoring. These problems are dealt with in other chapters.

## CARE ON RETURN TO THE SURGICAL WARD

### General procedure

On return to the ward, observation continues with regular hourly or two-hourly checks on pulse, blood pressure, respiratory rate and wound drains. In some patients hourly monitoring of urine volume will also continue. The surgeon gradually relaxes these measures as recovery continues and the patient stabilises. Thereafter the patient is visited by medical staff morning and evening to ensure that there is steady progression towards recovery without complication.

Awareness of the nature of the particular post-operative course and the common complications is important. Anxiety, disorientation and minor changes in personality, behaviour or appearance, are often the earliest manifestation of impending complications. Sleeplessness can be troublesome and depressing and it is important to recognise patients in need of quiet and rest. The general circulatory state and adequacy of oxygenation are noted and the pulse, blood pressure and respiratory rates checked from the nurses' chart. Enquiry is made concerning urinary and bowel function and whether the patient is coughing freely and expanding his chest.

The chest is examined physically and sputum inspected. The legs are inspected and examined for calf tenderness. Fluid balance must be carefully controlled in all patients recovering from a major operation. If an intravenous infusion has been established, the nature and amount of intravenous fluids and urinary volume are checked at least twice daily by the medical staff. Serum electrolyte concentrations are measured daily in all patients receiving intravenous fluid (see Chapter 8).

Once intravenous fluid therapy has been discontinued, oral fluid intake is monitored until it is clear that the patient can drink freely. Nutritional requirements are also borne in mind. A short period of a few days starvation causes little harm but if this is prolonged, nutritional support by parenteral or enteral means is required (see Chapter 10).

### The abdomen

In general surgical wards, many patients are recovering from an abdominal operation. The abdomen must be examined carefully each day seeking evidence of excessive distention, tenderness or drainage either from drain sites or wounds. The main abdominal complications are the slow recovery of intestinal motor function, anastomotic leakage and occult bleeding or abscess formation. Return of bowel sounds and the free passage of flatus reflect recovery of peristaltic activity.

If a nasogastric tube has been inserted, it should be kept open at all times and allowed to drain freely into a small plastic bag. The tube serves as an air vent but free drainage is usually combined with continuous or intermittent suction. Many surgeons do not allow patients to drink while a nasogastric tube is in place. Others permit the patient to drink measured small amounts of fluid at regular intervals. The time at which a tube is removed also is variable; many surgeons prefer to retain the tube until the volume of hourly aspirate suggests that gastric stasis has resolved.

### Soft tissue and wound care

Many patients in general surgical wards have had surgery involving soft tissue only. In general, complications are few and care of the wound and its underlying tissues are the main concern.

Bulky dressings are not normally used for incised wounds and the area can be inspected daily for signs of wound infection. Drains prevent accumulation of blood or fluid. Mild suction is usually applied and the amount of drainage measured daily. Once this falls to a few ml the drain is usually removed unless the surgeon has indicated that it should be retained for a longer period.

Traditionally, skin sutures remained in place until the wound was soundly healed. Early removal of skin sutures to prevent unsightly 'cross hatching' is now preferred by many surgeons. Replacement of sutures with adhesive strips (e.g. Steristrips) avoids tension and improves healing. If subcuticular sutures have been used, these may be left in until the skin is healed.

In the presence of wound infection, it may be necessary to remove one or two sutures prematurely to allow egress of infected material.

## COMPLICATIONS OF ANAESTHESIA

Nausea and vomiting are common after any anaesthetic and particularly after abdominal surgery. Anti-emetics, e.g. cyclizine or prochlorperazine, are useful; metoclopramide is of little value.

### Headache

Occasionally patients complain of severe post-operative headache, particularly after halothane anaesthesia. An analgesic should be prescribed. Spinal anaesthesia may also be associated with headache due to leakage of cerebrospinal fluid and it is advisable that the patient lies flat for 12 hours following an operation performed under this form of anaesthetic. If headache persists, it may be necessary to seal the injection site in the arachnoid by an injection of the patient's blood which will clot and close the leak (a 'blood patch').

### Sore throat

Passage of an endotracheal or nasogastric tube can cause trauma to the mucous membrane and a sore throat. Dryness of the mouth contributes to this. Symptoms are usually of short duration, although ulceration of the larynx with granuloma formation can cause persistent hoarseness.

### Vascular and neural complications

The intravenous administration of irritant drugs or infusions can cause bruising, haematomas, phlebitis or even venous thrombosis. The addition of heparin or hydrocortisone to the intravenous fluid is said to minimise these effects but is not of proven value.

Breakage of venous catheters can occur with carriage of the tip to great vessels, heart or lungs. Arterial cannulas and needle punctures are now the commonest cause of arterial injury and may lead to arterial occlusion, impaired circulation

and gangrene. Nerve palsies can be caused by stretching or compression of nerve trunks and the extra-vascular injection of irritant solutions. The nerves most commonly affected are the ulnar at the elbow joint, the radial in the upper arm or the brachial plexus at the shoulder. Care must also be taken to guard against nerve palsies when placing a patient on the operating table.

### Muscle pain

Myalgia affecting the chest, abdomen and neck may begin 24 hours after operation and last for 1–7 days. This is a specific complication of the administration of succinylmethonium compounds.

### Damage to teeth

Patients whose teeth are loose or old or who have crown and bridge work may suffer dental damage during intubation. They should be warned of this possibility before operation. Aspiration of a loose tooth into a bronchus is now a rare event.

### Damage to eyes

A patient whose eyes do not close during anaesthesia may develop corneal damage. In severe cases, this will lead to ulceration. This complication is usually prevented by the anaesthetist taping the eyelids during anaesthesia. An oily antiseptic solution or sulphacetamide eye ointment is used in patients who develop conjunctivitis.

## COMPLICATIONS OF SURGERY

### RESPIRATORY PROBLEMS

Respiratory failure in the immediate post-operative period due to hypoxia and airways obstruction has already been discussed. Once recovery from anaesthesia has occurred, the main respiratory problems are caused by lack of full expansion of the lungs and the accumulation of secretions. This leads to pulmonary collapse (atelectasis) and may progress to pulmonary infection. Pulmonary embolism is a complication of deep vein thrombosis and is considered separately.

## Pulmonary collapse

Inability to breathe deeply and to cough up bronchial secretions after surgery is the primary cause of pulmonary collapse. This is due to various factors which include paralysis of the cilia by anaesthetic agents, impairment of diaphragmatic movement and pain in the wound. As a result of the accumulation of secretions, the patient does not aerate his lungs fully and collapse may follow.

With complete obstruction of a major bronchus, air in the lung, lobe or a segment which it supplies, is absorbed, the alveolar space closes (atelectasis) and the affected portion of the lung contracts and becomes solid.

Pulmonary collapse after surgery thus varies from closure of a small segment to massive collapse of a lobe or, if a main bronchus is obstructed, the whole lung. In most instances, this occurs within 24 hours of operation.

The clinical signs of a lobar collapse include rapid respiration, slight cyanosis and tachycardia. Breath sounds are diminished and there is dullness over the affected lobe. Blood gas estimations reveal a low $Pa_{O_2}$ and an X-ray of the chest, areas of increased opacity. With massive collapse there is severe dyspnoea and the affected side of the chest is uniformly dull with absent breath sounds. The mediastinum is drawn over to the affected side and there is compensatory hyperinflation of the unaffected lung which is hyper-resonant on percussion.

*Management*. For the prevention of pulmonary collapse it is essential that the patient is encouraged to move around, to breathe deeply and to cough during the post-operative period. Regular visits by a physiotherapist should be arranged. Coughing and deep breathing are best encouraged after a small dose of analgesic or narcotic while the abdominal wound is supported with the hands or a temporary binder. Intermittent injection of local anaesthetic through an indwelling catheter in the epidural space of the mid-thoracic region may also be used to relieve pain. Inhalations of salbutamol relieve bronchospasm. Oxygen should be administered by nasal probes or mask if there is hypoxia.

In more severe cases, stimulation of the trachea with a catheter or instillation of 1–2 ml of sterile saline will encourage the patient to cough up secretions. Bronchoscopy may be required to suck out a plug of inspissated secretions. If hypoxia is severe, endotracheal intubation, artificial respiration and repeated bronchial aspiration may be required. Prophylactic antibiotic therapy is advised after sputum specimens have been sent for bacteriological culture and sensitivity determinations.

Posture is important. If collapse is extensive, the patient should be placed initially on the unaffected side so that he is forced to expand the affected lung. Thereafter, frequent changes of posture and intensive physiotherapy are essential aids to re-expansion.

## Pulmonary infection

Pulmonary infection commonly follows pulmonary collapse. Bronchopneumonia is common but lobar pneumonia occasionally results from infection of a collapsed lobe. Aspiration of gastric secretions is a potent and not uncommon cause of pulmonary infection. Pyrexia and a viscid green sputum are typical features. Pulmonary signs are those of collapse and consolidation with absent or diminished breath sounds. Bronchial breathing and coarse crepitations from surrounding areas of partial bronchial occlusion may be present. A chest X-ray usually demonstrates patchy fluffy opacities.

The patient must be encouraged to cough and antibiotics are indicated. The choice of antibiotic depends on the sensitivity of the likely infecting organism but ampicillin or cotrimoxazole are generally preferred. Oxygen administration is dictated by hypoxaemia, and more intensive respiratory support including bronchoscopy and assisted ventilation may be deemed necessary if respiratory function continues to deteriorate. Steroid therapy may be advised should aspiration of gastric contents be suspected.

## CARDIAC FAILURE

As indicated above, acute cardiac failure is most likely to occur in the immediate post-operative period. However, patients suffering from ischaemic or valvular heart disease, arrythmias, or severe trauma, are liable to develop cardiac failure in the subsequent recovery period. Excessive administration of fluid in the early post-operative period is a common predisposing cause which can be prevented by monitoring central venous pressure. Treatment with digitalis and diuretics is indicated.

Hypovolaemia or the complications of sepsis are major sources of cardiac insufficiency in patients during the recovery phase. Treatment is directed at the primary cause. Therapeutic measures include restoration of circulating blood volume, elimination of hypoxaemia, correction of acid-base balance and the use of inotropic agents to increase cardiac output.

## RENAL FAILURE

Acute renal failure after surgery results from protracted periods of inadequate perfusion of the kidneys. This may result from hypovolaemia, sepsis or anaphylaxis (e.g. mismatched blood transfusion). Patients with pre-existing renal disease or those who are jaundiced are more susceptible to the effects of poor perfusion and are more likely to develop acute renal failure following a less severe insult.

Acute renal failure can largely be prevented by adequate fluid replacement in the pre-, per- and post-operative phases so that urine volume is maintained at 40 ml per hour or more. Monitoring hourly urine volume after catheterisation is a necessary precaution in all patients having major surgery and in those considered at risk from renal complications. The early recognition and effective treatment of bacterial and fungal infections is also important.

The cardinal feature of acute renal failure is oliguria associated with a dilute urine (SG < 1010 urea < 300 mmol/l). Oliguria with a concentrated urine indicates that the kidney is functioning but is inadequately perfused. This is an indication to give more fluid and rapid infusion of 1 litre of normal saline should increase urine output. In this situation a careful check must be made for continued bleeding as a cause of hypovolaemia.

If oliguria is associated with dilute urine (the patient will be well hydrated and with a stable circulation) or should oliguria not respond to a saline infusion, 20–40 mg frusemide should be administered intravenously. If there is no response, acute tubular necrosis has probably occurred and treatment for renal failure is instituted.

Ischaemic renal lesions are usually reversible and the mainstays of treatment are replacement of observed fluid loss with a supplement of 600–1000 ml/day for obligatory insensible loss; restriction of dietary protein to no more than 20 g/day; avoidance of hyperkalaemia and acidosis. Haemodialysis is performed if conservative measures fail to prevent rapid rises in the concentrations of urea and potassium in the venous blood.

## THROMBOEMBOLIC PHENOMENA

These are described in detail in Chapter 21; management is summarised here for convenience.

### Deep vein thrombosis

Prophylaxis against deep vein thrombosis usually includes care to avoid compression of the leg veins during operation and in the post-operative period, the wearing of tapered support stockings and, in high risk patients, low dose subcutaneous heparin (calcium heparin 5000 units 12-hourly). Thrombosis is suspected clinically by the development of tenderness over the calf veins, by swelling of the foot or leg, or by the results of serial scintiscans. Under these circumstances, bilateral ascending phlebography is essential to confirm thrombosis and to determine whether the clot occludes the vein lumen and whether it is located in the ilio-femoral segment or in more distal veins. Some surgeons also perform a ventilation-perfusion (VQ) lung scan to establish a base-line for future reference should pulmonary embolism develop.

Confirmation of venous thrombosis on phlebography demands the following action.

1. Thrombosis confined to the calf vein carries a low risk of embolism and in a mobile patient is treated by support stockings and encouragement of mobility. If the patient is immobile and confined to bed, heparinisation may be considered.

2. Thrombosis in the ilio-femoral segment car-

ries a significant risk of embolism, particularly when the clot is non-occlusive. The patient is heparinised and confined to bed for 48 hours with the foot of the bed elevated. Thereafter, support stockings are fitted and the patient is mobilised. If phlebography shows a tail of non-occlusive thrombus, consideration may be given to insertion of a filter in the inferior vena cava.

*Heparinisation* is commenced with an intravenous bolus of 5000–10 000 units followed by 1000 units/h by continuous IV infusion. The whole blood clotting time is estimated at 6 hours and the dose is adjusted to maintain a clotting time of 2–3 times the control values. Heparinisation is usually continued for 7–10 days and is replaced by long-term oral anti-coagulant therapy. This is introduced during heparin administration by a dose of 20 mg phenindione followed by 5 mg/day. Further dosage depends on the prothrombin time which should be maintained at a ratio to normal of 2.0–4.0:1.

## Pulmonary embolus

Massive pulmonary embolus with severe chest pain, pallor and shock demands immediate cardio-pulmonary resuscitation, heparinisation (10 000–15 000 units intravenously as a bolus dose) and an urgent pulmonary angiogram. If the diagnosis is confirmed, the catheter may be left in the pulmonary artery so that pulmonary arterial pressure can be monitored. Arterial and CVP lines are also inserted to monitor pressures. If the patient's condition improves, heparinisation is continued. If deterioration occurs, the embolus must be removed, either by the administration of streptokinase to dissolve the clot or by pulmonary embolectomy under cardio-pulmonary bypass.

If a small pulmonary embolus is suspected by the occurrence of chest pain and haemoptysis, particularly when accompanied by tachypnoea and/or a pleural effusion, it is necessary first to confirm or refute the diagnosis. A chest X-ray and ECG are performed to rule out alternative causes and, if normal or if compatible with a pulmonary embolus, perfusion and ventilation lung scans are ordered. If one or more lobar or segmental defects are seen, the patient should be fully heparinised and carefully observed.

In all such cases, it is important to investigate the patient for the source of embolus by bilateral phlebography. If thrombosis is demonstrated with propagated clot lying loose in the vessel, a filter is inserted into the vena cava.

# 5. Special Problems in Operative Care

In discussing the care of patients before, during and after operation it was assumed that one was dealing with patients who generally were fit for anaesthesia and operation. However special problems may arise in particular groups of patients; these are considered in this chapter.

## THE EMERGENCY CASE

Time for detailed preparation (as outlined in Ch. 2) may not be available when patients admitted as surgical emergencies require urgent operation. Priority lies in correction of a life-threatening condition and relief of pain. However, the following must not be disregarded:

1. There must always be a full enquiry regarding conditions likely to affect anaesthesia, particularly cardiac, respiratory, metabolic and endocrine disease. The course of previous anaesthetics should be ascertained and a note made of drugs taken over the past 3 months. In the elderly man urinary problems are of particular importance as chronic retention and uraemia may be unsuspected hazards.

2. The cardiovascular and respiratory systems are always examined fully. Pulse rate and blood pressure are recorded, haemoglobin concentration is estimated, and ideally a chest X-ray is arranged. Arterial blood gas determination and $H^+$ concentration may be useful in patients who are shocked or who have respiratory problems.

3. The state of nutrition and hydration are assessed, and blood, urea and electrolyte concentrations are estimated in patients with overt or potential upset. For all major procedures, a sample of venous blood should be taken pre-operatively for blood grouping and cross-matching.

4. Obvious deficiencies or illness are corrected if possible before operation. Anaemia or blood loss are corrected by transfusion, congestive cardiac failure by digitalisation and diuretics, and dehydration by fluid and electrolyte replacement.

5. A nasogastric tube is passed before anaesthesia in all patients who have vomited, or who may have intestinal obstruction, peritonitis or perforated ulcer. A 4–6 hour fast is desirable before operation. If this is not feasible a nasogastric tube should be passed and the anaesthetist informed. In shocked patients a urinary catheter is passed to monitor urine volume. If large quantities of fluid or blood are being infused, central venous pressure is monitored.

6. Consent forms must be signed (children under 16 years require parental consent), the side of the operation should be marked, and the nursing staff should carry out their normal preparations. The type and dose of premedication is ordered only after discussion with the anaesthetist.

## THE NEONATE

The body of a newborn infant has a higher water content (700 mg/kg cf. 600 mg/kg in an adult): little fluid is normally required in the first few days of life. However, abnormal losses from the gastro-intestinal tract can produce *dehydration and electrolyte depletion* within a few hours and an intravenous infusion is an essential requirement for all infants undergoing surgery. The neonate has a blood volume of 88 ml/kg compared with

70 ml/kg in adults. He is very susceptible to *blood loss*. One unit of fresh blood should be cross-matched so that operative blood loss can rapidly be replaced. One mg of vitamin K₁ (phytomenadione) is injected before operation to compensate for possible deficiencies in clotting factors.

*Hypothermia* can develop rapidly, particularly in premature or dehydrated infants, due to the relatively large surface area of the newborn and his lack of subcutaneous fat. This must be corrected rapidly or acidosis, hypoglycaemia and hyperkalaemia can occur. Heat loss is reduced by placing the infant on a warming pad, and in an incubator set at 32°C after operation. Oxygen may be added to the air inflow and humidity is maintained at 90–100% to reduce insensible water loss from the skin and prevent crusting of bronchial secretions.

*Hyperthermia* may complicate anaesthesia in febrile infants with insufficient pre-operative fluid replacement. Rapid cooling is achieved in an ice-cooled alcohol bath.

*Overhydration* is readily produced postoperatively in premature babies. Provided operative blood losses are made good, postoperative intravenous infusion is probably unnecessary unless there are gastro-intestinal losses.

*Hypoglycaemia* may complicate neonatal surgery and is treated by infusion of 10% glucose for several days. Every effort should be made to recommence oral feeding soon after surgery; otherwise parenteral feeding is required.

Care is summarised in Figure 5.1.

## THE ELDERLY

A surgical operation has greater risk in the elderly than in younger patients. Although the increased mortality is associated with major operations, even the simplest procedure, e.g. hernia repair, may be hazardous. Because of structural and functional changes in the respiratory, cardiovascular and renal systems, and due to their changed metabolism, old people are less able to withstand an operation.

*Respiratory system.* Structural changes occur in the lungs and chest wall which reduce air space

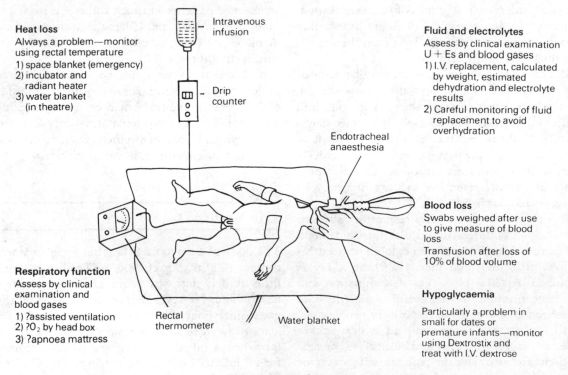

**Heat loss**
Always a problem—monitor using rectal temperature
1) space blanket (emergency)
2) incubator and radiant heater
3) water blanket (in theatre)

Intravenous infusion

Drip counter

**Fluid and electrolytes**
Assess by clinical examination U + Es and blood gases
1) I.V. replacement, calculated by weight, estimated dehydration and electrolyte results
2) Careful monitoring of fluid replacement to avoid overhydration

Endotracheal anaesthesia

**Blood loss**
Swabs weighed after use to give measure of blood loss
Transfusion after loss of 10% of blood volume

**Respiratory function**
Assess by clinical examination and blood gases
1) ?assisted ventilation
2) ?O₂ by head box
3) ?apnoea mattress

Rectal thermometer

Water blanket

**Hypoglycaemia**
Particularly a problem in small for dates or premature infants—monitor using Dextrostix and treat with I.V. dextrose

**Fig. 5.1** Neonatal surgery

and restrict ventilation. Lung capacity, forced expiratory volume and compliance are reduced; gas exchange is less efficient and $Pa_{O_2}$ falls. Rigidity of the pulmonary blood vessels produces imbalance between ventilation and perfusion. Relatively unoxygenated blood 'shunts' from pulmonary artery to vein which adds to hypoxia.

Elderly patients requiring elective procedures in whom respiratory impairment is suspected should have full investigation of the respiratory system before operation. This includes estimates of FVC, $FEV_1$ and blood gases. The sputum should be cultured and if positive an appropriate antibiotic given. Full oxygenation during and after operation is critical. Factors causing post-operative respiratory distress e.g. pain or nasogastric intubation are avoided. Intensive pre- and postoperative physiotherapy to the chest should be arranged.

*Cardiovascular system.* Atherosclerotic disease is common and thrombotic episodes frequent. Many old people have ischaemic heart disease and postoperative acute myocardial infarction may occur. A pre-operative ECG is essential in all patients over 55. Fatal postoperative myocardial infarction is more common in those with previous infarction and pre- and postoperative cardiac monitoring is instituted in those with ischaemic changes. An elective operation should not nor-mally be performed within 6 months of a proven infarct.

As vasomotor reflexes are defective, the elderly are intolerant to blood volume changes. Hypovolaemia is avoided by monitoring blood pressure and good control of fluid and electrolyte balance.

The risk of postoperative deep vein thrombosis and pulmonary embolism increase with age. Prophylactic measures should be taken (see p.281).

*Renal system.* The elderly are likely to have impaired renal function and are prone to develop acute tubular necrosis. Hypotension must be avoided. Urinary volume is monitored postoperatively so that oliguria can be promptly recognised and treated.

*Metabolic effects.* Body composition changes with age. Loss of cells, poor dietary intake, reduced caloric demands and endocrine hypofunction result in a chronic wasting disease. Serum proteins must be estimated pre-operatively. Specific deficiences are treated.

Drug metabolism is altered in the elderly and drug dosage should be carefully controlled. Oversedation of the elderly patient is bad as it may cause disorientation and unnecessary immobilisation.

Important points are summarised in Figure 5.2.

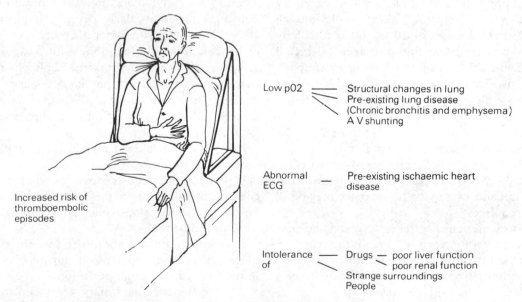

Increased risk of thromboembolic episodes

Low pO2 —— Structural changes in lung
Pre-existing lung disease
(Chronic bronchitis and emphysema)
A V shunting

Abnormal ECG — Pre-existing ischaemic heart disease

Intolerance of —— Drugs — poor liver function
poor renal function
Strange surroundings
People

**Fig. 5.2** Geriatric surgery

## THE PSYCHIATRIC PATIENT

All patients are anxious before operation. A calm and reassuring approach by ward staff and a truthful explanation of what is ahead can do much to allay fear. Tranquillisers are rarely necessary. If pre-operative anxiety is excessive operation should be postponed until a full psychiatric assessment has been arranged.

It must be remembered that psychiatric patients develop the same surgical diseases as 'normal' people. On the other hand, some hysterical patients produce a bewildering variety of symptoms in the hope of persuading a surgeon to operate. If careful investigation fails to elicit organic disease, a psychiatric opinion should be sought.

Abnormal psychiatric behaviour or a history of psychiatric disorder indicates the need for careful assessment by a psychiatrist during the pre- and postoperative periods. This should be undertaken by psychiatrist and surgeon. Drug therapy should be interrupted as little as possible during operation. Patients with suicidal and aggressive traits may require special supervision during their stay in a general hospital.

The management of postoperative mental disturbance includes recognition and treatment of precipitating factors, a sympathetic, calm and orderly approach to the patient, and if necessary sedation with diazepam (Valium — 15–30 mg daily in divided doses or 10 mg intramuscularly repeated in 4 hours) or chlorpromazine (Largactil starting with 25 mg t.i.d.; or 100 mg by suppository or 25–50 mg intramuscularly). Antidepressant therapy should not be given without psychiatric advice.

When treating mentally disturbed patients the following factors should be kept in mind:

1. Old patients in a strange environment often become disorientated, particularly at night. Adequate light and a sympathetic approach may be all that is required.

2. Disorientation may reflect hypoxia and may be resolved with oxygen and respiratory care.

3. Acute retention of urine in the elderly may cause abnormal behaviour. Catheterisation of a distended bladder will give relief.

4. Mental changes ('toxic psychosis') occur in septicaemia and may be the first sign of septicaemic shock. Patients who become confused must be examined for evidence of chest, wound or urinary tract infection. If an intestinal anastomosis has been performed leakage should be suspected.

5. Postoperative disorientation can occur from withdrawal of alcohol. Excessive alcohol intake may not have been suspected pre-operatively or may be denied by the patient. If in doubt his relatives should be consulted and treatment instituted (see p.53).

## THE JAUNDICED PATIENT

The risks of operation in the presence of jaundice are as follows:

1. *Impaired coagulation*. Bile salts in the intestine are necessary for absorption of fat-soluble vitamins (A, D, E and K). In jaundice, bile salts are absent or present in reduced amounts and absorption of vitamin K is impaired. Hepatic insufficiency leads to diminished hepatic synthesis of factors II, VII, IX and X.

The prothrombin time (PTT) monitors levels of these factors. If PTT is prolonged synthetic vitamin $K_1$ (phytomenadione) 10 mg intravenously or intramuscularly per day is given for several days before operation. If there is evidence of hepatocellular dysfunction, a full coagulation screen should be undertaken: Replacement of coagulation components may be necessary.

2. *Acute renal failure* ('Hepato-renal syndrome'). Risk of renal failure is increased in jaundiced patients as:

a. Dehydration is common and compounded by anorexia or vomiting.

b. Patients with obstructive jaundice excrete conjugated bilirubin in the urine which is believed to reduce glomerular perfusion and be toxic to tubular cells.

c. Disordered coagulation increases the risk of haemorrhage and hypotension during operation leading to reduced renal perfusion.

d. Infection of the biliary tree (cholangitis) commonly complicates biliary obstruction. Surgical manipulation of infected bile ducts can cause bacteraemia with toxic effects on the kidney.

Assuming that coagulation defects have been corrected, the most important prophylactic measure is to ensure full hydration of the patient before operation and monitor urine volume. The patient is catheterised and sufficient intravenous fluids are given to ensure a urinary output of at least 40 ml/h during operation and for 48 hours thereafter. Some administer diuretic agents such as frusemide or mannitol (100 ml 20% solution commencing 1 hour pre-operatively and given over 30 minutes) routinely during surgery but this is only necessary if adequate hydration fails to achieve adequate urine volumes. In patients with obstructive jaundice, the operation should be covered by antibiotic therapy. Cotrimoxazole (80 mg trimethoprim and 400 mg sulphamethoxazole in 5 ml diluted to 125 ml) 8 hourly or a cephalosporin are now preferred.

3. *Hepatotoxicity due to anaesthetic agents.* Many inhalation anaesthetics are hepatotoxic. The anaesthetist will choose that least likely to affect liver function e.g. cyclopropane, or may prefer epidural anaesthesia.

4. *Hepatitis virus.* Jaundiced patients with serum hepatitis constitute a potential danger to medical and nursing staff. All jaundiced patients undergoing surgery must have their serum tested for hepatitis B surface antigen and adequate precautions taken should this prove positive.

# THE MALNOURISHED PATIENT

Malnourishment presents special surgical hazards.

1. As blood volume is reduced, any further reduction by haemorrhage is not well tolerated;

2. Hypoproteinaemia leads to increased sequestration of fluid at the operation site and further reduces blood volume. The risk of pulmonary oedema following intravenous infusion of crystalloids is increased. If an intestinal anastomosis is performed, local oedema may impair patency and delay return of normal intestinal function.

3. Protein and vitamin deficiencies impair synthesis of collagen and delay wound healing. Wound dehiscence and anastomotic disruption are more common in patients who are malnourished.

4. Resistance to infection is reduced by impaired production of antibodies.

5. Protein reserves may be further depleted by the catabolic phase of the metabolic response.

The general nutritional state of the malnourished should be improved before operation if at all possible. If surgery cannot be delayed, full nutritional support must be given postoperatively.

Elemental minimal residue diets (Vivonex, Triosorbon and Flexical), are mixtures of synthetic carbohydrates, amino acids, fats (usually medium-chain triglycerides) and all essential vitamins and trace elements. They can be used as dietary supplements or to provide a complete daily intake of necessary foods in drinks of varying palatability. Alternatively, one can use various high-calorie low-residue food extracts which are available commercially. Some preparations are given in Table 5.1.

*Alimentary feeding.* Pre-operative nutrition is best provided by the alimentary route, using normal food if possible. A daily diet of 3000–3500 kcal with 100–120 g protein and added vitamins is ideally continued until body weight is within 15% of ideal.

If oral feeding is impracticable, e.g. in patients who cannot eat or in whom there is oesophageal or gastric obstruction, enteral feeding may be required. This can be given through a fine nasogastric tube or by gastrostomy or jejunostomy. The delivery of foodstuffs directly into the small intestine may cause diarrhoea and hyperosmolar solutions should be avoided. Gastrostomy and jejunostomy may cause local infection and may interfere with subsequent surgery.

*Intravenous feeding* ('parenteral nutrition') (see ch. 10). If oral intake is not possible or inadequate this is the best way to support those who are malnourished. Solutions of synthetic amino acids and of emulsified fats are now available and allow the intravenous administration of a balanced nutritional regime. Parenteral nutrition is particularly valuable in patients with excessive losses e.g. from intestinal fistulas.

**Table 5.1** Elemental diets.

| Fat | arachis oil |
|---|---|
| | corn (maize) oil |
| | sunflower oil |
| | coconut oil |
| | safflower oil |
| Protein | casein hydrolysates |
| | soya protein isolates |
| | carob seed flour |
| | whey protein |
| | synthetic amino acids |
| Carbohydrate | glucose, maltose |
| | glucose syrup solids |
| | polysaccharide polymers |
| | water-soluble dextrins |
| Minerals and vitamins | |
| | Mineral salts |
| | Vitamin preparations and synthetics |
| Examples | |
| *Vivonex*: | 1 sachet of 80 g |
| | Amino acids 6.18 g |
| | Carbohydrate (simple sugars) 69.0 g |
| | Minerals plus vitamins |
| | Energy: 300 kcals |
| | Six sachets daily |
| *Triosorbon*: | 1 sachet of 85 g |
| | Fat 19% |
| | Protein 19% |
| | Carbohydrate 56% |
| | Minerals plus vitamins |
| | Gluten free |
| | Energy: 400 kcal (1.67 MJ) |

## IMPAIRED HAEMOSTASIS

Haemostasis may be impaired by defective coagulation, disorders of the capillary endothelium, or platelet deficiency. The following are of surgical relevance:

### THE PATIENT ON ANTI-COAGULANT THERAPY

*Heparin* interferes with platelet aggregation and has antithrombin and antithromboplastin actions. A single intravenous dose of 5000 to 15 000 units prolongs clotting time to 2–3 times normal values for some 2 to 5 hours. Rapid reversion to normal follows stopping of therapy.

Protamine sulphate combines with heparin to form a stable complex without anticoagulant activity and is used to counteract heparin if urgent operation is required. A dose of 1.0–1.5 mg antagonises each 100 units of heparin. Protamine is given by *slow* intravenous injection. The quan-

tity of protamine required decreases rapidly with the time elapsed after heparin injection: after 30 minutes only about 0.5 mg is required to antagonise each 100 units injected. As low dose heparin therapy has been shown to prevent postoperative deep venous thrombosis, the heparinised patient requiring surgery is best treated by subcutaneous low-dose regime (5000 units prior to operation with 5000 units 12-hourly thereafter).

*Oral anticoagulants* of the coumarin and indanedione class act as substrate competitors with vitamin K, and depress manufacture of vitamin K-dependent clotting factors II, VII, IX and X. Provided that the prothrombin ratio is not greater than 1.5:1, major surgery can be performed without excessive bleeding.

As these drugs are bound to albumin and there is negligible renal excretion the duration of action is long. If liver function is adequate, 10 to 30 mg of synthetic vitamin $K_1$ (phytomenadione) given by intravenous or intramuscular injection will restore prothrombin time to normal within 24–48 hours. More rapid restitution can be achieved by natural vitamin $K_1$ (pylloquinone) or by transfusion of factor concentrates, plasma or blood.

## HAEMOPHILIA

Operations are potentially disastrous in haemophiliacs and close co-operation with a haematologist is essential. The level of anti-haemophiliac globulin (Factor VIII) must be maintained between 30 and 40% of normal by transfusion of concentrates of human anti-haemophiliac globulin or alternatively, fresh blood or plasma. Monitoring is by sequential estimates of Factor VIII (see p.98): the prothrombin time is normal in haemophilia.

The allied condition of Christmas disease (Factor IX deficiency) is less common and is usually less severe. Operation can be covered by transfusion of fresh frozen plasma or factor concentrate.

## THROMBOCYTOPENIA

Thrombocytopenia may be 'idiopathic' or secondary to such problems as drug reactions, hypersplenism, disseminated intravascular coagulation, or marrow destruction by radiotherapy or tumour.

Patients requiring multiple transfusions of banked blood may also develop thrombocytopenia; stored blood fails to replace platelet losses.

A platelet count of 40–50/ × 10⁹/l is normally adequate for haemostasis and platelet transfusions should be used to attain this level in thrombocytopenic patients requiring surgery. This can be given by a 'bolus' infusion immediately before operation.

## DISSEMINATED INTRAVASCULAR COAGULATION (DIC)

The causes of this rare syndrome include major trauma, septicaemia, hypoxia, transfusion reaction, metastatic carcinoma and amniotic fluid embolus. An unusual cause is transfer of peritoneal fluid to the systemic venous system by an artificial shunt as used in treatment of ascites. Coagulation systems are activated and platelet aggregation occurs within the vascular system, leading to thrombocytopenia, deficiencies of clotting factors and secondary activation of the fibrinolytic system. The level of fibrin-degradation products (FDP) is raised.

Surgically DIC is encountered most frequently in the post-operative period. Treatment is complex and may include steroids, heparin and epsilon aminocaproic acid. A haematologist should be consulted.

## FIBRINOLYSIS

*Primary* fibrinolysis is occasionally seen in patients with liver disease and metastatic carcinoma and is quite distinct from the *secondary* fibrinolysis of the DIC syndrome. The plasma fibrinogen level is diminished, platelet count is normal, thrombin time is normal or only slightly prolonged, and there is an early increase in plasma levels of fibrin-degradation products (FDP). Heparin is contra-indicated; epsilon aminocaproic acid acts as a fibrin substitute and is the treatment of choice. Its administration must be controlled by a haematologist.

---

## THE CARDIAC CASE

It has already been stated that all patients over 55 years or with cardiac symptoms must have a pre-operative ECG to detect arrhythmias and ischaemic change, and to serve as a baseline for postoperative comparison. If cardiac disease is present a cardiologist should be consulted pre-operatively.

Recent myocardial infarction seriously affects the response to surgery, and only emergency procedures are performed within 6 months of a proven infarct. Only after that time is the risk of a further infarct acceptable (Fig.5.3).

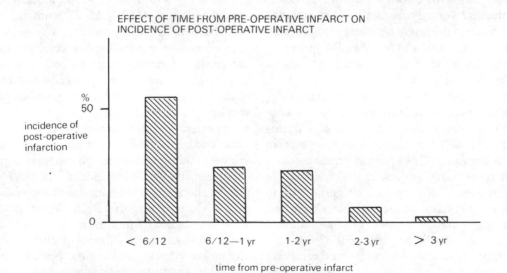

EFFECT OF TIME FROM PRE-OPERATIVE INFARCT ON INCIDENCE OF POST-OPERATIVE INFARCT

**Fig. 5.3** Risk of post-operative myocardial infarction in patients with pre-operative infarct

Patients with angina should be fully investigated before any operation. In mild cases of angina of effort, operation is safe provided anaemia is corrected and full and continued oxygenation of the blood is ensured during and after operation. Respiratory depression is avoided at all costs.

Wherever possible, operation is postponed in patients with severe angina particularly when it is of 'crescendo type'. In these circumstances coronary angiography and consideration for coronary artery revascularisation has priority.

Cardiac arrhythmias are corrected before surgery if possible. Pre-operative digitalisation may be required to control rapid atrial fibrillation, and lignocaine may be needed to suppress multiple ventricular ectopic beats.

Cardiac failure is an obvious risk factor. Occasionally a patient who requires surgery is found to have acute congestive failure. When possible, operation is delayed until failure is corrected by digitalisation and diuretics. The elderly hypertensive must be examined carefully for evidence of congestive failure; this again should be treated pre-operatively when possible.

Particular care is taken with fluid replacement in patients with congestive failure. Saline infusion is limited to approximately 500 ml daily, urine volume is monitored, and diuretics given as required. If large volumes of fluid or blood are required, monitoring of central venous pressure is essential.

Patients with valvular heart disease present particular problems. Not only are they liable to arrhythmias and failure, they may be taking drugs which can complicate the course of operation. Before other conditions can be treated by operation, surgical correction by valve replacement may be required.

Patients with some types of artificial heart valve are likely to be receiving anticoagulants. The dose should be reduced pre-operatively to give a prothrombin ratio of 1.5 to 1, or a low-dose heparin regime substitute. The normal anticoagulant regime is reinstituted as soon as the risk of acute bleeding is passed. Postoperative arterial emboli indicates the presence of intracardiac thrombus, and emergency cardiac surgery may be required to avert a fatal embolic episode.

Hypertensive patients are likely to be receiving antihypertensive agents. These drugs are now not normally withdrawn other than on the day of operation. Beta-adrenergic blockers are now the drugs most commonly used for the control of hypertension. As they impair normal cardiac responses, cardiac function must be monitored carefully during anaesthesia and in the postoperative period.

---

## CHEST DISEASE

---

## PRE-OPERATIVE ASSESSMENT AND MANAGEMENT

All patients requiring general anaesthesia are screened for chest disease by a careful history, physical examination and chest X-ray. Particular attention is paid to occupation and smoking habits, dyspnoea on exertion, and history of previous chest infection.

When impaired pulmonary function is suspected, forced expiratory volume over a standard one-second period ($FEV_1$) and forced vital capacity (FVC) are measured by spirometry. In obstructive airways disease the $FEV_1$ may be less than 1 litre and the ratio $FEV_1$:FVC is beneath the normal 80–85%. Arterial oxygen and carbon dioxide tension ($Pa_{O_2}$ and $Pa_{CO_2}$) bicarbonate [$HCO^-_3$] and pH [$H^+$] are determined as a baseline for future comparison. Normal values are $H^+$ 36–44 nmol/l, $Pa_{O_2}$ 12–15 kPa, $Pa_{CO_2}$ 4.4–6.1 kPa and plasma $HCO^-_3$ 21–27.5 nmol/l.

If the patient has a productive cough, a specimen of sputum is sent for bacteriological examination. If the sputum is green and purulent pre-operative antibiotic therapy is required; the antibiotic being selected on the results of culture and sensitivity determination.

Pre-operative physiotherapy helps clear the chest and gives valuable training in deep breathing and coughing for the post-operative period. Smoking should be forbidden. If possible the patient should stop smoking for at least two weeks before elective surgery. Bronchodilator therapy with salbutamol by mouth or by inhalation or by intravenous aminophylline is useful in obstructive airways disease and regular postural drainage should be instituted for patients with bronchiectasis or excess sputum.

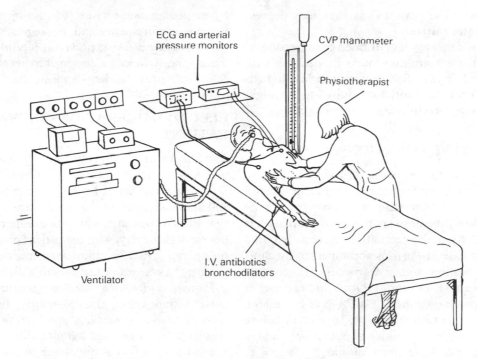

**Fig. 5.4** Post-operative care of patient with respiratory disease

Only life-saving operations should be undertaken in patients who are unable to maintain satisfactory ventilation and gaseous exchange at rest. Local or epidural anaesthesia should be considered as an alternative to general anaesthesia. If a general anaesthetic is unavoidable, pre-operative assisted ventilation may help clear the airways.

## POSTOPERATIVE CARE (Fig. 5.4)

Inhalation anaesthetics irritate the bronchial mucosa, inhibit ciliary action, increase bronchial secretions and reduce lung compliance. Wound pain impairs ventilation after thoracic and abdominal surgery. Sedation diminishes ventilation and prolonged deep sedation is contraindicated in patients with chest disease. Frequent small doses of narcotics are preferred to infrequent large doses.

The patient should expand his lungs fully by deep breathing every 30–60 minutes and clear accumulated secretions by coughing. This is facilitated by support of an abdominal wound by a physiotherapist or nurse placing her hands around the lower chest. Regular physiotherapy is essential to encourage the patient to clear his secretions. The patient must not be allowed to lie passively in bed taking shallow breaths. These fail to maintain lung expansion and allow accumulation of secretions resulting in increasing atelectasis and bronchopneumonia. The chest is examined clinically twice daily, and in the patient with chronic chest disease radiologically once daily. Respiratory efficiency is monitored by blood gas estimations.

If the patient is not able to co-operate, tracheal suction is used to clear the airway and stimulate coughing. Bronchoscopy may be required if significant airway obstruction persists.

Oxygen therapy is indicated for arterial hypoxaemia but should be given at a known concentration and its effect monitored by blood gas tension determination. A polymask or MC mask with a flow rate set at 4–6 l/min delivers approximately 60% oxygen. A ventimask or Edinburgh mask, which prevents rebreathing of expired $CO_2$, maintains inspired oxygen concentration below 35% when hypoxaemia is associated with hypercapnia. In these circumstances higher oxygen concentrations are avoided as they may depress the respiratory drive.

Antibiotic therapy is continued postoperatively. Bronchodilators are continued in patients with obstructive airways disease. Intravenous fluid administration is monitored carefully as even slight overload may precipitate pulmonary oedema.

## ASSISTED VENTILATION

Patients with severe chest disease may require assisted ventilation for hours or days after general anaesthesia. The anaesthetist will not remove the endotracheal tube until spontaneous ventilation is adequate. Assisted ventilation is required if a steady increase in $Pa_{CO_2}$ is accompanied by clinical deterioration and/or a rise in $H^+$ concentration to above 44 nmol/l. Other indications for ventilatory support include a $Pa_{CO_2}$ of less than 8 k Pa in a patient breathing 100% oxygen, failure to remove copious bronchial secretions, and a respiratory rate faster than 35/min.

There are two main types of respirator: volume-limited and pressure-limited. In the volume-limited type inspiration is terminated when a pre-set tidal volume has been delivered. Pressure-limited ventilators cycle when the peak tracheal pressure reaches a pre-set value.

A volume-limited respirator is preferred in patients with acute respiratory failure; high peak velocities compensate adequately for increased airway resistance and decreased pulmonary compliance. Oxygenation can be improved further by the use of positive end-expiratory pressure (PEEP) in which the ventilator is adjusted to provide positive pressure (5–10 cm $H_2O$) throughout the expiratory phase. This modification prevents alveolar collapse, decreases the diffusion distance for oxygen by thinning the alveolar wall, and encourages movement of fluids out of the alveoli and their adjoining interstitial space.

## THE DIABETIC

In pre-insulin days, diabetic patients undergoing surgery were exposed to considerable risk of developing fatal keto-acidosis. This risk is now reduced by meticulous supervision of insulin and carbohydrate requirements and by regular testing of blood and urine. As a general rule it is imperative to *avoid hypoglycaemia*; a degree of hyperglycaemia is acceptable provided keto-acidosis does not occur.

## ELECTIVE OPERATIONS IN DIABETIC PATIENTS

*Stable diabetics.* All diabetics must be admitted two to three days before operation to ensure that control is adequate. General anaesthesia can induce ketosis, and infection, starvation and trauma all increase the risk. Elective operations in diabetics are best carried out early in the day, with the patient placed first on the operating list. Specific management depends on the type of control of the patient's diabetes.

*Patients controlled by diet alone* require no particular action other than 4-hourly finger-prick blood glucose estimations and testing the urine regularly for sugar and ketones. Insulin may be needed temporarily if the blood glucose rises and ketosis develops.

*Patients whose diabetes is controlled by an oral hypoglycaemic agent* should omit their tablets on the morning of the operation and restart as soon as oral feeding recommences. Otherwise management is as for a patient controlled by diet alone.

*Patients whose diabetes is controlled normally by insulin* are easier to manage if soluble insulin rather than long-acting preparations are used. On the day preceding surgery the dose of depot insulin is halved and supplemented by soluble insulin later in the day. Hypoglycaemia is the major danger on the day of operation and no insulin is given prior to surgery.

Blood glucose is estimated pre-operatively. If less than 6.7 nmol/1, intra-operative hypoglycaemia is avoided by giving 25–50 g of glucose intravenously as a 10% solution. If the pre-operative blood glucose exceeds 11 nmol/1 (and this is unusual) one-third of the daily insulin requirement is given as soluble insulin *once operation has been completed*.

Following minor surgery the patient should be able to take carbohydrate orally. Drinks of 25 g glucose are given every 3 to 4 hours each covered by 12 units of insulin.

After major operations, it may be some days

before oral feeding is possible. Calorie requirements are covered by intravenous infusion of glucose (100 g/1) covered by soluble insulin (0.5 units/g) and monitored by twice-daily estimates of blood glucose. Postoperative complications increase the tendency to ketosis. Each specimen of urine must be tested for glucose and ketones: ketonuria indicates the need to increase insulin dosage. Arterial blood gases and $H^+$ concentrations will establish whether significant acidosis has developed. Electrolytes must be checked daily.

Once the patient is eating normally, he can revert to his usual insulin regime. A temporary increase in insulin requirements is common after major surgery.

## EMERGENCY OPERATIONS IN DIABETIC PATIENTS

An intravenous infusion is established and blood glucose, arterial gases and $H^+$ concentration are determined. The urine is tested for sugar and ketones. Glycosuria can usually be ignored *provided there is no ketosis*.

Keto-acidosis is an indication to defer surgery until acidosis and fluid and electrolyte abnormalities have been corrected by soluble insulin and intravenous fluids. Complete correction may not be possible until the precipitating surgical cause has been dealt with. Timely incision and drainage of an abscess may lead to considerable improvement in metabolic state. Considerable clinical judgement is required to decide the optimal timing of surgical intervention. The operation is usually performed under cover of an infusion of 10% glucose to avoid hypoglycaemia: postoperative carbohydrate and insulin requirements are determined by frequent testing of the blood and urine.

## THE ALCOHOLIC PATIENT

The following problems may arise:
1. The alcoholic is prone to malnourishment with hypoproteinaemia, chronic vitamin deficiency and poor liver function. Plasma proteins and liver function should be checked. Pre operatively the patient should have an adequate caloric intake and have daily injections of a multiple vitamin preparation (Parenterovite). If liver function tests are abnormal, the prothrombin time should be estimated. If prolonged, 20 mg synthetic vitamin $K_1$ (phytomenadione) is given daily by mouth or by intravenous or intramuscular injection.
2. The induction and maintenance of anaesthesia may require larger doses of anaesthetic agents than usual. The anaesthetist must be informed that the patient has an alcoholic history.
3. Withdrawal symptoms can pose problems particularly in the postoperative period. These consist of autonomic disturbances, hallucinations, sleep disturbance, tremor and various affective states. The mechanism is not understood. Possible fatal complications include epileptiform fits, hypovolaemia, circulatory collapse and hyperthermia.

## MANAGEMENT

The patient is nursed in quiet surroundings, isolated from the main ward. As he is likely to be dehydrated and liable to hypoglycaemia and hypomagnesaemia, intravenous infusions of saline, glucose, vitamins and magnesium are recommended.

Sedation is required. Chlormethiazole (Heminevrin) is commonly used. As the duration of the effects of alcohol withdrawal are not shortened by treatment a full 9-day course must be given. This consists of 1.5 g (three tablets of (500 mg) 6-hourly for the first 3 days; 1.0 g (two 500 mg tablets) 6-hourly for the next 3 days; and one 500 mg tablet 6-hourly for the final 3 days.

If the patient will not swallow, an 0.8% solution of chlormethiazole is administered by slow intravenous infusion. The solution is administered at a rate of 60 drops per minute (4 ml/min) until the patient is drowsy and then at 10–15 drops per minute (15 drops — 1 ml) to maintain sedation. Close and constant supervision is necessary and as soon as possible chlormethiazole tablets are substituted for the intravenous infusion.

Chlormethiazole is metabolised by the liver. Its activity may be prolonged in the alcoholic with liver decompensation.

Diazepam is now generally preferred to chlormethiazole. It is given initially by slow intravenous injection as an 0.5% solution, 150–250 $\mu$g/kg being given at a rate not greater than 5 mg/min. This is repeated if necessary in four hours or followed by an intravenous infusion to a maximum of 3 mg/kg over 24 hours. Oral medication (15–30 mg daily) may be continued.

Facilities for reversing respiratory depression must be available when using either regime.

## THE CONTRACEPTIVE PILL

Thrombo-embolic episodes are increased in women taking the contraceptive pill, particularly those which contain oestrogen. Most surgeons advise that the pill be discontinued for 6 weeks to 3 months before elective major surgery and this rule is inviolate if the patient has varicose veins, or if a non-urgent pelvic operation is required. If the pill is discontinued, advice must be given on the need for alternative methods of contraception. The ovulatory cycle may be upset by operation and adequate contraception is particularly important when the patient returns home.

Not all surgeons advise stopping the pill, maintaining that should pregnancy occur, the risks of subsequent venous thrombotic disease far outweigh those of an operation performed during administration of the pill. If the administration of the pill is continued full prophylaxis against deep vein thrombosis should be given (p.281).

## PREGNANCY

### PARTICULAR SURGICAL PROBLEMS

Pregnancy may influence surgical diseases in several ways:

1. Certain intra-abdominal conditions occur more frequently during pregnancy. Those of surgical importance are urinary tract infection, cholecystitis and intraperitoneal haemorrhage.

2. While acute abdominal inflammatory disease (e.g. appendicitis) is not more common in pregnancy, its course may be altered. The gravid uterus interferes with the normal walling-off of an infective lesion by bowel or omentum. The spread of infection is facilitated.

3. The altered position of the viscera and laxity of the abdominal wall can modify the signs of acute abdominal disease and lead to delays in reaching a correct diagnosis. Although the removal of a normal appendix during pregnancy should be avoided, it is equally important not to allow appendicitis to proceed to the point of perforation.

4. The need to avoid abdominal X-rays during the early months of pregnancy can increase diagnostic difficulties.

5. The altered hormonal background during a pregnancy may influence the course of disease outside the abdomen. For example, breast cancer occurring during the second half of pregnancy can be particularly fulminating.

## OPERATIONS DURING PREGNANCY

Elective surgery should be avoided during pregnancy. Operation is particularly dangerous during the first trimester; hypoxia and hypotension may cause developmental malformations in the fetus.

If operation during pregnancy is mandatory the anaesthetist must be forewarned. Drugs with teratogenic properties must not be given. As ovarian function is necessary for preservation of the fetus to the 16th week, ovaries should only be removed when there is no alternative.

Postoperatively the patient should be nursed in quiet surroundings. For most procedures the postoperative course is uneventful. If uterine pain, vaginal bleeding or vaginal discharge occur, an obstetrician must immediately be summoned. Various pharmacological agents, e.g. $\beta$ adrenergic stimulants, prostacyclines, which inhibit contraction are under review.

## THE ENDOCRINE CASE

The endocrine system consists of those glands which by virtue of their secretion of steroid, polypeptide or protein hormones, influence the function of a wide variety of 'target tissues'. Removal of a normal endocrine gland may have profound effects, and in the case of certain glands can prove fatal. Essential hormones must be replaced following ablative endocrine surgery.

Further illnesss, particularly if necessitating operation, can bring additional problems to patients with endocrine dysfunction.

## PITUITARY–ADRENAL SYSTEM

A particular problem is posed by those patients with pituitary or adrenal disorders in whom any additional stress may impose demands which cannot be met by secretion of glucocorticoid or mineralocorticoid hormones. This is particularly important in patients whose pituitary and adrenals have been removed; or when therapy with steroid hormones has resulted in suppression of normal endogenous secretion. Any operation or acute illness places such patients in danger of acute adrenal failure.

Normally these patients are aware of this problem, and have been warned to increase the dose of steroid maintenance therapy should these circumstances arise. In any patient requiring a general anaesthetic, steroid cover is best given as the soluble preparation cortisol (hydrocortisone) sodium succonate, 100 mg being given intravenously at the start of the operation. This dose may be repeated during the operation and further doses given by intravenous infusion (100 mg/500 ml saline per 4–6 hours and thereafter intra-muscular or oral administration of cortisol in reducing daily amounts will provide adequate steroid support.

Any surgical procedure is hazardous in patients with a catecholamine-secreting phaeochromocytoma of the adrenal medulla or paraganglionic tissue. Such patients have an extremely labile circulation and are prone to attacks of acute hypertension, hypotension and collapse. A history of paroxysmal adrenergic overactivity (hypertension, sweating, pallor, headache) or the discovery of hypertension in a young person should alert suspicion. If there is no opportunity for full and complete investigations pre-operatively, adrenergic blocking drugs should be available and the blood pressure carefully monitored during induction and maintenance of anaesthesia.

## THYROID

It is also important to assess thyroid status in patients requiring surgery. Thyrotoxicosis precipitates serious cardiac and metabolic effects and must be controlled before any operation. As there is a lag phase of up to 10 days before they exert their full inhibitory effect, the antithyroid drugs e.g. carbimazole are not helpful in the acute situation. The $\beta$-adrenergic blocking drugs rapidly antagonise the peripheral effects of thyroid hormone; propranolol t.i.d 10–30 mg should be given to the thyrotoxic patient in whom an emergency operation is required. The patient is sedated postoperatively and antithyroid medication started.

Equally important is the recognition that a patient is hypothyroid; cardiac arrythmias and arrest may develop during anaesthesia, and hypothermia and electrolyte deficiences may occur postoperatively. The careful administration of small doses of tri-iodothyronine supplemented by cortisol is accepted treatment, but must be carefully regulated. These problems are further discussed in Chapter 39.

# 6. Wounds and Wound Healing

A wound is a disruption of the normal continuity or contiguity of body structures caused by physical injury. The wounding agent may *penetrate* the surface epithelium, or give rise to a *non-penetrating wound* in which the integument remains intact while the force is transmitted to subcutaneous tissues or viscera. In both types of injury, inspection of the body surface may give little indication of the extent of damage to underlying structures.

Wounds may be classified according to the mode of damage:

1. an *incised* wound is caused by a sharp instrument, and when there is associated tissue tearing it is *lacerated*

2. an *abrasion* results from friction damage to the body surface and causes superficial bruising and loss of epithelium

3. a *crush injury* may be associated with massive tissue destruction without breaching the skin

4. *gunshot wounds* are caused by shotgun pellets or bullets. Bullets fired from high-velocity rifles cause much more tissue destruction than low-velocity bullets (see p.105)

5. *burns* are a distinct variety of wound due to heat, cold, electricity, irradiation or chemicals (see ch. 13).

---

## WOUND HEALING

### GENERAL PRINCIPLES

The essential features of the healing process are common to wounds of all tissues, and can be subdivided into three phases.

### Lag phase

The *lag phase* is characterised by the inflammatory response to injury. Capillary permeability increases and a protein-rich exudate forms in the wound, while inflammatory cells migrate into the area. Dead tissue is lysed and removed by macrophages, and bacteria are sought and destroyed by leucocytes. There is a delay of 2–3 days before fibroblasts begin to manufacture collagen from the protein-rich exudate, hence the term 'lag phase'.

### Incremental phase

The *incremental phase* is characterised by progressive collagen synthesis by fibroblasts and gain in tensile strength. The source of these cells is uncertain, but it seems likely that they arise from primitive mesenchymal stem cells in the injured area. A local stimulus to their formation may be high lactate levels consequent on ischaemia, and there is also evidence for a systemic factor in that collagen turnover remote from the wound increases. Synthesis of collagen increases as more fibroblasts appear, and the gain in tensile strength accelerates (Fig. 6.1). Old collagen in the area undergoes lysis while new collagen forms. Tensile strength is determined by the balance between these two processes. Macrophages lie adjacent to fibroblasts and may provide the amino acid building blocks needed for collagen synthesis. Collagen is synthesised within the endoplasmic reticulum of the fibroblast, and leaves the cell as tropocollagen. These monomer molecules polymerise between the cells to form cross-banded collagen fibrils.

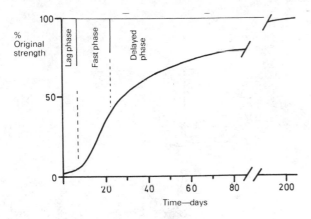

Fig. 6.1 Phases of wound healing

Proline and lysine are essential for collagen formation. Oxygen and ascorbic acid are necessary for their hydroxylation and incorporation into tropocollagen.

Collagen synthesis demands a continuing supply of energy. Ingrowth of capillary buds leads to formation of fragile capillary arches bringing oxygen and nutrients to the wound. In unapposed wounds new capillary formation is a major feature and the resulting mixture of capillaries, fibroblasts, macrophages and leucocytes is called *granulation tissue*. To the naked eye, healthy granulation tissue is red, granular and friable, and bleeds to the touch.

Fibroblasts have other important functions beside collagen manufacture. They synthesise *mucopolysaccharide* ground substance which forms an ideal environment for alignment and approximation of the tropocollagen monomers prior to polymerisation. The fibroblasts also contain microfibrils which enable them to pull in the wound margins. This *wound contraction* reduces the energy needed for wound healing by reducing the size of the defect in unapposed wounds. It must be distinguished from *contracture* which is the excessive shrinkage of fibrosis and which causes unsightly puckering and restricted mobility if the wound crosses a joint.

## Plateau phase

The *plateau phase* is characterised by levelling-off in the gain in tensile strength. In the final clear-ing-up process, excess collagen is removed and the number of fibroblasts and inflammatory cells declines. Collagen formation still proceeds more quickly than normal, but there is net resorption due to increased collagen lysis. However, the wound still gains in tensile strength from remodelling during this period, the collagen fibres being laid down as an interlocking network rather than as an amorphous mass. The wound continues to gain tensile strength for some 6 months, although the gain over the first 7–10 days is usually sufficient to allow removal of skin sutures without wound disruption. Remodelling never returns the wound to normal, and skin and fascia usually recover only 80% of their original tensile strength.

## HEALING IN SOME SPECIALISED TISSUES

### Skin

Skin healing requires restoration of epidermal continuity with restoration of strength in the supporting dermis. Meticulous apposition of the edges of a clean incised skin wound leaves a narrow epidermal defect which can be bridged easily (Fig. 6.2). The basal epidermal cells at the wound edges undergo mitosis and continuity of the basal layer is restored within a few days. This ideal method of healing requires minimal expenditure of energy, results in a fine hairline scar, and is known as healing by *first intention*.

If the wound edges are not apposed, the defect fills gradually with granulation tissue and restoration of epidermal continuity may take a considerable time. Continued basal cell division at the wound edges produces sheets of cells which migrate across the denuded area, but their advance is often hindered by infection. The process is known as healing by *second intention* and usually results in prolonged healing, excessive fibrosis, and an ugly puckered scar.

If a wound has begun to heal by second intention, it may be possible to compromise by freshening the wound edges and bringing them into apposition or by covering the defect with a skin graft.

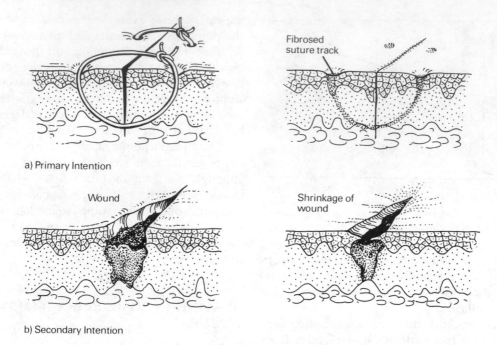

a) Primary Intention

Fibrosed
suture track

Wound

Shrinkage of
wound

b) Secondary Intention

**Fig. 6.2** Wound healing by primary intention and secondary intention

## Bone

Torn blood vessels produce a haematoma between the bone ends, and fibroblasts and capillaries grow into the ischaemic area to form granulation tissue. Leucocytes and macrophages are soon on hand to destroy bacteria and phagocytose debris. Cartilage forms within the granulation tissue and the resulting plastic connective tissue or *callus* binds the bone ends together. Dormant osteogenic cells in the periosteum become active osteoblasts and lay down a sheath of bone around the broken ends. At the same time, new bone forms in the medullary cavity. The cartilage in the callus calcifies and is replaced by a process of intra-membranous bone formation. The callus gradually shrinks and the new bone between the fractured ends becomes compact rather than spongy, with ultimate bony union. Extensive remodelling follows so that it becomes difficult to identify the fracture site. Strength returns gradually and, as with soft tissue injuries, the process continues for months.

The essential difference between healing of a fracture and soft tissue injury lies in the preliminary cartilage formation and subsequent conversion of fibrocartilage to bone. Nevertheless, the fibroblast retains central importance and its collagen provides a basic framework on which hydroxyapatite crystals condense to form bone.

## Nervous tissue

Wounds of the nervous system involve both neural and connective tissue. Neural tissue in the *central* nervous system cannot regenerate, and fibroblasts derived from glial or perivascular cells replace nervous tissue with collagen.

Damage to the *peripheral* nervous system is not so final. Cut axons degenerate distal to the injury but provided the neural body survives, the axons of the proximal stump attempt re-innervation by sprouting and crossing the gap to enter empty Schwann tubes. This endeavour is aided by fibroblasts forming a connective bridge, although this may prove self-defeating if it results in a dense collagen scar. Not all of the axons find their way into Schwann tubes; some find their way into the 'wrong' tube, and some perish as a result of entering tubes already occupied. Nevertheless, useful re-innervation is possible. Regenerating axons can grow as quickly as 4–5 mm a day, but on average the rate is approximately 1–1.5 mm a day.

## Intestine

Damage confined to gut mucosa, as in gastric erosion, is repaired by re-epithelialisation and leaves no scar. A return to normal becomes impossible when ulceration extends through the submucosa to involve underlying muscle, and a permanent fibrous scar is inevitable.

The stomach and small bowel have a plentiful blood supply and contain relatively small numbers of pathogenic bacteria. Leakage is uncommon following resection and anastomosis. Lysis of collagen occurs in the normal bowel on either side of the anastomosis as part of the inflammatory response, and at one week the anastomosis is usually able to withstand disruption as well as adjoining bowel.

The oesophagus has a weaker wall than the stomach and proximal intestine, and has less extensive blood supply. The distal colon also has a tenuous blood supply, and here the problems of healing are increased by the large numbers of pathogenic bacteria in the bowel lumen. Bacteria delay collagen synthesis and collagenase production can cause excessive lysis. Anastomotic disruption usually becomes manifest clinically by the fourth to sixth postoperative day.

Surgical technique is of fundamental importance in reducing the incidence of anastomotic leakage and wound infection after gastro-intestinal surgery (see below). The connective tissue of the submucosa is the strongest layer of the bowel wall and sutures or staples in this layer maintain apposition until sufficient tensile strength has been regained. In view of the dangers of anastomotic leakage, many surgeons leave drains at the site of anastomosis. This ensures free egress of infected material should disruption occur.

## FACTORS INFLUENCING WOUND HEALING

Many of these factors are interrelated, as for example the site of the wound, its blood supply, and level of tissue oxygenation. Some of the factors cannot be influenced (e.g. age), but many factors such as nutritional status, surgical technique and intercurrent disease can be influenced to promote wound healing.

## Blood supply

Wounds heal slowly in ischaemic tissue, are prone to infection, and frequently break down. Failure to heal by first intention is problematic in that the ischaemic wound may not be able to sustain the metabolic demand necessary for healing by second intention. Arterial oxygen partial pressure ($Pa_{O_2}$) is the important determinant of the rate of collagen synthesis and anaemia *per se* does not impair healing if the patient is normovolaemic and has normal arterial oxygen tension.

## Infection

The factors which determine whether a surgical wound becomes infected are:

*General patient factors.* These include increasing age, cardiovascular and respiratory status, nutritional status, and presence of intercurrent infection.

*Local wound factors.* Bacterial contamination of the wound is minimised by skin preparation and meticulous aseptic technique. The nature of the operation affects the degree of contamination anticipated. Wounds are classified as clean, clean-contaminated or dirty (see below).

Despite adequate precautions, at least some bacteria gain access to the wound during operation. They may enter from without, from internal foci of sepsis, or from the lumen of transected organs. In some cases, contamination occurs in the post-operative period.

Assuming that contamination is not gross, the wound is usually able to deal with bacteria without developing overt infection. Devitalised tissues, haematoma and the presence of foreign material (e.g. sutures and prosthetic materials) favour bacterial survival and growth outwith the reach of body defences. Hypoxia compromises the ability of leucocytes to kill bacteria and also favours the growth of potentially dangerous anaerobic organisms.

Infection of closed wounds is most likely when

contamination occurs during surgery, but the wound remains vulnerable for at least 3–4 days. The common infecting organisms are staphylococci, streptococci, *E. coli* and anaerobes such as bacteroides and anaerobic streptococci.

Overcrowding of surgical wards and excessive use of operating theatres increases the incidence of wound infection as the bacterial population of the atmosphere increases (see Ch. 3).

*Therapeutic factors.* Topical or systemic antibiotics or antibacterial chemicals are used increasingly in prophylaxis when wound contamination is anticipated. For example, one third of wounds used to become infected after appendicectomy for acute appendicitis. This incidence can be reduced to about 10% by topical antibiotics or the antibacterial agent, povidone iodine. Antibiotics are used widely to prevent infection during elective colon surgery and the current emphasis is on short courses of therapy to cover the period of operation (p.422).

## Age

Wounds heal less well with advancing age. This relates to a combination of diminished tissue response to injury, impaired blood supply, poor nutritional status, and a high incidence of intercurrent disease.

## Wound situation

Surgical incisions placed in the lines of least tissue tension are subject to minimal distraction and have the greatest chance of healing promptly to leave a fine scar. In the face, these lines form the lines of facial expression, and tend to run at right angles to the direction of underlying muscles.

Wounds of the head and neck heal quickly so that sutures or skin clips can usually be removed within 3–5 days. At the other extreme, wounds of the leg and foot heal slowly and sutures may have to be retained for 14 days. These differences reflect the importance of blood supply, and warm vascular areas are generally quicker to heal than the cool extremities.

## Nutritional status

A wound has high priority when competing with unwounded tissues for body resources. This means that malnutrition has to be severe before healing is affected. Protein availability is the most important factor, and wound dehiscence and infection are common when the serum albumin is low. As a rule of thumb, healing problems can be anticipated if recent weight loss involves more than 20% of original body weight.

Ascorbic acid is essential for proline hydroxylation and collagen synthesis, although the number of fibroblasts is not reduced in scorbutic states. Zinc is a component of enzymes involved in the healing process and its deficiency retards healing. Supplements of ascorbic acid and zinc are effective when these factors are deficient, but do not improve healing in normal subjects.

## Intercurrent disease

Cachectic patients with *severe malnutrition* (e.g. advanced cancer) have marked impairment of healing.

*Diabetes mellitus* impairs healing by reducing tissue resistance to infection and causing peripheral vascular insufficiency. Peripheral neuropathy may also contribute by diminishing peripheral sensation and allowing trauma to the healing wound.

Patients with a *haemorrhagic diathesis* are at increased risk of haematoma formation and wound infection.

*Obstructive airways disease* lowers $Pa_{O_2}$ and so affects healing. Abdominal wound dehiscence is commoner in patients with respiratory disease due to strain placed on the wound during coughing.

*Corticosteroid* therapy reduces the inflammatory response, impairs collagen synthesis, and reduces resistance to infection. The effect of steroids is most marked if they are given within 3 days of injury.

*Immuno-suppressive* therapy also impairs healing by depressing resistance to infection in patients already compromised by their underlying disorder.

## Surgical technique

*Skin incisions* are placed in the line of least tissue tension provided this allows adequate exposure. Meticulous aseptic technique is essential to avoid wound infection and poor healing. *Gentle tissue handling* is mandatory, and failure to achieve haemostasis, excessive use of diathermy and extensive dissection all contribute to wound devitalisation.

*Potentially infective sites*, such as the gut lumen during colonic surgery, should be isolated from the wound by additional sterile drapes and spillage of contents is avoided by correct use of occlusion and crushing clamps. Particular care is taken in areas where there is reduced resistance to infection (e.g. bone) or in areas where infection would have serious consequences (e.g. neurosurgery).

The choice of *suture materials* is important. The suture should be strong enough to provide support for the wound until tensile strength is sufficient to prevent breakdown. Absorbable materials are preferred but non-absorbable sutures may be essential in some situations, as for example in the aponeurotic layer of an abdominal paramedian wound. Any foreign material implanted in the body predisposes to infection, so that non-absorbable sutures should be inert, retain strength, and preferably be monofilamentous to avoid interstices which might favour bacterial growth.

Suture materials are designed to pass through the tissues with as little trauma as possible. To this end sutures are no longer threaded through a wide needle eye, but are usually bonded to the needle without any increase in bulk (the atraumatic suture). The needle may be round-bodied on cross-section when tissue resistance is low (e.g. intestinal suture), or triangular in section when sharp cutting edges are needed to facilitate passage through tough tissues such as skin.

To avoid wound devitalisation, sutures should not be placed too close together, too near the wound margin, or tied too tightly. When there is an increased risk of abdominal wound dehiscence, some surgeons reinforce closure with deep 'tension sutures' which pass through all layers of the abdominal wall, or all layers but peritoneum.

These sutures are of strong (gauge 1) non-absorbable materials and are threaded through a length of plastic tubing to avoid cutting into the abdominal wall. Most surgeons no longer use 'tension sutures' and prefer a mass closure technique in which non-absorbable sutures are placed through all layers of the abdominal wall except skin, or use a continuous suture of monofilament non-absorbable material to re-approximate the anterior rectus sheath.

*Accurate apposition* of wound edges keeps the task of healing to a minimum and favours healing by first intention. Dead space in the depth of the wound must be avoided if at all possible, as bleeding into the space and accumulation of exudate favours development of infection. When dead space cannot be avoided the wound may be left open and packed, or closed with insertion of a drain. Correct apposition of the deeper layers often allows the skin edges to fall together without tension so that skin apposition can be achieved by superficial sutures or Steristrips.

## Wound protection

Surgical closure does not close the door to wound infection. The risk of contamination from the surface is highest in the first 5 days and although the risk is usually small, it is customary to protect the wound by a sterile occlusive dressing or occlusive spray such as Nobecutane. If redressing is necessary an aseptic technique is essential.

Skin sutures and drains are potential portals for bacterial entry and should not be retained longer than necessary.

## PROBLEMS IN WOUND MANAGEMENT

## POST-OPERATIVE WOUND INFECTION

Surgical procedures can be classified according to the likelihood of contamination and wound infection.

*Clean* procedures are those in which wound contamination should not occur. A clean elective surgical incision should not become infected if no infective focus is encountered and no organ is entered which might contain pathogenic bacteria (e.g. colon). Subtotal thyroidectomy, parietal cell vagotomy, and meniscectomy are examples of clean operations in which the wound infection rate should be less than 1%.

*Clean contaminated* procedures are those in which no frank focus of infection is encountered, but a significant risk of infection occurs. Cholecystectomy, sub-total gastrectomy and prostatectomy are examples of operations in which wound infection occurs occasionally, but infection rates in excess of 5% denote breakdown in ward and operating theatre routine.

*Contaminated* or 'dirty' wounds are those in which gross contamination is inevitable and the risk of troublesome wound infection is high. Emergency surgery for perforated diverticular disease and drainage of a subphrenic abscess are examples of procedures likely to cause wound contamination.

## Clinical presentation

Post-operative wound infection usually becomes evident 3–4 days after surgery. In its common form it starts with superficial cellulitis around the wound margins or swelling of the wound with some serous discharge from between the sutures. In some cases of deep infection there are no local signs, although the patient may have pyrexia and increased wound tenderness.

Systemic upset is variable, usually amounting only to moderate pyrexia.

Fluctuation is occasionally elicited when there is an abscess or liquifying haematoma, and crepitus may be present if gas-forming organisms are involved. Toxaemia, bacteraemia and septicaemia can complicate serious wound infection.

The differential diagnosis includes other causes of post operative pyrexia, wound haematoma, and wound dehiscence.

*Wound haematoma* may result from reactive bleeding in the wound during the first 24–48 hours after operation. It causes swelling and discomfort with minimal pyrexia and few systemic signs. As a haematoma is liable to become infected, it should be evacuated.

*Wound dehiscence* will be considered separately (p.63).

## Treatment

Prevention is better than cure. The incidence of wound infection is reduced by adequate preparation of the patient, the prophylactic use of antibiotics in high-risk situations, and the observance of good operative theatre techniques. To avoid contamination, wounds should be dressed in a separate treatment or dressing room and not in the general ward.

Trivial superficial cellulitis can be managed expectantly. The area of redness is 'mapped out' with an indelible pen so that its extent can be monitored. Spreading cellulitis is an indication for antibiotic therapy.

Deeper and more serious infections can often be aborted by the removal of one or more skin sutures, to promote free drainage of infected material from suture track or wound. Failure to provide free drainage allows an infection to flourish in the hypoxic closed space and can lead to abscess formation. If the removal of skin sutures does not result in the free discharge of infected material, the wound should be probed gently with sinus forceps under aseptic conditions.

If pus is definitely suspected in the wound but adequate drainage has not been provided, the patient may have to be returned to theatre for full exploration of the wound under general anaesthesia.

The wound is left open and is usually packed lightly to prevent premature closure of the skin edges before infection has been controlled in the depths of the wound. In the presence of severe infection, the packing can be soaked in a bactericidal agent.

Many infected wounds heal rapidly without further surgery, particularly when the original skin incision was placed in one of the lines of least tissue tension. The problem is often one of keeping the wound open rather than one of achieving closure. If it appears that the wound will take a long time to close spontaneously, *secondary suture* or skin grafting can be considered to speed healing once it is clear that infection has been eradicated. The presence of clean healthy granulation tissue in the wound is usually a good indication that closure can be undertaken.

In all infected wounds a wound swab or a specimen of pus is sent routinely for bacteriological culture and sensitivity determinations. Although antibiotics are not usually necessary when the infection is not extensive and free drainage has been achieved, their use is indicated where there is spreading cellulitis, severe deep infection or persistent pyrexia. It is therefore important to know the sensitivity of the causative organism. In urgent cases a Gram-stain of a smear of material from the wound will give initial guidance to the initial choice of antibiotic.

## ABDOMINAL WOUND DEHISCENCE

Most surgical units have an overall incidence of abdominal wound dehiscence of about 1%. Wound dehiscence is a particular problem in obese patients, those with chest complications, those with abdominal distension due to ileus or ascites, and in patients with debilitating disease such as cancer. The incidence can be minimised by careful patient preparation, including preoperative chest care and cessation of smoking for at least 2 weeks before surgery, by meticulous attention to surgical technique, and by prompt treatment of postoperative respiratory tract infection. The value of deep tension sutures in preventing dehiscence is debated and many surgeons no longer employ them.

The signs of dehiscence are frequently delayed for 7–10 days after surgery. A *profuse* sero-sanguineous discharge of peritoneal fluid from the wound is often the first manifestation and indicates dehiscence unless proved otherwise. The patient may be unaware that dehiscence has occurred, or may have felt 'something go' after a bout of coughing or sudden exertion. The surface of the wound may appear intact, but disruption of the deeper layers can be demonstrated by contracting the abdominal wall by asking the patient to cough or lift his head from the pillow. In some cases, protrusion of bowel or omentum through the wound removes any doubt that dehiscence has occurred.

Immediate operative repair is mandatory when dehiscence is complete. Partial dehiscence of the deep layers can be treated conservatively if operation is contra-indicated by the patient's general condition. The patient is provided with an elastic or adjustable abdominal support so that it can be tightened by the patient during coughing or exertion. With careful management, the wound may then heal to allow discharge from hospital and return to work. However, an incisional hernia is inevitable and may require subsequent repair.

Abdominal wound dehiscence is repaired under general anaesthesia by 'through and through' sutures which pass through all layers of the abdominal wall.

## THE CONTAMINATED WOUND

The state of immunity against tetanus is determined and appropriate action taken (p.65). The wound is inspected carefully under good illumination so that contamination, degree of devitalisation and injury to vital structures can be assessed. A decision is made as to whether the wound can be dealt with under local (or regional) anaesthesia in the casualty department, or whether more extensive exploration and surgery is required under general anaesthesia in an operating theatre.

Small uncontaminated wounds are treated under local anaesthesia on an out-patient basis. The wound margins are cleaned with cetrimide solution and the wound irrigated copiously. Devitalised tissue is removed, deep tissues are sutured with absorbable material and the skin margins are closed.

More extensive, contaminated wounds usually require in-patient treatment with exploration and debridement under general anaesthesia. The wound and its margins are cleansed with cetrimide and pieces of grit, soil and other obvious foreign material are picked out. Once it is apparent that there is no injury to vital structures, the wound margins are excised with a scalpel (Fig. 6.3) and all devitalised tissue or tissue of questionable viability is removed. Damaged muscle should be trimmed back until bleeding occurs.

When contamination has been gross, primary closure should not be carried out. Wound infection and breakdown is inevitable and there is a risk of anaerobic infection which may threaten both life and limb. Under these circumstances *delayed primary suture* is employed. The wound is

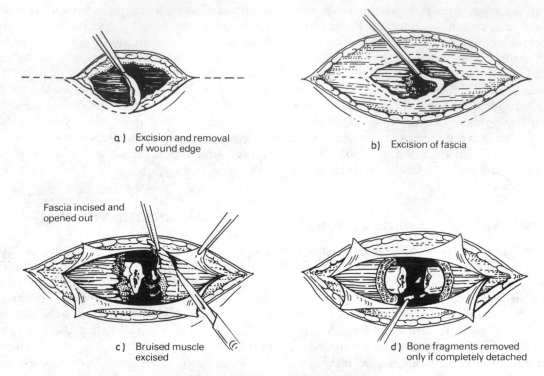

a) Excision and removal of wound edge

b) Excision of fascia

Fascia incised and opened out

c) Bruised muscle excised

d) Bone fragments removed only if completely detached

**Fig. 6.3** Technique of wound excision

packed with gauze soaked in an antiseptic, the dressing is changed daily (or more frequently if infection is severe), and closure is postponed for some days until it is obvious that infection has been eradicated and that the wound is filling with healthy granulation tissue.

Delayed primary suture can also be applied to wounds contaminated during surgery, as for example after emergency operation for perforated appendicitis or following resection of gangrenous bowel in a strangulated hernia. In these circumstances, the peritoneum and aponeurotic layer are closed but the skin and subcutaneous tissues are left open. Skin sutures may be inserted at this time, but are not tied until some days later when it is clear that infection has been avoided.

Antibiotic therapy is essential for grossly contaminated wounds. The choice of antibiotics is determined by the nature of the infection process but the aim is to achieve high tissue concentration as soon as possible. Crystalline penicillin (up to 5 mega units/day for 2 days) given intra-muscularly is preferred for traumatic wounds. Other antibiotics which achieve excellent concentrations in the wound include flucloxacillin and ampicillin and cephalosporins. Gentamicin, carbenicillin and oxacillin achieve only modest concentrations, and are used only when indicated by tests for bacterial sensitivity.

Following emergency surgery for faecal peritonitis, it has been popular to employ a combination of penicillin, gentamicin and lincomycin to reduce the dangers of peritonitis, wound infection and septicaemia. Metronidazole (Flagyl) is now used increasingly in this situation due to its ability to destroy anaerobes. Topical agents such as povidone iodine are also used in some centres to combat infection in contaminated wounds. Although antibiotic treatment is a valuable and important part of management, it must be stressed that it supplements but does not replace thorough surgical management. Radical excision of the wound margins, thorough mechanical cleansing, and delayed suture are the true foundations of successful management.

## MANAGEMENT OF DEVITALISED SKIN FLAPS

A common emergency problem is posed by the patient, usually an elderly female, who falls and raises a triangular flap over the surface of the tibia. As the base of the flap is usually situated distally, its circulation is likely to be impaired. In many cases the flap is blue-black in colour and obviously non-viable; in most viability is uncertain.

The wound is cleansed and non-viable tissue excised. The remaining flap should be 'defatted' before being sutured in place (Fig. 6.4). If the defect cannot be closed without tension, either the wound is allowed to granulate or a split skin graft is applied immediately. Grafting is unwise in the presence of gross contamination, when there may be no alternative to leaving the excised wound to granulate, and undertaking grafting as a secondary procedure. This involves a prolonged stay in hospital. When the wound is small, wound contraction may allow epithelialisation without grafting.

## GUNSHOT WOUNDS (see p.105)

Essential steps in management include excision of the missile and intruded foreign material, excision of devitalised tissues in the wound track, and excision of the entry and exit wounds. After thorough cleansing, the wound is left open and primary closure delayed whenever possible. Antibiotic prophylaxis is routine.

## SPECIFIC WOUND INFECTIONS

### TETANUS

The bacillus *Clostridium tetani* is found in large numbers in soil and faeces, and is a frequent contaminant of accidental wounds. Survival of all anaerobic bacilli in a wound is favoured by hypoxia, the presence of haematoma, and by devitalised tissue. Failure to debride and excise the wound coupled with ill-judged primary closure provides an ideal environment in which organisms flourish.

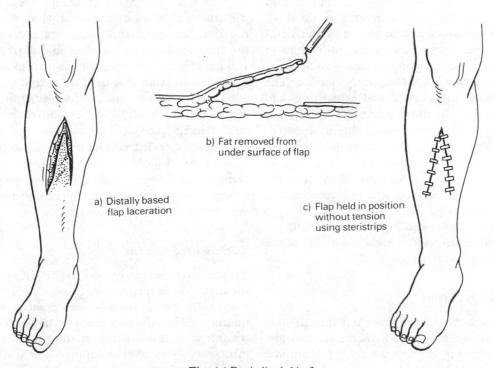

b) Fat removed from under surface of flap

a) Distally based flap laceration

c) Flap held in position without tension using steristrips

**Fig. 6.4** Devitalized skin flap

When infection is established, the tetanus bacillus causes little evidence of local wound inflammation. However, it produces an exotoxin which causes neuromuscular irritability and intermittent muscular spasm. In 30% of cases the initial injury may be a trivial puncture wound and may be so small as to be ignored by the patient.

The *incubation period* between injury and development of symptoms varies from a few days to 3 months, but most cases declare themselves within 2 weeks. The *onset period* denotes the delay between the first symptom and the onset of muscle spasms. The prognosis is better in patients with long incubation and long onset periods. The clinical presentation is insidious. Tingling, ache or stiffness in the original wound area is often the first symptom. Jaw movements become restricted (hence the traditional name, lockjaw), facial muscle spasms produce a sardonic grin (risus sardonicus), and the neck muscles become stiff. Dysphagia, laryngeal spasm and spasm of the chest wall muscles and diaphragm can compromise ventilation and threaten life. The risk of aspiration is reduced by use of an indwelling nasogastric tube. With severe infection, painful muscle spasm may become more widespread and increase in frequency and duration. Arching of the back muscles can produce a state known as opisthotonus. Sphincter spasm may cause difficulties in micturition. The patient remains conscious although consciousness is frequently clouded. The muscle spasms are painful and exhausting, and may be triggered by minor stimuli. The temperature may remain normal or only slightly elevated, despite profuse sweating and tachycardia.

It is important to realise that these are the clinical features of a severe attack. Many cases are mild and do not develop the full spectrum of muscle spasm.

Diagnosis is confirmed by the demonstration of club-shaped gram-positive rods in a biopsy of the devitalised wound tissue.

## Tetanus prevention

Tetanus is a preventable disease and although it is now uncommon in Western medicine, this low incidence can only be maintained by continued attention to prophylaxis.

a. *Active immunisation.* All children in Britain are now actively immunised against tetanus by three intramuscular injections (3 × 1 ml) of tetanus toxoid. The first and second injections are separated by an interval of 4–6 weeks, the second and 'booster' injections by an interval of 6 months to a year. Adults (except members and former members of the Armed Forces) are at present unlikely to have been immunised unless they have had previous injuries.

The state of immunity is checked when the patient first presents. Patients immunised within the last 10 years are given a booster injection of 0.5 ml of toxoid, although the need for this is debatable. A full course of immunisation is advisable if there is any doubt regarding immunisation in the past.

Passive immunisation by equine immune globulin (anti-tetanic serum, ATS) was popular before the move to active immunisation. However, there is an unacceptable incidence of hypersensitivity reaction and at best only transient immunity is produced. For these reasons, equine immune globulin should now be abandoned.

Human immune globulin is available but is only used in the management of neglected or contaminated wounds (e.g. gun-shot wound of the buttocks, agricultural accidents) as an adjunct to active immunisation and antibiotic treatment. It is given as 250 i.u. by intramuscular injection at a site distant from that used for toxoid.

b. *Wound excision and debridement.* Immunisation is not a substitute for careful excision and debridement (p.63).

c. *Antibiotics.* Intramuscular penicillin (at least 1 mega unit 6-hourly) is given routinely for all contaminated wounds, and is effective against the tetanus bacillus. In patients allergic to penicillin erythromycin may be substituted.

## Tetanus treatment

Treatment is intensive and begins the moment the diagnosis is made.

a. *Destruction of the infecting organism.* Human immune globulin has a more certain role in the treatment of established tetanus and is given intravenously as 5000 i.u. diluted in 500 ml saline over 6 hours on three successive days. The wound is excised, debrided, and is left open. Penicillin is administered to kill surviving bacteria and prevent further release of toxin.

b. *Life support.* The above measures should prevent continued liberation of exotoxin. The effects of toxin already liberated have also to be countered if the patient is to survive. The patient is nursed in a quiet, shaded intensive-care room and is well-sedated. Muscle spasms in severe tetanus are controlled by tubocurarine (or other neuromuscular blocking agent), necessitating ventilation. Curarisation apart, tracheostomy may be required to relieve respiratory embarrassment. Other agents sometimes used to depress excitability and control spasms include barbiturates, diazepam and chlorpromazine.

The patient is in a hypercatabolic state and nutrition must be maintained. Because of the inability to swallow, a nasogastric tube is passed to allow tube feeding. The patient must be turned regularly to avoid development of pressure sores.

Intense sympathetic activity has been troublesome in some cases of tetanus and arrhythmias may require beta-blocking agents for their control.

## CLOSTRIDIAL INFECTION

Six strains of clostridia can cause invasive infection of soft tissues in man, and produce a spectrum of changes ranging from superficial cellulitis to life-threatening gas gangrene. The organisms are saprophytes and form spores which are present in soil, faeces and clothing. They are strict anaerobes and their growth is favoured by failure to debride contaminated wounds.

The organisms produce a number of toxins including necrotising lecithinase, collagenase, hyaluronidase, protease, lipase and haemolysin. These toxins devitalise cells, destroy the local microcirculation and favour dissemination of infection. Their entry into the systemic circulation is heralded by clouding of consciousness, delirium, tachycardia, pallor and jaundice, progressing to circulatory collapse and death.

The organisms produce a brown seropurulent discharge with a characteristic autopsy room smell. The spectrum of local infection extends from superficial contamination of an open wound, through invasion of subcutaneous tissue, the production of *crepitant* clostridial cellulitis and localised painful myositis, to oedematous gangrene. Localised forms of infection do not produce systemic signs, or at most a mild systemic upset with fever and tachycardia. Diffuse myositis and oedematous gangrene produce profound systemic upset and threaten both life and the affected limb.

An infection typically takes 2–3 days to become manifest as an unexplained deterioration in the patient's general condition. The wound must be inspected, involving removal of plaster casts if need be. The brown sero-purulent discharge, odour, oedema and crepitus leave no doubt as to the diagnosis which is confirmed by a gram-stain of the discharge revealing Gram-positive rods.

### Prevention

As described for tetanus, correct primary wound care by excision and debridement are essential, and contaminated wounds must not be closed by primary suture. Penicillin remains the prophylactic antibiotic of choice. Polyvalent gas gangrene antitoxin is available but its efficiency is in doubt. Allergic reactions are common and it should not now be used.

### Treatment

An established infection is treated radically. The wound is opened widely, fascial compartments are freely incised, and dead tissue is excised. Muscle must be excised widely until bleeding tissue is encountered. In some cases amputation is obviously required.

Wounds are loosely packed and left open, to be closed only when they appear healthy. Wide tissue defects may require subsequent reconstruction with skin grafting. Amputation stumps are also left open in the first instance.

Antibiotic therapy is essential and penicillin is given in massive doses (e.g. 20–40 mega-units a day intravenously).

Hyperbaric oxygenation in a pressure chamber is useful but is not a replacement for adequate surgery. No increase in $Pa_{O_2}$ will get oxygen into dead tissues or eradicate established infection.

Hypovolaemia is common in gas gangrene, and multiple blood transfusions are needed.

A particular form of clostridial infection may follow penetrating injury to the colon or rectum, the source of infecting organisms being the bowel. In addition to wide debridement and free drainage, a proximal colostomy is essential.

## NECROTISING FASCIITIS

This denotes an invasive infection of fascial planes by multiple organisms such as microaerophilic streptococci, gram-negative bacilli, bacteroides and clostridia. Bacteria may have a synergistic effect on promoting spreading of infection. The infection causes thrombosis of vessels passing to the skin and produces widespread necrosis of the skin and subcutaneous tissues.

The organisms may enter through an apparently trivial wound, but spread rapidly and widely along fascial planes. The part becomes oedematous, crepitus may be elicited, and the skin becomes anaesthetic and discoloured. The patient usually shows clouding of consciousness, fever and tachycardia.

### Treatment

This consists of radical debridement with incisions placed in the long axis of the part. Fascia is more extensively involved than skin, and some skin can often be saved despite excision of underlying necrotic fascia. The muscle is not involved directly, but swelling can produce muscle ischaemia within osteofascial compartments. For this reason, fascia is incised widely to prevent muscle necrosis. It is vital that necrotising fasciitis be distinguished from clostridial myositis and gangrene; amputation should not be necessary in treatment of fasciitis.

Penicillin in massive doses is once again the mainstay of antibiotic therapy, but other agents such as gentamicin and metronidazole may be needed if culture shows the presence of gram-negative organisms and bacteroides.

Massive blood transfusions may be needed to sustain circulating blood volume. Hyperbaric oxygen therapy has been used but is less effective than in gas gangrene, and is no substitute for surgery and antibiotic therapy.

## SYNERGIC DERMAL GANGRENE

This is chronic progressive gangrene of the skin due to a synergic infection by aerobic and anaerobic organisms. It occurs predominantly in abdominal wounds, or around the perineum, buttock and scrotum. It may complicate the formation of a colostomy or an infection of the ischiorectal fossa.

The appearances are classical, there being a central black necrotic zone surrounded by an advancing serpiginous purplish area with a fading erythematous margin. Treatment is by intensive antibiotic therapy, radical excision of sloughs and, in severe cases, hyperbaric oxygen. The underlying subcutaneous tissues are not involved.

# 7. The Metabolic Response to Operation and Injury

Following accidental or deliberate injury, a series of changes occurs both locally and generally, which in due course serves to restore the *status quo*. The local response of inflammation is supported by the generalised response which conserves fluid and provides energy for repair. The generalised response is protean in its manifestations and is termed the *metabolic response to trauma*.

There is an *ebb* and *flow* phase following injury. The short *ebb phase* corresponds to the period of traumatic shock and is associated with general depression of enzymatic activity and oxygen consumption. The *flow phase* which follows is divided into two parts: (a) an initial *catabolic* phase with protein and fat mobilisation, with associated increased urinary nitrogen excretion and weight loss, which usually lasts 3–8 days; followed by (b) an *anabolic* phase lasting for some weeks during which protein and fat stores are restored and weight is regained (the recovery phase).

It is believed that the changes following injury are due to a complex neuro-endocrine mechanism designed to conserve body fluid volume, to mobilise amino acids from protein for gluconeogenesis and wound repair, and to mobilise fat for energy production.

The description that follows concentrates on the catabolic period of the *flow phase* as this is the period of most concern in the management of operated or injured patients.

## FACTORS INITIATING THE METABOLIC RESPONSE

The term 'injury' embraces a variety of causal factors, including trauma, haemorrhage and burns. Other factors which may induce or prolong the response include infection, myocardial infarction and pulmonary embolism.

## VOLUME DEPLETION

Volume depletion is much the most important single factor initiating the metabolic response to injury. Fluid loss is obvious in haemorrhage or burns. At the site of any injury or infection, there is local oedema due to excess fluid transudation from capillaries. This fluid sequestrates locally and is effectively lost from the circulating fluid volume. Changes in volume result in changes in plasma osmolality which further modify the response (see ch. 8). The general response in terms of volume conservation is summarised in Figure 7.1.

Catecholamines play an important part in volume conservation. They have vasoconstrictive effects on the kidney and circulation in general. They also affect intermediate metabolism of carbohydrate, fat and protein. The catecholamines have been described as the *front runner* hormones in the neuro-endocrine response to injury.

## AFFERENT NERVE IMPULSES

Afferent impulses, notably pain, play a lesser though significant role in the response. On reaching the hypothalamus, these impulses result in autonomic nerve stimulation and release of pituitary hormones. In some cases the injury may have been anticipated by the patient, and as a result the hypothalamic response triggered by impulses from higher centres before injury. In support of the significance of afferent nerve impulses, it has

VOLUME CONSERVATION IN RESPONSE TO OPERATION AND INJURY

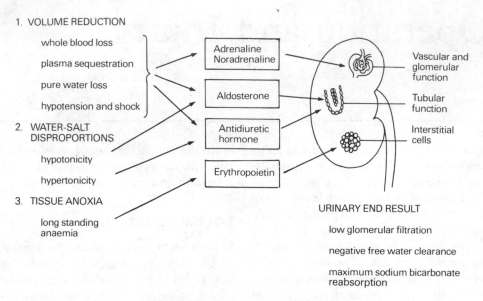

**Fig. 7.1** The volume conservation response

been demonstrated experimentally that the response to a standardised limb injury is much reduced by the section of nerves to that limb. Patients operated upon under spinal anaesthesia show a delayed response.

## TOXIC FACTORS

The role of toxic factors in initiating the metabolic response is not clearly defined. It is possible that they exert a modifying rather than initiating role. They may be two in number: *exogenous* or *endogenous*.

*Exogenous factors* e.g. exotoxin (e.g. from *Cl. welchii*) or endotoxin (Gram-negative organisms) may produce shock (see p.128) and initiate the response. *Endogenous factors*, e.g. particulate factors such as fat emboli or small platelet aggregates produced after injury, may generate afferent vagal stimuli and thus modify the response to injury. It has been suggested that non-particulate factors released from an injured site or hypoxic area (e.g. ATP, kinins, myoglobin) may initiate the response.

## FACTORS MODIFYING THE RESPONSE

Factors which modify the magnitude and duration of the metabolic response to injury include:

*Severity of injury:* the greater the injury, the greater the response;

*Nature of injury:* burns produce a greater response than other injuries of comparable size, probably because of greater heat loss from the burn area (see ch. 13);

*Infection* potentiates the metabolic response. The catabolic phase persists as long as infection remains;

*Other complications* such as deep venous thrombosis and pulmonary embolism potentiate the response;

*Nutritional status:* patients with poor nutritional status at the time of injury produce a smaller response than those with good nutrition. Starvation frequently occurs after operation or injury and has effects which complement the response (see p.74);

*Ambient temperature:* much of the increased

metabolism after injury is directed towards maintaining body temperature. This is particularly true of patients with thermal burns who lose energy due to evaporation of water from the burn. If the ambient temperature is raised from the usual 20°C or so in hospitals in temperate climates to 30–32°C, energy expenditure and consequent metabolic demand is much reduced after injury. This knowledge is utilised in specialised burns units.

*Corticosteroids* have an important permissive role in that a certain minimal level of circulating corticosteroids is necessary to produce the metabolic response. Adrenalectomised animals do not produce a metabolic response to injury unless given maintenance doses of corticosteroids;

*Age and sex:* the metabolic response is less pronounced in children and the elderly. However, there is some doubt whether children have a smaller response when body weight or lean body mass is taken into account. Premenopausal females appear to produce a smaller response than males of comparable age;

*Anaesthesia and drugs* may modify the response by affecting the vascular system and hormone production. For example, ether stimulates the output of catecholamines and ADH, morphine stimulates release of ADH, and spinal anaesthesia reduces the initial response by blocking afferent pathways.

Meticulous and gentle handling of tissue during operation reduces the amount of trauma and the post-operative metabolic demand. Prompt and adequate replacement of fluid loss limits liberation of catecholamines, aldosterone and ADH. In certain cases the phase of oliguria and sodium retention may be eliminated if replacement accurately balances loss. The provision of enough calories and nitrogen during the catabolic phase also modifies and occasionally prevents weight loss and negative nitrogen balance. However, it is doubtful whether this has a significant effect on wound healing or the duration of hospital stay in previously healthy patients undergoing elective surgery. In the undernourished patient or the patient with severe trauma or sepsis, the provision of adequate calories and nitrogen considerably influences recovery. In all patients prolonged post-trauma starvation adversely affects convalescence.

# CHANGES OCCURRING DURING THE METABOLIC RESPONSE

## PULSE AND TEMPERATURE CHANGE

Following injury the pulse rate rises temporarily due to catecholamine release. Frequently, there is a small rise in temperature lasting 24–48 hours, the so called *sympathetic fever*. This reflects a general increase in heat production, accompanied by an altered 'setting' of the temperature regulation centre under the influence of catecholamines. This rise in temperature is not due to infection and does not call for the use of antibiotics.

## WATER AND SALT RETENTION

Oliguria follows injury and normally lasts 48–72 hours. It is a consequence of release of antidiuretic hormone (ADH) and aldosterone.

ADH production is increased when *volume receptors* in the atria and hypothalamus are stimulated by blood volume reduction. Neural stimuli reaching the supra-optic nucleus from the injured part also result in ADH release. Any increase in osmolality stimulates *osmoreceptors* in the anterior hypothalmus causing further secretion of ADH. ADH acts principally on the collecting tubules of the kidney and to a lesser extent on the distal tubule to promote reabsorption of water. If excess water is administered to a patient during this phase, hypotonicity and hyponatraemia will result.

Aldosterone acts on the kidney to conserve sodium and so further reduces urine volume. Aldosterone secretion is increased by the following mechanisms, of which the renin-angiotensin mechanism is much the most important:

1. The juxtaglomerular apparatus of the kidney is sensitive to minor alterations in glomerular arteriolar inflow pressure, and secretes renin if inflow pressure falls. Renin acts with angiotensinogen to form angiotensin I. This is converted to angiotensin II, a substance which stimulates production of aldosterone by the adrenal cortex (see Fig.7.2). The macula densa is a specialised area of tubular epithelium immediately adjacent to the juxtaglomerular apparatus. It is sensitive to

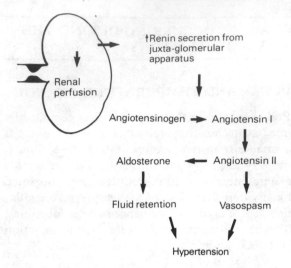

↑Renin secretion from juxta-glomerular apparatus

Renal perfusion

Angiotensinogen → Angiotensin I

Aldosterone ← Angiotensin II

Fluid retention          Vasospasm

Hypertension

**Fig. 7.2** Juxta-glomerular apparatus and aldosterone release

small alterations in the sodium concentration in the urine in the distal tubule. Reduction in sodium concentration activates renin release.

2. A minor role is played by receptors in the right atrium sensitive to volume decrease and receptors in the carotid artery sensitive to a fall in arterial pressure. Hypothalamic stimulation and release of corticotrophin (ACTH) results.

3. Aldosterone release may also be activated by a decrease in plasma sodium concentration or an increase in plasma potassium concentration reaching the adrenal cortex. Such changes in plasma concentrations occur frequently after injury.

Aldosterone acts principally on the distal renal tubules to promote reabsorption of sodium and bicarbonate, with increased excretion of potassium and hydrogen ion. Aldosterone also affects the exchange of sodium and potassium across all cell membranes, particularly those of cardiac and smooth muscle, possibly by modifying the effect of catecholamines on these cells. Large quantities of intracellular potassium are released into the extracellular fluid, which may cause a significant rise in serum potassium if renal function is impaired. The tendency to retain sodium and bicarbonate after injury may produce metabolic alkalosis with potentially adverse effects on delivery of oxygen to the tissues (see chapter on Shock).

In the absence of sweating, the only significant route of excretion of sodium and potassium in healthy people is in the urine. Approximately 50–80 mmol of each ion are excreted every 24 hours. Following injury, urinary sodium excretion may fall to 10–20 mmol/24 h for 2 to 3 days, depending on the severity of injury and the degree of fluid and electrolyte replacement. Potassium excretion may rise to 100–200 mmol/24 h for a similar period. This should be taken into account when calculating requirements for replacement after injury.

## CARBOHYDRATE, PROTEIN AND FAT METABOLISM

### Carbohydrate

In the absence of intake, body carbohydrate stores will supply needs for only 8–12 hours. Nevertheless, following injury there is a period of *hyperglycaemia*, the duration of which depends on the severity of injury and presence of complicating factors such as infection. The hyperglycaemia is produced by a combination of hepatic glycogenolysis and gluconeogenesis, and is initiated largely by catecholamine release and sympathetic overactivity.

Catecholamines increase glycogenolysis directly and also act indirectly by suppressing release of insulin and stimulating that of glucagon. Suppression of insulin release favours the release of aminoacids from muscle which are then available for gluconeogenesis. In addition, the effect of insulin on glucose metabolism is inhibited, possibly as a result of increased growth hormone levels. Glucagon is a potent stimulant of hepatic gluconeogenesis but does not significantly affect the efflux of aminoacids from skeletal muscle. Thyroxine can also accelerate gluconeogenesis but its precise role following trauma is not clear.

Increased breakdown of muscle protein and gluconeogenesis characterise the catabolic phase following injury and the resultant hyperglycaemia is sometimes called *the diabetes of injury*. The provision of exogenous glucose and insulin in injured patients may lessen this effect. Such therapy has been used in patients whose catabolic demands are excessive e.g. following severe burns.

## Protein

The daily intake of protein by a healthy adult is usually between 80 and 120 g (13--20 g of nitrogen). Of this, 2–4 g of nitrogen are lost daily in the stool, and 10–16 g in the urine. After injury the loss of urinary nitrogen increases. Following severe trauma or major burns it may reach three or four times normal. Nitrogen is lost in the form of urea and blood urea rises rapidly if renal function is impaired.

The rise in nitrogen excretion appears soon after injury. Following routine elective surgery it reaches a peak during the first week, returning to normal after 5 to 8 days. In major trauma, severe burns, or severe infection, the increase in nitrogen excretion may continue for many weeks. The patient is usually not capable of eating sufficient protein to match this loss, either because of intestinal ileus, or the anorexia associated with injury. During this phase he is in *negative nitrogen balance*. The provision of adequate calories and protein by the parenteral route may modify or obviate this negative nitrogen balance and is indicated if this is likely to last more than a few days (see ch. 10).

Negative nitrogen balance is associated with weight loss due to loss of muscle mass. The extent may be calculated from the formula:

1 g Nitrogen ≡ 6 g muscle protein ≡
30 g wet muscle mass.

A patient with a negative nitrogen balance of 15 g nitrogen a day thus loses approximately 450 g of muscle mass daily. The provision of adequate carbohydrate calories has a protein-sparing effect, reducing the degree of negative nitrogen balance by preventing the need for gluconeogenesis.

## Fat

Though energy derived from protein is important, the principal source of energy following trauma and during starvation is adipose tissue with its large triglyceride store. Catecholamines and glucagon activate adenyl-cyclase in the fat cells and produce cyclic adenosine monophosphate (cyclic AMP). This in turn leads to activation of triglyceride lipase and the breakdown of triglycerides to fatty acids and glycerol. Growth hormone and cortisol have a similar, though less important effect. Glycerol provides substrate for gluconeogenesis, while free fatty acids provide energy for all tissues and for hepatic gluconeogenesis. The decreased level of insulin following injury encourages lipolysis. A total of 200–500 g of fat may be broken down daily after severe trauma.

## ANABOLIC PHASE

Following the catabolic phase of metabolism the patient goes into an anabolic phase characterised by positive nitrogen balance, regain of weight and restoration of fat deposits. The turning point can often be recognised clinically in that the patient feels much better and his appetite returns, often quite suddenly. The hormones which contribute to anabolism are growth hormones, androgens and 17-ketosteroids.

The role of the various hormones affecting energy metabolism during the metabolic response to injury are summarised in Table 7.1.

## CHANGES IN BLOOD COAGULATION

After injury or infection, the blood may be hypercoagulable or hypocoagulable.

Hypercoagulation appears first and may contribute to the increased incidence of deep venous thrombosis and pulmonary embolism after operation or trauma. It is maximal in the first 12 hours after injury; increased secretion of ACTH and cortisol may be responsible by increasing the number of platelets and their adhesiveness. Noradrenaline also tends to increase coagulability.

Serum fibrinogen levels rise after injury. In patients with severe sepsis this rise is often long-sustained, and followed by a gradual fall. A rapid fall is associated with a poor prognosis.

Hypocoagulation follows hypercoagulation and is associated with increased fibrinolysis and reduction in serum fibrinogen. This can lead to generalised bleeding and, though not common, is seen most frequently after severe shock (particularly bacteraemic shock with disseminated intravascular coagulation), after operations on patients with disseminated carcinoma or extensive liver disease, or following cardiopulmonary bypass.

**Table 7.1** Effects of hormones on metabolism after injury

**Catecholamines - the stress hormones**

*Hyperglycaemia*
1. by action on liver — glycogenolysis
2. by action on muscle glycogen — lactic acid — glucose in liver (Cori cycle)
3. by action on pancreas — suppression of insulin (mainly alpha stimulation) stimulation of glucagon (beta stimulation)

*Increase in metabolic rate (beta-stimulation)*
*Mobilisation of free fatty acids*
1. Direct action on fat cells
2. Potentiated by low insulin levels

**Insulin — the storage hormone**
In non-stress states, insulin secretion in response to increasing blood glucose concentration facilitates the entry of glucose into many tissues with increased glycogenesis and lipogenesis. Low insulin concentrations after injury lead to:

1. accelerated triglyceride breakdown
2. increased release of amino acids from muscle
3. impaired entry of $K^+$ and P into cells

**Glucocorticoids, glucagon and growth hormone — the permissive hormones**

Glucocorticoids are released in response to elevated ACTH levels after injury or stress and have a permissive role, augmenting specific metabolic responses to stress:

1. hepatic gluconeogenesis is augmented by stimulating enzymes which increase direct conversion of 3-carbon fragments into glucose;
2. mobilisation of amino acids from the periphery is facilitated;
3. lipolysis is augmented.

Glucagon has actions on the liver opposed to those of insulin. Its major role after injury is strong stimulation of hepatic gluconeogenesis. It does not contribute to increased efflux of amino acids from muscle, but acts with catecholamines to stimulate lipolysis.

Growth hormone has effects in both the catabolic and anabolic phases:

1. the insulin response to altered blood glucose levels is 'reset';
2. free fatty acid release is augmented;
3. nitrogen retention is augmented, provided there is sufficient supply of non-protein calories.

# STARVATION AND ITS CONTRIBUTION TO THE METABOLIC RESPONSE

All patients who undergo surgery or receive an injury of magnitude will be starved for a period.

It is customary to starve the patient for about 12 hours before elective surgery, and he is unlikely to take any food on the day of operation itself. Patients undergoing operation on the alimentary tract may not be able to take food for 2 or 3 days post-operatively. Patients who develop complications may have to forgo food for days or even weeks. Further, patients with intra-abdominal disease, e.g. carcinoma of the alimentary tract, may have had an inadequate intake for weeks or months before operation.

If the trauma of surgery is relatively minor, and followed by only a short period of starvation e.g. cholecystectomy, vagotomy and drainage, the alterations in metabolism are similar to those of starvation alone; after major trauma there are marked differences.

In acute starvation, intermediate metabolism of protein, carbohydrate and fat is altered to preserve the supply of energy to the brain from 6-carbon compounds such as glucose by increasing hepatic glycogenolysis and gluconeogenesis.

Body energy is stored in the form of glycogen, protein and triglycerides. *Glycogen* is stored in the liver and in muscle in combination with water and electrolytes. In this state it provides only 2 kcal/g, as opposed to 4 kcal/g when dry. *Triglycerides* are not stored in combination with water, and 1 g of body fat produces just over 9 kcal of energy. *Protein* is stored principally in muscle, and is combined with water. Not all of this protein is utilised primarily as an energy source, some is used as a source of antibodies and enzymes, and structural and plasma proteins. Ingested protein in excess of that needed to replenish body stores is metabolised; any unused energy is stored as fat. In the absence of intake of food, protein provides energy through gluconeogenesis.

The total energy stores in a normal 70 kg male are shown in Table 7.2. The plasma proteins (210 g) potentially contribute 840 kcal to the stores. In short-term fasting the body can replenish plasma proteins at a rate equal to utilisation. However, in marked catabolism the rate of utilisation of plasma proteins exceeds that of liver synthesis. Unless exogenous proteins are provided hypoproteinaemia results.

In early starvation the basal energy requirement for a 70 kg adult is approximately 1800 kcal per 24 hours. The manner in which the body provides and utilises this energy is shown in Figure 7.3. The brain uses most of the available glucose, but some is broken down anaerobically in kidney and muscle to provide pyruvate and lactate which are recycled to provide further glucose by gluconeogenesis. The majority of body tissues use fatty acids and ketones as an energy source. If starvation is prolonged beyond a few hours, the glycogen stores in the liver and muscle become depleted. Muscle protein converted to glucose by gluconeogenesis maintains the brain's energy supply. This process cannot be continued indefinitely, and after 2–3 weeks the brain gradually

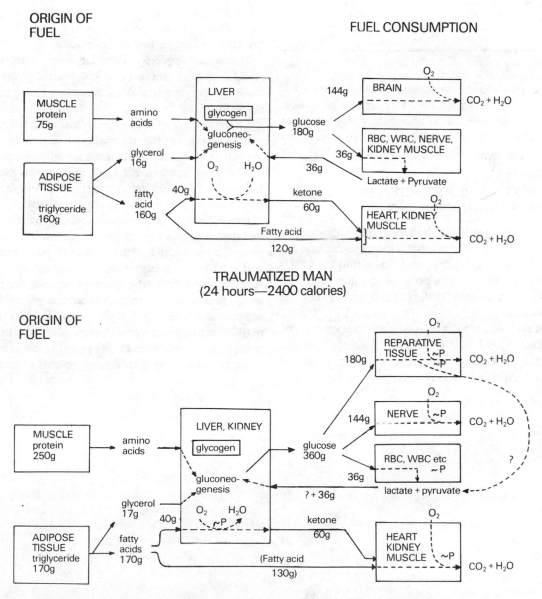

**Fig. 7.3** Utilisation of energy during starvation (From Cahill G.F. (1970) *N. Engl. J. Med.* 282: 668)

Table 7.2 Source of energy in 70 kg male. Assuming a basal expenditure of 1800 kcals per day, the fasting survival time would approximate 3 months.

|  | Weight of fuel | Energy produced kcals |
|---|---|---|
| Fat (adipose tissue) triglycerols | 15 kg | 141 000 |
| Muscle protein | 6 kg | 24 000 |
| Liver and muscle glycogen | 225 g | 900 |
| Circulating glucose, fatty acids, triglycerols etc. | 23 g | 100 |
|  |  | 166 000 |

reduces its glucose consumption and utilises ketones as an energy source. The amount of muscle protein utilised falls to about 20 g/day while fat consumption increases. The total energy requirement falls from 1800 kcal to about 1500 kcal/day.

## DIFFERENCES BETWEEN EFFECTS OF TRAUMA AND STARVATION

The general trend of the metabolic alteration in starvation is similar to that after trauma, but the combination of trauma and starvation *acclerates* utilisation of body stores of protein and fat. However, important differences exist between the two states.

*Protein metabolism.* In simple starvation the peak nitrogen loss is around 0.1 g/kg body weight per day. The losses are greater in post-traumatic catabolism and in severe injury and in sepsis may reach 0.4 g/kg body weight per day. The blood urea level normally falls in simple starvation, whereas following major injury the level is normal or elevated. The increases in urinary creatine excretion which occur after injury are not seen in simple starvation, and reflect differences in protein catabolism.

*Blood sugar.* During simple starvation, blood sugar levels fall and remain low, despite increased glucagon levels. Following trauma, blood sugar levels are elevated. In simple starvation, administration of glucose produces a rise in insulin secretion. This does not occur after trauma as long as the catecholamine level is increased.

*Hormonal response.* The increased output of ADH, aldosterone, catecholamines and glucocorticoids after trauma does not occur in simple starvation.

*Calorie-nitrogen ratio for tissue synthesis.* In simple starvation the optimal ratio of provision of *non-protein calories* to ensure that aminoacids are used for synthesis rather than energy provision is 100 kcal : 1 g nitrogen. After trauma, this ratio is increased to at least 200 kcal : 1 g nitrogen.

*Reversibility of metabolic changes.* The metabolic changes of simple starvation are rapidly reversed by feeding, either orally or parenterally, and positive nitrogen balance is easily achieved. After major injury, the changes are not reversed until increased hormone secretion reverts to normal and feeding by any route results in a marked wastage of nitrogenous products in the urine. However, it may be possible to achieve positive balance by giving large amounts of nitrogen rapidly.

# 8. Principles of Fluid and Electrolyte Balance in Surgical Patients

The majority of surgical patients with fluid and electrolyte problems cannot ingest fluid and so it must be administered intravenously. The effect of trauma on the secretion of antidiuretic hormone (ADH) and aldosterone necessitates careful control of fluid administration in the early postoperative period. Adequate amounts of water, sodium and potassium with anions, supplied as chloride, are routine requirements. In a few individuals, particularly those with chronic gastrointestinal tract loss, deficiencies of calcium and magnesium require correction.

## NORMAL WATER AND ELECTROLYTE BALANCE

In calculating fluid and electrolyte requirements it is essential to know how much the patient has lost so that accurate replacement maintains balance. The healthy individual loses fluid by three routes; the kidneys, the gastrointestinal tract, and the skin and respiratory passages. In a 70 kg adult approximately 1500–2000 ml urine are passed in 24 hours, 200– 300 ml of fluid is lost in faeces, and 800-1000 ml is lost as water vapour from the skin and respiratory tract (*insensible loss*) The onset of sweating (*sensible loss*) greatly increases water loss from the skin. Water is taken in as fluids and in solid food; an additional 100–200 ml/24 hours is provided endogenously by oxidation of fat.

In the absence of sweating, almost all the sodium lost is in the urine (50–80 mmol/day). Under the influence of aldosterone the kidney can reduce sodium loss to the order of 10–20 mmol/day.

The principal route of potassium excretion is also via the kidney, some 60–100 mmol being lost each day. The kidney cannot conserve potassium as efficiently as sodium but in severe potassium deficiency can reduce losses to 40 mmol/day. The normal daily losses and the requirements to maintain fluid and electrolyte balance are summarised in Table 8.1.

### Intravenous administration of normal requirements

When fulfilling these requirements by the intravenous route, sodium is normally provided as 0.9% sodium chloride, which contains 154 mmol sodium and 154 mmol chloride per litre. As it is isotonic with plasma it is traditionally called *normal* or *physiological* saline. For practical purposes, 500 ml of normal saline supplies the daily requirement of sodium. The remaining volume of water required (2.5 litres) is given as an isotonic non-electrolyte solution such as 5% dextrose. Potassium can be added either to saline or to dextrose from ampoules containing 1.5 g potassium chloride, (20 mmol of potassium and 20 mmol of chloride). Three ampoules supply a patient's daily need.

Instructions for the provision of the *normal* 24 hour fluid and electrolyte requirement are given in Table 8.2.

It is advisable that potassium is not administered in concentrations greater than 80 mmol/l except in severe potassium deficiency. Then continuous ECG monitoring is essential. Potassium should *never* be given as an intravenous bolus, as cardiac arrest will occur.

**Table 8.1** Normal losses.

|  | Volume | Na$^+$ | K$^+$ |
|---|---|---|---|
| Urine | 2000 | 80 | 60 |
| Insensible | 800 | – | – |
| Faeces | 300 | – | – |
| *Minus* Endogenous Water | 100 | – | – |
| Requirement | 3000 ml | 80 mmol | 60 mmol |

**Table 8.2** Provision of the normal 24 hour fluid and electrolyte requirement.

1.   500 ml 0.9% NaCl + 1.5 g KCl
2.   500 ml 5% dextrose
3.   500 ml 5% dextrose + 1.5 g KCl
4.   500 ml 5% dextrose
5.   500 ml 5% dextrose + 1.5 g KCl
6.   500 ml 5% dextrose
     4 hours per bottle

### Effect of sweating on requirements

Hyperventilation increases insensible water loss, and pyrexia also raises the water loss from the skin by approximately 200 ml/day per °C rise in temperature. The onset of sweating considerably increases fluid loss, which may reach a rate of 1 l/hour. Calculation of the amount of fluid lost by sweating is difficult and repeated weighing of the patient may be necessary. Sweat contains significant amounts of sodium (20–70 mmol/l) and potassium (10 mmol/l), and these losses must be taken into account when calculating requirements.

## EFFECT OF OPERATION ON FLUID AND ELECTROLYTE BALANCE

Following operation, release of antidiuretic hormone (ADH) conserves water by its action on the distal convoluted and collecting tubules. Oliguria results so that the urine volume is reduced to 1000–1500 ml for 2–3 days. Attempts to produce a diuresis by administration of water in the form of 5% dextrose are unsuccessful and only produce hyponatraemia and possibly water intoxication.

Aldosterone secretion conserves sodium and further contributes to oliguria. In the first two days the urinary excretion of sodium is reduced to approximately 30 mmol per day. Potassium excretion is increased during this period to approximately 120 mmol per day partly from the influence of aldosterone on the kidney and partly by the liberation of potassium from body cells generally. This is enhanced by cellular damage or by the infusion of stored blood. Serum potassium levels thus tend to rise in the early post-operative period, particularly if the glomerular filtration rate is reduced. For this reason intravenous potassium should not be provided in the first 48 hours after operation unless the patient is hypokalaemic or was potassium deficient pre-operatively.

Sequestration of extracellular fluid at the site of operation produces local oedema, and temporary loss of fluid from the circulation. Sequestration persists for approximately 48 hours, and may involve up to 4 litres of fluid, depending on the severity of the operation or injury. After partial gastrectomy 500 ml/day is the likely sequestration loss. Sequestration must be taken into account when calculating fluid and electrolyte requirements.

Not all patients require intravenous support following an operation. The majority tolerate 48 hours of fluid deprivation with only thirst and a possible increase in the risk of deep venous thrombosis. However, patients are more comfortable if fluid losses are replaced. If in doubt or if there is evidence of impaired renal or cardiac function, it is better to err on the side of underhydration rather than risk over-hydration with the induction of hyponatraemia and/or pulmonary oedema.

# FLUID AND ELECTROLYTE LOSS FROM THE ALIMENTARY TRACT

The majority of surgical patients requiring intravenous fluid and electrolyte therapy for sustained periods have continuing fluid loss from the gut. This may be due to the following circumstances.

## Intestinal obstruction

In general terms, the higher the obstruction in the intestine, the greater the fluid loss. This is due to failure of fluids secreted by the upper alimentary tract to reach the absorptive areas of the distal jejunum and ileum. Thus a patient with a high small bowel obstruction loses fluid more rapidly than one with a low small bowel obstruction. Major fluid loss from vomiting is not a feature of large bowel obstruction until very late in its course.

## Adynamic ileus

This condition, in which the small intestine ceases to function propulsively, may result from infection, from electrolyte imbalance (particularly potassium, calcium and magnesium deficiency) from hypoproteinaemia, from retroperitoneal trauma or haemorrhage, from hypoxia, from head injury or neurosurgical operations, and from shock due to different causes. Distension of the gut from swallowed air results in an increase in intestinal secretions and reduction of absorptive capacity. Unless the intestinal fluid is removed by naso-gastric aspiration, vomiting is persistent.

## Intestinal fistula

Fluid loss from an intestinal fistula may be considerable. As with obstruction, the higher the fistula the greater the fluid loss. Fluid loss is not often a major problem with fistulas of the large bowel.

## Diarrhoea

Fluid and electrolyte loss from diarrhoea may also be considerable. For example, in cholera and similar superinfections of the gut, some 6–10 litres may be lost each day resulting in fatal contraction of extracellular fluid volume.

*Management.* Table 8.3 gives approximate concentrations of electrolytes in some gastro-intestinal fluids and may be used to calculate losses over short periods. There is considerable variation in their constitution, and if gastrointestinal loss continues for more than 2–3 days, all the fluid and urine should be collected and sent to the laboratory for accurate determination of electrolyte content. Because of this variation in the constitution of intestinal fluids, the use of specially prepared fluids such as 'gastric solution' is not recommended.

An example of a patient's requirements is given in Table 8.4. In patients requiring replacement of fluid and electrolytes for more than 3–4 days, calculations such as those in Table 8.4 are likely to be inaccurate. The correction of acid-base imbalance and the provision of parenteral nutrition will have to be considered. The need for ions other than sodium and potassium should be considered if intestinal fluid loss continues, particularly magnesium (up to 1 mmol/kg body weight/day) and calcium (10–60 ml of 10% calcium gluconate/day = 4.5–27 mmol/day).

**Table 8.3** Approximate electrolyte concentrations in various gastro-intestinal fluids.

| | Volume (ml/24 hours) | $Na^+$ (mmol/l) | $K^+$ (mol/l) | $Cl^-$ (mmol/l) | $HCO_3$ (mmol/l) |
|---|---|---|---|---|---|
| Plasma | | 140 | 5 | 100 | 25 |
| Gastric Juice | 2500 | 50 | 10 | 80 | 40 |
| Intestinal fluid (upper) | 3000 | 140 | 10 | 100 | 25 |
| Bile + Pancreatic juice | 1500 | 140 | 5 | 80 | 60 |
| Mixed nasogastric aspirate | – | 120 | 10 | 100 | 40 |
| Ileostomy fluid — new | 700 | 125 | 20 | 110 | 30 |
| — mature | 500 | 50 | 5 | 20 | 25 |
| Diarrhoea (inflammatory) | – | 110 | 40 | 100 | 40 |

**Table 8.4** Example of daily fluid and electrolyte requirements in a patient with ileus.

Assume that a patient with ileus is in electrolyte balance and is losing 2 litres per 24 hours as naso-gastric tube aspirate, and 1.5 litres as urine. His 24 hour losses can be calculated:

|                                  | Vol. ml | $Na^+$ mmol | $K^+$ mmol |
|----------------------------------|---------|-------------|------------|
| urine                            | 1500    | 80          | 60         |
| nasogastric aspirate             | 2000    | 240         | 20         |
| insensible loss                  | 800     | –           | –          |
| minus endogenous water of oxidation | − 300 | –          | –          |
|                                  | 4000    | 320         | 80         |

Two litres of normal saline would supply 310 mmol of $Na^+$, which for practical purposes would satisfy his sodium needs, and the remaining two litres of water required would be supplied as 5% dextrose. Thus, in short term practice, provided urinary losses are normal, the replacement of the naso-gastric fluid volume for volume by normal saline gives the required sodium replacement, and the volume of urine plus 500 mls is replaced as dextrose. The patient requires 80 mmol of potassium, which would be supplied by four 1.5 g. ampoules of potassium chloride.

In patients requiring replacement for more than 3 or 4 days, such calculations are likely to be inaccurate and the need to correct potential acid-base imbalance and provide parenteral nutrition will have to be considered. The need for ions other than sodium and potassium should be considered if intestinal fluid loss continues, particularly magnesium (up to 1 mmol/kg body weight per day) and calcium (10–60 ml of 10% calcium gluconate per day = 4.5–27 mmol/day).

Patients who have pre-existing fluid and electrolyte deficiency, or who develop deficiencies under treatment should have the deficiency corrected by adding the calculated deficit to the normal requirement, usually spreading this replacement over 2–3 days.

Patients who have pre-existing fluid and electrolyte deficiency, or who develop deficiencies under treatment, should have these corrected by adding the calculated deficit to the normal requirement, usually spreading this replacement over 2–3 days.

## WATER IMBALANCE

### WATER DEPLETION

A reduction of 1–2% of total body water (350–700 ml) produces the sensation of thirst. Clinically obvious dehydration, with intense thirst, a dry tongue, and loss of skin elasticity (particularly over the clavicles) signifies a deficiency of at least 1.5 to 2 litres. *Pure water depletion is rare in surgical practice.* Water depletion is usually combined with sodium loss, the combination being generally referred to as 'salt depletion'. The combined loss of sodium and water results in contraction of the extracellular fluid volume (ECF) with circulatory changes (vasoconstriction and tachycardia) as well as the clinical features of dehydration. The most frequent cause of salt depletion is loss of gastro-intestinal secretions. Rapid infusion of normal saline is indicated.

## WATER EXCESS

In contrast to pure water depletion, water excess is not uncommon in surgical practice, particularly in the elderly post-operative patient who receives excess water in the face of persisting ADH activity. There is dilutional hyponatraemia, yet renal secretion of sodium continues despite the low serum levels. This contrasts with the patient who has hyponatraemia due to *sodium depletion*, whose urinary sodium is minimal and who also exhibits the clinical signs of reduction in blood volume. The patient with water excess looks comparatively well.

Inappropriate secretion of ADH may occur in a number of conditions including sepsis, severe pulmonary infection, ectopic secretion by tumours of lung or pancreas, and disease or trauma involving the brain and meninges.

### Treatment

If the condition of dilutional hyponatraemia due to water excess is recognised, the administration of water by mouth or intravenously (as 5% dextrose) should cease and the patient be allowed to 'dry out'. Electrolyte replacement should continue. In severe cases, where there is danger of water intoxication, hypertonic saline (3–5%) should be administered cautiously (100-200 ml over 2 hours) and the patient observed for rapid clinical improvement and a diuretic response. This therapy may be repeated after 12 hours.

# SODIUM IMBALANCE

Sodium is the principal extracellular cation, and changes in its total amount or its concentration affect the volume and tonicity of the extracellular fluid. The sodium concentration is the main indicator of extracellular fluid tonicity. The concentration of other ions e.g., $Cl^-$, $HCO_3^-$ and $K^+$ are also affected by acid-base change and by renal function, and therefore do not reflect dilutional change in the same way as sodium, which is relatively uninfluenced by these other factors.

In most clinical situations which involve sodium excess or deficit, there is a combination of volume and tonicity changes, either simultaneously or in sequence. It is artificial to consider changes in sodium without, at the same time, taking into account changes in its solvent, i.e., water. The significance of an elevated or low serum sodium is best determined from a study of the patient's history.

## SODIUM DEPLETION

### Causes

*Acute sodium loss* occurs in the following situations:

1. Haemorrhage or plasma loss
2. Acute gastric dilatation (the patient may lose up to 1 litre of ECF per hour over a period of 3–5 hours)
3. Massive diarrhoea, e.g., cholera, staphylococcal or pseudomembranous enterocolitis

*Chronic sodium loss* may occur in:

1. Chronic diarrhoea
2. Protracted ileus
3. Ileostomy
4. Chronic renal disease

As indicated above *dilutional hyponatraemia* can occur with a normal total body sodium but an excess of water. Causes include iatrogenic overdosage of ADH, or its inappropriate secretion by a tumour. Acute renal failure may produce a similar picture if the administration of water is continued in the face of oliguria. Chronic starvation may also produce dilutional hyponatraemia, due to excess production of water from the metabolism of body fat in the presence of elevated ADH levels. There is also an increase in aldosterone activity and total body sodium may actually be increased. A similar effect may be produced by chronic liver disease or congestive cardiac failure.

### Clinical features

As the fluid lost in these conditions is isotonic, there is contraction of ECF volume, along with the features of dehydration: thirst, oliguria and concentrated urine.

### Treatment

*Isotonic* fluid replacement is indicated. Should *water* or *hypotonic* solutions be administered either orally or intravenously, ADH will continue to conserve water so that excess water is not excreted. There is hypotonicity of the ECF and serum sodium concentration falls. If this becomes less than 110 mmol/l there is considerable danger of convulsions and water intoxication. Patients with major trauma or sepsis are likely to have persistent excess ADH activity and are particularly liable to this form of hyponatraemia.

Isotonic fluid replacement is continued while the patient is allowed to 'dry out'. Treatment with hypertonic saline is rarely necessary and should be considered only if the serum sodium has fallen to 110 mmol/l or should convulsions develop. Sodium level should be corrected slowly: too rapid changes may worsen the situation.

Mild dilutional hyponatraemia is harmless and does not call for the administration of sodium. In malnourished patients it is corrected by an adequate caloric intake.

Excess urinary loss of sodium in chronic renal disease may require an increased intake of sodium.

## SODIUM EXCESS

### Causes

True sodium excess is usually iatrogenic, and is due to the continued excess administration of sodium in the face of persisting aldosterone activity. This is particularly liable to occur in the postoperative or postinjury period. The volume of ECF is expanded with a risk of circulatory overload and pulmonary oedema.

Hypernatraemia associated with a true excess of sodium is relatively uncommon but it may occur in primary (Conn's syndrome) or secondary hyperaldosteronism. Hypernatraemia occurs more frequently as a result of abnormal loss of water or hypotonic fluids as follows:

1. *Pure water loss from skin or lungs*. The classic example is a shipwrecked sailor without access to water, who may compound the situation by drinking sea water (which is hypertonic). In clinical practice it may occur in patients supported on a ventilator without adequate humidification.

2. *Loss of hypotonic fluid*. Sweat is hypotonic, and if excess sweating is not compensated by taking fluid, hypernatraemia results. Gastrointestinal secretions may sometimes also be hypotonic, particularly in babies. Frequently the loss is replaced with drinking water which produces hyponatremia; if only isotonic saline is given true sodium overload with hypernatremia can develop.

### Clinical features

The consequences of hypernatraemia are:

1. thirst of great severity;
2. neurological symptoms: confusion proceeding to coma

The severity of the thirst is such that hypernatremia is rare in the conscious patient who has access to water.

### Treatment

Sodium excess is best treated by the administration of pure water or hypotonic solutions. The temptation to achieve rapid correction of the abnormal sodium concentration should be resisted as sudden changes in the tonicity of extracellular fluid can prove dangerous.

## POTASSIUM IMBALANCE

Potassium is the principal intracellular cation. Its intracellular concentration is 150 mmol/l. Only 60 mmol of the total body potassium of 3000 mmol is contained in extracellular fluid, where its concentration varies around 4.0 mmol/l. Levels below 2.5 mmol/l and above 6.0 mmol/l are dangerous and may cause cardiac arrest.

Increasing the intake or output of potassium produces only slow changes in serum potassium concentrations. Rapid equilibration of intra and extracellular potassium and efficient renal excretion guard against sudden flux in circulating concentrations. However, alterations in acid-base balance affect these exchanges and may produce rapid changes in extracellular potassium concentration.

### Acid-base changes and potassium balance

Derangement in acid-base balance causes changes in potassium balance within and outside the cell. Conversely, changes in potassium balance have secondary effects on acid-base balance.

*Acidosis*. Excess of hydrogen ions in the extracellular fluid causes the movement of $H^+$ into the cells in exchange for an equivalent amount of $K^+$ which moves out into the ECF. The serum potassium rises and there is increased excretion of potassium in the urine. If the acidosis continues, a considerable deficit in total body potassium results.

Should the acidosis be corrected rapidly without the provision of potassium ions, the potassium levels in the serum may fall catastrophically as potassium returns to the cells. This may take place within a few hours. This is a dangerous situation, which applies equally to metabolic and respiratory acidosis.

*In alkalosis* the exchange of potassium for hydrogen ions takes place in the opposite direction. Hydrogen ions $(H^+)$ move out of the cell in exchange for potassium ions $(K^+)$ which move in. Further, the kidneys conserve hydrogen ions $(H^+)$ at the expense of increased urinary loss of potassium. Hypokalaemia follows.

When the deficiency of potassium becomes

severe, the kidney will again allow the excretion of hydrogen ions ($H^+$) so that potassium is conserved. This paradoxical aciduria results in worsening of the alkalosis. In patients in this state, adequate replacement of potassium ions is an essential part of treatment.

*Effect of potassium imbalance on acid-base balance.* Potassium excess and deficiency have secondary effects on acid-base balance, due to the exchange of potassium for sodium and hydrogen ions across the cell membrane. Thus for every three ions of potassium withdrawn from the intracellular compartment there is replacement by two sodium and one hydrogen ion. States of potassium deficiency are associated with intracellular acidosis and extracellular alkalosis. Conversely, when there is potassium excess with an increase in movement of potassium into the cell, sodium and hydrogen ions are kept out leading to an extracellular acidosis.

## POTASSIUM DEPLETION

### Causes

Acid-base balance abnormalities apart, potassium depletion results from:

*Inadequate intake.* The kidney cannot conserve potassium as efficiently as it does sodium. Even in the absence of all potassium intake, urinary loss of potassium continues at the rate of approximately 40 mmol/day. This loss is borne primarily by the cells; the level of serum potassium is maintained until late in the deficiency state. The cellular component of urinary potassium is indicated by the ratio of potassium to nitrogen which is 3:1.

A special example of inadequate intake occurs in patients who are metabolically in an anabolic state, particularly when they are receiving intravenous nutrition. The formation of normal cellular components requires potassium which can be supplied only from the extracellular fluid. If potassium intake is not increased (up to 200–300 mmol/day) hypokalaemia may rapidly develop.

*Increased loss.* This is due to factors affecting the kidney or gastro-intestinal tract. These are:

1. Diuretics.

2. Aldosterone. This includes primary and secondary hyperaldosteronism and the response to stress.

3. Other adrenocortical steroids.

4. Chronic loss of gastrointestinal secretions, e.g., diarrhoea, malfunctioning ileostomy or the discharge of mucus from a villous papilloma.

In these cases the loss of potassium greatly exceeds that of nitrogen, indicating that it comes mainly from the extracellular fluid compartment. The potassium to nitrogen ratio in the urine may be as high as 10:1. Hypokalaemia develops more rapidly than that due to starvation alone.

### Clinical effects

The principal effect of hypokalaemia is impaired muscle contractility. There is generalised muscle weakness and ileus. The associated extracellular alkalosis may produce features of tetany with signs of neuromuscular irritability including a positive Chvostek's sign. Sensitivity to digitalis is increased, and this drug must be used with great care.

Electrocardiographic changes include an increased QT interval, depressed ST segment and inverted T waves. Should the serum potassium fall below 2 mmol/l cardiac arrest may occur.

### Treatment

Adequate replacement of potassium ions ($K^+$) is essential. In severe deficiency states the advised maximum rate of intravenous administration of 15 mmol/hour may be exceeded. Cardiac monitoring should be instituted. Adequate provision of chloride ions (as NaCl) is necessary to correct the alkalosis.

## POTASSIUM EXCESS

### Causes

*Excessive parenteral administration.* Potassium is lost from the body mainly through the kidney. Normal daily potassium intake and urinary excretion each approximate to 100 mmol. In the presence of normal renal function it is almost impossible to raise serum potassium levels by increasing *oral* intake. However, excessive or too rapid *parenteral* administration (in excess of 15 mmol/h may overwhelm the renal excretory mechanism and lead to hyperkalaemia.

*Renal failure.* Impaired renal function leads to a rapid rise in the serum potassium levels, even when exogenous intake of potassium is reduced or prevented. Endogenous release of free potassium continues through cell breakdown, a factor enhanced in the postoperative catabolic phase.

The rise of serum potassium which occurs in acute renal failure approximates 0.1–0.5 mmol/l per day.

### Clinical features

The clinical picture of hyperkalaemia is surprisingly similar to that of hypokalaemia. There is muscle weakness, loss of tendon reflexes and the development of paralysis. Electrocardiographic changes include peaked T waves, increase in the P-R interval and widening of the QRS complex.

Cardiac arrhythmias may develop. If the serum potassium exceeds 7.0 mmol/l these may proceed to ventricular fibrillation.

### Treatment

1. All administration of potassium is stopped.

2. Hyperkalaemia may be temporarily counteracted by the administration of other cations. In an emergency the intravenous administration of 50–100 ml 10% calcium gluconate, 100 ml M sodium bicarbonate or 100 ml 5% sodium chloride will improve the clinical features for an hour or two.

3. A slower but longer lasting depression of potassium levels in the serum may be achieved by the intravenous infusion of 250 ml 25% glucose with 20 units soluble insulin, given over 4 hours. This regimen 'drives' potassium back into the cells. It may be continued for up to 24 hours.

4. Ion exchange resins, which exchange three sodium ($Na^+$) for each potassium ($K^+$) ion are available for oral or rectal administration. 10 g of resin orally or 30 g rectally are administered each 6-hourly.

5. Should the serum potassium approach 7 mmol/l haemodialysis is indicated.

# ACID-BASE BALANCE

## METABOLIC ACIDOSIS

Metabolic acidosis is common in surgical practice, and is usually a consequence of impaired tissue perfusion (e.g. in shock). It is potentiated by renal failure. Metabolic acidosis can be suspected by the onset of deep rapid respirations in a depleted patient. The diagnosis is confirmed by measurement of arterial hydrogen ion ($H^+$), blood gases, and standard bicarbonate. Therapy is directed towards restoring tissue perfusion. Infusion of bicarbonate is only required when the plasma bicarbonate level is less than 15 mmol/l.

The amount of bicarbonate required to raise the standard bicarbonate level above 15 mmol/l may be calculated on the basis that 2 mmol of bicarbonate are necessary to raise the bicarbonate level of the extracellular fluid by 1 mmol/l, and that the ECF constitutes approximately 20% of body weight. For example, the amount of bicarbonate required to raise the plasma bicarbonate level from 10 mmol/l to 27 mmol/l in a 70 kg patient is:

$$(27 - 10) \times 70 \times 20/100 \times 2 = 476 \text{ mmol}$$

In practice only half of this amount is given slowly over 2 hours, and the standard bicarbonate level rechecked after 4 hours before further administration is considered. As an 8.4% solution of sodium bicarbonate contains 1 mmol of bicarbonate per ml the volume required can be calculated easily if an 8.4% or 4.2% solution is used.

Care must be taken not to overload the patient with sodium, and to correct the fall in serum potassium which tends to occur following bicarbonate therapy. As many such patients are potassium depleted, potassium replacement is an important consideration.

Acute renal failure and cardiac arrest produce severe metabolic acidosis and are considered elsewhere.

## METABOLIC ALKALOSIS

Transient metabolic alkalosis follows injury and may occur in shock, but the most frequent surgical cause of metabolic alkalosis is pyloric stenosis. The loss of acid from the stomach is compensated initially by renal conservation of hydrogen ion and associated increase in potassium output. Thus patients with metabolic alkalosis are always potassium-deficient, and many are severely hypokalaemic. Conversely, patients with potassium depletion from other causes often develop metabolic alkalosis.

The management of pyloric stenosis consists of prohibiting oral intake, hourly gastric aspiration, correction of dehydration by normal saline, potassium replacement, and surgical relief of the cause. The use of gastric lavage in the evenings, with intravenous administration of special 'gastric solution' is not recommended. Replacements should be tailored to the needs of the individual patient.

If a patient's standard bicarbonate level is greater than 35 mmol/l intravenous ammonium chloride has been recommended. This should not be used in the presence of potassium deficiency.

## RESPIRATORY ACIDOSIS

Respiratory acidosis is common in surgery, and may occur as a consequence of over-sedation, or post-operative chest complications. Management is directed towards relief of the underlying chest condition, supplemented if need be by assisted ventilation. The administration of bicarbonate is not indicated.

## RESPIRATORY ALKALOSIS

There are many causes of respiratory alkalosis. Those encountered in surgical practice are:

1. Hyperventilation on a mechanical respirator or under anaesthesia
2. Pain, apprehension or hysteria
3. Small areas of pulmonary atelectasis
4. Multiple pulmonary emboli
5. Central nervous system injury
6. Septicaemia (particularly Gram negative septicaemia)

The underlying cause should be sought and treated. Respiratory suppression using a drug such as phenoperidine is indicated occasionally. Sustained respiratory alkalosis has a poor progno-

**Table 8.5**

|  | $H^+$ | $PaCO_2$ | Standard $HCO_3$ |
|---|---|---|---|
| Metabolic Acidosis | ↑ | ↓ | ↓ |
| Respiratory Acidosis | ↑ | ↑ | normal |
| Metabolic Alkalosis | ↓ | normal or slight ↑ | ↑ |
| Respiratory Alkalosis | ↓ | ↓ | normal |

sis, usually because of the severity of the underlying condition.

## MIXED PATTERNS OF ACID BASE IMBALANCE

Many patients have a mixture of respiratory and metabolic components in their acid-base imbalance. Measurement of arterial blood gases, hydrogen ion and standard bicarbonate helps to reveal the contribution of the metabolic and respiratory components, and special nomograms are available for this purpose. The patterns of alterations in these parameters are shown in Table 8.5.

## MONITORING OF PATIENTS WITH FLUID AND ELECTROLYTE PROBLEMS

The following should be estimated daily:

1. Urine volume
2. Serum sodium, potassium, bicarbonate, and urea
3. Volume of losses from GI tract
4. Haemoglobin and haematocrit

In patients where the problems are complex, the following parameters should also be measured daily:

1. Arterial hydrogen ion, standard bicarbonate and partial pressure of carbon dioxide
2. Urinary sodium, potassium
3. Gastrointestinal fluid sodium, potassium
4. Body weight

Serum protein should be measured twice per week, and in special circumstances losses of magnesium and calcium should also be measured. Determinations of serum and urine osmolalities are useful in patients with severe disorders of hydration.

# 9. Blood Transfusion

The administration of blood in medical practice has been on record for at least 400 years. Early efforts often ended in disaster, primarily because the concept of blood group specificity was unknown. The definition of human ABO blood groups by Landsteiner in 1901 led to the recognition of many other blood groups and to the provision of safe compatible blood. An important recent development has been the introduction of blood component therapy in which different parts of a donation of blood are separated and concentrated for administration.

## EFFECTS ON BLOOD DURING STORAGE

As with all therapies, students must understand the basic properties of transfused blood. Particularly relevant are the changes which occur during storage.

Blood for routine transfusion is collected in citrate anticoagulant to which dextrose is added to prolong red cell viability. Many Blood Transfusion Services still use acid citrate dextrose (ACD); others add phosphate ions (CPD) or adenine (CPD-adenine) to further increase the life of the red cells. Approximately 425 ml of donated blood is added to 75–120 ml of anticoagulant mixture.

The changes which occur during routine storage at 2–6°C with ACD anticoagulant are summarised in Table 9.1. Red cell viability falls sharply after 4 weeks storage and for this reason the routine shelf-life of blood stored in ACD is 21 days (maximum permissible 28 days). Particular attention should be paid to the lability of certain haemostatic factors (notably platelets), to the increase in potassium and ammonia concentration in the plasma, and to the fall in pH during storage.

## SEROLOGICAL CONSIDERATIONS

Recent increase in our knowledge of blood group serology, affecting red cells, white cells, platelets and plasma proteins, has made blood transfusion a complex and highly technical procedure. However, the student must be familiar with the basic principles for clinical practice.

### RED CELL SEROLOGY

### ABO system

The most important red cell antigens are of the *ABO blood group system*. An incompatible ABO blood transfusion can cause immediate and fatal intravascular haemolysis. This occurs because many individuals have circulating natural (allo-) antibodies to ABO red-cell antigens (Table 9.2). The group O patient is at highest risk because his plasma contains both anti-A and anti-B antibodies. As approximately half of the patients who require transfusion are likely to be group O, the potential danger of a blood transfusion is considerable.

Antigens of the ABO system are present on all cells in the body. As they affect histocompatibility they are taken into account when selecting donors for organ or marrow transplantation (see Ch. 14). Both A and B antigens have sub-groups ($A_1$, $A_2$,

**Table 9.1** Mean changes in some characteristics of blood stored at $4 \pm 2°C$ in ACD.

| Parameter | Days stored | | | |
|---|---|---|---|---|
| | 0 | 7 | 14 | 21 |
| Red cell viability (%) | 95 | 90 | 84 | 75 |
| * Platelet viability (%) | 95 | 0 | 0 | 0 |
| † White cell viability (%) | 95 | 0 | 0 | 0 |
| ‡ Coagulation Factor V and VIII (%) | 95 | 30 | 30 | 30 |
| Free haemoglobin (g/L) | 0–0.10 | 0.25 | 0.50 | 1.0 |
| Lactic acid (g/L) | 0.20 | 0.70 | 1.20 | 1.40 |
| pH | 7.00 | 6.85 | 6.77 | 6.65 |
| Sodium (mmol) | 150 | 148 | 145 | 142 |
| Potassium (mmol) | 3.4 | 10 | 24 | 32 |
| Ammonia (μg %) | 50 | 260 | 470 | 680 |

* The fall in viability of platelets occurs in the first 48 hours.
† Figures refer to polymorphonuclear white cells: the fall occurs over the first 72 hours. A significant number of lymphocytes are viable at 21 days.
‡ All other coagulation factors are stable during storage.

**Table 9.2** The antigens and antibodies in each of the four main groups of the ABO system.

| Blood Group | Frequency in Population* (%) | Antigens on Red Cells | Natural ABO Antibodies | Compatible Donor Blood |
|---|---|---|---|---|
| O | 50 | Nil | Anti-A and Anti-B | *Only* O |
| A | 35 | A | Anti-B | A or O |
| B | 10 | B | Anti-A | B or O |
| AB | 5 | A and B | Nil | A, B, AB or O |

* These frequencies differ in other counries and even slightly within the United Kingdom. Asian people have an incidence of group B which is between 30–40%. This can create problems in Caucasian communities with pockets of immigrants.

*Notes:*
1. REMEMBER — O — the universal donor, AB — the universal recipient.
2. REMEMBER — the plasma in the transfusion of donor blood is so dilute that it rarely causes agglutination of the recipient's cells.
3. REMEMBER — blood should never be transfused without careful cross-matching except in the most extreme emergency; incompatibilities other than those due to the ABO system may cause reactions or sensitisations.

$A_3$, $B_1$, $B_2$ etc), and occasionally blood of an exact sub-group is required.

## Rhesus blood group system (Fig. 9.1)

This follows the ABO system in importance. There are five detectable antigens (D, C, c, E and e), but the most immunogenic, and therefore most relevant to transfusion, is D. For routine transfusions, only the D group is taken into account and patients and donors are classified as Rh(D) posi-

tive or Rh(D) negative; the most common combination of Rhesus antigens in Rh(D) negative individuals is cde.

The Rhesus system is important to the clinician for four reasons.

1. Although natural antibodies to the Rh antigen are rare, immune (iso-) antibodies can be generated which can cause compatibility problems and haemolytic reactions. These are usually less severe than from ABO incompatibility.

2. Rh(D) incompatibility is the most frequent cause of haemolytic disease of the new-born. *RhD*

RHESUS INCOMPATIBILITY

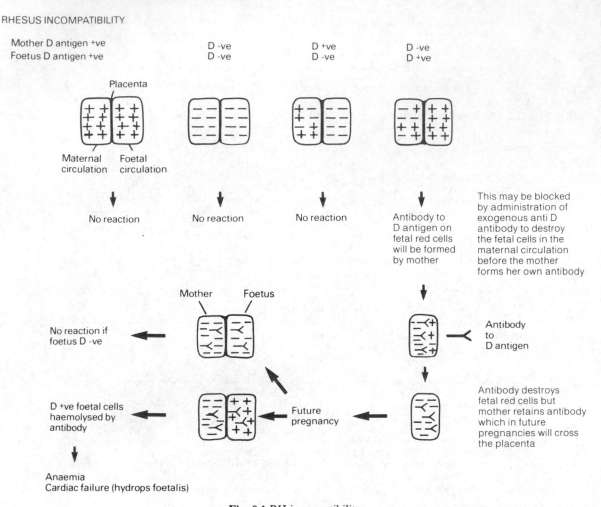

**Fig. 9.1** RH incompatibility

*negative women in the child-bearing age should not receive Rh(D) positive blood.*

3. Patients with circulating anti-D (i.e., an Rh negative patient who has received Rh positive blood) must receive Rh(D) negative blood. This can be difficult to supply, particularly when the patient has a rare ABO group (see Table 9.3).

4. The most common identifiable antibodies in acquired (autoimmune) haemolytic anaemia are Rhesus in specificity. Serious transfusion problems are frequently encountered.

## Other red cell antigens

Many other red cell antigen systems and specific antibodies have been identified, but their inci-

**Table 9.3** Availability of ABO Rh(D) negative blood in typical Caucasian community.

| O Rh(D) Negative | 10% |
| A Rh(D) Negative | 6% |
| B Rh(D) Negative | 2% |
| AB Rh(D) Negative | 0.5% |

dence is low. Such antibodies may cause clinical problems equal to those found with the Rh(D) system. Commonest are anti-E, anti-c and anti-e (of the Rh system), anti-K (Kell/cellano system), anti-Fy (Duffy system) and Jk (Kidd system). In such patients one must only give donations which do not contain the specific antigen.

## The universal donor

With the discovery of the Rhesus blood group system the concept of the 'universal donor' was extended to group O Rh(D) negative rather than just group O. The apparent advantage was that 'universal donor' blood could be given safely without the need for grouping and crossmatching.

However, there are considerable disadvantages to the use of uncrossmatched group O Rh(D) negative blood. Antibodies to other antigen systems may be present and cause transfusion reactions; some group O donations have high natural titres of anti-A which if the recipient is group A cause acute haemolysis; group O Rh(D) negative blood is rare and is essential for the transfusion of Rh negative women in the child bearing age. It should be used as universal donor blood only in dire emergency. If there is a shortage of O Rh(D) negative blood, O Rh(D) positive may have to be used.

In less extreme conditions (see Table 9.4) it is acceptable to use uncrossmatched but group-specific (homologous) blood. In all other circumstances only crossmatched blood of the appropriate group should be used.

## Practical considerations (Fig. 9.2)

The house-surgeon need no longer be familiar with the techniques of providing compatible blood for individual patients. However, he must be familiar with some of the procedures used in the Blood Bank and the principles underlying them.

1. The major cause of incompatible blood

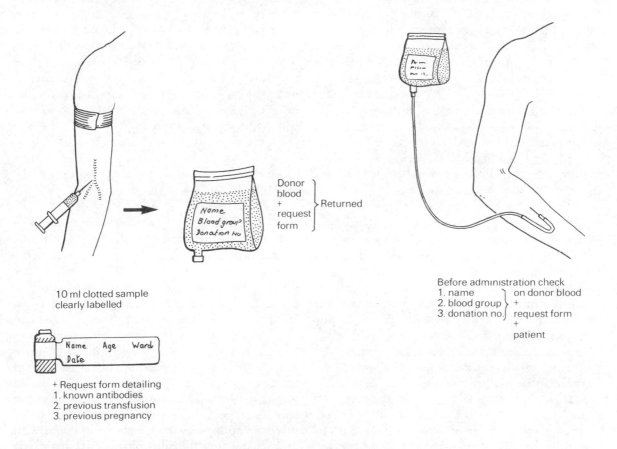

10 ml clotted sample
clearly labelled

Name    Age    Ward
Date

+ Request form detailing
1. known antibodies
2. previous transfusion
3. previous pregnancy

Name
Blood group?
Donation No

Donor
blood
+          } Returned
request
form

Before administration check
1. name        } on donor blood
2. blood group +
3. donation no. } request form
                    +
                    patient

**Fig. 9.2** Practical considerations

**Table 9.4** Response times* to requests for blood.

| Time | Product/procedure | Comments |
|------|-------------------|----------|
| Immediate | Not crossmatched (O Rh(D) Negative Universal Donor) | Use only in extreme life-threatening hae-morrhagic situations or when grouping and/or crossmatching facilities are not available (Obstetric Flying Squad) |
| 20–30 min | Not crossmatched (Homologous blood) ABO Rh(D) compatible) | Less extreme situations as described above. Also permissible in on-going mass-ive transfusion when crossmatching becomes academic (after 12 donations administered in 6 hours) |
| 1 hour (30 min in some Centres) | Emergency crossmatched | Limited technical procedures involved oc-casionally results in missing an antibody. |
| 2–3 hours | Fully crossmatched | Detection of antibodies can lead to further delay to identify the antibody and provide compatible donations. This can take sev-eral hours, days or weeks, depending on the rarity of the antibody or antibodies. |

* To these times must be added transport time, to and from the Blood Bank

transfusion is administration of wrong blood to the patient due to mistakes in documentation during the initial request (the blood in the tube does not correspond to the name on the label) or failure to check before administration that the *name, blood group* and *donation number* on every crossmatched donation corresponds exactly with those on the completed request form.

2. The house-surgeon should appreciate the time required to provide compatible blood for an individual patient (Table 9.4). He must also know the expected transport times and appreciate that these can vary in different localities.

3. Patients requiring repeated transfusions of blood require special consideration. Leucocyte, platelet and plasma protein antibodies apart (see below), red cell antibodies may be produced in the interval between the first and subsequent transfusions. A new serum specimen from the recipient must be provided each time a request is made. If during the administration of a transfu-sion compatible blood is held for more than 72 hours, a re-crossmatch should be requested against a fresh serum sample.

4. Delay in the provision of fully compatible blood can result from taking too small a sample of serum for cross-matching. For every unit re-quested at least 1 ml of blood is required. In practice it is advisable to take a 10 ml clotted sample: this will provide sufficient serum for

rechecking should a transfusion reaction occur.

5. In requesting blood, particular attention must be paid to the labelling of specimens and informing the Blood Bank personnel of known pre-existing immune antibodies, pregnancies and previous transfusions. They are then alerted to potential difficulties. If problems are known to exist, early consultation with the Blood Bank staff will facilitate correct therapy.

## WHITE CELL AND PLATELET SEROLOGY

Human white cells and platelets have genetically determined surface antigens which are part of the human leucocyte antigen (HLA) system. The HLA system is complex with a major histocom-patability role in organ and marrow transplants. Antigens of the HLA system are not expressed on mature red cells but are found on reticulocytes. Other (non-HLA) antigens specific to neutro-phils, lymphocytes or platelets have been recog-nised.

Routine blood transfusion, or pregnancy, can stimulate the development of leucocyte and/or platelet antibodies which may cause significant reactions during further transfusions. They may also impair the efficiency of subsequent transfusions of white cells or platelets and the function of transplanted organs.

## PLASMA PROTEIN SEROLOGY

Approximately one person in 2500 lacks IgA. If repeatedly transfused they may develop allo-antibodies directed against normal IgA, or against different determinants on the IgA molecule. Patients who have developed these antibodies may suffer reactions to subsequent transfusions of blood or blood products containing the specific plasma-protein antigen.

## COMPLICATIONS OF BLOOD TRANSFUSION

The morbidity and mortality of blood transfusion may be greater than that of general anaesthesia

(Fig.9.3). The list of potential complications is formidable:

### Febrile reactions

Pyrogens and minor bacterial contamination used to be a common cause of febrile reactions; this is no longer the case. The occasional febrile reaction now seen is more likely to be due to interactions between pre-existing recipient antibodies and transfused leucocytes, platelets or immunoglobulins. These are usually minor but as some are severe and even fatal all should be investigated. A significant number remain unexplained. They are best managed by stopping the transfusion and the intravenous administration of an antihistamine (chlorpheniramine sulphate, 20 mg) and hydrocortisone (sodium succinate, 100 mg). Further transfusions should be similarly covered, filtered, washed or frozen/thawed/washed/red cells (products with reduced white cells, platelets and plasma protein) may be necessary for patients who require continued transfusion or who continue to react despite antihistamine cover.

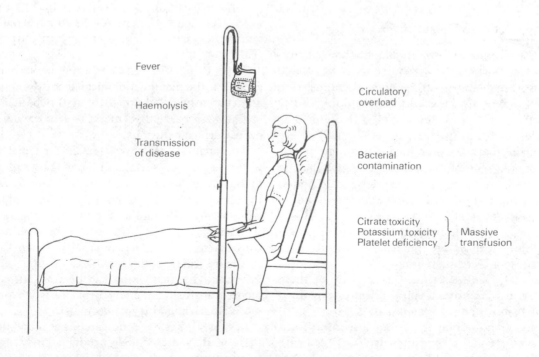

Fever

Haemolysis

Transmission of disease

Circulatory overload

Bacterial contamination

Citrate toxicity
Potassium toxicity  } Massive
Platelet deficiency  } transfusion

**Fig. 9.3** Complications of blood transfusion

## Bacterial contamination

Bacterial contamination of blood donations is rare. However, during donation a small number of skin bacteria can pass into the blood and if it is not stored at 4°C heavy growth may occur. Heavily contaminated blood is almost black and on transfusion causes sudden and severe endotoxaemia, which is usually fatal. Treatment is by intravenous infusions of antibiotics to cover both aerobic and anaerobic organisms and other supportive measures (see shock). The offending blood must be returned immediately to the Blood Bank for investigation.

## Circulatory overload

This complication occurs in severely anaemic elderly patients, particularly with cardiac insufficiency. Such patients should be transfused only with red cell concentrates. If blood loss and anaemia is not acute, only one unit of red cells should be given every 24 hours accompanied by 20 mg frusemide intravenously. In some patients exchange transfusion may be required.

## Haemolytic reactions

The most common form of immune (non-haemolytic) transfusion reaction is due to incompatible leucocytes, platelets or immunoglobulins (see above). The most sinister are those due to ABO incompatibility. Less than 50 ml of ABO incompatible blood can give rise to sudden and severe back pain, marked dyspnoea and profound hypotension. Haemoglobinuria and haemoglobinaemia occur and the patient becomes icteric in 24 hours. Within one hour of transfusion, acute renal failure may have developed. Disseminated intravascular coagulation (DIC), initiated by antigen/antibody complexes formed on the red cell membranes, may cause a bleeding diathesis.

General anaesthesia may mask many of these signs and symptoms, but sudden unexplained hypotension is an important marker.

Most other antibodies do not cause intravascular haemolysis: the antibody-coated red cells are destroyed more slowly by the reticulo-endothelial system, primarily spleen and liver. Jaundice usually develops, but renal failure and DIC are rare.

Massive haemolysis can follow administration of compatible blood which is heavily contaminated, accidentally frozen and thawed, or heated above 40°C.

It cannot be sufficiently stressed that *the most common cause of incompatible blood transfusions are mistakes made in the wards: errors in identification of crossmatching blood samples and/or failure to check blood prior to administration.*

Investigation and management of major intravascular haemolytic transfusion reactions are outlined in Table 9.5.

## Transmission of disease

Transmission of viral hepatitis remains the most serious and frequent complication of the administration of blood and blood products. A survey in the United Kingdom, before hepatitis (B surface antigen) testing became routine, indicated that the morbidity and mortality were 27 and 8 respectively per 10 000 units transfused.

Viral hepatitis from blood transfusions rarely arises from hepatitis type A (infectious hepatitis), cytomegalovirus (CMV) and Epstein Barr virus (EBV).

Type B hepatitis virus remains an important cause but the major aetiological agent is unknown and currently called non-A, non-B hepatitis.

The best preventive measure is to avoid unneccessary transfusions.

All donations are now screened for hepatitis B virus, using the surface antigen (HBsAg) as a marker. This reduces the overall risk of hepatitis by about 25%. Two blood products only are without risk: albumin and immunoglobulins.

All donations are also screened for syphilis. As spirochaetes have limited viability, blood stored for more than 4 days at 4°C is safe. Other infectious diseases which can be transmitted by blood transfusion include brucellosis, toxoplasmosis, malaria and trypanosomiasis.

Recent studies have indicated that blood donations and some blood products may rarely transmit an infectious agent which gives rise to the development of severe (often fatal) acquired

**Table 9.5** Management of intravascular haemolytic transfusion reactions.

| Investigations | Therapy |
|---|---|
| 1. Check for evidence of incompatible blood on bottle (bag) labels. Return suspect donation to Blood Bank for immediate investigation. | 1. Stop transfusion. |
| | 2. Hydrocortisone 100 mg I.V. |
| 2. Withdraw 30 ml blood and send to laboratories immediately. Inform Blood Bank medical staff. | 3. Insert urinary catheter, empty bladder and monitor urine flow. |
|    a. Serological investigations at Blood Bank (10 ml) | 4. 100 ml Mannitol (20%) and 100 ml of 0.9% saline. |
|    b. Blood Urea and electrolytes (10 ml) | 5. 150 mg Frusemide I.V. |
|    c. Coagulation screen (10 ml) | 6. If 2 hours after mannitol and saline the urine flow is less than 100 ml/h, then repeat 100 ml (20%) mannitol. If at the end of next 2 hours urine flow is less than 100 ml/h, assume acute renal failure and treat accordingly. |
| 3. Electrocardiogram. ? evidence of hyperkalaemia. | |
| 4. Coagulation and biochemical screens repeated 2–4-hourly until stabilised. | 7. If evidence of hyperkalaemia (clinical, ECG or laboratory evidence) institute resonium/insulin/glucose therapy. |
| | 8. If evidence of D.I.C., contact specialist for advice: patient may require systemic heparinisation. |

\* Every attempt must be made to avoid further blood transfusion until Blood Bank staff have checked compatibility of subsequent donations. In the meantime manage significant hypovolaemia with albumin solutions (SPPS), pooled plasma or artificial colloids.

immune deficiency (AIDS) in recipients. This problem is currently under intense investigation.

## Massive transfusion (Fig. 9.4)

If four units of blood are transfused consecutively into patients at a rate in excess of 100 ml/minute complications may arise. These include:

*Citrate toxicity.* Patients who are hypotensive or have liver or renal damage fail to metabolise or excrete the large load of citrate in transfused blood. It combines with ionised calcium leading to muscle tremor, tetany and cardiac arrhythmias. Citrate is also cardiotoxic.

*Potassium toxicity.* Potassium leaks out of red cells during storage. Rapid administration of large volumes of old blood may elevate the serum potassium to cardiotoxic levels. This is particularly liable to occur in patients with renal damage or severe crush injuries with extensive muscle damage. Excessive hydrogen ions in stored blood potentiate this effect.

*Platelet deficiency.* Stored blood has few viable platelets. Massive transfusions may lead to dilution thrombocytopenia and bleeding.

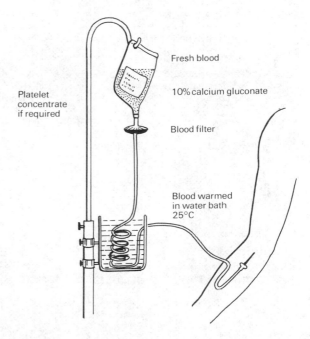

Fresh blood

10% calcium gluconate

Platelet concentrate if required

Blood filter

Blood warmed in water bath 25°C

**Fig. 9.4** Precautions with massive transfusions

These problems are prevented and/or treated by:

1. Warming blood (25°C) prior to transfusion. This will increase citrate metabolism and avoid the need for calcium adminstration. Otherwise, if more than 2 litres of blood have been administered, 10 ml of 10% calcium gluconate should be given for every two further units.

2. Using blood which is less than 5 days old and so reducing the risk of potassium toxicity.

3. Administering platelet concentrates if there is significant oozing due to failure of haemostasis.

Micro-aggregates of platelets and leucocytes are formed during the storage of blood and it has been suggested that when transfused in large amounts they may contribute to the adult respiratory distress syndrome. The use of in-line micro-aggregate blood filters has become popular but there is little evidence of their benefit, certainly in patients receiving less than 5 units of blood.

# BLOOD PRODUCTS AND THEIR CLINICAL USES

The introduction of plastic blood bags, large capacity centrifuges and plasma fractionation have permitted the production of several specific therapeutic products from blood donations. Low volume and highly concentrated derivatives, e.g. platelet and coagulation factor concentrates, can provide effective and specific treatment without the risk of circulatory overload. The use of such *blood component therapy* also reduces waste and increases safety (Table 9.6).

## BLOOD REPLACEMENT

### Acute haemorrhage

An average healthy adult can lose 500 ml of blood rapidly without ill effect. Provided circulatory

**Table 9.6** Examples of products which contribute to blood component therapy

| Blood product | | Shelf life | Main indications |
|---|---|---|---|
| Whole blood | | 21 days (ACD) 28 days (CPD) | Severe life-threatening haemorrhage: component of a transfusion policy (see text) |
| Red cell concentrates | | As Whole Blood | All routine transfusions; and part of a transfusion policy (see text) |
| White cell concentrates | | 12 hours | Severe leucopenia associated with life-threatening infection; ? to cover surgery in such patients |
| Platelet concentrates | | 72 hours | Non-immune severe thrombocytopenia |
| Transfer factor | | 5 years | Chronic mucocutaneous candidiasis |
| Interferon | | Not established | Virus infections and malignancy — not yet defined |
| Albumin | 5% | 4 years | Acute volume expansion |
| | 15–20% | 4 years | Severe symptomatic hypoproteinaemia |
| Factor VIII | Cryoprecipitate | 6 months | Haemophilia A management. von Willebrand's Disease. Hypofibrinogenaemia. Factor VIII Deficiency. |
| | AHF | 1 year | Haemophilia A management |
| Factor IX | II,VII,IX,X | 2 years | Haemophilia B factor replacement. Acquired deficiencies (liver disease, oral anticoagulant reversal) |
| | II,IX,X | 2 years | As above |
| Factor II (Fibrinogen) | | 1 year | Hypofibrinogenaemia when cryoprecipitate is unacceptable (see text) |
| Gammaglobulin Normal | | 4 years | Prophylaxis hepatitis A virus infection |
| Hyperimmune (anti-D) | | | Prevention Rh disease of newborn |
| (anti-Tetanus) | | | Prevention of tetanus |
| (anti-Vaccinia) | | | Prevention and treatment of vaccinia |
| (anti-Zoster) | | | Prevention and treatment of zoster |
| Fresh frozen plasma | | 1 year | Some bleeding conditions (see text) |

volume is maintained, with crystalloids and/or colloids, the loss of 1–2 litres of blood will not lead to irreversible hypotension. Children, the elderly and those with cardiopulmonary disease tolerate haemorrhage less well; they are also more susceptible to over-transfusion.

The assessment of blood loss is difficult, particularly following acute haemorrhage. Measurements of blood volume are time-consuming and often inaccurate, particularly in anaemic and/or debilitated patients. Estimations of haemoglobin and haematocrit are notoriously misleading when plasma and red cells are lost in the same proportion. Serial clinical observations of increasing pulse-rate, falling blood pressure, irritability, sweating, cold extremities, intolerance to exertion and frequent changing of posture are the best indications for blood transfusion in haemorrhage. Hasty action from a single clinical observation should be avoided unless additional information such as evidence of major internal haemorrhage into muscle or abdomen is available. A systolic pressure of less than 100 mm Hg following blood loss indicates a deficit of greater than 30% of the circulating volume, and the need for transfusion.

There is no need for specific action to replace coagulation factors, unless they are congenitally deficient, there is impaired liver function or the patient is on oral anticoagulant therapy. Rarely a deficit of 50% in coagulation factors may arise in severe haemorrhage, but this is still compatible with normal haemostasis. Release and resynthesis of coagulation factors by a normal liver readily compensates for losses associated with haemorrhage.

Oxygen-carrying capacity must be considered. In patients *without* cardiopulmonary disease an ideal balance between capillary flow and tissue oxygenation is achieved by a haematocrit of 30%. Because of the absence of fibrinogen, crystalloids and colloids are more beneficial to blood viscosity than plasma. Haematocrits below 30% are compatible with normal tissue metabolism, provided oxygen is also administered.

In planning a transfusion policy, it is no longer appropriate to replace blood loss ml for ml. If there is clinical evidence of hypovolaemia then up to 2 litres of crystalloid and colloid solutions should initially be transfused. Those which do not transmit hepatitis virus are ideal. Re-constituted freeze-dry plasma is an acceptable alternative, but its contained fibrinogen may increase blood viscosity and thus reduce capillary flow. It is also potentially icterogenic and its potassium content is high. Administration of red cell concentrates and whole blood can follow. The first two units can be red cell concentrates, but thereafter whole blood may be used. Useful guidelines are summarised in Table 9.7.

## Chronic anaemia

The risks associated with blood transfusion contraindicate its routine use for the treatment of chronic anaemia. Blood transfusion should only be considered when haematinics have failed. Impending and uncontrolled acute haemorrhage in the severely anaemic patient is potentially hazardous and every effort must be made to maintain the haemoglobin level above 7 g/dl, using blood transfusions. Delaying surgery, whilst awaiting a response to haematinics in preference to transfusion, may also be unacceptable.

Although successful major surgery can be performed on patients with haemoglobin levels of less than 5 g/dl with appropriate pre-operative transfusion, many surgeons and anaesthetists still prefer an initial haemoglobin of 10 g/dl before commencing an elective major operation. Provided surgical haemorrhage and pre-operative transfusions can be controlled and the pre-existing anaemia is asymptomatic a lower figure, eg. 7 g/dl, can be accepted. The blood product of choice for transfusion to the anaemic patient is red cell concentrate. Each donation (250 ml of concentrate) should raise the haemoglobin by 1.0 to 1.5 g/dl. Transfusion may be hazardous in the extremely anaemic patient (less than 5 g/dl), the elderly, or when significant cardio pulmonary disease is present. In these circumstances it is wise to cover each unit of concentrate with 20 mg frusemide i.v. Ideally, all pre-operative transfusions should be completed 24 hours before surgery.

## An overall transfusion policy

Over the last 15 years the administration of whole blood for most routine transfusions has been recognised as wasteful. The demand for special blood products, derived from plasma, now exceeds the requirement of red cells by a factor of almost two.

This problem can be resolved by the following policy:

1. Red cell concentrates should be used for all forms of chronic anaemia.

2. In acute haemorrhagic situations (including intra-operative blood loss following crystalloid administration) the first two donations of blood should be as red cell concentrates. This is followed by whole blood, as required, over the subsequent 24-hour period (see Table 9.7).

In paediatric cases and burns whole blood is more appropriate.

## BLOOD COMPONENTS

### Whole blood

Whole blood should be reserved for those patients with severe uncontrolled haemorrhage and clinical signs of hypovolaemia, and as part of a general transfusion policy (see above). Fresh (less than 6 hours old) whole blood to ensure haemostasis is no longer indicated: specific and more highly concentrated haemostatic components are preferred. Fresh whole blood should be administered to the bleeding patient with a systemic haemorrhagic diathesis only when specific concentrates are not available.

### Red cell concentrates

Red cell concentrates are prepared by removing plasma from donations of whole blood and resuspending the cells to give a haematocrit of 70%. They are the product of choice for routine transfusions and should account for 60–70% of all units transfused.

*Packed red cell concentrates.* This product has a haematocrit in excess of 90%. It is reserved for patients with severe anaemia and cardiac failure.

*Washed and frozen red cells.* Some patients (see p.91) may require donations with minimal leucocytes, platelets and plasma protein contamination. These are prepared by extensive saline washing of red cells. Washed red cells must be transfused within 12 hours.

A more effective but costly method is to use frozen-thawed-washed red cells. After thawing they are washed extensively to remove the cryoprotective agent, glycerol.

Frozen cells can be stored for many years and provide stocks of blood of rare groups.

*Filtered red cells.* Some patients require leucocyte poor or only red cell preparations. These are best prepared by filtration through special filters.

### Platelet concentrates

Platelet concentrates contain 60–70% of the platelets present in the original donation, suspended in approximately 40 ml plasma. An adult requir-

**Table 9.7** Transfusion options associated with haemorrhage.

| | |
|---|---|
| Previously healthy adults: | Begin with 1000 ml crystalloids; followed by 1000 ml colloids; followed by 2 Red Cell Concentrates; followed by Whole Blood as required |
| Elderly and/or significant cardio-pulmonary disease: | Begin with 500 ml crystalloids; followed by 500 ml colloids; followed by 2 Red Cell Concentrates; followed by Whole Blood as required. |

1. By using these regimes the majority of patients transfused for blood loss associated with elective surgery will not require *blood* transfusion.
2. Dextrans and gelatin solutions are the colloid preparations of choice. They are contra-indicated in patients with a pre-existing systematic haemostasis failure and plasma or albuminoid should be used.
3. Patients with severe liver disease or those on full doses of oral anticoagulants should receive 500 ml fresh frozen plasma (FFP) along with the 2 Red Cell Concentrates. Further doses of FFP may be required.

ing this form of therapy usually needs a pool of platelets from 5–6 donations to achieve haemostasis. Platelet concentrates should be administered as rapidly as possible (within 15 minutes).

Platelet therapy is indicated in patients with an active haemorrhagic diathesis due to thrombocytopenia (less than $20 \times 10^9/l$) or those with clinical evidence of platelet malfunction. Platelet concentrates are also of value following massive transfusion of stored blood in which the platelets are non-functioning (Table 9.1 and page 93). They are of little value in patients with immune thrombocytopenia or those with obvious splenomegaly, for they are rapidly removed from the circulation before they can exert their haemostatic effects. Prophylactic platelet therapy (5–6 donations per day) aids patients receiving intensive chemotherapy.

As platelet concentrates are contaminated by small amounts of red cells, it is advisable, but not essential, to provide ABO Rhesus compatible donations. Efficiency is best assessed by clinical observation: post-transfusion platelet counts are unreliable. Repeated transfusions of platelet concentrates should be avoided; patients develop an immune refractory state. Should this arise platelets from HL-A compatible donors can be given. This is very expensive.

## White cell concentrates

The number of granulocytes required to achieve a therapeutic effect is approximately $2–5 \times 10^{10}$ cells. They are prepared by an extracorporeal device known as a Blood Cell Separator, which continually removes the buffy coat from the circulating blood of a single donor. An ABO and HL-A compatible donor is preferred, usually a relative.

In surgical practice granulocyte transfusions are indicated only in patients with an uncontrolled infection and leucopenia of less than $1.0 \times 10^9/l$. They are given daily in a volume of 150–200 ml for 3–4 consecutive days. Donor leucocytes are an important source of a new range of blood products. Transfer factor, extracted from normal leucocytes, may enhance cellular immune mechanisms in certain deficiency states. Interferon is obtained from virus-stimulated leucocytes and is currently under clinical investigation for the treatment of viral and malignant disease.

## Fresh frozen plasma

Plasma separated from fresh blood and stored at $-30°C$ contains all coagulation factors. Thawing takes approximately 60 minutes. The thawed plasma should be used within 4 hours as coagulation factors V and VIII deteriorate rapidly. Fresh frozen plasma should be ABO compatible with the recipient.

Fresh frozen plasma is not a panacea for all bleeding states. Its main indication in surgical practice is when patients on anticoagulant therapy or with severe liver disease require emergency operations or continue to bleed. 800 ml (four donations) are infused in 60 minutes. In elderly patients, circulatory overload may be prevented by frusemide (40 mg i.v.). Fresh freeze-dried plasma is available in some parts of the world. It has the advantage that it can be stored in a domestic refrigerator. Before use it is redissolved in a small volume of distilled water.

## Outdated (freeze-dried) plasma

This is prepared from a pool of 10 donations of varied ABO blood groups. It can be administered to a recipient of any blood-group. One unit is made up with 400 ml distilled pyrogen-free water. As the potassium content is high (up to 30 mmol/l) it should be given with caution in patients with renal impairment. The risk of hepatitis is increased by pooling.

Outdated freeze-dried plasma once had a major role in the management of hypovolaemia; with the introduction of safer colloids (dextrans, gelatins) and preparations of human albumin, its use has declined. Its main indication now is in the management of burns; but even then it may be replaced by albumin preparations.

As freeze-dried outdated plasma can be stored for up to 5 years it is still useful as an acute volume expander in countries without facilities for plasma fractionation. In concentrated form (made up in 150 ml distilled water) it provides a useful source of coagulation factors, except the labile factors V and VIII.

## Factor VIII concentrates

There are two available concentrates of human factor VIII; cryoprecipitate and antihaemophilic fraction (AHF). When fresh plasma is frozen to $-40°C$ and then allowed to thaw at $4–8°C$, a precipitate forms which contains 20–80% of the Factor VIII, fibrinogen and Factor XIII of the original plasma. It also contains clinically significant quantities of the factors which stimulate synthesis and release of Factor VIII and increase platelet adhesion in patients with von Willibrand's disease. The cryoprecipitate from each donation is stored at $-30°C$ in a small volume (20–50 ml) of the plasma supernatant. It dissolves rapidly at $37°C$ and should be used within 4 hours of reconstitution. Material from several donations is usually pooled prior to administration. Each donation of cryoprecipitate contains 50–150 units of Factor VIII.

Antihaemophilic fraction (AHF) is obtained as a freeze-dried product of plasma fractionation. It has significant advantages over cryoprecipitate: a standard and stated dose is available, it can be stored in a domestic refrigerator, and its administration is much more convenient. Currently, it is more expensive than cryoprecipitate. As it is prepared from large plasma pools it carries a high risk of transmitting hepatitis.

The main use of these preparations is in the management of haemophilia. Minor episodes of joint or muscle pain usually require a single intravenous dose of Factor VIII; more serious haematomas need to be treated for 2–4 days. If major surgery is required Factor VIII must be administered 8-hourly for the first two days and 12-hourly for the next 10–14 days. Major surgery on an adult haemophiliac may require the Factor VIII content of over 1000 donations.

Home therapy is a recent development in the management of haemophilia. The patient or relative administers a small dose (250–500 units) of Factor VIII concentrate as soon as pain is felt in a joint or a muscle, thus aborting a more serious bleed and subsequent hospital admission. AHF is ideal for this form of treatment. All Factor VIII concentrates carry the risk of transmitting hepatitis: As there are trace amounts of anti-A and anti-B in most preparations large doses occasionally cause mild haemolysis in those of group A, B or AB.

## Factor IX concentrates

There are two types of Factor IX concentrates available. Both are fractionation products and available as freeze-dried preparations. One is a mixture of coagulation factors II, IX and X and the other of II, VII, IX and X. They are used primarily in the management of hereditary coagulation factor deficiencies, particularly Factor IX deficiency (Christmas disease or haemophilia B). The principles of replacement therapy in Christmas disease are similar to those in haemophilia A.

More recently these concentrates have been used to reverse excess oral anticoagulant therapy and to prepare patients for liver biopsy. However, this practice should be avoided, if possible, in view of the risk of hepatitis.

Factor IX concentrates carry the same risk of transmitting hepatitis as concentrates of Factor VIII. Some preparations may be thrombogenic, particularly in patients with severe liver disease. Thrombogenic activity increases if the concentrates are left standing after reconstitution with distilled water. They should be used immediately.

## Fibrinogen concentrates

Large pool fractionated concentrates of fibrinogen are still available, but cryoprecipitate, available as a single donation (0.1–0.3 g of fibrinogen per pack), has considerably less risk of transmitting hepatitis. This form of therapy is used in patients with hereditary fibrinogen deficiency and is only rarely indicated in surgical practice for patients with disseminated intravascular coagulation.

## Albuminoid preparations

Preparations of human albumin are available in two forms. A 4.5–5% solution (stable purified protein solution, S.P.P.S., salt content approximately 140 mmol/l), used for acute volume expansion; and a 15% or 25% solution poor in salt (salt poor albumin; S.P.A.), used to correct hypoproteinaemia.

Human albumin preparations are heated to

destroy hepatitis viruses: some have a significant kinin content which may produce transient hypotension. Such reactions are rare and invariably benign.

Preparations of human albumin are very expensive. The 5% preparation costs at least 10 times as much as colloid volume expanders such as dextrans. S.P.P.S. should be reserved for those hypovolaemic patients likely to develop significant hypoproteinaemia (i.e. crush injuries, septic peritonitis, severe acute pancreatitis, prolonged intestinal obstruction and mesenteric vascular occlusion) and those with systemic failure of haemostasis in whom artificial colloids are contraindicated. S.P.P.S can be used in the management of hypovolaemia associated with burns, but many still prefer plasma with its content of biologically active proteins.

Albumin infusions should not be used to supply nutritional requirements. Albumin must be broken down to amino acids before incorporation into body proteins and this process is slow (half-life 18 days). Moreover, the essential amino acid content is poor (particularly tryptophan) and infused albumin increases the catabolic rate. Its main value in hypoproteinaemia is as an acute oncotic agent.

Patients are at risk from low oncotic pressure when total serum protein falls below 52 g/l (albumin less than 25 g/l). Salt-poor albumin should be administered in amounts calculated as 2 × (desired - actual albumin level) × (plasma volume), assuming a plasma volume of 40 ml/kg. This calculation allows for the extravascular deficit which will consume approximately half the administered dose.

## Immunoglobulin preparation

Immunoglobulin preparations consist of IgG with only trace amounts of IgM and IgA. The concentration of protein is usually 15 g/100 ml, but antibody content is variable and depends on the donors used. Immunoglobulin preparations are usually administered intramuscularly, do not transmit viral hepatitis, and only rarely cause untoward reactions. There are two types.

1. Human normal immunoglobulin (HNI) is prepared during routine fractionation of large pools from over 2000 ordinary donations. It is used as replacement therapy in hypogammaglobulinaemia and for passive protection against hepatitis A infection or measles.

2. Human specific immunoglobulin (HSI) is produced by fractionation of donations known to have particularly high titres of a specific antibody. They include anti-D, anti-tetanus, anti-vaccinia and anti-varicella (zoster), anti-HBV and anti rabies fractions.

*Anti-D* immunoglobulin has proved outstandingly successful in preventing immunisation against the Rhesus D antigen during pregnancy. It is also indicated if Rh(D) positive blood is transferred accidentally to a Rh(D) negative recipient. The dose is 10 *μg/ml of red cells administered.*

*Anti-tetanus* fraction is available as a 250 i.u. dose for prophylactic therapy. It should be given to patients who have not had appropriate active immunisation (full initial course or a booster) within 5 years, and who present with a dirty (soil-contaminated) wound, or one which has not received medical attention for over 72 hours. A more concentrated preparation (5000 i.u.) is available for use in established tetanus.

*Anti-HBV.* Current evidence suggests that prophylactic use of this specific immunoglobulin can diminish the severity of hepatitis B viral infections. The recommended dose is 10–20 mg/kg body weight given within 5 days of exposure. The material is inevitably in short supply and most frequently used for health service staff who accidentally inoculate themselves with the body fluids of a patient known to be HBs-Ag positive. This occurs from needle pricks or from splashes onto cuts or mucous membranes.

*Anti-rabies.* This preparation is now available as prophylactic therapy for those who receive animal bites in continental countries.

# 10. Parenteral Nutrition in Surgical Patients

The importance of metabolic factors in the response to surgery has been emphasised. A well nourished patient withstands surgery better than one poorly nourished, wound healing is more efficient and resistance to infection is greater. Surgery and injury impose considerable catabolic demands, and starvation adds an important component to post-traumatic catabolism, particularly when continued for more than 3–4 days after surgery. The avoidance of starvation is of particular importance in chronically ill patients with intestinal disease, and in patients with severe trauma, burns or sepsis.

The recommended daily basal requirements for adults are summarised in Table 10.1.

In the starved patient, non-protein calories must be provided in the ratio of at least 100 kcal/g nitrogen if protein is to be used to replenish stores rather than as an energy source. After injury, this ratio is 200 kcal/g nitrogen. Table 10.2 indicates approximate nitrogen and calorie requirements in the fasting state, and after operation or injury. A patient's requirements are usually estimated on the basis of his clinical condition, but replacement may be calculated more accurately by measurement of urinary urea or nitrogen excretion.

The most efficient way of feeding a patient is to give him palatable food to eat. However, many surgical patients have anorexia or mechanical problems such as ileus and are unable to eat enough to match requirements. This problem may be tackled in four main ways:

## Elemental diets and dietary supplements

Elemental diets consist of preparations of amino acids and appropriate non-protein calories in the form of fat and simple sugars, supplemented in some cases with alcohol (which provides approx. 7 kcal/g). Such diets are expensive, hyperosmolar, often unpalatable, and patients are rarely persuaded to take more than 7 g nitrogen and 1400 kcal

**Table 10.1** Daily basal requirements for 70 kg man

|  | Per kg BW | Per 70 kg patient |
|---|---|---|
| Water | 35 | 2450 |
| Non-protein calories | 30 | 2100 |
| Carbohydrate (gram) | 2.0 | 140 |
| Fat (gram) | 3.0 | 210 |
| Protein (gram) | 0.7 | 50 |
| Nitrogen (gram) | 0.1 | 7 |
| Sodium (mmol) | 1.0 | 70 |
| Potassium (mmol) | 1.0 | 70 |
| Vit B (mg) | 0.5 | 35 |
| Vit C (mg) | 0.1 | 70 |

**Table 10.2** Nitrogen and caloric needs in various states.

|  | Nitrogen gm/kg | Nitrogen gm/70 kg | Energy kcal/70 kg |
|---|---|---|---|
| Starved | 0.1 | 7.0 | 1400 |
| After moderate injury (e.g. partial gastrectomy) | 0.2 | 14.0 | 2800 |
| Hypercatabolic (multiple injury, major burn, severe sepsis) | 0.3–0.5 | 21–35 | 4000–7000 |

a day in this way. Elemental diets can be used to supplement other diets, and to prepare patients for large bowel surgery, as they leave minimal residue in the colon.

## Nasogastric or nasojejunal feeding

A patient who is unconscious or unable to eat because he is on a mechanical ventilator but has a normally functioning gastro-intestinal tract may be fed a proprietary diet (e.g. Clinifeed) down a nasogastric tube to maintain nutritional status. Patients will tolerate, for long periods, a very fine nasogastric tube (Plexitron) which does not have the risks of oesophageal ulceration or chest complications associated with larger tubes.

## Gastrostomy or jejunostomy

Patients who are unable to swallow because of oesophageal obstruction may be fed through a gastrostomy. This technique was once used to prepare patients for oesophageal resection, but is no longer favoured as it interferes with subsequent surgery. It still has a place, however, for patients with long benign oesophageal strictures who are considered inoperable or who refuse surgery.

A feeding jejunostomy is a means of nourishing patients with gastric or high intestinal obstruction or patients with fistula being prepared for surgery. It is now used less frequently:

1. Because the feed may produce intestinal hurry and diarrhoea, although this is minimised by attention to its composition and osmolality;

2. Due to the incidence of local complications such as infection

3. Due to the advent of parenteral nutrition.

## Parenteral nutrition

Parenteral (intravenous) nutrition is now widely used as an excellent method of providing nutritional support. It may be continued for weeks or months if necessary with appropriate care of the catheter site and the use of special catheters.

# PRINCIPLES OF PARENTERAL NUTRITION

Parenteral nutrition employs the intravenous route to provide the patient's requirements of protein, calories, electrolytes and vitamins within the limit of his volume requirement or capacity to accommodate. The limitation on volume means that concentrated solutions of carbohydrate, fat and amino acids are used. Concentrated carbohydrate and amino acid solutions are thrombogenic, and catheters have to be placed in central veins. They are also hyperosmolar, and may produce hyperosmolar diuresis and acute hyperosmolarity problems (see p. 103). The solutions available for parenteral nutrition are numerous, but may be summarised as follows:

*Carbohydrate solutions* are available in concentrations from 20–50%. Glucose solutions are the cheapest. Fructose, or sorbitol (which is converted to fructose in the body) have the theoretical advantage that one step in glucose breakdown for energy provision is omitted, but in practice this advantage is not apparent. Further, fructose preparations have a tendency to produce lactic acidaemia. One litre of 50% glucose provides 2000 kcal.

*Fat emulsions* are now mainly prepared from soya-bean oil, in concentrations from 10% to 20%. These emulsions are nonthrombogenic and are not osmotically active. One litre of 20% fat emulsion provides 2000 kcal. It is recommended that not more than 50% of the patient's calorie requirements be provided from fat, to reduce the possibility of ketosis.

*Amino acid solutions* provide the 'raw material' for protein synthesis and are available either as casein hydrolysates or as synthetic l-amino acids. Preparations are now available which provide up to 17 g of nitrogen/l (110 g of protein). For maximum utilisation of nitrogen 200 kcal are required to be given from non-protein sources.

*Alcohol* provides an energy source (7 kcal/g) and is easily metabolised. It is rarely given because of its sedative side effects.

*Mixed solutions* are available which provide the optimum ratio of non-protein calories to nitrogen (200 kcal/g N). They have the advantage of simplicity. Having determined the amount of nitrogen required, one administers a mixed solution of appropriate nitrogen concentration over a 24-hour period, within the limits of the patient's volume restriction. However, patients' electrolyte requirements differ, and it is important not to opt for simplicity to the disadvantage of the patient.

In deciding on an appropriate regimen the following factors should be considered:

1. nitrogen and consequently non-protein calorie requirements;

2. volume of fluid required;

3. electrolyte requirements, particularly sodium and potassium, bearing in mind that the need for magnesium, phosphorus and zinc also increases after injury. The sodium requirements of the patient frequently determine the type of amino acid preparation to be used;

4. the post-operative increase in the requirement for vitamins A, B and C. This can be met by vitamin preparations such as Parentrovite or Solivito.

### Example

A patient requires 14 g of nitrogen per 24 hours, with a volume limitation of 3 litres. At least 2800 non-protein calories are required to ensure utilisation of the nitrogen. His parenteral regime could read:

1 litre amino-acid solution (14 g N)
1 litre 50% glucose (2000 kcal)
1 litre 10% fat solution (1000 kcal)

High volume losses can be replaced by using larger volumes of less concentrated carbohydrate solution, while larger electrolyte losses may be replaced by adding saline to the daily fluid intake.

Supplements of electrolytes or vitamins should not be injected into solutions used for parenteral nutrition for fear of precipitating amino acids or de-emulsifying fat preparations. Supplements should be injected into saline, or infused separately.

It is now common practice to make up the patient's daily requirements in a '3-litre bag' under strict sterile conditions. This is infused over 24 hours using a simple pump, thus obviating the need to change bottles.

### Sites for insertion of cannula for parenteral feeding

A long radio-opaque intravenous cannula can be inserted by a percutaneous technique so that its tip lies in the superior vena cava. The inferior vena cava route is contra-indicated because of the greater risk of thrombosis, particularly in the presence of intra-abdominal sepsis. The position of the catheter should be checked radiologically after insertion.

The sites most frequently used for insertion are:

1. the internal jugular vein, entered between the two heads of sternomastoid, one inch above the clavicle;

2. the subclavian vein, entered either by the supraclavicular route or the infraclavicular route at the mid-clavicular point;

3. the basilic vein, entered in the antecubital fossa. This site is now less popular.

## INDICATIONS FOR PARENTERAL NUTRITION

Parenteral nutrition costs up to £70 per day, and carries certain serious hazards. It should not be instituted without careful consideration of its necessity.

### PRE-OPERATIVE INDICATIONS

The principal indication is malnutrition. The classic example is the patient with dysphagia from an obstructing oesophageal carcinoma. Two to three weeks of parenteral nutrition before operation may improve the chances of survival after oesophageal resection. The patient with pyloric stenosis is rarely so malnourished as to require pre-operative parenteral nutrition and attention is directed to correction of fluid and electrolyte deficiency, and restoration of haemoglobin and plasma protein levels with a view to early operation. In late cases, however, parenteral nutrition may also be needed and should be continued in the postoperative period.

Patients with severe malabsorption who require surgery should receive parenteral nutrition, as should those who require operation after sustained chronic protein and fluid loss from inflammatory bowel disease.

## POSTOPERATIVE (OR POST-INJURY) INDICATIONS

The majority of patients undergoing elective surgery who pursue an uneventful postoperative course do not require parenteral nutrition. There is no evidence that their progress would be improved and they should not be exposed unnecessarily to the attendant risks and expense. The principal indications are:

*Protracted ileus.* Intestinal motility is impaired after abdominal surgery and after some operations on the spine, chest, or brain, usually returning to normal after 48 hours. If there is no sign of peristalsis after 3 days, parenteral nutrition may be instituted while the underlying cause of the ileus is determined and dealt with.

*Hypercatabolic states.* In certain conditions, the metabolic demands are so high that parenteral nutrition should be instituted immediately. These situations include:
1. multiple injury
2. major burns
3. severe sepsis
4. some patients with head injury or after certain neurosurgical operations
5. tetanus

*Small bowel fistula.* Oral feeding is usually withheld during the management of a small bowel fistula to decrease the amount of intestinal secretion. In the absence of distal obstruction, or a local disease process such as carcinoma or Crohn's disease, it is anticipated that the majority of these fistulae will close on conservative management with parenteral nutrition.

## COMPLICATIONS OF PARENTERAL NUTRITION

*Thrombophlebitis.* A frequent complication is thrombo-phlebitis. This rarely results in major pulmonary embolism, but can cause local disability and oedema of the arm before the collateral venous circulation develops. Even then, some patients are left with exercise claudication in the arm. Concentrated carbohydrate solutions are usually responsible, but the risk is also related to the length of the intravenous catheter and its constitution. Thus thrombophlebitis is more common when the catheter is inserted in the antecubital fossa and when non-siliconised catheters are used.

*Infection.* Infection and septicaemia are the most serious complications of parenteral nutrition. The usual organisms are coliforms or staphylococci, but the incidence of fungal infection has increased, possibly because many patients requiring parenteral therapy are already receiving broad-spectrum antibiotics.

The insertion site should be dressed on alternate days, an antiseptic cream applied, and the drip tubing changed daily. Great care should be taken to avoid contamination when changing bottles, and injection of additives into high calorie fluids should be avoided. The 3-litre bag system described above makes these manoeuvres unnecessary. If redness appears at the catheter site, the catheter should be removed, its tip sent for culture, the insertion site swabbed and cultured, and blood cultures taken. If a patient receiving parenteral nutrition develops an unexplained fever, similar action should be undertaken.

*Problems of insertion.* Pneumothorax may occur during insertion of the catheter by the subclavian route. With experience, this complication is rare. Occasionally, a catheter tip penetrates from the lumen of the innominate vein or the vena cava, and infusion fluid enters the thorax to produce an increasing pleural effusion.

*Catheter embolism* due to breaking off a portion of the catheter is rare with modern cannulas.

*Osmotic diuresis.* Osmotic diuresis occurs as a result of renal overspill of hyperosmolar solutions after too rapid infusion. It can be minimised by gradually increasing the infusion rate to 1 1/8 hours. The urine should be checked for sugar 6-hourly and the infusion slowed if glycosuria occurs.

*Hyperglycaemia and reactive hypoglycaemia.* Severe hyperglycaemia and an acute hyperosmolar syndrome may be produced by over-rapid infusion of concentrated carbohydrate solutions. This may be avoided by maintaining a slow infusion rate (infusion rates should never be increased to 'catch up' if the infusion has fallen behind schedule), and administering insulin concurrently (one unit of soluble insulin per 10 g of glucose). Hypoglycaemia may occur when parenteral feeding is discontinued abruptly. Additional glucose is then given.

*Metabolic acidosis.* Metabolic acidosis may develop during parenteral nutrition. This may occur during infusion of amino acids or fructose, particularly when administered with alcohol.

*Hypophosphataemia.* Hypophosphataemia may occur in patients receiving parenteral nutrition and can be prevented by appropriate additives.

*Fat overload.* Allergic reactions to fat emulsions are now rare. Some patients, particularly those with sepsis, may be unable to clear fat emulsions from their circulation at normal rates and thrombocytopenia may develop.

*Liver disease.* Patients with severe liver disease may deteriorate if fat emulsions are administered, and may show increases in blood ammonia levels in response to amino acid infusion. Parenteral nutrition in such patients should be supervised with great care.

## ALTERNATIVE REGIMES OF PARENTERAL NUTRITION

The risks associated with conventional parenteral nutritional techniques have prompted the surgeon to use alternative means of sparing protein.

*Peripheral administration of amino acids.* Dilute amino acids (e.g. 3% freamine) are not thrombogenic and may be administered through a peripheral vein. 90 g of amino acids in water may be administered in 24 hours. It has recently been claimed that this results in nitrogen equilibrium and occasionally positive nitrogen balance. If the body has adapted to the starved state it will utilise its own fat stores for energy and utilise less endogenous protein for gluconeogenesis. Carbohydrates should be avoided in this regimen as they tend to increase insulin secretion and inhibit lipolysis.

The value of this technique has still to be assessed.

*Alpha-keto acids.* Parenteral nutritional regimes in the past have provided amino acids themselves as the 'building blocks' for protein synthesis. However, it has been recognised that the distinction between essential and non-essential amino acids results from the body's inability to synthesise the carbon skeleton of the essential amino acids. If these carbon skeletons could be supplied the body would be able to synthesis essential amino acids by utilising endogenous waste nitrogen such as urea and thus spare the protein pool.

Such alpha-keto acids may be particularly applicable to patients with uraemia or liver disease, but at present they are extremely expensive.

# 11. Multiple Injury

## INTRODUCTION

Road traffic accidents are the outstanding cause of severe multiple injury in Britain and constitute as great a problem as industrial, domestic and recreational accidents and crimes of violence taken together. Each year some 7000 people are killed and 350 000 injured on British roads. Blood alcohol levels exceed the legal limit in one-third of road users who are fatally injured. Restraining seat belts, crash helmets, stricter legislation on alcohol consumption, and improved vehicle design have reduced the incidence and severity of injury.

More than one region of the body is injured in 80% of those who die compared to 20% of those who survive road traffic accidents. Injuries of the head are the most frequent cause of death, but the chest is affected in half and the abdomen in one-quarter of fatal cases. Spinal or pelvic fractures and fracture-dislocations are present in one-fifth of those who are killed. Limb fractures are even more common.

Many of the advances in care have stemmed from the lessons of warfare. Improved on-the-spot resuscitation, efficient transportation, and intensive hospital care have progressively decreased the hospital mortality of battle injury from 8% in World War I, to 4.5% in World War II, and to less than 2% in Vietnam.

## MECHANISM OF INJURY

### CLOSED INJURY

Non-penetrating or blunt injury results from road traffic accidents, falls and violence from fists or blunt weapons. In road traffic accidents the victim's chest or abdomen may be crushed by the collision, seriously impairing ventilation or rupturing abdominal viscera. Fracture of ribs and pelvis are common after crush injury. Alternatively, sudden deceleration may tear viscera from their vascular pedicles, transect the aorta or duodenum at points of fixation, or fling the viscera against unyielding internal surfaces with bruising, laceration and disruption.

### PENETRATING INJURY

Knife wounds cause damage confined to their track. Evaluation of the extent of internal damage may be difficult unless exploration of the wound is undertaken.

As a missile traverses the body its kinetic energy is expended in shock waves which radiate from the track (Fig. 11.1). The resultant tissue damage is proportional to missile velocity. Most revolvers and machine-guns fire low-velocity bullets travelling at less than the speed of sound; modern rifles fire high-velocity missiles.

Bullets may be deflected in their course through the tissues, and pieces of clothing, bony splinters, and fragments of bullet may act as secondary missiles, increasing the extent of tissue damage. A single entry wound indicates that the missile is lodged in the body. High velocity missiles usually traverse the body and characteristically produce a large exit wound. Shotguns fire a hail of pellets which cause extensive soft tissue injury at close range.

### BOMB INJURY

Bombs cause injury in a number of ways:
*Shrapnel and flying debris* are the commonest

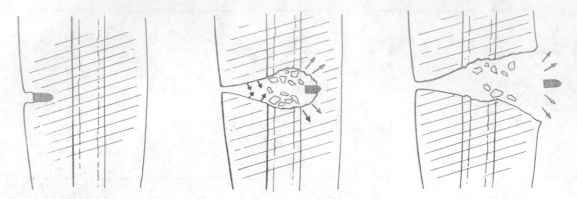

**Fig. 11.1** Missile with shock waves from track — note that the exit wound is larger than the entry wound

cause of injury and produce penetrating and non-penetrating injury with bruising, lacerations and fractures. The wounds are characteristically multiple and grossly contaminated.

The *flash* of an explosion causes extensive superficial burns of exposed areas and clothing frequently catches fire.

*Blast injury* is less common. It gives rise to lung damage as the shock wave traverses the chest wall. Alveolar haemorrhage and pulmonary oedema lead to respiratory distress and derangement of gas exchange. Thereafter, the patient develops increasing dyspnoea, audible moist sounds throughout the chest, and diffuse interstitial oedema on chest X-ray. Hypoxaemia and hypercapnia can be severe. Blast injury may also perforate the eardrums and occasionally ruptures abdominal viscera.

## PRIORITIES IN MANAGEMENT
(Table 11.1)

The first objective is to deal effectively with conditions which pose an immediate threat to life. Confirmation of diagnosis and treatment are often inseparable as for example in management of tension pneumothorax. Preservation of function can receive attention once the threat to life has been averted.

The essentials of first aid are to ensure that the airway is patent, that external haemorrhage is controlled, and that the patient is placed semi-prone rather than supine. Fractures can be immobilised temporarily by splints. The patient should

**Table 11.1** Priorities in management of multiple injury.

| | |
|---|---|
| FIRST PRIORITY — deal with any *immediate threat to life* | |
| Ensure patent airway | |
| Maintain ventilation | relieve tension pneumothorax |
| | seal open chest wounds |
| | assist ventilation |
| Maintain the circulation | control haemorrhage |
| | relieve cardiac tamponade |
| | monitor and treat shock |
| Relieve increased inracranial pressure | |
| SECOND PRIORITY — treat conditions which *ultimately threaten life* | |
| Debride cerebral wounds | |
| Repair gastro-intestinal perforations | |
| Explore thoracic and abdominal wounds | |
| — treat conditions which pose an *urgent threat to function* | |
| Relieve pressure on the spinal cord | |
| Repair vascular injuries | |
| Reduce, debride and immobilise compound fractures | |
| Immobilise single fractures | |
| THIRD PRIORITY — treat conditions *not threatening life or posing urgent threat to function* | |
| Reduce dislocations | |
| Reduce closed fractures | |
| Debride soft tissue injuries ± closure | |
| Repair peripheral nerve injuries | |

be transported to hospital as quickly as possible and should not be left unattended. When spinal injury is suspected the patient is not moved until the extent of injury has been determined. If spinal fracture is believed likely, the spine is kept extended as flexion may allow the unstable spine to damage the cord irreparably (Fig. 11.2).

### Establish and maintain a patent airway

The brain can withstand ischaemia for only 4–6 minutes. Lesser periods of hypoxia may cause irreversible brain damage even though the patient

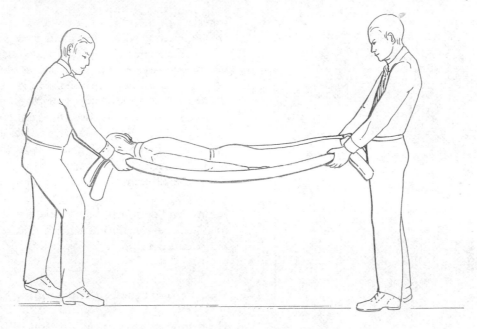

**Fig. 11.2** Method of transport of a patient with an injured spine

survives. There is no point in maintaining a circulation which is not transporting oxygen. Attention to the airway takes precedence in management.

The unconscious patient is never left unattended. He is best nursed semi-prone to ensure that the tongue falls forwards and that material cannot pool in the pharynx and be aspirated into the respiratory tract (Fig. 11.3). A finger is swept through the back of the mouth to remove food, dentures, clotted blood, and suction is used to keep the mouth and pharynx empty.

An oropharyngeal airway is inserted in the first instance, but it is replaced by a cuffed endotracheal tube if there is continued anxiety about the airway (Fig.11.4). The inflated cuff prevents

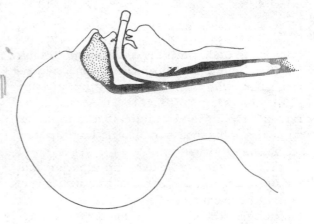

**Fig. 11.4** Cuffed endotracheal tube

aspiration of material alongside the tube. Oxygen can be administered more effectively, ventilation can be assisted, and regular bronchial suction is facilitated. Emergency tracheostomy is indicated in the rare event that airway obstruction cannot be controlled by endotracheal intubation.

### Maintain ventilation

Open sucking chest wounds are occluded by a sterile pad; tension pneumothorax is relieved by

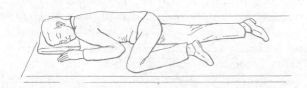

**Fig. 11.3** Nursing of an unconscious patient in the semi-prone position

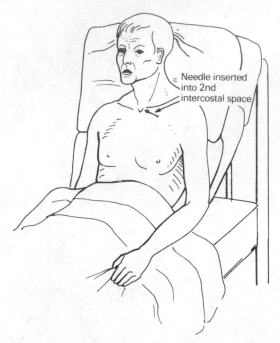

Needle inserted into 2nd intercostal space

**Fig. 11.5** Emergency decompression of a tension pneumothorax (if air escapes a drain and water seal should be inserted)

inserting an underwater sealed drain; and unstable flail chest injuries are managed by endotracheal intubation with intermittent positive pressure ventilation (see p. 255). All of these conditions can kill rapidly and require urgent treatment without wasting time on radiological confirmation of the clinical diagnosis.

It is important to note that tension pneumothorax can occur in the absence of external signs of injury. Immediate insertion of a wide-bore needle through the second interspace in the midclavicular line is demanded should there be unilateral hyper-resonance, absent breath sounds and tracheal deviation (Fig. 11.5).

## Maintain the circulation

External haemorrhage is controlled by direct pressure with a sterile pad pending definitive treatment in an operating theatre. Internal abdominal or thoracic bleeding may require urgent operation. Bleeding into the soft tissues can cause considerable blood loss which requires prompt

transfusion. Blood is withdrawn for grouping and cross-matching when the patient arrives in hospital and an intravenous line is established. If blood loss has been massive, universal donor blood (O-Rh neg) is used until matched blood becomes available (Chapter 9). In the majority of cases, colloid and crystalloid solutions are used to maintain the circulation until matched blood arrives. Blood warming devices should be used if rapid transfusion of stored blood is needed. The management of shock is detailed elsewhere (Chapter 12).

Cardiac tamponade may complicate chest trauma and seriously impair the circulation. Immediate pericardiocentesis is life-saving (see p.256 and p.118).

## Relieve increased intracranial pressure

Head injuries may cause intracranial bleeding or cerebral oedema leading to increased intracranial pressure and cerebral compression (see p. 109). The signs of cerebral compression usually develop after an interval but some patients present at a stage when immediate decompression is needed to save life. It is important to monitor all head injury patients from the time of admission and not to delay transportation of the severe or complicated head injury to an appropriate centre.

Once it is apparent that a patient is not in immediate danger from impaired ventilation, circulatory failure or cerebral compression, a detailed history can be obtained and the full extent of injury can be assessed by physical examination.

## HEAD INJURY

Head injury of sufficient severity to warrant admission to hospital occurs in 200 per 100 000 persons per year. Twelve (6%) of these are serious injuries, producing coma. Road traffic accidents account for half of all head injuries and three-quarters of all serious injuries. Two-thirds of road traffic accident victims have injury to the head.

## MECHANISM OF HEAD INJURY AND ITS CONSEQUENCES

*Primary brain damage* at the time of injury commonly results from displacement and distortion of brain tissue. The extent of damage depends on the plane and direction of the applied force and on its velocity and magnitude. The brain is suspended within the cranium and can move along an antero-posterior axis whereas lateral movement is limited by the falx cerebri and falx cerebelli. It follows that blows to the front or back of the head produce maximal displacement of the brain, the cerebral hemispheres being displaced relative to the less mobile brain stem. The resulting tearing and shearing can cause loss of consciousness, and may prove fatal if extensive damage results.

Concussion is a disordered state of consciousness due to disruption of function without discernible brain damage. More severe injury causes contusion or laceration of brain substance at the point of impact or at the diametrically opposed pole as the brain is driven against the skull or dural septum ('contre-coup' injury) (Fig. 11.6), as well as diffusely distributed shearing lesions in the white matter. Gross brain damage may occur if the force tears the small vessels of the brain stem, leading to ischaemia and interruption of nervous pathways.

Injuries from penetrating missiles are much less common than closed head injuries. Missiles traversing the brain drive bone fragments along their path and produce widespread brain damage. A tangential missile path can cause a 'gutter' fracture, driving bone fragments into the brain, and producing profuse bleeding from torn vessels.

*Increased intracranial pressure* within the unyielding cranium leads to cerebral compression, and is a major cause of death in patients who survive the primary injury. The pressure increase may be due to intracranial bleeding, brain swelling, or a combination of the two. Intracranial bleeding may be extradural, subdural, subarachnoid, intracerebral or intraventricular (see Chapter 21).

*Skull fractures* are produced by compression, local indentation, or tangential injury. Compression fractures are usually closed and linear, forming fissures which pass through the thinner areas of the skull and skirt bony buttresses (Fig. 11.7). Linear fractures of the vault frequently extend into the base of the skull, and may cross foramina to damage cranial nerves or become compound to the middle ear, air sinuses and cribriform plates. Such compound fractures can allow passage of cerebrospinal fluid and air through the ear (CSF otorrhoea) or nose (CSF rhinorrhoea), and permit entry of infection.

Depressed fractures produced by indentation of the vault may be compound or closed, depending on whether the scalp remains intact (Fig. 11.8). Compound fractures are complicated by infection in 5–10% of cases. The inner table of

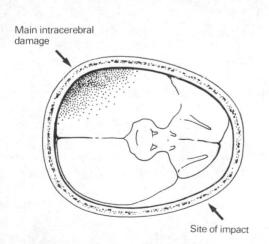

**Fig. 11.6** Mechanism of contre-coup injury

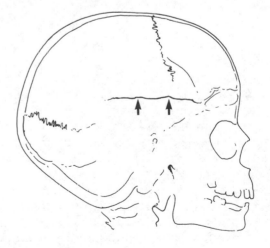

**Fig. 11.7** Fissure fracture of skull

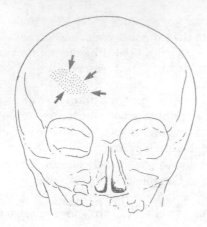

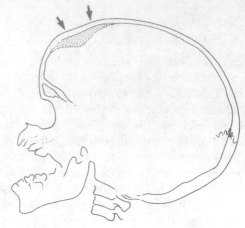

**Fig. 11.8** Depressed fracture of skull

the skull is driven through the dura to lacerate and contuse the underlying brain in 50% of cases. There is an increased risk of epilepsy if the depressed fracture has been complicated by haemorrhage or infection.

Tangential injury may produce wide separation of large fragments of skull and lift them off the underlying dura (Fig. 11.9). There may be little or no primary brain damage despite alarming X-ray appearances. It must be stressed that any type of skull fracture may occur without significant brain damage. Conversely, the absence of a fracture on X-ray does not exclude brain injury or compression.

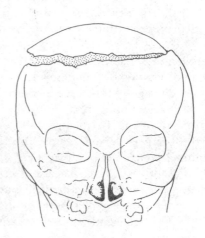

**Fig. 11.9** Effect of tangential injury

## PRINCIPLES OF MANAGEMENT

### Immediate management

Adequate ventilation is of prime importance. Hypoxia, present in 30% of comatose head injured patients, increases brain swelling and intracranial pressure. If the patient is deeply unconscious an endotracheal tube should be passed and ventilation assisted as necessary. Blood pressure, heart rate and peripheral circulation should next be assessed and immediate measures taken to treat shock, which is present on admission in 15% of severely head-injured patients. In view of the risk of aspiration, a nasogastric tube should be passed in the unconscious patient to keep the stomach empty. Conscious patients are not given anything by mouth until it is certain that operation is not needed.

### Initial assessment of injury

The cause and time of head injury are established, and the level of consciousness assessed by separately noting the eye opening, motor and verbal responses. Valid assessment of conscious level cannot be made in patients who are shocked or hypoxic. The patient may have remained conscious since the accident, remained unconscious, or suffered a transient loss of consciousness followed by recovery. Rapid recovery does not imply trivial injury. On the contrary, recovery may be short-lived and the patient becomes unconscious again after a 'lucid' interval. This sequence of events suggests cerebral compression from intracranial haemorrhage, but can be due to early post-traumatic epilepsy.

Continuing assessment of the level of consciousness is the key to the early diagnosis of cerebral compression, and sedation must be avoided. Care must be taken if the patient has had drugs or alcohol as depression of the level of consciousness may be wrongly ascribed to these agents. When in doubt, always assume that depression of consciousness is due to brain injury.

The head and neck are examined carefully and the neurological evaluation is completed. The size, shape and light response of the pupils is established. Limb movements, power, deep tendon reflexes and plantar responses are determined. Pulse rate, blood pressure, respiration rate and temperature are recorded. Regular re-assessment at 15 or 30 minute intervals is essential if neurological deterioration is to be detected in time to allow effective surgical treatment. A head injury chart is commenced on admission and the following parameters monitored (Fig. 11.10).

*Level of consciousness.* As indicated above, repeated monitoring of the level of consciousness is essential to the recognition of improvement or deterioration in the patient's condition. Various scales have been used to record this. The Glasgow coma scale has been officially accepted as the international standard for assessment of conscious level, and has now been adopted in many Accident and Emergency departments (see Table 11.2).

*Size and reaction of pupils.* Unilateral cerebral compression causes an initial brief constriction of the pupils on the side of the lesion, followed by dilatation, loss of light response and ptosis. These changes are caused by prolapse of the temporal lobe through the tentorium, with irritation followed by compression of the oculomotor nerve on the side of the lesion (Fig. 11.11). As intracranial pressure continues to rise, similar changes develop in the pupil of the opposite side. Bilaterally fixed and dilated pupils indicate advanced cerebral compression. Bilateral, small fixed pupils are an indication of intrinsic brain stem damage.

*Movement, muscle tone and reflex function.* Pressure on the motor cortex causes muscle twitching followed by progressive paresis on the opposite side of the body. With herniation of the temporal lobe through the tentorium the ipsilateral cerebral peduncle is distorted and contralateral paresis is followed by extensor or 'decerebrate' rigidity. In

**Table 11.2** Glasgow Coma Scale.

| Eyes | Open | spontaneously | 4 |
|---|---|---|---|
| | | to verbal command | 3 |
| | | to pain | 2 |
| | No response | | 1 |
| Best motor response | To verbal command | obeys | 6 |
| | To painful stimulus | localises pain | 5 |
| | | flexion withdrawal | 4 |
| | | flexion abnormal (decorticate rigidity) | 3 |
| | | extension decerebrate rigidity | 2 |
| | | no response | 1 |
| Best verbal response | | oriented and converses | 5 |
| | | disoriented and converses | 4 |
| | | inappropriate words | 3 |
| | | incomprehensible sounds | 2 |
| | | no response | 1 |
| Total | | | 3–15 |

some instances, e.g. when there is a chronic subdural haematoma, the brain stem is forced against the opposite edge of the tentorium, compressing the contralateral motor tract and causing hemiplegia on the side of the lesion.

*Pulse, blood pressure, respiration rate and temperature.* Further increases in pressure force the midbrain through the tentorium (midbrain coning) and the medulla oblongata and portions of cerebellum are forced through the foramen magnum (Fig. 11.12). This process eventually distorts vital centres in the medulla. This produces an increase in blood pressure, bradycardia and decreased respiration rate. These signs therefore appear late in the coma of brain compression. Damage to the hypothalamus or pons leads to hyperpyrexia.

**Aids to assessment**

Skull X-rays are ordered routinely with antero-posterior, right and left lateral, and Towne's views. Towne's views are taken antero-posteriorly with the head extended so that the X-ray shows the occipital bone (Fig. 11.13). Open mouth X-rays to demonstrate the odontoid process and facial views to show the sinuses and any fractures may also be required. X-rays detect fractures and foreign bodies. If the pineal gland is calcified it may be displaced from the midline by

........................................................HOSPITAL

NAME

UNIT No

D. of B.

**NEUROLOGICAL OBSERVATION CHART**

CONSULTANT

WARD

| DATE | | | | | | | | | | | | | | | | | | | | | | | | | | TIME |
|------|---|---|---|---|---|---|---|---|---|---|---|---|---|---|---|---|---|---|---|---|---|---|---|---|---|---|------|

**C O M A   S C A L E**

| | | | | | |
|---|---|---|---|---|---|
| Eyes open | Spontaneously | 4 | | | Eyes closed by swelling = C |
| | To speech | 3 | | | |
| | To pain | 2 | | | |
| | None | 1 | | | |
| Best verbal response | Orientated | 5 | | | Endotracheal tube or Tracheostomy = T |
| | Confused | 4 | | | |
| | Inappropriate Words | 3 | | | |
| | Incomprehensible Sounds | 2 | | | |
| | None | 1 | | | |
| Best motor response | Obey commands | 6 | | | Usually records the best arm response |
| | Localise pain | 5 | | | |
| | Normal Flexion | 4 | | | |
| | Abnormal Flexion | 3 | | | |
| | Extension to pain | 2 | | | |
| | None | 1 | | | |

COMA SCALE TOTAL 3 – 15

INTRACRANIAL PRESSURE

Pupil scale (m.m.)

1, 2, 3, 4, 5, 6, 7, 8

Blood pressure and pulse

240 230 220 210 200 190 180 170 160 150 140 130 120 110 100 90 80 70 60 50 40

Respiration 30 26 22 18 14 10 6

Temperature °C

40 39 38 37 36 35 34 33 32 31 30

| **PUPILS** | right | Size | | | + reacts |
| | | Reaction | | | − no reaction |
| | left | Size | | | c. eye closed |
| | | Reaction | | | |

| **L I M B   M O V E M E N T** | **A R M S** | Normal power | | | Record right (R) and left (L) separately if there is a difference between the two sides. |
| | | Mild weakness | | | |
| | | Severe weakness | | | |
| | | Extension | | | |
| | | No response | | | |
| | **L E G S** | Normal power | | | |
| | | Mild weakness | | | |
| | | Severe weakness | | | |
| | | Extension | | | |
| | | No response | | | |

**Fig. 11.10** Head injury chart

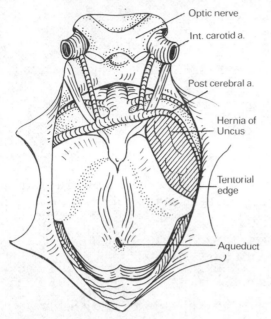

Fig. 11.11 Temporal lobe prolapse — cause of IIIrd nerve irritation and palsy

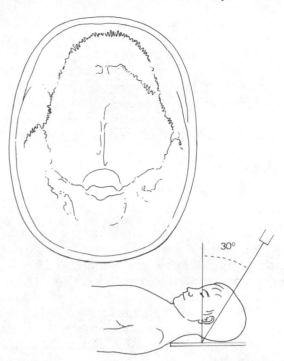

Fig. 11.13 Towne's view to demonstrate the base of the skull

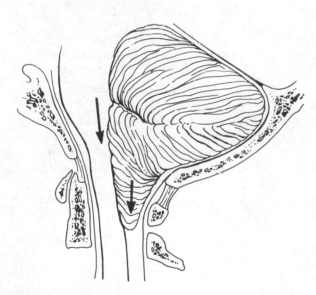

Fig. 11.12 Foraminal coning

unilateral pressure increase (pineal shift). In the comatose patient a lateral film of the cervical spine should also be taken.

*Echo-encephalography* is a simple, rapid, safe, non-invasive but unreliable technique. The ultra-sonic echoes detect asymmetry of the ventricular system and shift of the midline falx cerebri.

*CT-scanning* (computerised axial tomography) has revolutionised the diagnosis of intracranial lesions. The technique is non-invasive and cere-bral oedema and intracranial haemorrhage can be demonstrated readily (see Chapter 22). The patient must remain absolutely still and general anaesthesia is required if the patient is restless. Serial examinations can be performed.

*Pressure monitors.* The pressure within the su-barachnoid space is a useful monitor of increasing intracerebral pressure. Continuous recording can be arranged by screwing a threaded bolt into a small burr-hole in the skull.

*Carotid arteriography* is rarely used nowadays to diagnose intracranial lesions after head injury.

*Exploratory burr holes* are seldom employed nowadays, being indicated only when neurologi-cal deterioration due to suspected intracranial haemorrhage is extremely rapid or when CT-scan or angiography are unavailable (Chapter 21). The dura and brain surface are visualised so that extra-cerebral haemorrhage can be detected and dealt with.

*Pneumo-encephalography, ventriculography and electro-encephalography* have no place in the assessment of acute head injury. *Lumbar puncture* has little place in the management of head injured patients; by reducing the pressure in the spinal subarachnoid space the procedure facilitates coning when intracranial pressure is high. The only indication for lumbar puncture is when meningitis is suspected.

## MANAGEMENT OF THE UNCONSCIOUS PATIENT

*Restraint* by bandages or straps may be needed as sedation must be avoided. The patient must never be spreadeagled in a supine position and should always be restrained on his side (Fig. 11.14). Prophylactic *anticonvulsants* are given to patients with intracranial haematomas or contusion. The skin over *pressure points* is protected by frequent changes of posture, and by the use of ripple mattresses and soft sheepskins.

Hyperpyrexia is common and should be corrected as it promotes brain swelling and increased intracranial pressure. It is controlled by surface cooling with fans, wet sheets or ice packs, or administration of the antihistamine, promethazine.

The *bladder* should be drained by an indwelling Foley catheter. This avoids retention of urine, keeps the bed dry and, most important of all, allows accurate monitoring of fluid balance. Involuntary micturition at a later stage can be managed by attaching a length of Paul's tubing around the penis and leading it into a collecting bag.

A *nasogastric tube* keeps the stomach empty and is used for feeding if coma is prolonged for more

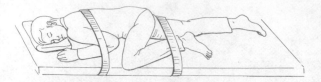

**Fig. 11.14** Patient in the semi-prone position with restraining straps

than three or four days. *Intravenous fluids* are used to maintain fluid balance. Care must be taken to avoid overhydration. Brain swelling is frequent when serum sodium falls below 120 mmol/l.

## MANAGEMENT OF SPECIFIC PROBLEMS

### Scalp injuries

Scalp lacerations bleed profusely but heal well. Temporary haemostasis is achieved by compression of the wound edge. The area is shaved and the wound is debrided, cleaned with an antiseptic, and sutured (Fig. 11.15).

### Skull fractures

Simple fractures of the vault do not require treatment but all patients are admitted for observation to exclude intracranial bleeding.

Depressed fractures of the vault are compound to the exterior in 90% of cases. The surface wound is usually small and can be debrided and closed. If there is extensive skull depression on X-ray, a formal skin flap is reflected so that the fracture can be fully exposed (Fig. 11.16). Loose pieces of bone are removed or elevated. The dura is left intact unless intracranial bleeding is sus-

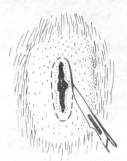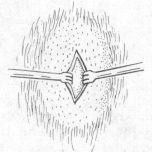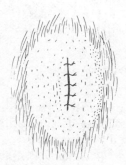

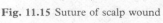

**Fig. 11.15** Suture of scalp wound

Simple depressed fractures can be left un-treated provided the inner table is only depressed a few millimetres. Depressed fractures which overlie a major venous sinus are also treated conservatively as operative interference can cause major bleeding.

Fractures of the base of the skull that are compound into the ear or nose are managed conservatively at first with antibiotic cover. If discharge of cerebro-spinal fluid persists for more than one or two weeks, the torn dura is repaired by a fascial graft.

### Extradural haemorrhage

Extradural bleeding results from tearing of the middle meningeal vessels during temporal bone fracture in 70% of cases (Fig. 11.17). In the remainder the haematoma is located frontally or in the posterior fossa. Primary brain damage is usually not severe and the classical history is one of transient loss of consciousness followed by an apparent return to normality. A bruise or 'boggi-ness' in the temporal region with an underlying fracture on X-ray should always signal the possi-bility of extradural bleeding. Following the 'lucid interval' there is gradual deterioration in the level of consciousness and signs of tentorial herniation

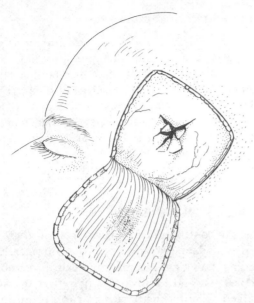

**Fig. 11.16** Exposure of a depressed skull fracture

pected. If the dura has been breached the wound is cleaned and devitalised brain tissue is removed by suction. The dura is closed if possible, larger bone fragments replaced as a mosaic and the scalp flap sutured without drainage. Extensive skull defects may be restored 3–6 months later by plates of acrylic resin.

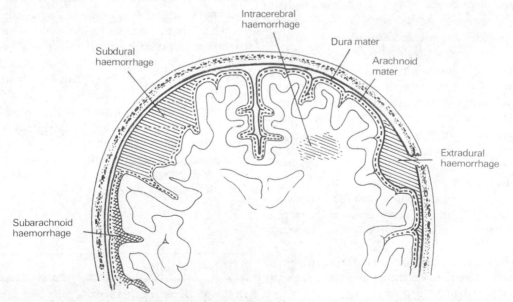

**Fig. 11.17** Sites of intracranial haemorrhage

appear, followed by slowing of the pulse and respiration rate, and an increase in blood pressure. By this stage, urgent surgical intervention is required. This 'classical' picture is seen in a minority of cases, however, and the best aid to detection is a high index of suspicion in all patients with skull fracture, awake or in coma. In young children the skull is thin and pliable enough to permit extradural haemorrhage without a fracture.

At operation, the clot is evacuated through a temporal burr-hole. The opening is enlarged and the bleeding point is coagulated.

Extradural haemorrhage can also follow injury to dural venous sinuses, in which case the clinical course of the syndrome is protracted.

## Subdural haemorrhage

Subdural haematoma is more common than extradural. Veins passing from the cerebral hemispheres to venous sinuses are torn during displacement of the brain at the time of injury (Fig. 11.17). This form of subdural bleeding is commoner in older patients, possibly because brain atrophy facilitates displacement. The other principal source of subdural haemorrhage is cerebral laceration, usually at the temporal poles.

Cerebral compression may be acute, subacute with compression of the brain by solid clotted blood, or it may be delayed for weeks or months with formation of a liquid chronic subdural haematoma. Little force is needed to tear the veins and the initial injury may be trivial. In its acute form, subdural haematoma simulates extradural bleeding but skull fracture is less common. Craniotomy is required for removal of the mass of subdural blood clot and location and arrest of the source of haemorrhage.

Headache, apathy and gradual deterioration in conscious level are associated with localising signs and evidence of generalised increase in intracranial pressure in cases of chronic subdural haematoma.

Bilateral parietal burr-holes allow evacuation of the liquid chronic haematoma and the prognosis is excellent provided surgery is undertaken before severe compression occurs.

## Subarachnoid haemorrhage

The commonest cause of subarachnoid haemorrhage is trauma. Subarachnoid bleeding does not produce a circumscribed haematoma (Fig. 11.17). Blood in the cerebrospinal fluid is irritant and produces headache, neck stiffness, photophobia and irritability. Conservative management is indicated, but the possibility of confusing this clinical picture with the similar syndrome due to meningitis must be remembered.

## Intracerebral haemorrhage

Cerebral contusion can prove fatal if there is extensive damage and profuse intracerebral bleeding. A large haematoma causes cerebral compression and localising signs reflect the area involved. The haematoma may rupture into the ventricular system. Surgery is indicated only if compression occurs or CT scan shows a large haematoma. The clot is evacuated and devitalised brain tissue is removed.

## Brain swelling

Brain swelling can increase intracranial pressure and cause clinical deterioration without localising neurological signs. It is usually due to congestive distension of cerebral blood vessels. Brain oedema is much less common, and after head injury is usually limited to the zones of the brain in the vicinity of extra- or intra-cerebral haematomas or brain contusions. The diagnosis may be suspected after head injury, but is only accepted after intra-cranial bleeding is excluded by CT brain scan or carotid arteriography. Brain swelling is best managed by hyperventilation and intravenous mannitol (0.5–1.0 g/kg body weight as a rapid intravenous infusion). Glucocorticoid therapy has little or no place in the management of brain swelling after head injury.

# CHEST INJURY

In this section the general principles of the management of the chest injury are discussed. For further details of specific conditions, reference should be made to Chapters 19 and 20.

Injuries to the chest occur as a result of penetrating (bullet and stab) wounds and blunt trauma. Crush injuries of the chest are particularly common in accidents involving motor vehicles either because the driver is compressed against the steering wheel or the victim is 'run-over'. In all injuries, attention must first be paid to the adequacy of the airways and to ensure that ventilation of the lungs is unimpaired.

The rib cage is commonly injured and single or multiple fractures of the ribs occur with all significant blunt trauma. Multiple fractures may produce an unstable segment of the chest wall which loses its attachment to the rest of the rib cage forming a so-called 'flail chest' (Fig. 11.18). Unlike the rest of the chest wall, which expands on inspiration, the flail segment is sucked in, and there is 'paradoxical movement' and impaired ventilation.

Laceration of the pleura by penetrating injury or by the sharp end of a fractured rib may cause pneumothorax with collapse of the lung. A valve-like effect may allow air to enter but not leave the pleural cavity producing a 'tension pneumothorax' which impairs ventilation and venous return with potentially fatal consequences. Alternatively, there may be bleeding into the pleural cavity; a 'haemothorax'. Contusions and lacerations of the lung may also cause pulmonary oedema and allow escape of the air into the pleural cavity (pneumothorax) or soft tissues (surgical emphysema).

Severe trauma to the chest can have even more serious effects. Laceration of the trachea or main bronchus not only causes sudden and massive pneumothorax but because of the rigidity of the structures, the hole will not seal and leakage of air continues despite decompression of the pleural cavity. The heart also is prone to injury and myocardial contusion or bleeding into the pericardial sac can have dangerous consequences. Rising pressure within the pericardium causes the condition of 'cardiac tamponade' which impairs venous filling of the heart to the extent of cardiac failure and death. Rupture of the aorta may occur with rapid deceleration and the oesophagus, thoracic duct or diaphragm can be damaged in any severe crushing injury.

## EVALUATION

The severity of chest injury can readily be underestimated and a thorough examination must be carried out in all cases. Signs of respiratory distress include dyspnoea, stridor and cyanosis. All clothing must be removed and chest movement carefully observed noting asymmetrical expansion, paradoxical movement and indrawing of the intercostal muscles. Bruising is sought and may point to the severity of the trauma. For example, the imprint of the hub of a steering wheel over the sternum should alert one to a potentially serious injury to mediastinal vascular structures.

Gentle palpation may reveal tenderness over rib fractures, unstable segments of chest wall, or the 'crackling' sensation of subcutaneous emphysema. Percussion may detect hyper-resonance or dullness due to air or blood in the pleural cavity. Auscultation is performed in all cases. Coarse crepitations indicate accumulation of secretions; diminished or absent breath sounds indicate areas of under-ventilation or of fluid in the pleural cavity.

If respiratory distress is present, arterial blood is withdrawn for blood gas estimations.

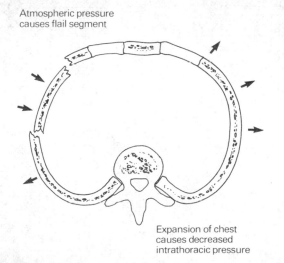

Atmospheric pressure
causes flail segment

Expansion of chest
causes decreased
intrathoracic pressure

**Fig. 11.18** Flail chest injury

## IMMEDIATE ACTIONS

Attention to the airways has first priority (see above). Should respiratory distress, hyper-resonance or inaudible breath sounds and tracheal displacement suggest a tension pneumothorax, the pleural cavity must be immediately decompressed by insertion of a wide-bore needle through the second intercostal space in the mid-clavicular line (see Fig. 11.5). If air escapes under pressure, the clinical diagnosis is confirmed and a tube can be inserted either at the needle site or laterally in the 4th space with underwater sealed drainage to allow continued escape of air from the pleural cavity and expansion of the lung (Fig. 11.19).

If a flail segment of chest wall is associated with paradoxical respiration, the patient is immediately turned on to the injured side, temporarily fixing the unstable chest wall while preparations are made to insert a cuffed tube into the trachea to allow assisted ventilation.

Falling arterial blood pressure, distended neck veins and diminished heart sounds are signs of cardiac tamponade and urgent needle aspiration is indicated. With the patient supine, a wide-bore needle is inserted between the junction of the left lower costal cartilage and xiphisternum passing at 45° to the skin and directed towards the tip of the right scapula (Fig. 11.20). An ECG lead can be attached to the needle to monitor damage to the cardiac muscle. If blood is obtained the pericardial sac is aspirated completely and a tube inserted into it.

### Chest X-ray

Provided these life-threatening events are excluded, a postero-anterior X-ray of the chest is

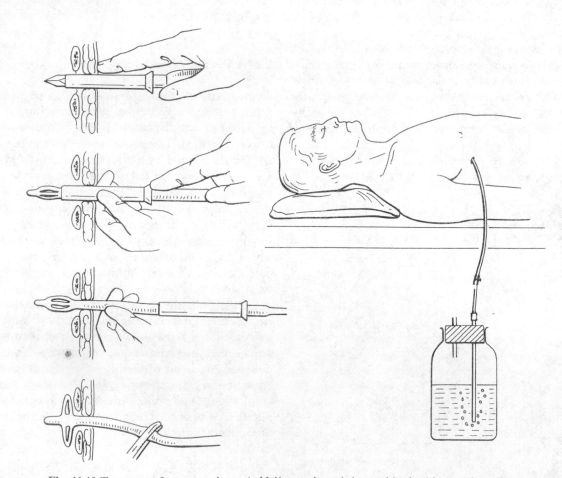

**Fig. 11.19** Treatment of a pneumothorax (a Malécot catheter is inserted in the 4th space laterally)

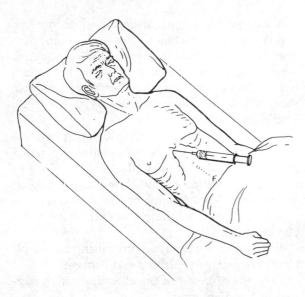

**Fig. 11.20** Pericardial aspiration

obtained and scrutinised as follows:

1. The rib cage is examined rib by rib. Additional local views are requested if fracture is suspected. Surgical emphysema may be detected as streaks of air in the tissue planes of the chest wall.

2. Evidence of a pneumothorax should be sought in all cases. Lung markings may be absent or the edge of a partially collapsed lung seen. Shift of trachea or mediastinum to the opposite side associated with a pneumothorax indicates tension. Accumulation of fluid in the pleural cavity first causes opacification of the costophrenic angle but as much as 500 ml of fluid can accumulate without radiological abnormality. Larger amounts of fluid cause more extensive opacification.

3. Mediastinal widening, particularly if associated with pleural fluid, suggests bleeding from major vessels and urgent angiography is required. Mediastinal emphysema (air streaks) and surgical emphysema in the tissue planes of the neck suggest damage to the oesophagus.

4. An enlarged cardiac shadow suggests tamponade. However, as little as 50 ml of blood in the pericardial sac can obstruct venous return and this will not be radiologically visible.

5. Foreign bodies may be detected if radio-opaque.

6. Loops of air-filled bowel in the chest indicate rupture of the diaphragm.

## Definitive management

The management of the various complications of chest injury are described in Chapter 20.

---

## ABDOMINAL INJURY

---

## MECHANISM AND CONSEQUENCES OF INJURY

*Non-penetrating trauma* of the abdomen is more common than penetrating injury, and considerable judgement is needed to assess the likelihood of internal injury. Even minor blows can cause serious injury if the anterior abdominal muscles are relaxed at the moment of impact, or if the viscera are distended or pathologically enlarged. There may be few outward signs of internal injury.

*Penetrating trauma* can also prove deceptive in that the full extent of injury may only become apparent when the abdomen is explored. Penetrating wounds of the chest, loin, flank, buttocks and perineum may all extend into the abdomen.

Sudden deceleration or direct compression are the common causes of blunt injury to viscera. The spleen and liver are relatively protected by the rib cage, but direct trauma to the lower chest may cause rib fractures and so rupture these organs. The kidneys are frequently damaged by blows in the loin, and the full bladder is particularly liable to damage from falls or blows to the lower abdomen. Pelvic fractures are commonly associated with bladder injury.

The gut and its mesentery may be damaged directly by penetrating injury or torn by the shearing forces of sudden deceleration. The gut tears most frequently at the junction of fixed and mobile parts e.g. the duodeno–jejunal flexure.

Bleeding is the main danger after trauma to solid organs, whereas peritoneal contamination is the prime danger after rupture of hollow viscera. Trauma to the pancreas can cause massive bleeding, pancreatitis and pseudocyst formation.

## EVALUATION OF ABDOMINAL INJURY

Repeated examination of the abdomen and regular monitoring of vital signs are the basis of assessment of injury and determine the need for surgery.

*Abdominal pain* may be due to bruising of the abdominal wall or to peritoneal irritation by blood or intestinal contents. On occasions, abdominal pain may be referred from spinal or chest wall injury. The absence of pain or lessening of its severity does not rule out serious injury as pain may be masked by associated neurological injury or shock. Pain at the shoulder tip suggests diaphragmatic irritation and is most often due to intraperitoneal bleeding following rupture of the spleen or liver. Rupture of a hollow viscus may give surprisingly little pain in the early stages. Analgesia should be withheld if possible until the abdomen has been examined by the surgeon responsible for the further care of the patient.

*Bruising* of the abdominal wall is a useful guide to the site and severity of injury. If the pattern of clothing, seat belt or steering wheel is imprinted on the bruised area, severe compression has occurred.

*Tenderness and guarding* are the most reliable signs of injury, but their absence does not exclude intra-abdominal damage. Increased muscle tone is a reflex response to peritoneal irritation and is one of the few signs preserved in unconscious patients. Board-like rigidity, such as occurs with a perforated peptic ulcer, is uncommon after abdominal trauma.

*Abdominal distension* may reflect major haemorrhage. Sequential measurement of girth is often advised but is of doubtful value. Leakage of bowel content, pancreatitis, retro-peritoneal haematoma and spinal cord injury can all produce distension from intestinal dilatation due to ileus.

*Digital rectal examination* may reveal bogginess in the pouch of Douglas due to blood. Peri-rectal surgical emphysema is occasionally detectable and suggests colonic or rectal injury. Blood on the examining finger raises the suspicion of contusion or laceration of the bowel.

*Urinalysis* is essential. Haematuria indicates urinary tract injury (p.125).

*X-rays of the chest and abdomen* are ordered unless massive bleeding demands immediate operation. The standard supine antero-posterior view of the abdomen does not disturb the patient: lateral decubitus views are preferred to erect views when there is anxiety about moving him. Useful radiological signs include:

1. Free intra-peritoneal gas indicating perforation of a hollow viscus or, less commonly, penetration of the abdominal wall.

2. Retro-peritoneal gas (shown by streaking) signifies duodenal, colonic or rectal injury.

3. Obliteration of the psoas outline by retro-peritoneal bleeding.

4. Fracture of the lower ribs raising the suspicion of hepatic, splenic or renal damage.

5. Loops of bowel in the chest indicating rupture of the diaphragm.

6. Demonstration of radio-opaque foreign bodies.

Intravenous pyelography is essential if renal damage is suspected; a gastrografin meal or enema may be useful if there is doubt regarding the integrity of the gastro-intestinal tract. Many surgeons now regard selective arteriography as mandatory if rupture of liver or kidney is suspected.

*Laboratory aids* are seldom of diagnostic value in the early course of abdominal trauma. The haemoglobin concentration and haematocrit reflect blood loss only after blood volume has been restored by haemodilution which may take several hours or days. An elevated serum amylase level is helpful in indicating trauma to the pancreas or duodenum.

*Abdominal lavage* is now performed in many centres to determine whether there has been leakage of blood or alimentary fluid into the peritoneal cavity. 500 ml of sterile saline is run into the peritoneal cavity through a needle or tube inserted in the midline beneath the umbilicus. The fluid is recovered by lowering the container below the level of the abdomen. The presence of bile or significant amounts of blood (obscuring vision through the effluent fluid) indicates the need for exploration (Fig. 11.21). Although false positive or false negative results are rare with peritoneal lavage, clinical examination retains basic importance in assessing the need for exploration.

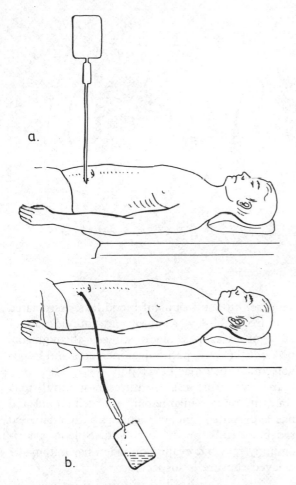

**Fig. 11.21** Abdominal lavage. (a) 500–1000 ml of normal saline run into abdominal cavity. (b) Saline allowed to reflux back into bag, and the presence of blood noted.

## PRINCIPLES OF MANAGEMENT OF ABDOMINAL INJURY

### Resuscitation

Massive intraperitoneal bleeding requires urgent laparotomy as blood volume can only be restored after the source of bleeding has been controlled. In most patients there is time for resuscitation before laparotomy but, if continuous bleeding is suspected, operation should not be unduly delayed.

### The decision to operate

Careful and repeated assessment of the patient is the key to management. Small and apparently trivial penetrating injuries can be explored under local anaesthetic in the operating room. In contrast to former teaching, isolated stab wounds are now treated expectantly unless there are specific indications for laparotomy. Larger wounds in association with multiple injury require laparotomy followed by debridement and excision of the penetrating wound. When there is gross wound contamination the superficial tissues should be left open and delayed primary suture performed at 72 hours.

Laparotomy is indicated in cases of blunt abdominal trauma (1) if there are signs of major blood loss or peritoneal irritation; (2) if there are localising signs within the abdomen; or (3) if free gas is shown on abdominal X-ray films. Laparotomy is also indicated (4) if there is unexplained clinical deterioration in a patient with minimal abdominal signs, or if the requirements for resuscitation exceed those suggested by the known extent of injury. If the integrity of the abdominal viscera is in doubt, it is usually better to operate than to await further clinical deterioration. Otherwise one may miss the opportunity to deal effectively with the problem before complications ensue.

### Essentials of operation

The abdomen is opened through a long midline or paramedian incision. If blood is present it is removed from the peritoneal cavity so that bleeding sites can be identified and clamped. Open intestinal wounds are occluded with light clamps.

Injuries are then dealt with systematically; the injured spleen is removed, the injured liver is repaired or partially resected, and the injured gut is repaired, resected or exteriorised. A final careful palpation and inspection of all organs and viscera including the pancreas is carried out to make certain that no injury has been missed. If the peritoneal cavity has been contaminated, it is lavaged with saline and the abdomen closed with appropriate drainage.

## SPECIFIC ABDOMINAL INJURIES

### Haematoma formation

Intraperitoneal haematomas are evacuated and bleeding vessels ligated. Insertion of a drain is

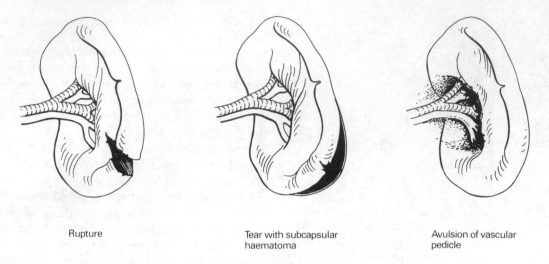

Rupture                     Tear with subcapsular          Avulsion of vascular
                            haematoma                      pedicle

**Fig. 11.22** Types of splenic injury

advisable if oozing continues or if there is a large traumatised area. Retroperitoneal haematomas are left undisturbed unless surrounding the duodenum or pancreas when exploration is necessary. Aortography may be indicated post-operatively to determine further management if bleeding continues.

### Injury to the spleen

The spleen is one of the organs most frequently damaged by abdominal trauma. It is particularly susceptible to injury when pathologically enlarged, e.g. by infective mononucleosis or malaria. The degree of splenic damage varies (Fig. 11.22). It may be (1) ruptured; (2) avulsed from its pedicle; or (3) torn beneath the capsule which remains intact with a subcapsular or intrasplenic haematoma. Rupture and avulsion are the common forms of injury. They cause immediate intraperitoneal bleeding with related clinical signs. Delayed rupture occurs in approximately 5% of splenic injuries and is thought to be due to gradual enlargement of a subcapsular haematoma which then bursts through the capsule. In such cases, rupture and free bleeding usually occurs within two weeks of injury but this can be delayed for months or even years.

The classical clinical features of splenic rupture are pain, tenderness and guarding in the left upper quadrant of the abdomen, pain in the left shoulder-tip, and signs of blood loss. Associated fracture of the lower left ribs are found in about 20% of cases. As blood spreads through the peritoneal cavity, peritonism increases and hypovolaemic shock may develop.

In doubtful cases, ultrasonography may confirm splenic enlargement or haematoma and has superseded splenic scans with $^{51}$Cr-labelled red blood cells or $^{99m}$Tc colloid. Splenic arteriography may aid evaluation when haematoma or delayed rupture is suspected.

Splenectomy is the standard form of treatment for all forms of splenic rupture, but in view of the risks of splenectomy in children there is a growing tendency to conserve splenic tissue by partial splenectomy or by suture of small capsular tears.

### Injury to the liver

*Blunt trauma* is a more common cause of damage to the liver than is penetrating injury. Superficial lacerations may have stopped bleeding by the time of laparotomy and need no more than abdominal drainage. Alternatively, there may be extensive hepatic disruption which is difficult to visualise, particularly when the superior and posterior surfaces of the organ are affected (Fig. 11.23). Haematomas within the liver substance often escape detection, and selective angiograms are useful when haematoma formation is suspected.

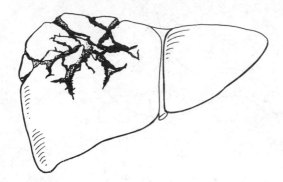

**Fig. 11.23** Severe hepatic lacerations

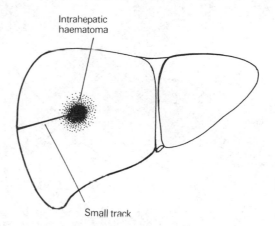

**Fig. 11.24** Intrahepatic haematoma

Severe bleeding can sometimes be controlled temporarily by occlusion of vessels in the free border of the lesser omentum, but bleeding from torn hepatic veins cannot be controlled in this way. Packing of the torn liver is only justifiable for temporary control during laparotomy, or if the patient has to be transferred to a centre capable of dealing with his injury.

The principles of management consist of adequate exposure, if necessary by extending the abdominal wound into the chest or anterior mediastinum, debridement with removal of devitalised tissue, and suture-ligation of torn vessels and bile ducts. Extensive hepatic damage may require hepatic lobectomy. Multiple abdominal drains are essential after all forms of hepatic trauma and prevent collection of blood and bile which may become infected.

*Penetrating liver trauma* due to stab wounds and low velocity bullets can be managed by abdominal drainage provided the liver wound is not bleeding actively at laparotomy but the possibility of residual intrahepatic haematomas must be kept in mind (Fig. 11.24). Damage to a large vessel is managed by direct suture of the affected vessel whenever possible, and buttresses of ox fibrinogen are a useful means of preventing sutures from cutting through the liver substance. High velocity bullet wounds cause extensive liver damage and hepatic resection is usually required.

Operations for all forms of hepatic trauma may be complicated by jaundice due to temporary hepatic insufficiency or biliary obstruction, hypoalbuminaemia, hypoglycaemia and coagulation disorders.

## Injury to the biliary tract

Biliary tract damage is a rare complication of penetrating trauma. Gallbladder damage is treated by cholecystectomy, while bile duct injuries are repaired if possible by direct suture and temporary T-tube drainage. Extensive bile duct injury may necessitate choledocho-jejunostomy.

## Injury to the gastro-intestinal tract

Injury to the *stomach* is rare and is usually due to penetrating injury. Blunt trauma occasionally causes rupture if the stomach is distended. Escape of gastric juice causes peritoneal irritation as in perforation of a peptic ulcer. In most cases the gastric wound can be excised and sutured.

Damage to the *duodenum* is more serious and usually follows severe crushing trauma which also affects the pancreas. Rupture of the duodenum is often retroperitoneal and is easily overlooked at laparotomy unless the duodenum is formally mobilised. Small wounds may be excised and repaired; larger defects can be occluded by a loop of jejunum acting as a patch (Fig. 11.25), while duodenectomy and partial pancreatectomy may be needed for extensive damage.

The *small bowel* may be damaged at several sites by penetrating trauma. Rupture due to blunt trauma most often occurs at the duodeno-jejunal flexure. Clinical signs of injury may be minimal in the early stages and a high index of suspicion is required. Wounds of the small bowel are sutured after debridement, but resection is needed if the

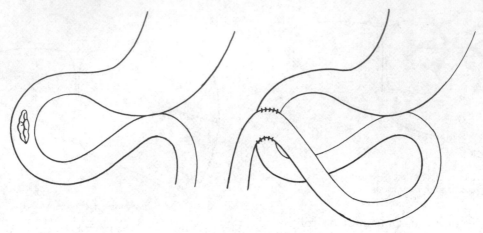

**Fig. 11.25** Jejunal patch for duodenal tear

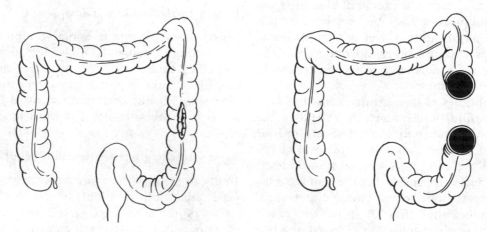

**Fig. 11.26** Treatment of a large bowel laceration

damage is extensive or if the bowel has been devitalised by tears in its mesentery.

*Large bowel* injuries frequently follow penetrating wounds of the abdominal wall or perineum. Faecal contamination of the peritoneum is usual and the traumatised bowel is often devitalised. Primary suture is justified only if the wound is small, as in a knife wound, and the damaged bowel is usually resected with exteriorisation of the cut ends (Fig. 11.26). Intestinal continuity is restored at a later date following appropriate bowel preparation.

### Injury to the pancreas

The pancreas may be damaged by penetrating or blunt abdominal trauma. Because of its fixed position as it crosses the vertebral column, the gland is at risk in blunt trauma to the upper abdomen and is especially vulnerable in the region of its neck (Fig. 11.27). Blood and enzymes escape into the retroperitoneal tissues and may produce a palpable swelling. Injuries to other organs may divert attention from the pancreas, but its close relationship to major blood vessels makes haemorrhage the major cause of death in pancreatic trauma. Pancreatic injury is a particular risk of crush injuries in childhood.

*Diagnosis.* Diagnosis of pancreatic trauma may be difficult and abdominal signs are sparse in the early stages. The indication for laparotomy is often haemorrhage or rupture of another viscus. During the laparotomy it is vital that the pancreas is mobilised and carefully inspected. A rise in

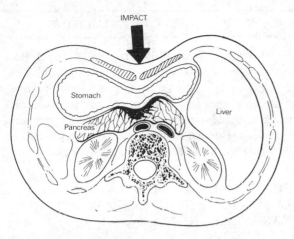

**Fig. 11.27** Pancreatic rupture

serum amylase after abdominal trauma suggests pancreatic injury and in association with increasing abdominal signs should be regarded as an indication for laparotomy. Sometimes the diagnosis of pancreatic trauma is missed, and the patient presents later with a pseudocyst.

*Surgical treatment.* Haemorrhage is first controlled to allow adequate examination of the gland. Further management then depends on whether there has been major duct injury.

1. *No duct injury* — Adequate drainage of peripancreatic tissue should be provided.

2. *Duct injury* — If the duct is damaged in the body and tail, distal pancreatectomy is indicated. If the head of the pancreas is badly damaged pancreatico-duodenectomy may be needed, particularly if there is major associated damage to the duodenum. If the duodenum is intact and haemorrhage can be controlled, it may be wiser simply to provide adequate drainage to the region and assess progress. In many such cases the gland heals without serious dysfunction and further operation is unnecessary.

### Injuries to the urinary tract

Blunt trauma to the flank may cause contusion, laceration or rupture of the kidney. Sporting injuries are a common cause of renal trauma and, in motor traffic accidents, rapid deceleration, by throwing the kidney forward, may tear or transect the renal pedicle. Penetrating wounds of the kidney are relatively rare. On the other hand, damage to the ureter, although rare, is almost exclusively due to this cause.

The urinary bladder is susceptible to injury when distended. The degree of trauma required is usually severe and will have caused associated fractures of the pelvis. Rupture of an over-filled bladder may occur with relatively minor trauma.

Rupture may either be into the peritoneal cavity (intra-peritoneal) or into the pelvic tissues (extra-peritoneal) when extravasation of urine spreads along the tissue planes and is limited only by fascial attachments. Eighty per cent of extraperitoneal ruptures are associated with fracture of the pelvis. Laceration or rupture of the male urethra also may complicate a fractured pelvis. This commonly affects either its prostatic or membranous portions. Injury to the anterior urethra is less common and follows direct damage to the penis or perineum, classically as a result of a straddle injury. Unlike injuries to the bladder, extravasation of urine is not prominent unless the sphincteric mechanism is disrupted.

The management of injuries to the urinary tract is fully discussed in Chapter 40.

## INJURY OF THE EXTREMITIES

Most injuries to the extremities do not pose an immediate threat to life and, unless complicated by major haemorrhage, they have a low priority in management.

Penetrating wounds of the extremities are cleansed, debrided and explored. Meticulous cleansing minimises the risk of infection, wide debridement prevents tetanus and gas gangrene, and exploration uncovers unsuspected injury to major vessels, nerves and tendons. The principles of wound management are covered in Chapter 6.

## VASCULAR INJURY

Ninety per cent of vascular injuries follow penetrating trauma. If major, they may threaten life by haemorrhage or threaten limb survival by devascularisation.

Injury to an artery may result in contusion, laceration, or transection. Contusion with occlusion of flow is due to a damaged intima and is the most common. Arterial lacerations usually continue to bleed, as the intact portion of the vessel prevents retraction. With transection, retraction can occur and bleeding may cease.

Venous injury may follow penetrating trauma or the vessel may be compressed and occluded by adjacent arterial bleeding or soft tissue injury. Oedema and distal venous congestion may then obstruct arterial inflow and lead to gangrene. Penetrating wounds involving arteries or veins often lead to an arteriovenous fistula.

It is important in all injuries involving limbs to evaluate the state of the peripheral circulation. This includes an assessment of peripheral pulses, temperature, pallor and capillary and venous filling. The cold, pale, pulseless limb due to interruption of arterial blood supply is readily recognised.

However, it should be remembered that the peripheral circulation is reduced by shock and that repeated assessment after resuscitation is essential if vascular injuries are to be detected. Haematomas are common after all injuries. If expanding or pulsatile, arterial injury must be suspected.

The principles of management of suspected vascular injuries are as follows:

1. Control bleeding by the application of direct pressure to the wound.

2. Resuscitate to relieve shock.

3. Evaluate the vascular state of the limbs.

4. If there is evidence of ischaemia, arrange urgent angiography unless a) fractures and dislocations are present which may contribute to arterial damage, or (b) there is a penetrating wound when immediate reduction of fractures and/or exploration of the wound is essential. In other cases, angiography will determine the need for action.

5. In closed injuries which are associated with ischaemia and fractures or dislocations, an angiogram should be performed after reduction of the fracture to ensure that the vascular supply is intact.

Details of the types and management of individual vascular lesions is given in Chapter 21.

# FRACTURES AND DISLOCATIONS

Fractures and dislocations have a relatively low priority in the management of multiple injuries. Associated blood loss usually poses a more immediate problem and temporary splinting of fractures provides pain relief while more pressing injuries are assessed and treated. Exceptions can be made in the following circumstances.

## FRACTURES AND DISLOCATIONS COMPLICATED BY NEURAL OR VASCULAR INJURY

While these injuries do not threaten life, they may constitute a serious threat to limb survival and function. Treatment is undertaken as soon as life-threatening injuries have been dealt with.

## COMPOUND FRACTURES

Compound fractures are those in which the fracture communicates directly or indirectly with a body surface. All such fractures are potentially infected. Fractures are common following bullet wounds and despite the small entry wound must be regarded as compound and treated as such.

Treatment of compound fractures has high priority after attending to life-threatening conditions (see Table 11.1). Delayed or inadequate treatment may allow infection of the wound and fractured bone, leading to delayed or non-union and osteomyelitis.

The principles of management include extensive debridement and wound cleansing. Primary skin closure is preferred unless the viability of deeper tissues is in doubt or the wound is grossly contaminated. Reduction and immobilisation of the fracture can usually be achieved immediately, but internal fixation is inadvisable because of the risk of infection. Antibiotics are given routinely and tetanus prophylaxis is essential.

# PERIPHERAL NERVE INJURIES

Peripheral nerve injuries occur most often as a result of penetrating trauma, but can occur in association with fractures and dislocations. Nerve injury may take the following forms.

## Neuropraxia

This consists of transient loss of physiological function after slight injury. There is no loss of nerve continuity and no degeneration. The prognosis is excellent and recovery within six weeks is usual.

## Axonotmesis

This more serious injury follows compression or traction damage. The continuity of the nerve sheath is maintained but there is Wallerian degeneration of nerve fibres distal to the point of injury. Recovery requires that the axons regenerate and grow down the intact sheath, and this may take several weeks or months. Although the axons grow distally down their sheath at a rate of 3 to 4 mm a day, excessive fibrosis may hinder growth so that reinnervation is delayed and the final functional result less than perfect.

## Neurotmesis

Neurotmesis denotes division of a nerve. It commonly follows penetrating trauma but may result from fracture in blunt injury. Fibrous tissue forms between the divided nerve ends and although the divided axons attempt to grow distally, reinnervation of end organs is unusual.

Complete interruption of nerve function causes loss of cutaneous sensation and flaccid paralysis in the area supplied by the affected nerve.

## MANAGEMENT OF PERIPHERAL NERVE INJURIES

*Neuropraxia* and *axonotmesis* are managed by passive exercises and careful splinting to prevent fixed contractures. Protection of anaesthetic skin is essential. Sequential electrical testing of muscle activity and nerve conduction are used to monitor progress of return of function after these types of injury.

*Neurotmesis* demands operative intervention if function is to be restored. Clean lacerations are repaired immediately by end-to-end suture of the nerve sheath. If there has been contamination of the wound, delayed nerve suture is preferred. The cut nerve ends are marked with non-absorbable sutures and secondary nerve suture is undertaken once the original wound has healed soundly, usually within two to three weeks. Nerve suture gives variable results in that fibrous tissue formation hinders growth of the axons, while many axons are deviated from their course and fail to enter an appropriate neurilemmal sheath. Taking account of the various periods of delay during initial recovery of nerve cell function and restoration of myoneural activity, the overall time for recovery is unlikely to be less than one day for each mm of growth required.

## LIMB REPLANTATION

Using microsurgical techniques it is now possible to attempt replantation of an entire limb or one of its constituent parts. Digital replantation can be carried out, and the big toe can be transferred to the hand to replace a severely damaged thumb.

Replantation of the arm or leg is also feasible. The severed limb is immersed in a container of iced water to reduce metabolism, the arteries are perfused with a combination of low molecular weight dextran, heparin and saline, and operation is performed as soon as possible after resuscitation.

These procedures are highly specialised and best results are achieved by teams specifically trained in their application.

# 12. Shock

## DEFINITION

Shock may be defined as an acute alteration of the circulation leading to *reduced cellular perfusion* with resultant generalised cellular hypoxia and vital organ damage. Reduced cellular perfusion is common to all patients in shock regardless of the cause.

## CAUSES

Shock may result from a variety of causes, the majority of which are associated with a reduced cardiac output. The consequent reduction in tissue perfusion is compounded by the action of catecholamines liberated in response to the stress of the initiating cause.

### HYPOVOLAEMIA

Hypovolaemia is an important cause of shock, a low venous return leading to a reduced cardiac output. In surgical practice hypovolaemia may result from:

1. *Haemorrhage*
2. *Loss of gastro-intestinal fluid*, as in intestinal obstruction, small bowel fistula, or diarrhoea
3. *Trauma and infection*. Injury or infection increases capillary permeability and leads to local sequestration of fluid and oedema
4. *Burns*. Fluid loss results from direct surface loss (weeping or blistering), tissue sequestration and the loss of normal waterproof action of the skin

5. *Renal loss*. Excessive water and electrolyte loss from the urinary tract, e.g. in sodium-losing chronic nephritis, tubular necrosis, diabetic ketosis or Addisonian crisis is an occasional cause of prostration and shock (see p. 132).

### PUMP FAILURE

Primary impairment of cardiac action can cause shock by abruptly reducing cardiac output. This may result from myocardial infarction, acute ventricular arrhythmia, acute cardiomyopathy, or acute valvular lesions caused by aortic dissection or by trauma producing severe incompetence. Secondary impairment of cardiac action may result from cardiac tamponade producing constriction of the heart, or from major pulmonary embolism producing severe obstruction to right ventricular outflow.

In all shock states myocardial performance is affected adversely as a result of reduced coronary arterial perfusion, and in some cases due to the additional depressant effect of circulating peptides released from the site of infection or injury.

### BACTERAEMIA

Bacteraemic shock is most frequently associated with Gram-negative bacillary infection, though Gram-positive organisms or fungi are sometimes responsible. The most frequent sources of infection are the urinary tract, the biliary tract, and the large bowel.

Bacteraemic shock is more complex than hypovolaemic or cardiogenic shock. The bacteria concerned produce toxins, most frequently endotoxins, which participate in an antibody-complement reaction from which substances are produced which profoundly affect the heart and peripheral vasculature. In contrast to hypovolaemic or cardiogenic shock, cardiac output is frequently high, but perfusion is reduced as a result of the opening of many peripheral arteriolar-venular shunts.

## ANAPHYLAXIS

Anaphylactic shock closely resembles bacteriogenic shock, in that an antibody complement complex is of central importance in the development of the clinical picture.

## NEUROGENIC FACTORS

True neurogenic shock follows spinal transection or brain stem injury with loss of sympathetic outflow below the site of injury, and consequent vasodilation. The rapid increase in size of the vascular bed 'soaks up' the cardiac output so that venous return falls, and cardiac output is reduced.

Pain makes a potentially important contribution to shock in patients with trauma, particularly those with fractures. Pain increases the output of catecholamines, with adverse effects on the microcirculation. Immobilisation (not necessarily reduction) of fractures should be assured early in the management of patients with multiple trauma.

The example of neurogenic shock most frequently cited is the vaso-vagal attack, or faint, in which intense vagal activity produces a marked bradycardia and fall in cardiac output. The circulation rapidly returns to normal with the involuntary assumption of the horizontal position. This condition is of physiological interest but its transient nature removes it from the true spectrum of shock.

## ENDOCRINE FACTORS

Although adrenal failure is by itself a potent cause of the shock syndrome, due to sudden withdrawal of circulating cortisol and aldosterone, the role of the adrenal cortex in the production of shock by other causes is debatable. In Addisonian states, due to chronic adrenal insufficiency, the loss of salt and water from kidneys and bowel leads to hypovolaemia. Acute adrenal failure may occur as a complication of septicaemia (Waterhouse-Friedrichsen's syndrome), but this is usually regarded as a terminal event.

## PATHOPHYSIOLOGY OF SHOCK

The factors producing shock initiate the 'metabolic response' discussed fully in Chapter 7. Release of large amounts of catecholamines in the early stages has important effects on both the macrocirculation and the microcirculation. Failure to rectify the initiating factor results in persistence of the normal response with reduced tissue perfusion resulting in generalised cellular hypoxia and consequent metabolic changes. Different organs vary in their susceptibility to impaired perfusion, and individual organ failure may become manifest.

## MACROCIRCULATION

Diminished venous return activates baro-reflexes which increase cardiac rate and cause peripheral arteriolar constriction. These reflexes are supplemented by the rising level of blood catecholamines. The increase in cardiac rate improves cardiac output, while increased peripheral resistance raises arterial blood pressure. Thus a normal blood pressure may be maintained for a time, but tissue perfusion may not improve, and may even be reduced further by the peripheral vasoconstriction.

Peripheral vasoconstriction is more marked in the vessels of the skin and extremities than in central organs. This tendency to preserve flow in central organs has been described as the 'sympathetic squeeze'. The characteristic picture of shock is one of cold pale skin due to peripheral vasoconstriction, and the associated sweating is due to sympathetic sudomotor activity.

Patients in bacteraemic shock present a different clinical picture. The circulation is often hyperkinetic, the cardiac output is higher than normal, and the extremities are warm. The explanation of this 'warm shock' presentation is not entirely certain, but it is due in part to arteriovenous shunting induced by kinins from the infected area. The low A-V oxygen difference in these patients supports the shunting theory, and indicates that the cells are not utilising (or receiving) oxygen.

Myocardial function or contractility is adversely affected and the capacity of the heart to deal with an increased load deteriorates as shock continues. Much of the impairment is a consequence of low coronary arterial flow and myocardial cellular hypoxia. Local and generalised metabolic acidosis, together with alterations in plasma electrolyte levels, alter cardiac contractility and cause further deterioration by provoking arrhythmias.

## MICROCIRCULATION

Peripheral cellular perfusion is further affected by constriction of precapillary sphincters under the influence of catecholamines. As a consequence less blood enters the capillary bed, the *vis a tergo* is reduced further and capillary flow becomes sluggish.

In normal conditions only about one third of the capillaries are open at one time. Normally capillaries open in response to hypoxia and close when flow through them has restored tissue oxygen tension. In the sluggish flow conditions of shock the capillaries remain open longer than normal and more capillaries open, further expanding the capillary bed. Consequently, flow in individual capillaries becomes even slower and there is a tendency for blood to sludge in the capillaries. Coagulation time is shortened in shock and the combination of sludging and slow flow encourages endovascular coagulation leading to further impairment of flow, worsening hypoxia and local metabolic acidosis, and local cell death. Extensive endovascular coagulation depletes coagulation factors in the blood and may lead to haemorrhage, particularly in subcutaneous tissues and mucous membranes (disseminated intravascular coagulation — DIC).

The post-capillary capacitance vessels in shock may be either constricted or dilated. Constriction may briefly improve venous return, but will ultimately impair capillary flow by providing obstruction. Dilatation of the post-capillary capacitance vessels results in reduced venous return.

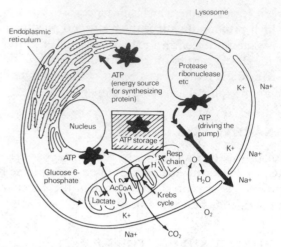

**Fig. 12.1** Energy supply in the cell (after Thal & Wilson, in: *Current Problems in Surgery*, Chicago, 1965)

## CELLS

In order to function normally cells require to extract energy from glucose. This process occurs in the mitochondria and provides energy for storage in the form of adenosine triphosphate (ATP) and releases free hydrogen. Oxygen is necessary to remove the majority of the freed hydrogen in the form of water (Fig 12.1). Energy is easily released from ATP and is necessary for cellular protein and enzyme synthesis, for maintenance of the sodium pump, and for cell reproduction.

In shock, oxygen is deficient, so that other hydrogen receptors in this chain become saturated. Energy transformation in the Krebs cycle is impaired, and lactic acid cannot be dehydrogenated to pyruvate and thus accumulates. The cell has to rely on anaerobic glycolysis for energy production, with a poor yield of ATP compared with aerobic glycolysis (Fig 12.2). Consequently, vital cellular functions deteriorate; protein and enzyme synthesis fails, sodium leaks into the cell while potassium leaks out, and plasma potassium levels rise. The lysosomal membranes eventually break down, with intracellular release of proteases, esterases and phosphatases and cell death occurs. If such changes are widespread, the patient will not recover (Fig. 12.3).

## ACID-BASE BALANCE

Accumulation of lactic acid from anaerobic cellular metabolism leads eventually to generalised

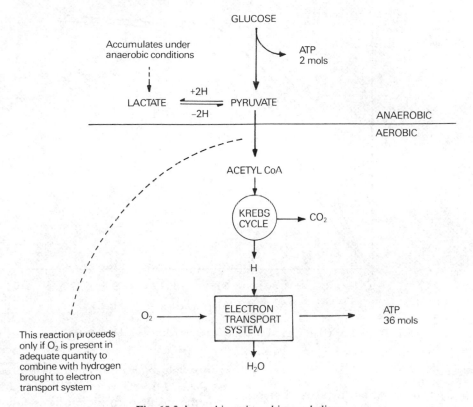

Fig. 12.2 Anaerobic and aerobic metabolisms

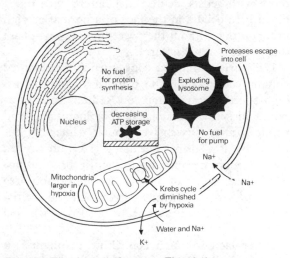

Fig. 12.3 The sick cell (Source as Fig. 12.1)

metabolic acidosis. This is compensated by buffers, and by respiratory and renal mechanisms, until the acid load becomes too great. Renal compensation is impaired in shock as a result of reduced renal blood flow; the development of renal failure greatly increases the tendency to acidosis.

Some patients in shock develop alkalosis, which may be respiratory or metabolic or a combination of the two. Respiratory alkalosis due to hyperventilation is more common. Metabolic alkalosis can result from impaired renal handling of bicarbonate and this may be important in patients receiving large transfusions of stored blood (citrate is metabolised to bicarbonate in the body). Alkalosis shifts the haemoglobin oxygen dissociation curve to the left (Fig 12.4). This, while improving the 'take-up' of oxygen in the lungs, impairs its release in the tissues.

## INDIVIDUAL ORGANS

The 'sympathetic squeeze' reduces the effects of shock on the vital organs at the expense of the periphery. However, this sparing is relative, and important effects on individual organs are recognisable.

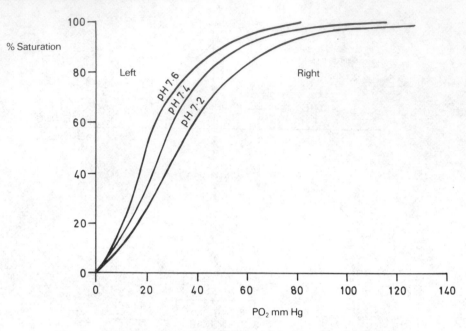

**Fig. 12.4** Shifts of the oxygen dissociation curve in response to pH changes

### Nervous system

The earliest sign of cerebral hypoxia is restlessness which may give way to stupor and coma. If respiratory alkalosis is present, cerebral blood flow is reduced and this, together with the effect on the haemoglobin oxygen dissociation curve, increases the tendency to anaerobic metabolism. The effects of cerebral hypoxia are usually rapidly reversible in all but the elderly, unless hypoxia has been prolonged.

### Kidneys

Renal failure was once a frequent cause of death in shock. Increasing knowledge of the mechanisms of derangement of renal function and more sophisticated management have reduced the incidence of death from this cause.

A fall in urinary output is much the most frequent effect of shock on the kidneys. Initially this results from reduced glomerular filtration due to reduced renal blood flow, together with the volume-conserving actions of antidiuretic hormone and aldosterone. If the shocked state continues, however, chemical and structural damage to renal tubular cells ensues. *Oliguria* is defined as the production of less than 400 ml of urine in 24 hours, while *anuria* is defined as the production of less than 20 ml of urine in 24 hours. As recovery from the insult occurs oliguria is followed by a marked diuresis. In some patients, particularly those with sepsis, acute renal failure with rising blood urea occurs in the face of a normal or high urine output without the preceding oliguric phase (high output renal failure).

If oliguria is simply a consequence of attempted volume conservation the urine has a normal-to-high specific gravity and low sodium concentration. This situation is managed by increasing fluid administration. Extensive tubular damage is denoted by low urine specific gravity, increasing urinary sodium concentration and a urine osmolality close to that of plasma. A rising blood urea in the presence of adequate hydration and arterial blood pressure indicates acute renal parenchymal damage.

Other factors which contribute to oliguria in shock include tubular necrosis, tubular blockage by debris, intravascular coagulation, jaundice, hyperkalaemia, and nephrotoxic drugs such as the aminoglycoside antibiotics.

Acute renal failure is usually reversible, and fluid restriction and dialysis allow recovery provided the primary cause of shock is controlled.

## Lungs

Acute respiratory failure (synonyms: adult respiratory distress syndrome, shock-lung syndrome) is an important cause of death in shock. The development of secondary bronchopneumonia leads to a mortality rate of approximately 50%.

Two principal groups of patients are recognised:

1. *Wet lungs*. Pulmonary oedema is the principal component resulting from acute cardiac failure, or overhydration particularly with crystalloid solutions. Pulmonary vein constriction, however, may contribute to the onset of oedema, and pulmonary capillary permeability is increased in shock possibly as a result of release of histamine or bradykinin. Gas exchange is less impaired than in the second group and the prognosis is better.

2. *Dry lungs*. This situation may be preceded by pulmonary oedema, but gas exchange is severely impaired due to *atelectasis* resulting from plugging of small bronchioles aided by *reduction in surfactant activity*. Shallow breathing encourages the development of atelectasis. Gas exchange is further impaired by the formation of *hyaline membranes*. A further problem in these patients is an *increase in pulmonary vascular resistance* which may be more profound and persistent than the rise in peripheral vascular resistance. The cause may include vascular compression from atelectasis, and capillary plugging by platelets, leukocytes, fat embolism, or solid particles in blood or plasma infusions. Acidosis and hypoxia also increase pulmonary vascular resistance, and fibrinopeptides released during endovascular coagulation produce further sustained pulmonary hypertension. These changes are usually seen in patients with severe sepsis, and the prognosis is poor.

## Heart

Myocardial performance is adversely affected in shock as a result of reduced coronary arterial perfusion. Hypoxia limits aerobic metabolism in the myocardium, and acidosis causes problems by depleting myocardial stores of noradrenaline. In addition contractility and left ventricular function in haemorrhagic and septic shock are further impaired due to humoral agents acting directly on the myocardium.

## Liver

The liver is the major site for conversion of lactate to pyruvate and increasing levels of lactate indicate severe impairment of hepatic function, principally due to low liver blood flow and portal venous oxygen desaturation. Routine tests of hepatocellular function show deterioration, and jaundice is a not infrequent accompaniment of shock.

## Gastro-intestinal tract

The splanchnic blood flow is markedly reduced in shock and adynamic ileus is a frequent complication. In patients with atheromatous mesenteric vessels, ischaemic colitis may develop but haemorrhage from the small bowel is not common.

Superficial ulceration of the stomach or duodenum — *stress ulceration* — may produce major haemorrhage especially in septic shock. Excess corticosteroid secretion or administration, and bile reflux have been suggested as the cause.

## Adrenals

The adrenal glands play a fundamental role in the response to injury or infection, and the production of corticosteroids and catecholamines is normally well maintained throughout the shock state (see Ch. 7). Acute pathological changes occurring in the adrenals are rare in shock, although necrosis may occur in meningococcal septicaemia (Waterhouse-Friedrichsen's syndrome).

## Reticulo-endothelial system

The reticulo-endothelial system plays a protective role in shock by an undefined but probably non-specific response. For example, exposure of animals to repeated doses of endotoxin protects them against the effects of shock induced subsequently not only by endotoxin, but also by trauma or haemorrhage.

In the shocked patient, the impairment of normal reticulo-endothelial responses may be demonstrated by depression of detoxification, phagocytosis and antibody formation. The susceptibility of the shocked patient to infection is well recognised clinically. This impairment of reticulo-endothelial function may relate to reduction in blood flow through liver and spleen.

## CLINICAL SYNDROME OF SHOCK

The classical appearance of the shocked patient is seen after haemorrhage and is due to intense sympathetic stimulation. The patient is pale with a rapid thready pulse and cold extremities. The peripheral veins are contracted due to reduced filling and sympathetic venoconstriction. Capillary filling is slow, as judged by return of colour after pressure on the nail-beds or ear-lobes. Sweating occurs due to sympathetic sudomotor stimulation. The patient becomes restless as a result of cerebral hypoxia, proceeding to apathy as hypoxia becomes more severe.

Initially the blood pressure is maintained or even raised, particularly in young patients. This is due to increased peripheral vascular resistance. Nonetheless tissue perfusion is markedly reduced with induction of the metabolic changes associated with shock. Arterial hypotension develops sooner or later in all shocked patients, and accentuates the impaired perfusion. Central venous pressure falls as return from the capillary bed is reduced. This fall occurs well before the drop in arterial pressure and may precede tachycardia.

Respiratory rate increases as a result of baroceptor stimulation initially complemented by the development of hypoxia and metabolic acidosis.

Urinary output is low.

The overall picture of haemorrhagic shock is one of low cardiac output. This classic picture is modified in cardiogenic shock, where central venous pressure is elevated due to acute cardiac failure. In bacteraemic shock, the cardiac output may be normal or elevated, the extremities warm, and the pulse full. The high flow through inflamed areas is associated with peripheral arteriovenous shunting, but the high metabolic demand in the tissues is not satisfied by this apparent increase in flow. As the patient responds to treatment, the clinical appearances return towards normal. The value of simple clinical assessment cannot be over-emphasised.

## PRINCIPLES OF MANAGEMENT

Restoration of adequate perfusion at the cellular level is the essential aim in the treatment of shock. The principles of management are:

### RESTORATION OF TISSUE PERFUSION

In the majority of patients this is achieved by adequate *intravenous infusion of fluid*. Patients with clinical evidence of myocardial dysfunction will require inotropic drugs to improve function, and certain patients with persisting abnormalities of peripheral vascular tone will need vasoactive drugs.

### ADEQUATE OXYGENATION

All shocked patients become hypoxic, and oxygen administration is routine. Patients with respiratory difficulty or a developing acute respiratory distress syndrome require intermittent-positive pressure ventilation.

### TREATMENT OF THE PRECIPITATING CAUSE

Haemorrhage is arrested, and infection treated by appropriate antibiotics, drainage of abcesses, or removal of the source (e.g. ruptured appendix).

### MONITORING

The response of the patient to therapy is the guide to whether treatment is appropriate or adequate. The response is assessed at frequent intervals following the initial 'base-line' assessment.

*General appearance.* Note pallor, sweating,

restlessness, venous filling and temperature of extremities.

*Cardiovascular parameters.* Measure pulse rate, arterial blood pressure and central venous pressure. More sophisticated assessment of parameters such as cardiac output, left ventricular function, and pulmonary and peripheral vascular resistance is necessary in some patients. ECG monitoring is required for patients with primary cardiogenic shock or secondary myocardial dysfunction.

*Urinary output.* Catheterise and measure hourly urine volume and specific gravity. Measurement of urinary osmolality supplements information obtained from determination of the specific gravity.

*Haematological and biochemical measurements.* Haemoglobin, haematocrit, urea and electrolyte levels are required for base-line and progress assessment. Arterial blood gas and pH measurements to assess hypoxia and acid-base balance are essential. Blood lactate levels give a good indication of cellular hypoxia and hepatic function.

In the initial stages of management, clinical and cardiovascular assessments are made every few minutes. The frequency of assessment decreases as the patient responds. Continuous recording of cardiovascular parameters is valuable in some patients in the early stages. Haematological and biochemical indices require to be measured hourly in some patients. In the majority less frequent determinations are necessary.

The peripheral circulation in shock has been likened to a marshy swamp in contrast to the normal running stream. The object of treatment is to get the stream running. Early and adequate therapy based on the principles outlined will achieve this without major cellular damage, and with prompt recovery of organ function. If treatment is delayed or inadequate, it may be possible to restore satisfactory circulation, but at the expense of residual organ dysfunction, e.g. of kidneys, lungs and the liver. Specific management of such organ failure will be required. More generalised cellular damage, resulting in failure of the sodium pump, with leakage of potassium from cells — the sick-cell syndrome — is of serious import. Patients who reach this stage are usually refractory to treatment.

# MANAGEMENT OF SPECIFIC SITUATIONS

## HYPOVOLAEMIC SHOCK

Haemorrhage is the most frequent cause of hypovolaemic shock, and the management of haemorrhagic shock exemplifies the approach to all shocked patients.

1. The general condition of the patient is noted, and peripheral perfusion assessed by noting the temperature of hands and feet, return of colour after blanching the nail bed and the state of filling of the veins on the dorsum of the hands and feet

2. An adequate airway is ensured and oxygen given.

3. External injuries and obvious fractures are noted, and continuing bleeding is stopped by direct pressure.

4. The pulse rate and arterial blood pressure are recorded.

5. An intravenous infusion is started and blood drawn from the needle or cannula for grouping and cross-matching, and for base-line determination of haemocrit and urea and electrolytes. If haemorrhage is not associated with obvious injury, the platelet count and prothrombin time should be determined. In severely shocked or traumatised patients more than one infusion line should be set up.

The preferred site for initial infusion is the antecubital fossa. If suitable veins are not available here or elsewhere in the arm, the alternatives are to cannulate the subclavian or internal jugular vein. Alternatively a cut-down to a suitable vein e.g. long saphenous may be performed. The initial infusion fluid should be crystalloid (either normal saline or buffered Ringer lactate solution), and one litre should be given as rapidly as possible (10–15 minutes). If one is close to a blood transfusion centre, grouped blood can be available for infusion in 10 minutes. The provision of grouped and cross-matched blood requires approximately 1 hour. If a long delay is anticipated, infusion may be continued with albumin (25-50 g/l of normal saline) or hepatitis-free plasma. Dextran may cause difficulties with subsequent cross-matching, and may provide coagulation problems. If haemorrhage is continuing group O Rh-negative blood may be used direct from store until adequately cross-matched blood arrives. Once the infusion is running, a central venous line is inserted to allow central venous pressure measurements.

6. The patient is best kept level. The head-down position adversely affects respiration and reduces cardiac output.

7. Pain relief is important to reduce further catecholamine production. Obvious fractures of long bones are immobilised by splinting. Appropriate analgesics are administered intravenously and the dose noted. Restlessness due to cerebral hypoxia requires restoration of cerebral perfusion, not sedation.

8. The patient is catheterised, and hourly urine output and specific gravity recorded.

9. At this stage a rough assessment of the blood loss associated with obvious injury may be made (see chapter on multiple injury).

The rate and volume of fluid and blood replacement is determined by the patient's response to infusion rather than to any rule of thumb. Individual patients vary greatly in their response to haemorrhage.

The colour and peripheral perfusion of the patient is noted, the changes in arterial pressure and pulse rate recorded. The trend in central venous pressure is monitored. As these parameters return to normal the rate of infusion is slowed. Failure to improve them or deterioration after initial improvement is evidence of continuing haemorrhage, and an indication for urgent operation.

Urinary output should reach a minimum of 50 ml/hour. A lower volume with high specific gravity indicates the need for more infusion, while oliguria with low specific gravity suggests the onset of acute renal failure. If the patient's clinical state suggests that he has been adequately infused, the use of diuretics at this stage may prevent acute renal failure. Frusemide (up to 1000 mg IV) is preferred to mannitol. It will initiate a diuresis within 20 minutes unless there is acute renal failure, when specific management is instituted.

Once the circulation is stabilised, the investigation and definitive management of the source of haemorrhage is undertaken.

## BACTERAEMIC SHOCK

In addition to the principles of management of hypovolaemic shock, it is necessary:

1. to determine the source of infection
2. to determine the organisms responsible
3. to treat the infection.

Serial blood samples are sent for culture, as are specimens of urine and sputum. Swabs are taken for culture from all wounds. Investigations to determine the presence of intrathoracic or intra-abdominal infection or abscesses are initiated. Patients receiving total parenteral nutrition may become infected from the venous catheter — if this is suspected the catheter should be removed and the tip sent for culture.

In the absence of specific bacteriological information, treatment is commenced which will cover both Gram-negative (the more likely) and Gram-positive organisms. A combination of gentamicin (80 mg b.d.) and metronidazole (500 mg 8-hourly) is suitable. Infected wounds and abscesses are drained. A recognised source of contamination, e.g. perforated appendix, empyema of gall bladder, stones in the common bile duct, is treated by appropriate surgery.

Antibiotic therapy will not be successful in the presence of a continuing source of contamination and suspected sources of bacteraemia must always be investigated, and if confirmed, eradicated or drained.

## CARDIOGENIC SHOCK

Fluid infusion in cardiogenic shock requires great caution and central venous pressure monitoring is mandatory. Attention is directed to three areas:

*The management of cardiac failure.* Digitalisation is usually indicated. Hypokalaemia potentiates the effects of digoxin and care must be taken to avoid induction of arrhythmias. Stimulating drugs such as isoprenaline or dopamine are often used when there is secondary myocardial dysfunction in other types of shock. Again, there is a risk of induction of arrhythmia, particularly in the older patient.

Mechanical support using intra-aortic balloon counter pulsation has been used recently, and may be combined with partial left ventricular by-pass.

*The management of arrhythmia.* Acute arrhythmias are managed by drugs appropriate to the arrythmia. β-blocking drugs or quinidine-like drugs are useful in many situations, but electrical cardioversion may be required. Expert cardiological advice should be sought.

*Correction of mechanical factors.* Cardiogenic shock may be precipitated by mechanical factors such as tamponade, valve rupture or massive pulmonary embolism. Drainage of tamponade, and consideration of valve replacement or embolectomy will be necessary.

## NEUROGENIC SHOCK

Neurogenic shock may follow high spinal injury or brain stem injury. Adequate ventilation and fluid replacement is necessary. Vasoconstrictor drugs may be indicated in this type of shock.

## PERSISTING INADEQUATE TISSUE PERFUSION

In some patients, despite adequate fluid infusion and management of myocardial and respiratory dysfunction, persisting metabolic acidosis and lactic acidaemia indicate that tissue perfusion remains unsatisfactory. Persisting vasoconstrictor catecholamine activity is usually implicated, and is an indication for the use of α-blocking vasodilators such as phenoxybenzamine, either alone or in combination with β-stimulants such as dopamine or isoprenaline.

Drugs of this type result in a large expansion of the peripheral vascular bed, and one must be prepared to infuse large volumes of fluid to ensure adequate venous return. Ideally when such drugs are being used the patient should be continuously monitored with frequent determination of cardiac output and peripheral vascular resistance.

## RESPIRATORY SUPPORT IN THE SHOCKED PATIENT

Hypoxia is invariable in shock. Mild hypoxia is an indication for humidified oxygen by nasal catheter or mask (6 l/min); concentrations approaching 100% may be achieved if a tight-fitting mask is used.

If hypoxia is severe, or progressing on oxygen therapy, an endotracheal tube should be inserted and positive pressure ventilation instituted. This may expand atelectatic alveoli while humidification reduces secretion viscosity and allows ventilation of obstructed segments of lung. Secretions are aspirated through the endotracheal tube.

Tracheostomy will be necessary if it is envisaged that ventilation will be required for more than 4–5 days. Ventilation is adjusted to maintain an arterial $Pa_{O_2}$ of 70–90 mmHg (9.3–12.0 kPa) and a $Pa_{CO_2}$ of 30–40 mmHg (4.0–5.3 kPa). In some patients it will not be possible to maintain adequate oxygenation without significant hypocarbia and the prognosis is poor. The use of an extracorporeal membrane oxygenator may be considered at an early stage for such patients. A diuretic such as frusemide should be given to reduce interstitial and pulmonary oedema, and digitalisation is indicated if pulmonary oedema is established.

Patients with the acute repiratory distress syndrome frequently develop pulmonary infection, and broad-spectrum antibiotics should be given.

## MANAGEMENT OF ACUTE RENAL FAILURE

Once acute renal failure is established, it is imperative not to overload the patient with fluid, and input must be carefully equated with fluid loss.

*Dialysis.* Peritoneal dialysis or haemodialysis is indicated when the blood urea rises at a rate of 7–10 mmol/l per day. It prevents the development of severe metabolic acidosis, potassium intoxication and the gastro-intestinal, cerebral and cardiovascular effects of severe uraemia. Haemodialysis requires heparinisation, and is best avoided in patients with major soft tissue trauma, or high risk of gastro-intestinal bleeding. Peritoneal dialysis is not suitable for patients with intraperitoneal sepsis, recent gastro-intestinal resection, or intra-abdominal vascular grafts.

*Potassium levels.* Potassium intake must be restricted, and the high levels of potassium in banked blood and crystalline penicillin should be remembered. Emergency measures which reduce a high serum potassium level include:

1. The administration of sodium bicarbonate ($NaHCO_3$) corrects metabolic acidosis and reduces serum potassium by encouraging transfer into cells

2. Intravenous administration of 50 g glucose

with 20 units soluble insulin also favours transfer of potassium into cells

3. Intravenous calcium gluconate (2–4 g in 500 ml 5% dextrose) should be given over 4 hours if cardiotoxicity due to hyperkalaemia is present or imminent

4. Potassium ion exchange resins may be given orally or as retention enemas, and will extract approximately 1 mmol of potassium per gram of resin. The usual dose is 50–100 g in each 24 hours.

*Diet.* A high-calorie diet is given to ensure protein sparing. Approximately 40 g protein should be given each day, with 60–70 kcal/kg body weight as non-protein calories. Most patients are unable to take this amount orally and parenteral supplementation is necessary.

*Acidosis.* Metabolic acidosis can occur in shock without evidence of renal failure. Improved tissue perfusion corrects the situation and is the primary objective of treatment.

If standard bicarbonate levels fall below 15 mmol/l, it is advisable to correct the base deficit. The amount of sodium bicarbonate required is calculated from the following formula: dose in mmol = 0.2 × body weight (kg) × (27-standard bicarbonate mmol/l )

Half the calculated dose is given initially, and subsequent doses determined by the patient's response.


## NON-SPECIFIC DRUGS IN SHOCK THERAPY

The role of *steroids* in the managment of shock remains debatable. If they are to be effective they must be given in high dosage (e.g. dexamethasone 2–6 mg/kg body weight 4–6 hourly for 48 hours), but objective clinical evidence for their efficacy remains elusive. Among the advantages claimed for high-dose steroid therapy are improved myocardial function, reduced peripheral vascular tone, stabilisation of mitochondrial membrane and reduced intracellular release of lysosomal enzymes, protection against development of severe pulmonary changes, and protection against the action of sensitised antibody-complement complexes in bacteraemic and anaphylactic shock.

The use of *Trasylol* (aprotinin), an antikallikrein agent, has recently been advocated in shock. In theory, Trasylol blocks kinin release and avoids the potentially harmful effect of these substances on myocardial and peripheral vascular function. The value of Trasylol has not been confirmed in practice.

*Glucagon* has actions akin to β-adrenergic drugs, and improves cardiac performance, even in fully digitalised patients. Infusion of 3–5 mg per hour has been used in shock, and benefit reported in a few cases. In theory glucagon would also improve hepatic blood flow.


## DISSEMINATED INTRAVASCULAR COAGULATION

In shock, as in other stress situations, the blood becomes hypercoagulable and some degree of intravascular coagulation occurs. This may be extensive and disseminated (DIC), and coagulation factors consumed to such an extent that a bleeding tendency results and massive haemorrhage may occur. Platelets, prothrombin, fibrinogen and factors V and VIII become depleted, and as a result of accompanying fibrinolysis, fibrinopeptides and fibrin-degradation products (FDPs) appear in the blood. The laboratory tests to confirm DIC are based on these changes.

The prime objective of therapy is management of the underlying cause, and with successful treatment DIC will resolve. Heparin infusion has been advocated to prevent progression of DIC and though clinical results have been disappointing, its use may be justified when DIC progresses rapidly and is associated with severe haemorrhage. In some patients, a secondary fibrinolysis becomes the dominant feature, and the use of epsilon-aminocaproic acid (EACA) to inhibit fibrinolysis is advised in addition to heparin. Heparin and EACA must be used with caution and dosage is difficult to control. Direct replacement of platelets and clotting factors is safer and provides some control while the underlying cause is managed.

# 13. Burns

As burns affect principally the skin, a knowledge of the structure and functions of skin is central to an understanding of burn injury.

## STRUCTURE AND FUNCTIONS OF SKIN

Skin consists of epidermis and dermis. The epidermis is a layer of keratinised, stratified squamous epithelium (Fig. 13.1). The hair follicles, sweat glands and sebaceous glands are epidermal appendages within the dermis. Due to their deep location the appendages often escape destruction in superficial burns, and are a source of new cells for reconstitution of the epidermis. The skin area is approximately 0.25 m² at birth, and is 1.5–1.9 m² in adults. Skin accounts for some 15% of lean body mass and is one of the largest organs of the body. It prevents excessive water loss, helps control body temperature and provides a barrier against infection.

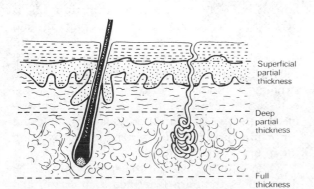

**Fig. 13.1** Diagram of skin showing categories of burn depth

For further details of skin anatomy see Chapter 17.

## TYPES OF BURN

Burn injuries cover a wide spectrum of severity. Severe burns pose a major threat to life, involve a long stay in hospital, and carry a risk of permanent disfigurement or impairment of function. The majority of burns follow accidents in the home and could be prevented by basic safety precautions.

### Injurious agents

Burns may be caused by flames, hot solids, hot liquids or steam, or by physico-chemical agencies such as irradiation, electricity or chemicals. Toddlers are particularly liable to scalding by hot liquids or steam in kitchen accidents, and unguarded fires are a threat to all children. Severe disfigurement of the face and neck can result from clothing catching fire, although the incidence of this type of injury has been reduced by use of non-flammable clothing materials. Impaired mobility, poor co-ordination and diminished awareness of pain increase the incidence of burns in the elderly and infirm.

Sunburn is the commonest irradiation injury but is rarely a major problem. Industrial accidents account for most physico-chemical burns, although accidental or deliberate ingestion of caustic or corrosive chemicals is still an occasional cause of domestic burn injury. The extent of injury caused by electrical burns is easily underestimated as surface damage may be small despite extensive deep injury.

## THE EFFECTS OF BURN INJURY

### Local effects

The local effects result from damage to the epidermis and the inflammatory response of underlying tissues. Destruction of the epidermis allows loss of electrolyte-free water, the magnitude of which depends on the extent of injury. Instead of the normal insensible loss of 15 ml/m² body surface per hour, as much as 200 ml/m² per hour may be lost after full-thickness skin destruction.

In its least severe form the dermal inflammatory response consists of capillary dilatation, as in the erythema of sunburn. Following more severe burns, the capillaries become permeable to protein, and an exudate forms with a protein content only slightly less than that of plasma. Lymphatic drainage fails to keep pace with the rate of exudation and interstitial oedema results. An increase of 2 cm in the diameter of a lower limb represents accumulation of over 2 litres of interstitial fluid. Exudation is maximal in the first 12 hours, capillary permeability returning to normal within 48 hours. With more severe injury, the epidermis and dermis are converted into a coagulum of dead tissue termed *eschar*. Far from providing a barrier to infection, eschar provides an ideal environment for bacterial growth. Contamination may occur at any time and wound care should commence at the time the patient is first seen. Sepsis delays healing, increases the patient's caloric needs, and forms a new threat to life just when the dangers of hypovolaemia have been overcome.

### General effects

The general effects of burns are hypovolaemia, dehydration and increased catabolism. Circulating plasma volume falls as exudate accumulates and excessive amounts of water evaporate from the burned surface. Some red cells are destroyed by the burn, and many more are damaged but not destroyed immediately. However, red cell losses are small in comparison to plasma loss in the early period and haemoconcentration is reflected in a rising haematocrit. Hypovolaemic shock ensues if plasma volume is not restored. It goes without saying that the severity of these changes depends on the extent of the burn injury. The rising haematocrit is associated with movement of water and electrolytes into the bloodstream from the interstitial tissues of unburned areas of the body. The effects are ultimately shared by all body tissues as water moves out of the cells to balance changes in the surrounding interstitial fluid.

Excessive water loss from the burned surface causes expenditure of calories as heat of evaporation. In severe burns some 7000 kcal may be expended daily and weight loss of 0.5 kg/day is not unusual.

## CLASSIFICATION OF BURNS

Burns are classified according to their depth as partial- or full-thickness. A partial-thickness burn is one in which sufficient epidermal cells survive to restore the epidermis. Full-thickness burns destroy the epidermis completely.

### Partial-thickness burns

The most superficial injuries involve only the epidermis. Pain and swelling subside within 48 hours and the superficial epidermis peels off within a few days. New epidermal cover is provided from undamaged cells of the basal germinal layer (Fig. 13.1), and the final cosmetic result is perfect. In more severe injury, the epidermis and superficial dermis are destroyed. Restoration of the epidermis then depends on intact epithelial cells within the epidermal appendages. Pain and swelling are marked, but complete healing without scarring can be anticipated within approximately two weeks. Infection delays healing and can cause further tissue destruction, converting the injury to a full-thickness one.

When only the bases of the appendages escape destruction, the burn is termed *deep dermal* and epithelialisation takes 3–4 weeks, even in the absence of infection. The resulting epidermis is thin and readily traumatised, and the cosmetic result is often less than perfect.

## Full-thickness burns

A full-thickness burn destroys the epidermis and underlying dermis, including the epidermal appendages. The destroyed tissues undergo rapid coagulative necrosis and form an eschar which usually begins to lift off the underlying tissues within 2–3 weeks. Unless the raw area is cleaned and grafted, epidermal cover can only occur through laborious inward movement and growth of cells from the intact skin around the burn margin. Fibrosis and ugly contracture are inevitable in all but small injuries.

## Determination of burn depth

There is no foolproof method for determining the depth of a burn in the early period after injury, and even experienced plastic surgeons may not be able to make an accurate assessment for days or even weeks following the injury.

Scalds usually produce partial-thickness injury, whereas burns due to electricity or contact with hot metal are usually full-thickness.

*Erythema* denotes that epidermal damage is superficial. *A dead white appearance* frequently indicates full-thickness injury, although at least some of these burns prove to be deep dermal. *A dry leathery mahogany-coloured* skin with visible thrombosed veins denotes full-thickness destruction.

*Intact cutaneous sensation* implies that the epidermal appendages have survived, as they lie at the same level as cutaneous nerve endings in the dermis. In practice, anaesthesia to pinprick can be a misleading guide to burn depth.

*Blisters* are accumulations of fluid at the junction of epidermis and dermis and while they indicate partial-thickness damage after scalding, they are a notoriously unreliable sign in burns resulting from contact with hot solids or flame. Blisters appearing many hours after injury are often due to infection and give no indication of burn depth.

## PROGNOSIS AFTER BURN INJURY

Prognosis depends on the following factors:

*Age and general condition.* Infants, the elderly, alcoholics, and those ill from other disease fare less well than healthy young adults.

*Extent of the burn.* Extent can be estimated using the 'rule of nines' (Fig 13.2) but tables are available for more accurate calculation. The rule of nines cannot be used in children because of the relatively large size of the head. The head and neck account for 19% of body surface at birth, whereas each lower limb accounts for only 13%. Hypovolaemic shock is anticipated if more than 15% of the surface is burned in an adult, or more than 10% in a child. At one time burns greater that 30% were generally fatal; this is no longer the case.

*Depth of the burn.* Partial-thickness burns of the trunk and limbs (excluding the hands and feet) which involve less than 10% of the body surface seldom constitute a threat to life or function. Full-thickness burns always take longer to heal and may require grafting.

*Site of the burn.* Burns involving the face, neck, hands, feet or perineum may threaten cosmetic appearance or function. They require in-patient management.

## MANAGEMENT OF THE BURNED PATIENT

### FIRST AID

Prompt effective action prevents further damage, may save life, and may avoid months of suffering. The principles of first aid are to arrest the burning process, ensure an adequate airway, and avoid wound contamination.

*Arrest the burning process.* Burning clothing is extinguished by smothering the flames in a coat or carpet. The victim must be placed flat on the ground to avoid flames rising to burn the head and neck with inhalation of smoke and fumes. The heat within clothing can continue to burn the body for many seconds after flames have been extinguished, so that clothing must be removed

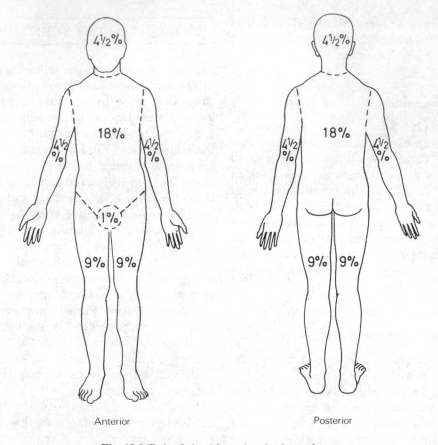

**Fig. 13.2** 'Rule of nines' for estimating burned area

immediately or doused in cold water. Similarly, clothing soaked in boiling water will scald for some 30 seconds unless cold water is applied liberally. A burned hand or arm is best placed under the cold tap to dissipate heat and give pain relief. Chip pans are a common cause of domestic accident. It is dangerous to remove the burning pan from the kitchen. The source of heat is turned off and the top of the pan covered with an asbestos or fibreglass fire mat (if available) or damp dish towel to exclude air and extinguish flames.

Chemical burns require copious irrigation with water for several minutes. If the eyes are involved, prompt and prolonged irrigation may save the patient's sight.

Electrical burning is arrested by switching off the current source, not by pulling the patient free. If this is not feasible, the patient is pushed free from the contact with a non-conductor such as a wooden chair.

*Ensure an adequate airway*. The patient should be moved into a smoke-free atmosphere. Smoke and fumes irritate the respiratory tree and can precipitate respiratory arrest. Mouth-to-mouth ventilation is commenced if necessary. Cardiac arrest may follow electrocution and the appropriate procedure should be instituted.

*Avoid wound contamination*. The burn is covered by a clean sheet and on no account should traditional 'household remedies' be applied. At best they are messy and interfere with subsequent care; at worst they are positively destructive, converting partial to full-thickness injuries.

## TRANSFER TO HOSPITAL

The patient should be transferred to hospital as soon as possible, unless the burn is obviously trivial. Severe burns are best treated from the outset in a specialised burn unit. Hypovolaemia takes time to become manifest, and it is easy to misjudge the severity of injury, thus missing the opportunity for uncomplicated transfer. Patients embarking on journeys expected to take more than 30 minutes should ideally be accompanied by a trained person. An intravenous infusion is commenced if the burn is extensive.

Full-thickness burns are often relatively painless. Partial-thickness injuries can be excruciatingly painful and opiates may be needed for pain relief. Analgesics should be given intravenously and the dose and route of administration must be recorded.

## ARRIVAL IN THE ACCIDENT AND EMERGENCY DEPARTMENT

### Adequate ventilation

Maintenance of an adequate airway remains the first priority. A patent airway on admission is no guarantee that the patient will remain free from airway problems. Respiratory tract injury is suggested by dyspnoea, coughing, hoarseness, cyanosis and coarse crepitations on auscultation. Burns of the head and neck can obstruct the airway by oedema, although this usually takes some hours to develop. Endotracheal intubation is advisable if there is anxiety about airway patency. Tracheostomy is never undertaken lightly in view of the danger of infection of burned tissues around the stoma.

### Initial assessment and management

Once airway patency is assured, the time of injury, type of burn and its previous treatment are established. The extent and depth of the burn are assessed to determine whether shock can be expected. If the burn is over 15% in extent, an intravenous infusion is commenced, and blood is withdrawn for cross-matching, haematocrit, urea and electrolyte determination. Blood gas analyses are performed if there is concern about the airway. Establishing an intravenous infusion takes priority over a detailed history or full physical examination. Vasoconstriction is often marked and it may be necessary to insert a cannula into the internal jugular or subclavian vein. Intravenous therapy may be required for many days

but the number of available veins is often reduced by the extent of injury. Veins must be treated with great respect as they are precious in burned patients. Once intravenous infusion is established, regular recording of pulse, blood pressure and hourly urine output is commenced.

Severe pain is relieved by intravenous injection of opiates. Tetanus can complicate burns and if the patient has not recently received tetanus toxoid this should be given. In general, patients with burns involving more than 10% of the body surface should be admitted to hospital, as should all patients whose site of injury poses particular management problems.

## GENERAL MANAGEMENT OF THE BURNED PATIENT

### BURN SHOCK

The aim of management is to prevent shock by prompt fluid replacement. Assessment and management of the shocked patient is discussed in general terms in Chapter 12. With regard to burned patients, various 'formulae' are available to help calculate requirements. The Brooke Army Hospital formula (Table 13.1) is one of the best known, and aims to provide plasma (or plasma substitute), electrolytes and water. It is a compromise between two schools of thought, the one stressing the importance of colloid replacement, the other the need for balanced electrolyte solu-

**Table 13.1** Brooke Army Hospital formula: Estimated fluid requirements in first 24-hours after burn injury

Colloid (plasma, plasma substitute, dextran)
  0.5 ml/kg/percentage of body surface burned

Electrolyte solution (Ringer lactate)
  1.5 ml/kg/percentage of body surface burned

Water (5% dextrose in water) 2000 ml for adults (correspondingly less in children)

Note: a. burns greater than 50% of body surface are calculated as 50% burns
  b. colloid and electrolyte requirements in second 24 hours are approximately half of those estimated for the first 24 hours

tions. The need for fluid is greatest in the early hours, and half of the amount calculated for the first 24 hours is given in the first 8 hours. Many centres do not use burn formulae in resuscitation, preferring to rely on continued monitoring to dictate fluid needs.

*Colloid replacement.* Little or no colloid is needed in patients with partial-thickness burns, whereas full-thickness burns require amounts of the order suggested by the Brooke formula. Dextran (MW 70 000) is generally less satisfactory than plasma or albumin. It is metabolised more rapidly and may upset clotting mechanisms when more than 1 litre is infused.

*Crystalloid replacement.* Infusion of saline or Ringer lactate is used to replace losses of crystalloid. Despite renal retention of sodium after injury there is a tendency to hyponatraemia in the first 2 or 3 days due to ADH secretion and sequestration of sodium in interstitial oedema. As inflammatory oedema is reabsorbed, the serum concentration returns to normal, and unless water intake is maintained there is a danger of hypernatraemia. Tissue destruction releases large amounts of potassium into the ECF, but hyperkalaemia is largely prevented by increased renal excretion of potassium as part of the metabolic response to injury (ch. 7). Once the first few days have passed, continuing potassium losses can produce hypokalaemia in a patient unable to eat and drink normally.

*Water replacement.* A 5% dextrose solution is used to replace losses of electrolyte-free water by evaporation. Excessive evaporation continues until the burn has re-epithelialised, and a high water intake must be maintained. Although most burned patients are thirsty, paralytic ileus is common and oral fluids may cause gastric distension, vomiting and aspiration. The majority of patients are able to drink normally after 48 hours.

*Blood transfusion.* Blood is seldom needed in the first 48 hours, but continuing red cell destruction in deep burns often leads to anaemia, and haematocrit is monitored daily.

## ORGAN FAILURE COMPLICATING THE MANAGEMENT OF BURN SHOCK

The problems of organ failure in shock have been discussed in detail in Chapter 12 and only those respiratory and renal problems specific to burn shock are considered here.

### Respiratory problems

The patient with head and neck burns is best nursed sitting up to encourage dispersal of oedema. Physiotherapy is essential to clear bronchial secretions after inhalation of smoke and fumes. Continued observation is mandatory, and blood gases and chest X-rays are repeated regularly in patients with ventilation problems. Arterial hypoxaemia is proof of inadequate ventilation. Assisted ventilation and oxygen therapy may be needed and antibiotics should be prescribed. Tracheostomy may be unavoidable despite the problems associated with its management. Encircling slough impairing chest expansion is incised or excised.

### Renal failure

Acute tubular necrosis is a common complication of extensive deep burns. The risk is especially high in the elderly, those with pre-existing renal disease, and patients developing haemoglobinuria or myoglobinuria. These pigments appear in the urine after massive red cell destruction or extensive muscle damage (particularly after electrical injury) and can damage the tubules and obstruct urine flow by forming pigment casts.

Hourly urine output should be maintained above 50 ml an hour. A falling output reflects inadequate resuscitation or the onset of renal failure. Measurement of urine specific gravity and the response to small test infusions will distinguish between them. Diuretics are used only if oliguria persists after adequate fluid replacement.

## NUTRITIONAL MANAGEMENT

Evaporation from open wounds is the major cause of excessive caloric expenditure following severe burn. Wound sepsis increases the patient's energy expenditure. Energy losses are reduced if the patient is nursed in an environmental temperature of 30–32°C. A high caloric intake is impracticable during the period of hypovolaemic shock, but is encouraged as soon as the patient can drink. Even with full patient co-operation, it is difficult to maintain a daily oral intake of more than 5000 calories and 150 g of protein. Parenteral nutrition is avoided if possible because of the risks of sepsis, but may be necessary if insufficient calories can be taken orally. Vitamin supplements must be provided after severe injury.

## SEPSIS

Septicaemia is a constant threat to the burned patient until skin cover has been fully restored. Resistance to infection is low, the wound provides a continuing reservoir of infecting organisms, and intravenous cannulae, indwelling urinary catheters and tracheostomy wounds are all potential sources of infection. The incidence of septicaemia has been reduced by use of topical antibacterial agents but *Pseudomonas aeruginosa* remains a problem and mortality from this type of Gram-negative septicaemia is still high. Prophylactic systemic antibiotics are advisable in patients with severe burns: systemic penicillin will combat streptococcal infection, but carbenicillin or gentamicin may be needed if wound swabs reveal that Gram-negative organisms are responsible for significant sepsis.

Blood is taken regularly for culture if there is severe wound infection, or if the patient becomes confused, disorientated, and hypotensive. A positive culture is an absolute indication for systemic antibiotic therapy.

## CURLING'S ULCER AND STRESS ULCERATION

Acute ulceration of the duodenum (Curling's ulcer) and multiple gastric erosions (stress ulceration) may follow major burns. The $H_2$ receptor antagonist, cimetidine, is prescribed prophylactically.

## LOCAL MANAGEMENT OF THE BURN

Care of the burn wound begins at the time of injury and continues until epithelial cover has been restored. Infection poses the major problem, and is the main threat to life once the first 48 hours have passed.

## PRINCIPLES OF WOUND MANAGEMENT

### Initial cleansing and debridement

The burn is cleaned meticulously with soap and water as soon as possible after admission, and adherent clothing or loose devitalised tissue are removed. An aseptic technique is essential, cleansing being carried out in an operating theatre or clean dressing room. Blisters should be punctured and serum expressed. General anaesthesia is best avoided and pain is controlled by intravenous morphine if necessary. In shocked patients, the wound is covered by a clean drape, and further care is postponed until resuscitation is underway.

### Prevention of contamination

The burned patient is particularly susceptible to infection. The protective epidermis is destroyed by full-thickness injury, thrombosis of cutaneous vessels impairs the normal response to infection, and both cellular and humoral immune mechanisms are depressed. Organisms readily colonise the burn wound, multiply rapidly, and soon invade the surrounding tissues.

Haemolytic streptococci were once a major cause of death but improved wound care and topical antibacterial agents have greatly reduced the risk of burn sepsis. Streptococci, staphylococci, coliforms, bacteroides and proteus organisms can usually be controlled although *Pseudomonas aeruginosa* remains troublesome in most burn units. Mechanical protection against infection can be provided in a number of ways. The following methods are not mutually exclusive and more than one technique may be employed as the needs of the patient alter. All personnel coming into contact with the burned patient must wear a cap and mask, and all dressings are performed with meticulous aseptic technique.

*Dry occlusive dressings.* Partial-thickness burns of the extremities excluding the hands and feet, and involving less than 10% of body surface, are often suitable for outpatient treatment by occlusive dressing. The dressings prevent contamination, absorb exudate and provide comfortable support. After the initial cleansing, the burn is covered by a layer of Sofratulle, a layer of coarse mesh gauze, a bulky layer of fluffed gauze, and an outer retaining bandage of gauze or stockinette. Compression by an elastic bandage fails to prevent exudation, may constrict the limb and is best avoided. The dressing is reviewed daily and although it can often remain in place for 4–5 days, it must be changed immediately the exudate soaks through all layers. Bacteria traverse a soaked dressing in hours.

Occlusive dressings are also used to protect burns during patient transfer, to prepare wounds for grafting after separation of eschar, and when patients have to be nursed in an environment where contamination is likely. The drawbacks of occlusive dressings are that frequent debridement is difficult, escape of pus is hindered and topical antibacterial agents cannot be used. Furthermore, they can provide an excellent culture medium rather than a barrier to infection unless managed carefully.

*Exposure.* Following initial cleansing and debridement, the burn is exposed to the air. Sterile sheets are impracticable and unnecessary. The patient is allowed to form his own barrier against infection. In partial-thickness injury this consists of encrusted exudate, whereas after full-thickness damage the wound is covered by a thick layer of eschar. Exposure is particularly useful for burns of the face and neck, and can be used for burns of the trunk and extremities. Epithelialisation proceeds under the crust of partial-thickness burns, the crust separating spontaneously 2–3 weeks later with a perfect cosmetic result. Unless the eschar covering full-thickness burns is excised early, it should soften and begin to lift spontaneously at about 3 weeks. Once eschar has been removed, exposure is abandoned and the burned surface is occluded in preparation for grafting.

*Topical antibacterial agents.* Mafenide acetate (Sulfamylon : 4-amino 2-methyl-benzene sulphonamide acetate) inhibits growth of both Gram-positive and Gram-negative bacteria when applied as a 2 to 3 mm layer of cream and can penetrate eschar to achieve this effect. The layer of mafenide cream also reduces evaporative water loss. The cream is applied every 4 hours during the first few days, but application 8-hourly becomes adequate as the rate of exudation

decreases. It is washed off completely each morning and the burn is inspected before re-application. A burning sensation is common after application, but analgesia is seldom needed.

Mafenide inhibits carbonic anhydrase and can cause metabolic acidosis if applied frequently and extensively. Hyperventilation is a valuable warning sign, and is an indication to interrupt treatment, check acid-base status, and give bicarbonate if required. Provided this limitation is borne in mind, mafenide cream has made a major contribution to reducing the incidence and severity of infection in burn wounds.

*Silver nitrate solution.* Silver nitrate is bacteriostatic and does not inhibit epithelial growth when used as an 0.5% solution. Thick gauze dressings are soaked in silver nitrate and held in place by stockinette. The dressing is kept moist by adding fresh silver nitrate every 2–3 hours, and the dressings are changed completely every 12–24 hours.

Silver nitrate stains black when exposed to air, and its use is only feasible in specialised units. Dangerous depletion of sodium and chloride can follow this method of treatment, and can occur rapidly, especially in small children. Potassium and calcium depletion have also been reported.

*Biological dressings.* Xenografts such as porcine skin are now available in the freeze dried state and can be reconstituted for use as a temporary occlusive 'biological' dressing.

## Relief of constriction

The dangers of progressive respiratory embarrassment from eschar in encircling burns of the chest have already been mentioned. Severe oedema or encircling eschar in the limbs may imperil the circulation and require appropriate relieving incisions.

## Restoration of epidermal cover

Full-thickness burns of less than 10% are suitable for primary excision of eschar under general anaesthesia within a few days of the accident. The exposed surface is either grafted immediately or prepared for grafting 3–4 days later. Primary excision and grafting is not feasible for more extensive burns; and delayed grafting is usually employed. Eschar begins to separate spontaneously after some 2 weeks, the process being accelerated by infection. Topical antibacterial agents delay separation by inhibiting bacterial growth. In any event, separation is usually completed surgically under general anaesthesia during the 3rd or 4th week. The exposed surface may then be grafted immediately although some preparation is normally needed. Blood loss may be considerable during excision of eschar unless spontaneous separation has been well advanced.

The recipient site must be sufficiently vascular to nourish the graft, and be free from debris and infection. Occlusive dressings, changed frequently, are used to prepare surfaces for grafting, and excessive granulation tissue should be excised. The β-haemolytic streptococcus is a troublesome cause of graft lysis, and systemic penicillin (intramuscular) is given routinely for 24 to 48 hours before attempting skin grafting. Significant contamination of the surface by other organisms may necessitate specific antibiotic therapy.

Avascular sites such as bone, tendon, fat and fascia may not provide sufficient nourishment for free grafts, and special techniques involving pedicle grafts may be needed. There is normally no difficulty in finding enough skin when the burn involves less than 20% of body surface area. Temporary cover for more extensive injuries can be provided by pig skin xenografts.

Free skin grafts may be full-thickness or partial-thickness (split skin), and are cut with a long-bladed knife or electric dermatome. *Partial-thickness grafts* are used extensively in burned patients. They are approximately 0.25mm thick and include the basal layer of the epidermis but not the epidermal appendages. The donor site forms a new epidermis from remaining islands of epithelium and more skin can be harvested after 14 days. Excess skin can be stored at 4°C for up to 4 weeks.

Full-thickness grafts are used in cosmetically important areas where contraction has to be avoided, or in areas such as the palms of the hands, which are subjected to repeated trauma. A graft will not 'take' if there is movement between it and the recipient area, or if the graft is floated off by accumulation of blood or serum. Large flat surfaces are covered by sheets or strips of skin held in place by occasional sutures. Accumulation beneath the graft is prevented by multiple small perforations or by daily expressing serum from the edges of the sheet. Alternatively, the graft is cut into small 'postage stamp' squares which are extremely tenacious, but do not give such a good cosmetic result.

The graft is exposed if feasible, but in many areas a bulky firm dressing is needed to prevent loss of adherence. Immobilisation of the part within a padded plaster cast is inadvisable when burns extend over joints.

## Functional and cosmetic result

Wound closure is not necessarily the end-point in management. Many months of staged reconstructive surgery may be needed for an optimal functional and cosmetic result. Attention to detail during the early weeks will prevent many problems, and the value of correct positioning and physiotherapy cannot be over-emphasised.

The patient who survives a major burn constitutes a challenge in rehabilitation. Emotional support, physiotherapy and occupational therapy are essential at every stage during healing if morale and function are to be preserved. With an energetic programme it is usually possible to restore skin cover to even the most extensive injury within three months. The patient should then be encouraged to return to his normal environment, returning to school or work as the case may be. Regular out-patient assessment is essential to reassure, to advise and to support morale. Scar hypertrophy is often worst in the early period after discharge, but tends to improve over the next few months. Function generally takes precedence over cosmetic problems if staged reconstructive operations are necessary. Contractures must be corrected as early as possible. Ultimately, the patient and his surgeon may have to come to terms with an optimal rather than perfect functional and cosmetic result.

# 14. Organ Transplantation

The transplantation of simple and relatively inert tissues from one human to another is now an established technique. Avascular tissues such as cartilage and cornea survive well in a new host and are used freely by plastic and ophthalmic surgeons. More complex tissues e.g. arteries and bones survive initially but are slowly rejected or degenerate. For this reason non-biological materials e.g. silicone polymers, nylon and terylene which elicit no reaction are preferred for the provision of a conduit, valve or supporting structure.

Organ transplantation is much more complicated. To be successful, not only must the organ be accepted in its new environment, but it must also remain capable of normal function. Although organ transplantation theoretically can be used to treat all manner of organ failure, technical and biological constraints limit practicability to the kidney, liver and heart.

In this chapter the general principles of organ transplantation as applied to the kidneys will be discussed. The current status of liver, heart and other organ transplants will be noted.

## RENAL TRANSPLANTATION

In the treatment of chronic renal failure, long-term dialysis and transplantation are complementary. In most renal centres, transplantation is regarded as the prime method of management. It allows the full rehabilitation of the patient in that reliance on a machine is unnecessary and the chance of long-term survival is greater than in those treated by chronic dialysis. Transplantation is also cheaper, demands less manpower, and frees dialysis machines for the long-term support of patients unsuitable for transplantation.

Sufficient donors are not yet available to meet the needs of all potential recipients. As a result many suitable patients are denied the opportunity of transplant.

Successful renal transplantation depends on a number of factors. These include: a good kidney, technical expertise, meticulous post-transplant care of the patient, prompt recognition and management of complications, and control of the homograft reaction.

## A GOOD KIDNEY

*Renal ischaemia.* The more complex an organ, the less it can withstand deprivation of its blood supply. The time of deprivation is termed the 'total ischaemic time'. This is inversely proportional to the likelihood of rapid return of function following revascularisation.

The effect of ischaemia is markedly reduced by lowering the temperature of the organ, and cold storage or cold perfusion can be used. After the organ is removed from the donor it is cooled rapidly, usually by a combination of extreme cooling and a short period of perfusion with 20 ml of 0.5% lignocaine together with 250 i.u. heparin at room temperature to relieve vessel spasm and prevent clotting. Ice-cold saline electrolyte or dextran solution is then infused through the renal artery until the venous effluent is blood-free and the surface of the kidney pale.

The simplest method of storing the ischaemic kidney is in a plastic container, immersed in saline or dextrose solution. This is kept at 5°C by placing the container in crushed ice (Fig. 14.1).

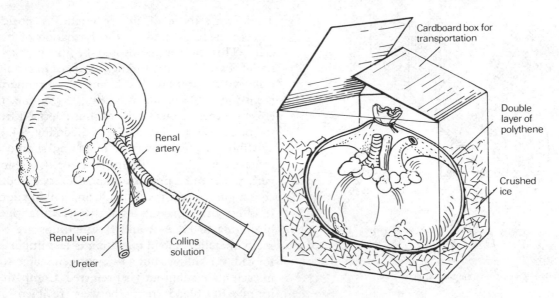

**Fig. 14.1** Storage and perfusion of kidney

Alternatively the renal artery may be connected to a perfusion machine which allows continuous pulsatile hypothermic perfusion with suitable colloid (usually albumin) to which nutrients and electrolytes are added. The preferred solution is 4.5% albumin with added hydrocortisone, benzyl penicillin, magnesium, potassium and glucose at a flow rate of 100 to 300 ml per minute and temperature of 8°C. As these machines are portable cold perfusion can be maintained during transport of the kidney.

The total ischaemic time is thus composed of a period of 'warm ischaemia' — that from donor cardiac arrest to the time cold perfusion is started, and a period of 'cold ischaemia' — that from the start of the cold perfusion to connection of the graft to the recipient. Restoration of renal function is possible after a maximum of 1 hour of warm ischaemia and four days of cold ischaemia. For early onset of graft function (i.e. within 3 days of transplantation) the warm ischaemic time should not exceed 40 minutes, or the cold ischaemic time 8 hours. The transportation of kidneys from a donor in one city to a recipient in another is now commonplace.

*Removal of kidney from donor.* The type of donor and manner of his death affects the warm ischaemic time and state of the kidney. Preferably a donor should be young, fit, and not suffering from any condition likely to impair renal function. Most suitable donors have been involved in road traffic accidents.

For many years British practice determined that potential donors had to be pronounced dead from circulatory failure before the transplantation team could remove the kidney. This led to delay and in many instances the limits of warm ischaemic time were exceeded. For this reason the success rates of renal transplantation in this country were relatively poor. With the legal acceptance of 'brain death' (see appendix) and continuation of circulatory support until the donor organ is removed, ischaemic time should now be minimal.

## THE RECIPIENT

Before dialysis was readily available a recipient for renal transplant was often in poor general condition and liable to overhydration, anaemia, hyperkalaemia and acidosis. Dialysis now ensures that recipients are in better condition although fluid and electrolyte disturbances are still a problem.

The operation itself is technically not difficult. The new kidney is implanted in an extraperitoneal pocket in the iliac fossa, the renal artery is anastomosed end-to-end with the internal iliac artery, the renal vein is implanted into the side of

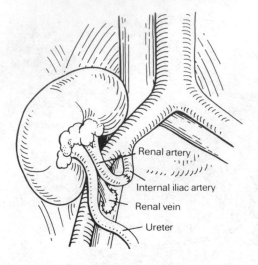

**Fig. 14.2** Renal transplantation technique

the external iliac vein, and the ureter is implanted into the bladder (Fig. 14.2). If the recipient has bilateral renal failure associated with hypertension or chronic bilateral renal infection, bilateral nephrectomy precedes transplantation.

## THE HOMOGRAFT REACTION

The main obstacle to the earlier application of renal transplantation was the homograft reaction which, if uncontrolled, led to rejection of the organ. Foreign antigens from donor kidney cells sensitised the host who then mounted a cell-bound and humoral attack on the foreign organ. In the absence of continuous immunosuppressive therapy, a transplanted organ will survive only if identical in antigenic composition to the host tissues. This situation is found only in consanguineous twins.

Although blood group antigens of ABO type are carried on all cells and affect graft survival, the main histocompatibility antigens are of the HLA series. These first four loci have been defined (A, B, C, D) each of which carries many separate alleles. In all some 150 different antigens have been recognised. Most belong to the HLA-A and HLA-B subgroups. Specific typing sera are obtained from parous women and are used to determine HLA type of recipient and donor (Fig. 14.3).

Tissue incompatibility can also be recognised by culturing lymphocytes from the prospective donor with those of the recipient. A positive reaction is recognised by the formation of blast cells. This can be monitored be the uptake of radioactive [$H^3$] thymidine. By treating donor cells with mithramycin-C, and thus rendering them incapable of incorporating thymidine, the effect on the recipient cells of those derived from the donor can be selectively studied (Fig. 14.4).

Although ideally perfect matching should be achieved in all cases, the number of tissue antigens makes this a practical impossibility except in consanguineous twins. When using a living donor it is essential that at least two HLA antigens belonging to HLA-A and B subgroups are correctly matched. Good matching is less important for cadaver kidneys but a two-antigen match (one in each main subgroup) is preferred. Compatibility of ABO blood groups between recipient and donor is always sought.

## IMMUNOSUPPRESSION

The drugs used to suppress immune reaction in the recipient are azathioprine (Imuran) and prednisone. Azathioprine inhibits lymphocyte proliferation and suppresses both cellular and humoral immunity. It is given in large doses (5 mg/day) for the first few days after transplantation and then gradually reduced to a maintenance dose of around 2 mg/day. The dose of azothiaprine is adjusted to keep white cell counts around 8000 per $mm^3$. Overdosage leads to diminished graft function.

Glucocorticoids have a complementary effect and many consider that prednisone is the most important adjunct to clinical transplantation. Immunoglobulin synthesis is inhibited and the effect of antigen-antibody complexes on the enzyme systems of the transplanted organ reduced. The initial dose of 200 mg per day is gradually reduced to a maintenance dose which should be kept as low as possible (10–15 mg/day). Other methods of enhancing the immunosuppressive effect of azathioprine include antilymphocytic serum, antilymphocytic globulin and extracorporeal irradiation of the recipient's blood. A new immunosuppressive agent with greater specificity for inhibiting the homograft reaction is cyclosporin-A.

Following transplantation a grafted kidney

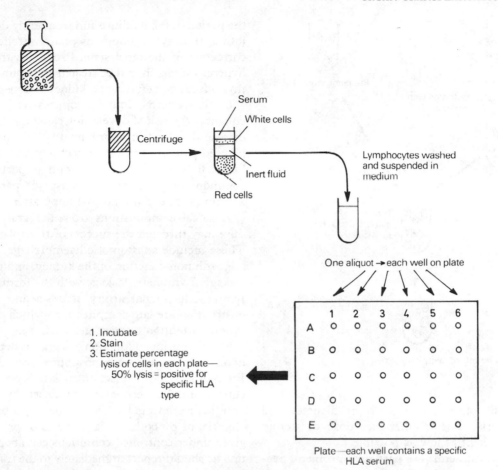

**Fig. 14.3** HLA typing

does not function for a few days. Copious quantities of dilute urine are then passed as the graft gradually resumes full function. Provided maintenance immunosuppressive therapy is satisfactory, function should continue for many years. 'Rejection crises' may occur from time to time and are treated by short-term high-dose parenteral steroid therapy (see below).

## COMPLICATIONS OF RENAL TRANSPLANTATION

Renal transplantation has complications. These mainly relate to the previous ill-health of the patient and the need for continuous immunosuppressive therapy.

1. Bacterial, viral and fungal infections are frequent and occur at some time in 40% of transplanted patients. Early recognition and prompt treatment are essential.

2. As many of the patients accepted for transplantation have systemic arterial disease and advanced uraemia, cardiovascular and cerebrovascular complications occur in 25% of cases and account for one third of deaths. Pulmonary embolism is also common. For some reason this is more frequent when the warm ischaemic time has been prolonged.

3. Gastro-intestinal complications include peptic ulceration, gastro-intestinal haemorrhage, pancreatitis and hyperamylasaemia. Patients with a previous history of peptic ulceration should have prophylactic reduction of acid secretion by the $H_2$-receptor blocker cimetidine.

4. Like other patients receiving long-term steroid therapy renal transplant patients develop

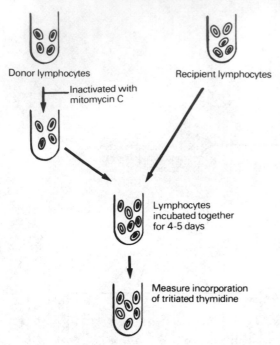

Donor lymphocytes

Recipient lymphocytes

Inactivated with mitomycin C

Lymphocytes incubated together for 4-5 days

Measure incorporation of tritiated thymidine

**Fig. 14.4** The mixed lymphocyte test

metabolic complications such as diabetes and osteoporosis. The maintenance dose of steroid should be kept as low as possible.

5. Hypercalcaemia is a particular problem. Secondary hyperparathyroidism is common during the period of renal failure and frequently develops into a 'tertiary' autonomous phase unrelieved by correction of the renal state. Patients with severe hypercalcaemia should be treated by subtotal parathyroidectomy before a new kidney is transplanted.

6. Long-term immunosuppressive therapy enhances the risk of developing cancer. Malignant disease develops in approximately 7% of transplanted patients and may affect any site. Reticulum-cell lymphoma of the brain is particularly common: its incidence in transplant patients is 250 times that of the normal population.

7. Local complications from the graft procedure may threaten the success of transplantation. These include anastomotic haemorrhage, ischaemia with non-function of the kidney, and ureteric leakage. Lymphatic leakage with the formation of lymphoceles, renal artery stenosis and outflow obstruction are late complications which demand prompt attention to avert graft failure.

8. The continued function of a graft is dependent upon continued immunosuppressive therapy. From time to time a rejection crisis may occur. The patient usually recognises its onset by feeling unwell, fevered and flu-like; by the development of oliguria, or by both. As large doses of prednisone given under controlled conditions can abort rejection he should report immediately to the transplant unit where creatinine estimations are carried out.

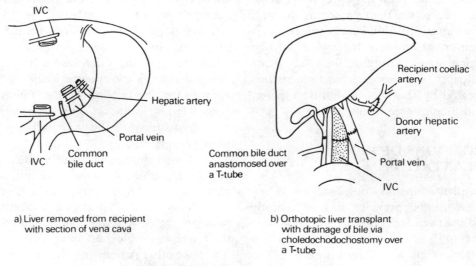

a) Liver removed from recipient with section of vena cava

b) Orthotopic liver transplant with drainage of bile via choledochodochostomy over a T-tube

**Fig. 14.5** Liver transplantation technique

## RESULT OF RENAL TRANSPLANTATION

The results of renal transplantation in any centre depend on the availability of good kidneys with minimal periods of warm ischaemia, recipients in good health and reasonable matching. Overall, with cadaveric transplantation, approximately 40% of grafts survive for one year and 20% for five years. Better results are obtained with related living donors. If the function of a graft is well stabilised at three years (and this occurs in 50% of cadaver transplants) there are excellent prospects of pro-longed survival, particularly with a patient under 50 years of age and without cardiovascular disease.

## LIVER TRANSPLANTATION

There is no easy way of removing nitrogenous substances from the circulation in patients with liver failure. Attempts have been made to remove these by dialysis over dextran-coated charcoal but the results are disappointing. Alternatively an animal liver can be connected extracorporeally to

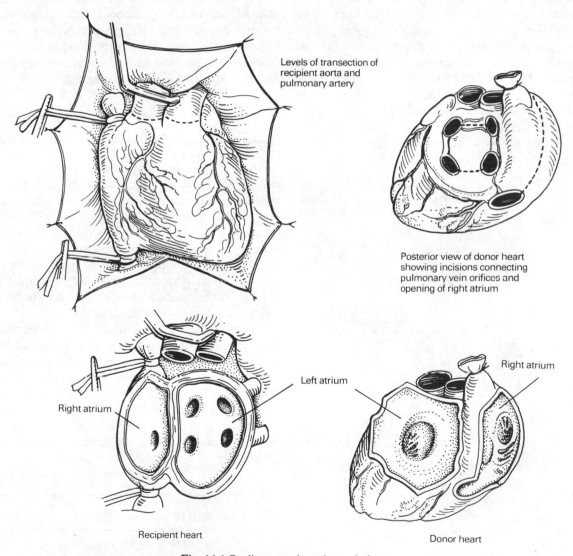

Levels of transection of recipient aorta and pulmonary artery

Posterior view of donor heart showing incisions connecting pulmonary vein orifices and opening of right atrium

Right atrium

Left atrium

Right atrium

Recipient heart

Donor heart

**Fig. 14.6** Cardiac transplantation technique

the patient to serve as a 'dialysis machine'. Experimentally, baboon livers have been shown to carry out both synthetic and excretory functions on prolonged perfusion without immunological or other clinical reaction. Limited studies in man have been encouraging. Other approaches include the establishment of cross-circulation with a living baboon, with a human volunteer, or with a cadaver human liver. Surprisingly, the lack of an effective 'artificial liver' has not proved to be a serious limiting factor in the development of liver transplantation. Despite technical difficulties, several hundreds of liver transplants have now been performed and some 50 patients are known to be alive with functioning liver transplants. The indications for transplantation are benign parenchymatous disease causing liver failure in the young, and to a lesser extent cholangio-carcinoma. Liver transplantation is now rarely performed for hepatocellular carcinomas, which are more commonly resected. The regenerative powers of the liver are great. Small remnants attain normal liver function speedily.

Because of its size a liver transplant is best placed orthotopically, i.e. in the bed of the excised liver (Fig. 14.5). A particular problem is the prevention of biliary stasis with formation of biliary sludge or a biliary fistula.

## HEART TRANSPLANTATION

Transplantation of the heart has only recently been regularly practised in this country (Fig. 14.6). The heart must be removed from the donor whilst still beating and until recently this was not allowed in Britain. Although in experienced hands the results of heart transplants are surprisingly good, many doubt that transplantation is economically justified while there are waiting lists for simpler forms of cardiac surgery.

## PANCREAS

In the insulin-dependent diabetic patient insulin therapy controls the day-to-day needs for carbohydrate. Its use prolongs life but it does not prevent the long-term complications of the disease. It is believed that this is due to failure to restore the control of homoeostatic responses which require variations in the secretion of insulin over short periods of time. In experimental animals with induced diabetes this fine balance can be restored by pancreatic grafts.

A pancreatic graft must drain its endocrine secretions into the liver and this poses formidable technical problems. The transplantation of a whole pancreas necessitates the transfer of a considerable bulk of foreign tissue whose exocrine secretory function is not required. There is thus interest in methods of isolating the islets of Langerhans from fresh pancreas and transplanting them into the liver by injection into the portal vein (Fig. 14.7).

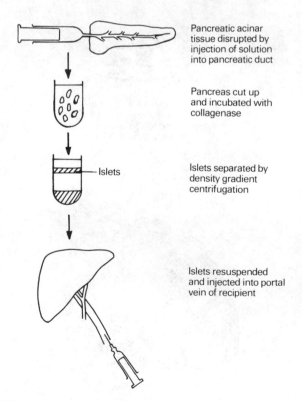

Pancreatic acinar tissue disrupted by injection of solution into pancreatic duct

Pancreas cut up and incubated with collagenase

Islets separated by density gradient centrifugation

— Islets

Islets resuspended and injected into portal vein of recipient

**Fig. 14.7** Pancreatic islet transplantation technique

## BONE MARROW TRANSPLANT

The experimental finding that mice could be protected against lethal irradiation by an intra-

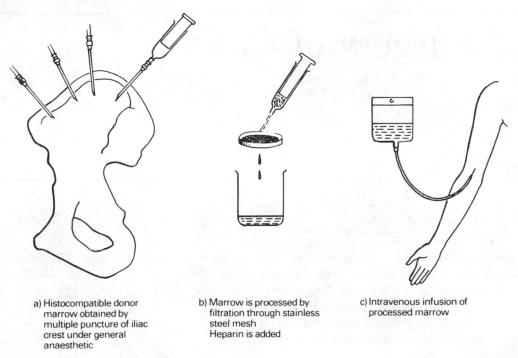

a) Histocompatible donor marrow obtained by multiple puncture of iliac crest under general anaesthetic

b) Marrow is processed by filtration through stainless steel mesh Heparin is added

c) Intravenous infusion of processed marrow

**Fig. 14.8** Bone marrow transplantation

venous infusion of marrow cells suggested that bone marrow transplant might be used for victims of radiation accidents and patients with immunological deficiency disorders. They are also used to treat severe aplastic anaemia and to facilitate the treatment of leukaemia by whole-body irradiation or high-dose chemotherapy. As bone marrow contains immunologically competent cells the problems of histocompatability are compounded by reaction of donor cells against host tissues. This syndrome of graft-versus-host disease may affect the skin, gastro-intestinal tract and liver. It presents as a skin rash, followed in a few days by diarrhoea, abdominal pain and distension, and an increase in liver enzymes. Diagnosis is confirmed by skin biopsy.

The bone marrow cells are obtained by multiple aspirations from the iliac crests of histocompatible donors and are sieved to make a single cell suspension. Following intravenous injection the cells colonise the marrow and function in 10–20 days. During this period, platelet transfusion may be required and, because of susceptibility to infection, patients are kept in sterile conditions. If available granulocyte infusions may also be given (Fig. 14.8).

Patients with an immunodeficiency syndrome require no immunosuppressive preparation but all others require immunosuppression in the form of cyclophosphamide administered for four days before the transplant and intermittent methotrexate therapy thereafter. Graft-versus-host disease is treated by methotrexate and antilymphocyte serum.

# 15. Surgery of Cancer

## NATURE OF A NEOPLASM

A neoplasm or new growth is a mass of cells which proliferate in an atypical and relentless way, and serve no useful function. The mechanism by which this abnormal activity is induced is not known; a prime event is the induction of change in genetic composition by virus or other carcinogens.

Neoplastic transformation of cells does not necessarily result in a tumour. Transformations occur continuously, but because of immune surveillance or simple wastage, i.e. loss of cells from the surface, mutant cells are destroyed before they proliferate. For persistence of growth these protective mechanisms must also break down to allow the neoplastic cells to reproduce within the tissues of their host. It may also be that for the formation of a tumour the stem cells must be transformed so that they can constantly replicate in mutant form (Fig.15.1)

The host environment is important in 'promoting' tumour growth. For example 'hormone-dependent' cancers of the breast, prostate and endometrium require a correct balance of hormones for continued growth (Fig.15.2).

### Benign and malignant neoplasms

Neoplasms are benign or malignant. The essential difference is the capacity to invade and metastasise. The cells of benign tumours do not invade surrounding tissues but remain as a local conglomerate. Malignant tumours are invasive, and their cells enter blood and lymphatic channels to be deposited in remote sites. These deposits form

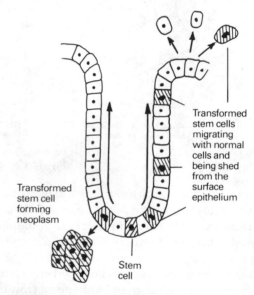

**Fig. 15.1** The nature of a neoplasm: the concept of cells transforming and either being released to the surface or forming a tumour

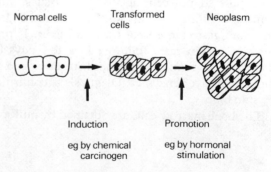

**Fig. 15.2** Induction and promotion

'secondary' or 'metastatic' tumours similar in cell type to the original 'primary' site. Malignant tumours are fatal because of their ability to metastasise.

Spread via { 1. Lymphatics  4. Cerebrospinal spaces
2. Blood vessels  5. Epithelial surfaces
3. Coelomic spread  6. Iatrogenic

SURGERY OF CANCER   157

## Mechanism of spread

Traditionally a malignant tumour was believed to spread initially by local *permeation* i.e. by direct centrifugal extension along tissue spaces and 'embolisation' of lymphatics to the regional lymph nodes. Metastasis in these regional lymph nodes was the first step in the dissemination of a tumour. The second step, that of dissemination by the bloodstream, followed (Fig.15.3).

It was this theory which led to the general belief that cancer was 'curable' provided that it had not spread beyond the regional nodes; and to the performance of 'curative' radical operations designed to eradicate the primary tumour and all malignant cells in its related lymph nodes.

This theory is no longer tenable. It is now believed that even at its earliest stage a tumour spreads simultaneously by lymphatics and by the bloodstream to form widespread micrometastases. Regional lymph node involvement is no longer regarded as a stage in the progression of the disease, but as an indicator of widespread dissemination (Fig.15.4). It is this concept which has led to a reappraisal of the role of local treatment, and to recognition of the need for systemic control.

The mechanisms of invasion and of metastasis are obscure (Fig. 15.5). Malignant cells can secrete a number of factors which may determine their biological behaviour and allow continued growth both at primary and metastatic sites. Examples are the 'angiogenesis factor' which stimulates surrounding capillary growth, proteolytic enzymes which digest surrounding fibrous tissue, and prostaglandins which induce osteolysis and allow development of skeletal deposits.

The natural history of a tumour is also related to its growth rate. Some tumours grow rapidly and quickly outpace the resistance of normal tissues. Others are slow-growing and years may pass before deposits reach a size which threatens the normal function of surrounding tissue. The reason for this difference is ill-understood but the degree of differentiation of the tumour cells is one factor. Tumours which histologically are composed of primitive 'anaplastic' cells are more aggressive than well-differentiated tumours.

## Types of tumour

The distinction between simple and malignant tumours is fundamentally clinical, and is usually confirmed by histopathological examination.

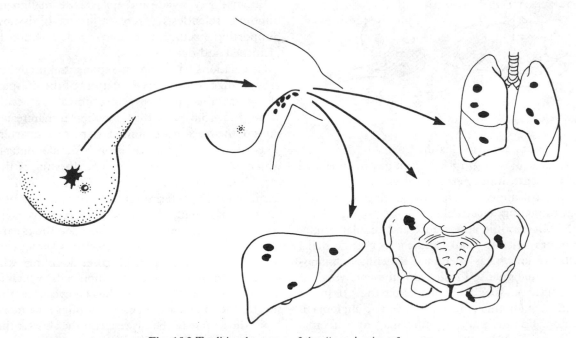

**Fig. 15.3** Traditional concept of the dissemination of cancer

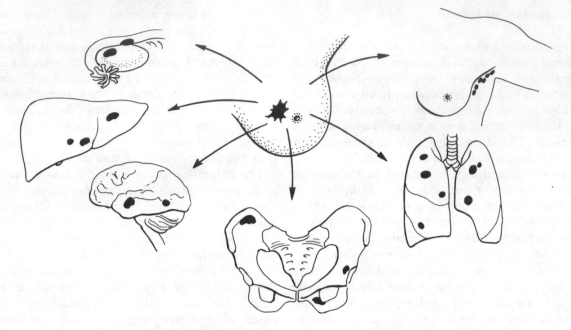

**Fig. 15.4** Modern 'explosive' concept of cancer dissemination

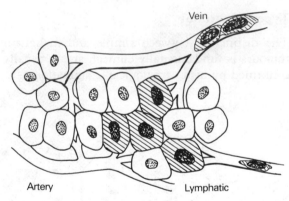

**Fig. 15.5** Invasion

Tumours are also classified by:

1. Tissue of origin : e.g. skin, gastro-intestinal tract, breast, lung, nervous system etc.

2. Gross appearance e.g. ulcerating, proliferating, fungating, cicatrising.

3. Microscopic appearance and cellular origin: tumours arising from epithelial or endothelial cells are known as adenomas if benign, carcinomas if malignant; those from mesenchymal or connective tissues are named after their tissue of origin e.g. lipoma, fibroma, myoma, angioma if benign; liposarcoma, fibrosarcoma, myosarcoma, angiosarcoma if malignant.

## Natural history and estimate of cure

Benign tumours rarely threaten the life of the patient. They are usually self-limiting but may cause functional abnormalities.

Because they invade and metastasise, malignant tumours relentlessly replace normal tissues. Supporting structures are destroyed, function is disturbed and death results.

Calculations based on an exponential model of growth suggest that three-quarters of the lifespan of a tumour is spent in a 'preclinical' or occult stage (Fig. 15.6), and that the clinical manifestations of the disease are limited to the final quarter. The number of cell divisions (or doublings) which can take place is finite. The duration of the 'doubling time', i.e. the time for each cell to duplicate itself, determines the total duration of a tumour, assuming that this time remains constant. It is estimated that 45 doublings are required for a single cell to become a tumour of 1 cm diameter; and that 15 further doublings will result in a tumour of 1 kg (1 billion cells) which is likely to be fatal. The faster the cell cycle, i.e. the shorter the time between each doubling, the more rapid the course of the disease and the shorter the duration of life.

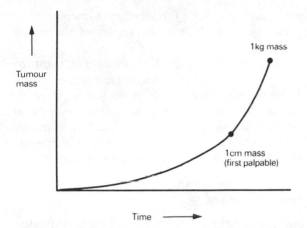

**Fig. 15.6** Exponential model of tumour growth

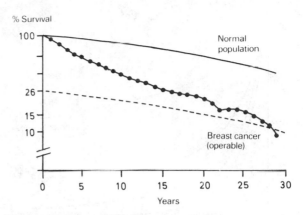

**Fig. 15.8** Cumulative survival curve (---- is parallel to normal survival) (from Brinkley D & Haybittle J L)

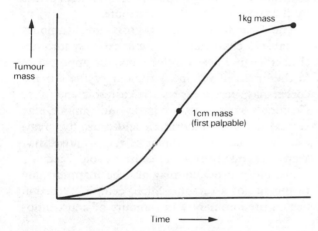

**Fig. 15.7** Alternative model for tumour growth: Gompertzian

These considerations do not take account of the variations which may occur as a result of periods of accelerated or retarded growth. It is now believed that the best mathematical model for tumour growth is 'Gompertzian' (Fig. 15.7).

## Cure

For cure every malignant cell must be eradicated. Not only should there be no recurrent tumour during the patient's lifetime, but there should be no evidence of residual tumour at death. This rigid definition of curability can rarely be applied. A normal duration of life without further evidence of disease is generally accepted as evidence of cure.

Cure rates of individual cancers are assessed by survival rates. Cumulative survival curves (life-tables) of patients with the disease are compared with those of age-matched healthy subjects of the same population (Fig. 15.8). Divergence of these two curves indicates that patients with cancer are dying faster than their normal partners; when they become parallel patients with the disease are dying at no greater a rate than their age-matched controls. The time from primary treatment when these two curves become parallel is the time at which cure can be assumed.

Cure rates vary according to the aggressiveness of the disease and the success of treatment. In some cancers, e.g. stomach and lung, metastases grow rapidly and cause death within a few years of clinical evidence of the disease. In others, e.g. breast and melanoma, many years may elapse before spread is evident and even when metastases have occurred life may be long (Fig 15.9). Five-year survival rates cannot provide a satisfactory estimate of cure for all tumours.

Many regard the treatment of a malignant tumour as a matter of extreme urgency. When one considers the duration of the natural course of cancer, a week or two spent in careful investigation and planning of treatment is good practice. Naturally, this period must not be unduly delayed: patients with cancer are worried and wish to have their initial treatment completed within a reasonable time.

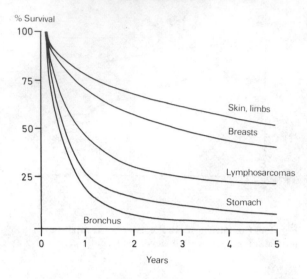

**Fig. 15.9** Survival curves for different cancers

## MANAGEMENT OF CANCER

There are three steps in the management of the patient with cancer:

1. Diagnosis of the disease
2. The determination of its extent
3. Treatment.

### DIAGNOSIS

Benign tumours often remain unrecognised during life or may cause symptoms due to local effects.

Malignant tumours vary in their clinical effects. Some cause a rapidly progressing and debilitating illness; in others local effects predominate.

#### Local effects

A tumour which lies on the body surface or within a hollow viscus may bleed, or discharge excess mucus or pus. In the gastro-intestinal tract diarrhoea is often a manifestation.

A hollow viscus or duct may be obstructed. Bronchial obstruction and pulmonary collapse can be caused by a tumour of lung, intestinal obstruction by a tumour of bowel, jaundice by a tumour of the bile ducts or pancreas.

A tumour within a closed space may cause pressure symptoms. Increased intracranial pres-

sure may complicate intracerebral tumours; paraplegia may result from a tumour of the spinal cord.

Invasion of an organ by tumour may compromise its normal functions and cause organ failure. Invasion of tissues such as pancreas, bone or nerves can cause severe pain. A cancer can also mimic the pain of benign disease. For example, cancer of the stomach can produce dyspeptic symptoms similar to those of a benign ulcer.

#### Systemic effects

Anorexia, asthenia, lassitude and general debility are classical symptoms of cancer. In part these may be explained by chronic anaemia or inanition, but elaboration of abnormal proteins and peptides by the tumour may also contribute.

The secretory products of some tumours produce characteristic clinical syndromes (Fig. 15.10). These products may be appropriate to the organ of origin. A tumour of the adrenal cortex may secrete excess corticosteroid and cause Cushing's syndrome; a parathyroid tumour may secrete excess parathormone and cause hypercalcaemia; an islet cell tumour of the pancreas may secrete excess insulin and cause hypoglycaemia.

Secretory products may also be inappropriate to the site of a tumour. Such 'ectopic' secretion occurs predominantly in tumours of neuroendo-

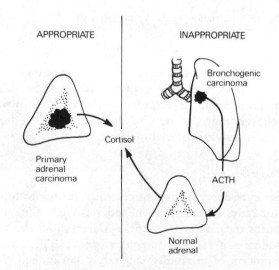

**Fig. 15.10** Examples of appropriate and inappropriate tumour secretion

**Table 15.1** Ectopic hormone production by neoplasms

| Syndrome (type of endocrine activity) | Neoplasms responsible | Main clinical features |
|---|---|---|
| ACTH — MSH (adrenocorticotrophic hormone — melanocyte stimulating hormone) | 1. Oat-cell ca. lung<br>2. Non beta islet-cell carcinoma<br>3. Carcinoma of pancreas<br>4. Thymomas<br>5. Carcinoid tumours<br>6. Other: tumours of thyroid, adrenal cortex, liver, prostate, breast, ovary, parotid, phaeochromocytoma, para-gangliomas, gangliomas | Cushings syndrome: hypertension, hypokalaemia, oedema, acne and hirsutism (in women), impaired glucose tolerance, occasionally obesity and striae. Dark pigmentation. |
| LH (luteinizing hormone) | 1. Hepatoma<br>2. Mediastinal teratoma<br>3. Various lung tumours | Precocious puberty in children. Gynaecomastia in men |
| ADH (anti-diuretic hormone) | 1. Carcinoma of lung<br>2. Carcinoma of duodenum<br>3. Carcinoma of pancreas | Weakness, confusion, incoordination, nausea and vomiting; hyponatraemia (part dilutional, part secondary to increased urinary sodium loss; plasma osmolality <260 mmol/l) |
| PTH (parathyroid hormone) | Carcinomas of: lung, pancreas, liver, colon, adrenal, parotid, ovary, vagina, uterus, bladder and kidney | Lethargy, weakness, nausea, vomiting, confusion, coma progressing to death; short Q-T interval on ECG and arrhythmias; peripheral neuropathy; rarely, bone resorption and renal calculi |
| TSH (thyroid-stimulating hormone) | 1. Choriocarcinoma<br>2. Hydatidiform mole | symptoms of hyperthyroidism, e.g. tremor, tachycardia, sweating, weight loss etc. |
| Insulin | 1. Malignant bronchial carcinoid<br>2. Fibrosarcoma; liposarcoma | Attacks of tachycardia, sweating, tremor, loss of concentration and diplopia especially during fasting; relieved by carbohydrate ingestion |
| Erythropoietin | 1. Phaeochromocytoma<br>2. Hepatoma<br>3. Cerebellar haemangioma | Raised red-cell mass features of polycythaemi, headache, high B.P., ruddy face, DVT |

crine origin and produces a variety of endocrine syndromes (Table 15.1).

## Clinical signs

A tumour on the surface of the body is visible; those within a body cavity or hollow viscus may be seen through an endoscope. Tumours of subcutaneous tissues or superficial organs, e.g. the breast, may form a visible swelling but are more likely to be found by palpation.

Many tumours are without clinical signs. Lying deep within the body, they are diagnosed by imaging techniques. Simple radiology may demonstrate a soft tissue tumour e.g. of the lung or bone, but for tumours affecting the stomach or intestine barium and/or air contrast techniques are necessary. For some deep-seated tumours e.g. pancreas or brain other methods of imaging are required. These include angiography, radioactive scintiscans, ultrasonography and computerised tomography (see Ch. 1).

Tumours may also be recognised by functional disturbances. This may be demonstrated by physical (e.g. electroencephalographic) or biochemical abnormalities. Abnormal liver function may indicate invasion of the liver by tumour.

These various diagnostic procedures have been fully discussed in Chapter 1.

## Pre-symptomatic diagnosis

It is recognised that by the time a tumour is first clinically apparent it may already be far advanced.

This has led to the presymptomatic diagnosis of tumours by 'screening'. Air contrast barium studies and endoscopy can be used to detect mucosal cancers of the stomach, mammography to detect impalpable breast cancer, cytological examination of urinary deposits to detect cancer of the bladder and the cytology of vaginal secretions to detect cancer of the cervix. Screening is costly and effectiveness must be critically evaluated before routine use.

## Histological diagnosis

Neoplastic disease can be detected cytologically e.g. by the demonstration of malignant cells in secretions, in washings, or in needle aspirates. However a definitive histological diagnosis must be made in all cases of suspected cancer. A surgeon must never perform a major mutilating procedure for cancer without histological proof of malignant disease. The suggestion that a preliminary biopsy can facilitate the spread of cancer is not supported by fact and punch, needle and drill biopsies are now established techniques (Ch. 1).

Initial histological diagnosis allows the further investigation and treatment of the disease with knowledge of its proven diagnosis.

## STAGING

The objective of 'staging' is to define the extent of the disease and its likely prognosis. The International Union against Cancer (UICC) has described a system of clinical staging by which the tumour (T), regional lymph nodes (N), and metastatic spread (M) are documented separately. Clinical, radiological and endoscopic investigations are used (Table 15.2).

Although clinical staging is still important in defining the extent of the local disease and allowing comparisons between series of patients, its value in detecting the extent of metastatic spread is limited. The palpability of regional lymph nodes is a poor indicator of their involvement by tumour. Impalpable nodes may still contain metastases; palpable nodes are not necessarily involved by tumour. Reactive hyperplasia in regional lymph nodes is associated with many tumours.

**Table 15.2** TNM pre-treatment classification, post treatment histopathological classifications have also been defined

*T — Primary tumour*
The following general definitions are used throughout:

| | |
|---|---|
| Tis | Pre-invasive carcinoma (carcinoma-in-situ) |
| T0 | No evidence of primary tumour |
| T1, T2, T3, T4 | Evidence of increasing degrees of size and/or local extent of primary tumour |
| TX | The minimum requirements to assess the primary tumour cannot be met |

*N — Regional lymph nodes*
The following general definitions are used throughout:

| | |
|---|---|
| N0 | No evidence of regional lymph node involvement |
| N1, N2, N3 | Evidence of increasing degrees of involvement of regional lymph nodes |
| N4 | Evidence of involvement of juxta-regional lymph nodes (where applicable) |
| NX | The minimum requirements to assess the regional lymph nodes cannot be met |

*M — Distant metastases*
The following general definitions are used throughout:

| | |
|---|---|
| M0 | No evidence of distant metastases |
| M1 | Evidence of distant metastases |

The category M1 may be subdivided, according to the following notation:

| | | | |
|---|---|---|---|
| Pulmonary: | PUL | Bone Marrow: | MAR |
| Osseous: | OSS | Pleura: | PLE |
| Hepatic: | HEP | Peritoneum: | PER |
| Brain: | BRA | Skin: | SKI |
| Lymph Nodes: | LYM | Other: | OTH |

| | |
|---|---|
| MX | The minimum requirements to assess the presence of distant metastases cannot be met |

Small deposits of tumour in viscera and bones cannot be detected by routine radiology. Even the resolution of radio-isotope scintiscans, ultrasonography and CT scans is insufficient to detect small deposits. Many patients who, on clinical and radiological grounds, are believed to have localised (Mo) disease have unrecognised widespread microscopic deposits of a tumour.

Biochemical 'markers' to detect functional abnormalities from invasion of organs or tissues are seldom helpful (Table 15.3). Although metastases in the liver may cause elevation of liver enzymes and metastases in bone elevation of the urinary excretion of collagen breakdown products (hydroxyproline), such tests are rarely of value in detecting occult metastatic disease. One requires a specific 'marker' of tumour burden by which the presence of residual tumour following the removal of the primary site can be recognised.

**Table 15.3** Some tumour markers.

| Marker | 'Relative Tissue Specificity' |
| --- | --- |
| Human chorionic gonadotrophin (HCG) | Chorion Testis |
| Acid phosphatase | Prostate |
| Carcinoembryonic antigen (CEA) | Colon and rectum Breast Liver Bronchus Pancreas |
| Fetoprotein | Liver Testis |
| Thyrocalcitonin | Thyroid |
| Tyrosinase | Melanoma Breast |
| Creatine-kinase BB | Prostate Breast |
| B-glucuronidase | Leptomeningeal |
| Breast-cyst fluid protein (BCFP) | Breast |
| Pancreatic oncofoetal antigen (POA) | Pancreas |

These are available for prostatic cancer (acid phosphatase), testicular and chorionic cancer (gonadotrophins), neuroblastoma (catecholamines) and, to some extent, colon (CEA) and liver (alphafetoprotein) cancers. CEA and alpha-fetoprotein are two of the so-called 'oncofetal antigens'. These are secreted by fetal tissues and some tumours. Other 'markers' reflect the turnover of nucleoproteins e.g. the levels of polyamines and methylated nucleosides in the urine. However, the main value of all such estimates is not in early disease but to monitor the progress of recurrent disease by serial assay.

Currently the most reliable indicator of the extent of a malignant tumour is the histology of the regional lymph nodes. Lymphangiography may be of value in detecting metastases from some tumours, e.g. melanoma, lymphoma, testicular tumours, but in general histological evidence is the only certain method. Even more accurate staging is possible by additional surgical procedures. The assessment of lymphomas now includes bone and marrow sampling and a full laparotomy at which the spleen is removed for histological examination and biopsies are taken of retroperitoneal lymph nodes and liver. In some tumours, e.g. bladder and large bowel, the histological assessment of the depth of mural penetration is also an important index of extent and prognosis.

The prognosis of a tumour is also affected by its biological characteristics. Its size, contour, degree of nuclear and cellular anaplasia and the extent of lymphocytic infiltration all influence outcome. Lymphomas with cell surface receptors for immunoglobulins respond better to systemic chemotherapy than those without; breast cancers which contain cytoplasmic protein with a high affinity for binding oestrogen (oestrogen receptors) are more likely to respond to hormonal measures and have a better prognosis than those without.

The degree of reactivity of regional lymph nodes to the tumour, as indicated by the appearance of sinus histiocytosis, is also correlated with prognosis. Tumours associated with marked changes fare better than those associated with inactive lymph nodes. This reactive change may represent a host-tumour response.

## TREATMENT

### Local disease

*Benign tumours.* Provided sufficient surrounding tissue is excised to ensure its complete removal a benign tumour is cured by local excision. In some benign tumours, e.g. pleomorphic adenomas of the parotid, extension occurs beyond their apparent macroscopic limits. Removal of the gland or organ is the only sure way to cure (Fig. 15.10).

*Malignant tumours.* Some malignant tumours grow slowly, have little tendency to recur and may be cured by local excision. In many cancers however, local treatment has as its main objective control of local disease and the reduction of tumour burden. Control of the disease as a whole also requires systemic treatment.

The extent of the local treatment required for a malignant tumour depends on knowledge of its natural history, in particular the likelihood of local recurrence and of multi-focal deposits. The anatomy of the part involved is an important consideration as damage to nearby tissues must be avoided. The establishment of a balance between relief of symptoms and morbidity is difficult; the quality of life is as important as survival.

The general objective is to excise the primary tumour with as wide a margin of normal tissue as is practicable. In most sites this requires removal of the organ of origin.

During an operation for cancer care is taken to try to avoid spillage of malignant cells. In some sites, e.g. testes, large bowel, many surgeons ligate the main vessels draining the tumour region before it is mobilised so that the shedding of malignant cells into the circulation is avoided.

Before handling a tumour of the bowel, a ligature is placed proximally and distally to prevent spillage of cells into the lumen of remaining bowel, a cause of recurrence at the anastomotic site. Many surgeons now irrigate a wound or body cavity with 1:500 cetrimide to destroy 'free floating' cells and minimise the likelihood of local recurrence, but there is little evidence that this is of value.

*Radiotherapy* is a useful alternative to surgery in some forms of cancer. The development of high-energy irradiation with megavoltage X-rays, accelerated electrons and beams of heavy particles permits more effective radiation of the tumour with less damage to the skin and surrounding tissues (Fig. 15.11). Techniques to increase tumour sensitivity to X-rays are under study. These include hyperbaric oxygenation and radio-sensitising drugs. However, many tumours are resistant to all forms of radiation.

Radiotherapy is also used to increase the local control achieved by surgery. An example is the treatment of the chest wall with postoperative radiotherapy in breast cancer (Fig. 15.11).

*Lymph nodes.* The management of regional lymph nodes varies according to the site and type of a tumour. With some tumours, e.g. of the gastro-intestinal tract, breast and testes, regional lymph nodes are routinely resected or irradiated irrespective of their involvement. In others, e.g. malignant melanoma, head and neck cancer, regional lymph nodes are treated only if they are proven to contain metastatic growth. This variation in practice has arisen from considerations of technique and morbidity rather than from any logical plan of management. In general it is those nodes which can readily be removed in continuity

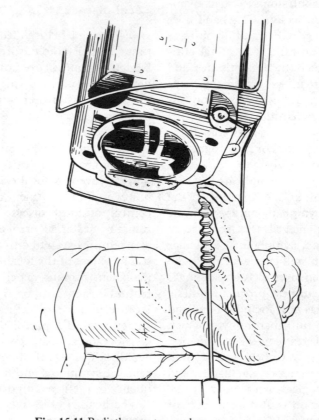

**Fig. 15.11** Radiotherapy to supplement mastectomy

with the primary tumour which have been treated by primary en-bloc excision. Removal of uninvolved nodes has no therapeutic advantage. By contrast removal of involved nodes is a rational way to reduce tumour burden and prevent progression of regional disease. Prior sampling of lymph nodes for histological examination is a rational development particularly in sites where node dissection causes severe morbidity e.g. the neck and groin.

Radiotherapy may also be used to treat regional lymph nodes and so prevent the continued growth of lymphatic deposits. Such irradiation of nodes is used routinely for some tumours e.g. seminoma testis.

### Systemic therapy

'Adjuvant' systemic chemotherapy is now advised for many types of cancer. Its objective is the control of occult metastatic disease. Effective agents are still lacking, particularly in solid tumours, and controlled therapeutic trials to assess the value of chemotherapeutic agents are an essential pre-requisite to their routine use. Chemotherapy is toxic; morbidity and the quality of life must always be considered before advising this form of treatment.

Recognition that different chemotherapeutic agents may act at specific points in the cell cycle has led to combinations of cell cycle-dependent and independent drugs. Such regimes, which may be administered for months or even years, have revolutionised the management of lymphomas but as yet are of little proven value in solid tumours.

Other methods of systemic therapy, e.g. suppression of circulating hormones or stimulation of the immune system, are under study. Some of these methods necessitate surgical procedures such as the removal of endocrine glands.

---

## PALLIATION OF ADVANCED CANCER

The terminal stages of malignancy can be prolonged and pain and other distressing symptoms are frequent. Effective palliation is achieved by

1. local and/or systemic therapy to induce tumour regression
2. non-specific treatment which does not affect tumour growth but relieves symptoms.

## SPECIFIC THERAPY

Tumour regression can be achieved by local radiotherapy or by systemic hormone or chemotherapy. The choice of treatment varies according to tumour type. Surgery has little place in the palliation of advanced malignant disease. However, local excision of an ulcerating or fungating tumour may prove worthwhile: the palliative resection of gastric or rectal tumours spares considerable discomfort. Surgery may also relieve functional upsets caused by tumours e.g. dysphagia, intestinal obstruction or impending paraplegia.

When a palliative operation is performed the patient and his relatives should understand that its object is to prevent additional suffering and not to attempt cure.

## SYMPTOMATIC CARE

### Pain relief

A wide range of analgesic and narcotic drugs are available to relieve pain. The choice depends on the type of pain, its severity and the stage of illness. The aim is to achieve complete analgesia without impairing mental clarity or inducing side effects. Some commonly used agents are shown in Table 15.4.

The patient must never 'wait' for his next dose of analgesia. Schedules of administration are planned to prevent rather than treat pain. When pain is severe narcotic drugs should be used; fear of addiction is irrelevant.

The best narcotic mixture is morphine sulphate (starting with 5–10 mg) and prochlorperazine (5 mg) in chloroform water. This is as effective as the traditional Brompton cocktail and doses of morphine up to 60 mg four-hourly can be given in this way. For parenteral therapy diamorphine is the drug of choice. The initial dose is 5 mg four hourly; this is increased as required.

Other measures may aid pain relief. That due

**Table 15.4** Analgesics used in cancer therapy.

| | Preparations | Dosage | Contraindications | Side effects |
|---|---|---|---|---|
| **MILD AND MODERATE PAIN** | | | | |
| *Non-narcotics* | | | | |
| aspirin | tabs 300 mg | 300–900 mg 4-hourly | peptic ulcer anticoagulants | gastric irritation |
| paracetamol (Panadol) | tabs 500 mg syrup 120 mg/5 ml | 500 mg–1 g 4-hourly | hepatic impairment | hepatotoxic |
| naproxen (Naprosyn) | tabs 250, 500 mg syrup 125 mg/5 mg suppositories 500 mg | 250 mg 6-hourly | – | mild |
| mefanamic acid (Ponstan) | caps 250 mg tabs 500 mg | 500 mg tid | hypersensitive states | diarrhoea dizziness |
| ibuprofen | tabs 200, 400, 600 mg syrup 100 mg/5 ml | 2 g daily | – | mild gastrointestinal upset |
| *Narcotics* | | | | |
| codeine phosphate | tabs 15, 30 mg syrup 25 mg/5 ml injection 60 mg/ml | 10–60 mg 4-hourly | hepatic impairment respiratory disease | constipation dizziness |
| dihydrocodeine tartrate (DF 118) | tabs 30 mg | 30 mg 4-hourly | hepatic impairment respiratory disease | constipation dizziness |
| pentazocine (Fortral) | caps 50 mg tabs 25 mg injection 30 mg/μl suppository 50 mg | 25–100 mg 4-hourly | | hallucinations |
| dextropropoxyphene hydrochloride | tabs 32.5 mg plus paracetamol 325 mg (Distalgesic) | tabs 2 3– daily | | respiratory depression |
| **SEVERE PAIN** | | | | |
| *Narcotics* | | | | |
| Methadone hydrochloride (Physeptone) | tabs 5 mg injection 10 mg/μl | 5–10 mg 6-hourly | – | constipation nausea |
| pethidine hydrochloride | tabs 25.5 mg injection 50 mg/ml | 50–150 mg 4-hourly | renal impairment | nephrotoxic |
| phenazocine hydrochloride (Narphen) | tabs 5 mg | 5 mg 4-hourly | poor respiratory reserve mono-amine oxidase inhibitor therapy asthma increased intracranial pressure | constipation nausea respiratory depression urinary retention |
| buprenorphine (Temgesic) | tabs 200 μg (Sublingual) injection 300 μg/ml | 200 μg 8-hourly — 400 μg | poor respiratory reserve mono-amine oxidase inhibitor therapy asthma increased intracranial pressure | constipation nausea respiratory depression urinary retention |
| diamorphine hydrochloride (heroin) | tabs 5, 10 mg injection 5 mg/10 mg per ml suppositories 10 mg | 5–10 mg 4-hourly | poor respiratory reserve mono-amine oxidase inhibitor therapy asthma increased intracranial pressure | constipation nausea respiratory depression urinary retention |
| morphine | tabs 10 mg 30 mg injection 10, 30 mg/ml elixir 8.4 mg/ml suppositories 15 mg | 10–20 mg 4-hourly | poor respiratory reserve mono-amine oxidase inhibitor therapy asthma increased intracranial pressure | constipation nausea respiratory depression urinary retention |

to intracerebral or nerve root compression can be helped by dexamethasone (8 mg daily in divided doses). Pain may also be reduced by neurosurgical procedures (see Chapter 22). Supplementation of analgesics with anti-emetics — prochlorperazine (Stemetil) 5– 10 mg— and tranquillisers —chlorpromazine(Largactil) 25–50 mg— prevents nausea and relaxes the patient.

## Other symptoms

*Vomiting* is caused by mechanical obstruction of stomach or intestine, by drug toxicity, or by anxiety and fear. Reassurance, attention to diet, sedatives and anti-emetics may help. Obstructive vomiting may require surgical relief.

*Dysphagia* due to oesophageal obstruction is distressful as the patient cannot swallow his saliva. Relief can be provided by the insertion of a prosthetic tube. Gastrostomy and jejunostomy do not relieve dysphagia but add to the patient's discomfort. They are seldom indicated.

*Dyspnoea* can be helped by a bronchial dilator e.g. salbutamol or aminophylline. Diffuse lymphangitic permeation of the lungs can cause severe respiratory distress which may be helped by prednisone therapy (10–15 mg t.i.d). Purulent sputum may indicate the need for antibiotic therapy. Episodic bouts of acute dyspnoea terrify a patient, particularly at night. Adequate sedation is essential. Excess bronchial secretions may be controlled with atropine.

*Thrush*. The majority of patients with terminal cancer develop a monilial infection. Nystatin suspension gives considerable improvement in appetite and well-being. Sucking a slice of fresh pineapple is a good way to cleanse the mouth.

The smell of a *fungating lesion* is distressing, and may be minimised by isolation in a well-ventilated cubicle with deodorant aerosols or fumigators and frequent dressings of eusol, 4% povidone (Betadine) in liquid paraffin or proflavine emulsion. Adequate *sleep* is essential. Nitrazepam (Mogadon) is best except for the elderly when chlormethizole (Heminevrin) is preferred.

## CARE OF THE DYING

Death from malignant disease is usually a gradual process of withdrawal. A sympathetic doctor can greatly help the patient and his relatives. A dying patient must never feel abandoned on a surgical ward; doctors and nursing staff must be prepared to spend time to help the patient die with dignity.

It is not usual to tell patients that they are dying from malignant disease but relatives must be kept informed. In some circumstances frank but kind discussion with the patient and relatives can do much to restore confidence and prepare for the inevitable outcome.

The attention of a doctor must not cease after the death of a patient. A few words of sympathy by a member of the surgical staff can give comfort to the bereaved relatives.

# 16. The Acute Abdomen

Many conditions produce acute abdominal pain. Comprehensive coverage of each is not feasible but the principles of assessment and management of the patient with acute abdominal pain will be defined, and certain problem areas considered. Specific causes of the acute abdomen are considered in detail elsewhere.

## PRINCIPLES OF ASSESSMENT AND DIAGNOSIS

### THE HISTORY

Patients with acute abdominal pain may present at any time of the day or night demanding prompt assessment and treatment without recourse to many of the usual diagnostic aids. There is no substitute for experience in the management of these patients, and a *full history and physical examination* is fundamental.

### ABDOMINAL PAIN

#### Innervation of abdomen

The perception of abdominal pain is subserved by both autonomic (*visceral* pain) and somatic nervous systems (*somatic* pain).

*Visceral afferents* run from nerve endings in the muscle of the intestine and other abdominal organs along the path of the sympathetic nerves, joining the pre-sacral and the splanchnic nerves to cross to the sensory roots through rami communicantes to enter the lumbar (L1–2) and thoracic (T6–12) regions of the spinal cord (Fig. 16.1). The nerve supply to those viscera which have developed from the primitive gut which, embryologically, is a midline structure, is bilat-

eral. The nerve supply to paired organs such as the kidneys and testicles, is unilateral. Visceral pain is abolished by division of the splanchnic nerves or by blocking their conduction by local anaesthesia. The *vagus nerve* has no role in the appreciation of abdominal pain.

*Somatic afferents* supply the abdominal wall including its lining of parietal peritoneum. These accompany the segmental nerves and gain access to the spinal cord through the appropriate dorsal root (T5–L2). The peritoneum under the diaphragm is an exception in that it is supplied by the phrenic nerve (C3,4&5) which descends with the diaphragm from the neck (Fig. 16.2).

#### Perception of pain

*Visceral pain.* Pain arising in a hollow organ such as the intestine is evoked by distension or excessive contraction. Local ischaemia may also contribute to intestinal pain and in some conditions, e.g. mesenteric vascular occlusion, may be the dominant component. Obstruction of a hollow viscus causes bouts of excruciating, cramping pain as increased muscle contractions attempt to overcome the blockage. This is called 'colic'. The frequency of the bouts of pain varies according to the viscus involved (Fig. 16.3).

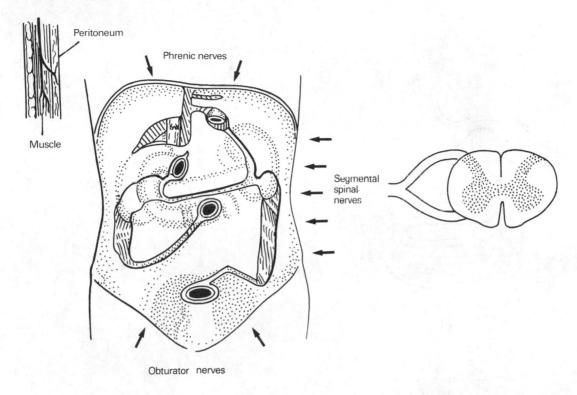

**Fig. 16.1** The sensory innervation of the abdominal cavity. (a) Parietal peritoneum.

The pain of peptic ulceration is due to muscular spasm and/or direct irritation of exposed nerve endings by acid. Handling, cutting or clamping the intestine does not cause pain unless the mesentery is dragged upon and stretched.

Pain arises from a solid organ as a result of pressure and/or congestion. There are variations between organs. The liver, spleen and kidney are insensitive to pressure or incision unless inflamed, while the testis and the renal pelvis normally are sensitive to pressure alone. Thus acute hepatitis is painful as is compression injury to the testis.

Visceral pain is dull, deep-seated and cannot be precisely localised. That arising from the intestine and its outgrowths (liver, spleen, pancreas) is felt in the mid-line. Pain from the foregut (e.g. peptic ulcer pain) is epigastric; that from the mid-gut (e.g. obstruction of small bowel or appendix) is peri-umbilical; and that from the hind-gut (e.g. colonic obstruction) is hypogastric.

The unilateral pain which arises from paired organs (kidney and testis) is also perceived in the embryological position of the organ. Pain from the testis is often felt low in the abdomen, rather than in the scrotum.

*Somatic pain.* The visceral peritoneum is insensitive. The parietal peritoneum, lining the abdominal wall, is sensitive to tactile, thermal or chemical stimuli. It cannot be cut, cauterised or handled painlessly. Potent chemical irritants include bile, escaped intestinal contents, enzyme-rich exudates and bacterial inflammation.

Somatic pain is sharp (knife-like), and readily localised to its site of origin. The exception is that which arises from the diaphragmatic peritoneum which is perceived in the shoulder region (Fig. 16.3). Painful stimulation of the parietal peritoneum is associated with reflex muscle guarding, rigidity and hyperaesthesia. Diffusion of the products of inflammation through the peritoneum into the overlying muscle may contribute to some of these effects.

*Mixed pain.* Some abdominal conditions cause both visceral and somatic pain. For example, an attack of acute appendicitis may start with

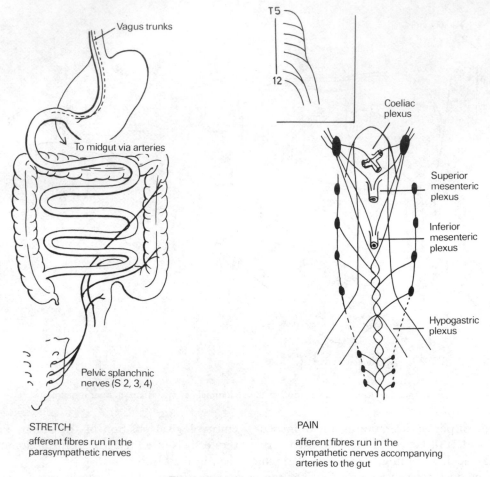

**Fig. 16.1** (b) Abdominal viscera.

visceral pain due to obstruction of the appendix. This is dull, diffuse and experienced in the region of the umbilicus. Once the inflammatory process has spread through the wall of the appendix and irritates the parietal peritoneum, the pain becomes somatic and is sharp and well-localised.

## Other factors

The *mode of onset* of the pain is important. Explosive onset of excruciating abdominal pain suggests a vascular accident or perforation of a hollow viscus. Colic due to obstruction of the biliary tract, gut or urinary tract may also have a sudden onset, but this is not often described as explosive. Pain which starts gradually and worsens progressively is typical of peritonitis.

The *severity* of pain is difficult to define objec-

tively as patients vary greatly in their reaction. Excruciating pain which is unrelieved by conventional doses of narcotics usually indicates a vascular catastrophe. The severe, intermittent pain of colic, and the severe pain of acute pancreatitis or perforation of a peptic ulcer, are usually more amenable to relief by narcotics. Pain which arises as a consequence of progressive peritonitis without initial perforation (e.g. acute appendicitis) is typically dull, gradually increases in severity, and becomes less well localised with the passage of time.

The *localisation* of visceral pain is imprecise (see above). While localisation of parietal pain is precise, it is complicated by the spread of peritonitis. *Referral* of pain to other areas can confuse unless interpreted correctly. Thus, irritation of the diaphragmatic peritoneum by blood, air or

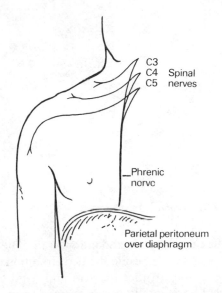

Fig. 16.2 The shared sensory innervation of the shoulder and the diaphragm

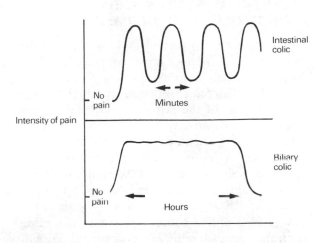

Fig. 16.3 The differing patterns of intestinal and biliary colic

gastro-intestinal content, may give pain and hyperaesthesia in the shoulder tip. Pain from the biliary tract may be referred to the right scapular region; the pain of ureteric colic may radiate into the groin. A *shift* of pain may also aid diagnosis. The classic example is acute appendicitis where the initial central abdominal colic of appendiceal obstruction eventually gives way to pain in the right iliac fossa as parietal peritonitis develops. Gradual spread of pain throughout the abdomen usually indicates development of diffuse peritonitis.

It is important to appreciate that a lessening of pain does not necessarily indicate that the underlying condition has resolved. The excruciating pain of mesenteric vascular occlusion may wane despite the presence of gangrenous bowel. Following perforation of a peptic ulcer there is frequently a 'period of illusion' where pain diminishes temporarily despite progressive peritonitis. Diminution of pain may also occur in the terminal stages of peritonitis, regardless of cause.

## ANOREXIA, NAUSEA AND VOMITING

These are common symptoms in patients with acute abdominal pain, but are not always present.

Anorexia is particularly common in acute appendicitis, while nausea, retching and vomiting are prominent features of acute pancreatitis, high intestinal obstruction and obstruction of the biliary tract. Gastroenteritis can simulate an acute surgical condition, but the nausea and vomiting frequently *precede* the onset of colic which is associated with diarrhoea.

## ALTERATION IN BOWEL HABIT

Many acute abdominal conditions develop so rapidly that there is no time for alteration in bowel habit to become apparent. With complete intestinal obstruction inability to pass flatus or faeces eventually occurs, but in the initial stages there may be one or more bowel movements as the gut distal to the obstruction is evacuated by strong peristaltic waves passing on beyond the site of obstruction. Diarrhoea is a marked feature in gastroenteritis or colitis but can also occur as a manifestation of pelvic sepsis, as for example in acute pelvic appendicitis. Blood is present in the stool in some cases of mesenteric vascular occlusion, but repeated bloody diarrhoea is much more likely to be due to ulcerative colitis or dysentery. It must not be forgotten that bleeding from the upper gastro-intestinal tract may produce massive melaena without haematemesis.

## MENSTRUAL STATUS AND GYNAECOLOGICAL DISEASE

The frequency of menstruation and date of the last menstrual period must be established in female patients.

The Graafian follicle normally ruptures 14 days after the start of the last menstrual period, and release of the ovum may be complicated by bleeding. This is the cause of the lower abdominal pain which occurs half-way through the menstrual cycle, notably in young girls: 'mittelschmerz' (middle-pain). The follicle then becomes a corpus luteum which degenerates before the start of the next period unless conception occurs. Bleeding from the corpus luteum is an occasional cause of pain in the late stages of the menstrual cycle.

Females of child-bearing age should be asked about contraceptive practice and the likelihood of pregnancy. Rupture of an ectopic pregnancy is an acute abdominal condition which demands prompt treatment. Lower abdominal and shoulder-tip pain (due to blood irritating the diaphragmatic peritoneum) is characteristic and 'withdrawal bleeding' due to cessation of hormone production following death of the embryo is frequent. This is scanty and dark, and follows the pain, in contrast to the profuse bright red bleeding which precedes the pain of abortion.

Low abdominal pain and tenderness can also be caused by acute salpingitis. A history of purulent vaginal discharge may provide a useful clue.

## EXAMINATION

### ABDOMINAL EXAMINATION

Physical signs may be reduced in the elderly, grossly obese, gravely ill, and in patients on steroid therapy. As sedation also obscures pain and tenderness, it is best avoided until a decision on management has been made. This rule is relaxed when pain is severe, or in young children, in whom abdominal examination may not be practicable without sedation.

Abdominal examination is carried out with the patient lying flat and the abdomen uncovered from xiphisternum to groin. Flexing of the thighs

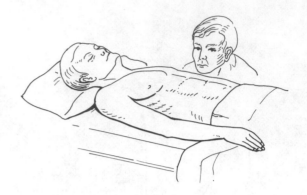

**Fig. 16.4** Inspection of the abdomen

will relax the anterior abdominal wall. The clinician sits or kneels beside the bed (traditionally on the right side) so that his arm and hand can be extended horizontally across the abdomen.

### Inspection

Inspection is the essential first step (Fig. 16.4). The presence of scars, the bulging of hernias or other abnormal masses may be seen. A note is made of whether the abdomen moves freely with respiration and the patient should be asked to 'blow out his abdomen' so that the flaccidity of the abdominal wall can be assessed. The abdominal contour is assessed.

The abdomen is distended in most cases of intestinal obstruction, whereas it is indrawn and scaphoid in the early stages of perforation of a viscus. Following a perforation the patient usually lies still with the abdomen rigid for fear of exacerbating the pain by movement, whereas patients with colic are restless and may not be able to lie still during examination. Patients with acute pancreatitis sometimes find that sitting forwards relieves their pain, and are uncomfortable when lying flat. Peristalsis is occasionally visible in intestinal obstruction.

### Palpation

Palpation follows inspection. It is first carried out gently to detect tenderness and muscle guarding. Tenderness is sought by gentle palpation with all of the fingers of one hand, holding them extended at the interphalangeal joints and gently flexing

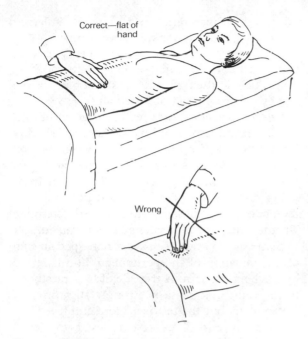

Fig. 16.5 Palpation of the abdomen

and extending the metacarpophalangeal joints (Fig. 16.5). Tenderness is sought first in those areas furthest from the patient's pain. Inflammation of the parietal peritoneum causes a reflex increase in overlying muscle tone which is detected on palpation as *guarding* of the muscles concerned, and in its extreme form as board-like *rigidity* of the abdominal wall.

Inflammation of the peritoneum lining the anterior abdominal wall is easy to detect. Direct tenderness and guarding are obvious on abdominal examination. Detection of peritonitis affecting other areas of the abdominal cavity may prove more difficult. Pelvic peritonitis may produce little or no tenderness or guarding on examination of the abdomen, though digital rectal examination is very painful. Inflammation of the diaphragmatic peritoneum does not cause abdominal guarding or tenderness. Shoulder-tip pain is present but radiological screening is needed to reveal restricted diaphragmatic movement. Peritonitis involving the posterior parietal peritoneum may produce few signs on abdominal examination. It is for this reason that the symptoms of acute pancreatitis and retrocaecal appendicitis overshadow the abdominal signs.

Guarding and rigidity of the muscles of the anterior abdominal wall usually denotes peritonitis. However, it may also occur in renal colic, rare neurological disorders, and hysteria or malingering. In renal colic, rigidity is confined to the muscles of the affected side while the voluntary spasm of hysteria can be overcome if the examining hand remains on the abdomen while the patient is asked to breathe deeply, or when his attention is distracted by questioning.

*Deep palpation.* Once gentle palpation has defined areas of tenderness and guarding, deep palpation is used to detect abdominal masses. In the acute situation, these include intra-abdominal abscesses, empyema of the gallbladder, diverticulitis, aortic aneurysms, twisted ovarian cyst, and intussusception.

It is also important to palpate each organ in turn, seeking enlargement of liver, spleen and kidneys.

## Percussion

Percussion is used to delineate abdominal organs and abnormal masses, and to determine the cause of abdominal distension. The percussion note is tympanitic when distension is due to gas, as in intestinal obstruction, and dull when distension results from fluid, as in ascites or a full bladder. The situation of the dullness (whether in the flanks or suprapubically) and whether it shifts on change of posture is noted. Free air rises within the peritoneal cavity so that perforation of the gastro-intestinal tract may be associated with diminution or absence of liver dullness as air accumulates beneath the diaphragm.

Gentle percussion may also be used as a means of detecting rebound tenderness in inflammatory disease.

## Auscultation

Auscultation is an essential routine, and it should be carried out centrally to detect bowel sounds and over masses and arterial sites (aorta-epigastrium, renal, iliacs) to detect vascular bruits. It should be remembered that the normal heart sounds may be heard in a distended abdomen. Auscultation may have to be prolonged and repeated when there is doubt about the presence or frequency of bowel sounds (peristaltic activity). Peristalsis is increased in mechanical intestinal obstruction, by gastroenteritis, and by the presence of blood in the bowel lumen. Activity ceases in paralytic ileus but bowel sounds may still be heard in the initial stages of mesenteric vascular occlusion. The detection of a bruit during auscultation may indicate vascular disease.

### Examination of the groin

Examination of the groin is important yet easily forgotten. Many experienced clinicians begin their examination in this area. Detection of a small inguinal or femoral hernia may be particularly important in intestinal obstruction. The patient may be unaware that he had a hernia and the central localisation of abdominal colic may focus attention away from the region.

Pus tracking down the psoas sheath is a rare cause of groin swelling. A colonic neoplasm may occasionally perforate retroperitoneally and cause crepitus and erythema in the groin.

The femoral pulses must be palpated routinely during examination of the groin. In the male the testes and scrotum are also examined (see Chapter 37).

### Digital rectal examination

Digital rectal examination is mandatory and performed by a strict routine (Fig. 16.6). Tenderness on rectal examination may be the only sign of pelvic appendicitis. Cervical tenderness may be associated with salpingitis and abnormalities of the male prostate should be sought. Faecal impaction can be detected and a specimen of stool can be tested for occult blood so that the need for proctoscopy or sigmoidoscopy can be assessed.

Should disease of the uterus, fallopian tubes or ovaries be suspected, a vaginal examination is also performed.

### Special clinical tests

*Murphy's sign* is a sign of peritoneal tenderness in acute cholecystitis. The patient is asked to take a deep breath while the examiner palpates over the region of the gallbladder. A catching of breath at the zenith of inspiration occurs as the inflamed gallbladder contacts the examiner's fingers.

*Rovsing's sign* is present in some cases of acute appendicitis. Deep palpation in the left iliac fossa causes pain in the right iliac fossa. In practice the sign is inconstant and of little value.

*Rebound tenderness* denotes a resurgence of pain as the examiner's hand is withdrawn sharply while palpating the abdomen. It indicates parietal peritonitis but its value is controversial. Overzealous attempts to elicit rebound tenderness inflict unnecessary pain, and light percussion of the abdominal wall is a better way to determine whether the parietal peritoneum is inflamed.

*Cutaneous hyperaesthesia* is a non-specific sign of inflammation of the peritoneum and is tested by pricking the skin. A triangle of hyperaesthesia in the right iliac fossa is strongly suggestive of appendicitis but the test is seldom employed.

*Ilio-psoas test.* This test is used to detect restriction of movement of the iliacus and psoas major muscles. The patient lies on his side with the side to be tested uppermost and the ilio-psoas muscle is stretched by fully extending the thigh (Fig. 16.7). Restriction of movement may be elicited when there is retrocaecal inflammation e.g. from appendicitis or a perinephric abscess. When inflammation is advanced the patient sometimes lies with the hip flexed on the affected side to relax the irritated psoas muscle. The ilio-psoas test cannot be interpreted when there is rigidity of the abdominal wall muscles.

*Obturator test.* This is a method of detecting pelvic peritonitis irritating the obturator internus muscle. Deep-seated pain occurs when the thigh is flexed at right angles to the trunk and the leg internally rotated (Fig. 16.8).

The ilio-psoas and obturator tests are little used today.

## INTERPRETATION OF VITAL SIGNS

The *temperature* is often normal in the early stages of peritonitis. Elevation denotes infection, but not necessarily within the abdomen. In the severely shocked patient it may be normal or subnormal despite advanced infection.

*Tachycardia* is present in most acute abdominal conditions. The pulse rate may be increased by

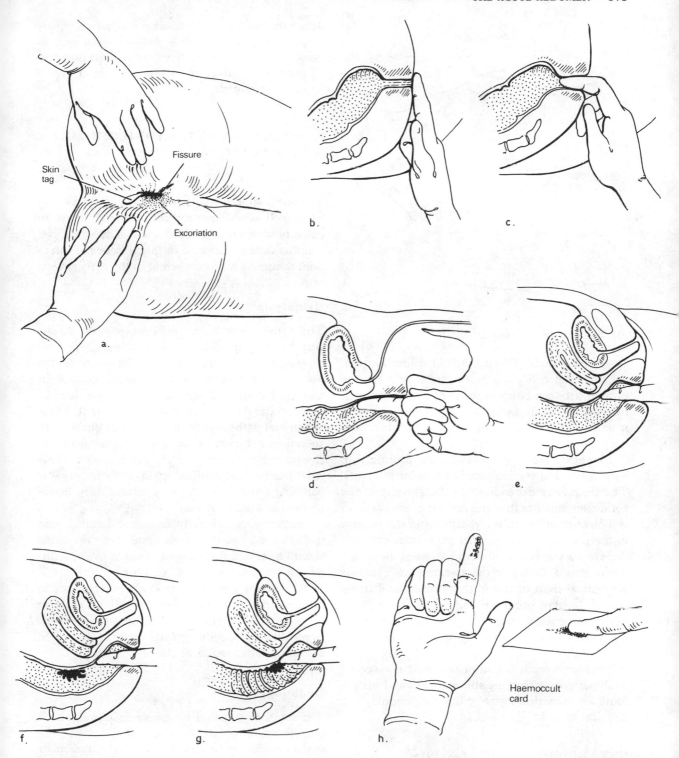

**Fig. 16.6** Rectal examination. (a) Inspection. (b) & (c) Introduction of the finger. (d) Palpation of the prostate. (e) Palpation of the cervix. (f) & (g) If a lesion is outwith the reach of the examiner's finger, then asking the patient to strain may be of assistance. (h) Always test for faecal occult blood.

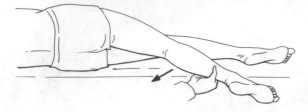

**Fig. 16.7** The psoas test

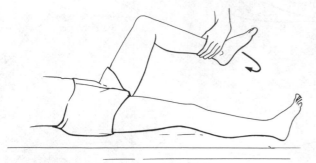

**Fig. 16.8** The obturator test

severe pain alone. When the pain is intermittent, e.g. in renal colic, the pulse rate may return to normal between bouts of pain. The pulse must be monitored in all cases. A progressive increase usually indicates infection or circulatory insufficiency.

The *blood pressure* is determined routinely on admission, and is monitored at regular intervals. The frequency depends upon the severity of the condition and whether the patient is shocked.

The *respiration rate* is typically rapid and shallow in the presence of abdominal pain. Intra-thoracic disease can produce abdominal pain, but high fever, cough, flaring of the alae nasi and cyanosis are typical signs of respiratory problems. Flaring of the alae nasi occurs in abdominal disease only when movement of the diaphragm is impeded. Hyperventilation is an early sign of septicaemic shock.

Thorough examination of the chest is essential in all patients with acute abdominal pain. Laparotomy in a patient with basal pneumonia is a classical mistake.

## ESTABLISHING A DIAGNOSIS

Once a full history and physical examination has been completed an attempt should be made to define the nature of the disease process responsible, and to identify the organ or organ system involved (Table 16.1). A working diagnosis and its likely alternatives are made and further investigations arranged.

## LABORATORY AND RADIOLOGICAL AIDS TO DIAGNOSIS

### Haematology

The haemoglobin concentration, haematocrit and white cell count are routine determinations in patients with an acute abdomen. The white cell count is usually elevated in the presence of infection, though it may be normal in the early stages.

### Urinalysis

The urine must be tested routinely for sugar, acetone, protein, bile and urobilinogen. Testing for sugar is essential for the detection of the undiagnosed diabetic and to assess control in known diabetics. Diabetic patients are just as likely to develop an acute abdomen due to intra-abdominal pathology as non-diabetics but require special care during the operative and post-operative period (see Chapter 5). Diabetic keto-acidosis may produce abdominal pain without organic pathology and in such cases unnecessary laparotomy must be avoided.

Porphyria occasionally causes abdominal pain (p.181) and in those with a family trait the urine should be tested for porphobilinogen by the addition of Ehrlich's aldehyde reagent.

Microscopy will reveal pus cells and bacteria in urinary tract infection, and red blood cells in patients with renal colic. Measurement of urine osmolality or specific gravity may be useful in assessing dehydration or shock.

### Radiology

A chest X-ray should be taken on admission. It may show (1) primary chest pathology; (2) secondary chest pathology e.g. pleural effusion or pulmonary aspiration; (3) evidence of cardiac failure; or (4) free gas under the diaphragm. Where obstruction is suspected, erect and supine

**Table 16.1** Some non-traumatic causes of acute abdomen.

| Pathological process | Organ commonly involved | Disease | Page reference |
|---|---|---|---|
| Inflammation | Appendix | Acute appendicitis | 407 |
| | Gall-bladder | Acute cholecystitis | 490 |
| | Colonic diverticula | Acute diverticulitis | 427 |
| | Meckel's diverticulum | Acute diverticulitis | 396 |
| | Fallopian tube | Acute salpingitis | 180 |
| | Pancreas | Acute pancreatitis | 503 |
| Obstruction | Small intestine | Acute intestinal obstruction | 447 |
| | Colon | Acute intestinal obstruction | 447 |
| | Ureter | Ureteric colic | 595 |
| | Urethra | Acute retention of urine | 589 |
| Ischaemia | Small intestine (hernia) | Volvulus (strangulation) | 518 |
| | Mesenteric artery thrombosis | Intestinal infarction | 404 |
| | Ovarian cyst | Torsion | 179 |
| Perforation | Duodenum | Peforated peptic ulcer (peritonitis) | 377 |
| | Gall-bladder | Biliary peritonitis | 534 |
| | Colonic diverticulum or tumour | Faecal peritonitis | 428 |
| | Ectopic pregnancy | Haemoperitoneum | 179 |
| Arterial rupture | Spontaneous — splenic artery aneurysm | Haemoperitoneum | 544 |

abdominal films should be taken and may show distension and fluid levels. Otherwise, a supine film is satisfactory unless one is seeking evidence of an intestinal perforation, or wishes to exclude an aortic aneurysm when a lateral decubitus film is also taken. Radiological signs include localised ileus in such inflammatory conditions as appendicitis and pancreatitis, radio-opaque opacities in some patients with gallstones and urinary calculi, vascular calcification in aortic aneurysms. Abnormal enlargement or displacement of abdominal organs may point to the site of disease.

Gastro-intestinal perforation is not always associated with radiological evidence of free air in the peritoneum. In cases of doubt a gastrografin meal may be indicated. As gastrografin is water-soluble, it does not irritate the peritoneum. Gastrografin meals and enemas can also be used in the investigation of suspected intestinal obstruction.

Ultrasonography is the key investigation in the assessment of patients thought to have biliary tract disease. Intravenous pyelography is invaluable in the diagnosis of urinary tract obstruction or trauma. Angiography is used occasionally to investigate severe gastro-intestinal bleeding and genito-urinary haemorrhage. Ultrasonography is now preferred to aortography if a ruptured aortic aneurysm cannot be excluded on clinical examination.

**Peritoneal lavage**

Peritoneal lavage has an established place in assessing blunt abdominal trauma (see Chapter 11). Its value is less certain in acute abdominal conditions. Lavage is contra-indicated if distension or scarring are present. False negative (and to a lesser extent false positive) results may be misleading and most surgeons prefer to undertake laparotomy when a surgical cause for an acute abdomen cannot be excluded by conventional clinical examination.

**Clinical chemistry**

Urea and electrolyte determinations are seldom of diagnostic significance, but are essential in the assessment of fluid and electrolyte needs. The result of liver function tests are seldom available in time to influence initial management, but the earliest opportunity should be taken to establish a baseline, particularly in patients with liver and biliary tract disease. The serum amylase is a valuable aid when acute pancreatitis is suspected provided its limitations are borne in mind (see Chapter 31). Arterial blood gases, hydrogen ion concentration and standard bicarbonate should be measured in all shocked patients, and those with respiratory problems.

## COMPUTER-ASSISTED DIAGNOSIS

Computer-assisted diagnosis has been shown to improve the accuracy of diagnosis of acute abdominal pain to over 90%. The clinician alone will achieve an accuracy of only 70 to 80%. However, in the final analysis, the diagnosis and determination of the need for laparotomy are still based primarily on the history and interpretation of the physical findings (see Table 16.1).

## INSTITUTION OF TREATMENT

All patients suspected of having acute abdominal disease should be confined to bed, given nothing further by mouth, and wherever possible, analgesics withheld until a firm decision has been taken on the likely diagnosis and proposed management. If the patient has vomited, or upper gastrointestinal disease, obstruction or perforation is suspected, a nasogastric tube should be passed, and the stomach kept empty by regular or continuous aspiration. Patients requiring urgent laparotomy who have eaten within the past 4–6 hours should also have a tube passed so that the stomach is empty when anaesthesia is induced.

An intravenous line is inserted when there is blood loss, dehydration, shock or electrolyte disturbance or if these are anticipated. A fluid balance chart is essential. The bladder should be catheterised in shocked patients and when urinary retention is suspected. Pulse and temperature are recorded regularly in all cases, and regular recording of blood pressure, central venous pressure, and hourly urine output are essential in shocked patients.

The prescription of antibiotics should not be routine when infection is suspected but should await specific indications. For example, the majority of patients with acute pancreatitis or perforated peptic ulceration do not require antibiotics. Antibiotics are usually (but not invariably) prescribed in acute cholecystitis and are essential if peritonitis is thought to be due to colonic perforation. If antibiotic treatment is started before operation, blood samples for culture should be taken before the first dose is given.

Assessment of the need for laparotomy is an important objective of the surgeon's evaluation of the acute abdomen, but must never become the sole objective. One should always first construct a list of differential diagnosis, and attempt to define the diagnosis of greatest probability. The nature of the disease process and the organ or system involved should wherever possible be recorded in writing in the case notes.

The timing of operation is determined by the balance between the nature of the underlying disease process, the patient's general condition and the need for pre-operative resuscitation. Considerable delay may have elapsed before the patient is first seen by the surgeon, and as a general rule, conditions requiring surgery do deteriorate with time. However, while delay may be disastrous for a patient with a ruptured aortic aneurysm, adequate pre-operative resuscitation may prove life-saving for the grossly dehydrated patient with mechanical intestinal obstruction.

In many patients, the diagnosis and the indications for operation are uncertain at presentation and regular re-examination over the next few hours will clarify the position.

There are many instances when the surgeon must balance the risk of needless surgery against the danger of not operating promptly. For example, the penalty of not operating early in acute appendicitis far outweighs the dangers of laparotomy in mesenteric adenitis. To await signs which would make the clinical diagnosis of appendicitis certain would inevitably increase morbidity and mortality from gangrene and perforation. For this reason some surgeons will accept that the appendix may be normal in as many as 20% of emergency appendicectomies.

## SURGICAL CAUSES OF ACUTE ABDOMEN

The surgical causes of the acute abdomen have been listed in Table 16.1. They include obstructions, inflammatory disease (most commonly appendicitis, cholecystitis, diverticulitis and pancreatitis), perforation and strangulation and mesenteric ischaemia. All of these may lead to peritonitis and are considered in detail elsewhere (for reference see Table 16.1). Gynaecological and non-surgical causes are discussed in this chapter.

## GYNAECOLOGICAL CAUSES OF THE ACUTE ABDOMEN

### RUPTURED ECTOPIC PREGNANCY

The fertilised ovum implants at abnormal sites once in every 200 pregnancies. The fallopian tube is by far the commonest site, possibly on account of delayed transit of the ovum as a result of previous tubal infection, such as gonococcal salpingitis. If the erosive trophoblast penetrates the wall of the tube it may rupture, usually after about six weeks of pregnancy. Alternatively, the conceptus may be extruded from the fimbrial end of the tube.

#### Clinical features

In many cases, bouts of cramping pain in one or other iliac fossa associated with fainting attacks and vaginal bleeding, point to an abnormal pregnancy. With rupture, there is excruciating pain, blood loss and circulatory collapse. The abdominal pain is generalised and there is shoulder pain which may become apparent on elevating the foot of the bed. A missed period is noted in the majority of patients but the menstrual history may be confused by bleeding at the time of implantation or following death of the embryo.

Signs of pregnancy such as enlargement of the breasts and uterus are not usually present but cervical softening and tenderness are apparent on gentle pelvic examination. Should a haematoma form between the layers of the broad ligament, a tender mass may be palpable.

Pregnancy tests are unhelpful in detecting an ectopic pregnancy prior to rupture due to inadequate placental production of chorionic gonadotrophin. Laparoscopy and culdoscopy are used as diagnostic aids.

#### Treatment

A diagnosis of ruptured ectopic gestation demands urgent surgery. Following rapid resus-citation to compensate for blood loss, laparotomy is performed and the involved tube removed. Following an ectopic pregnancy, there is a 10% chance of an ectopic pregnancy occurring in the remaining tube.

### RUPTURE OF FUNCTIONAL OVARIAN CYST

Bleeding from either a ruptured Graafian follicle or corpus luteum may cause abdominal pain.

#### Clinical features

The patient is usually between 15 and 25 years of age and complains of sudden pain in one or other iliac fossa. Nausea and vomiting may be present but there are no systemic signs and the pain usually settles within a few hours. Tenderness and guarding in the right iliac fossa can mimic acute appendicitis and a few patients bleed sufficiently to suggest rupture of an ectopic pregnancy. On rectal examination there may be tenderness in the recto-vaginal pouch.

#### Treatment

The patient is observed and laparotomy advised only when acute appendicitis or ruptured ectopic pregnancy cannot be excluded.

### TORSION OF AN OVARIAN CYST

Benign ovarian cysts are common in women under 50 years of age and may undergo torsion (Fig. 16.9). Although a minority (10%) of ovarian cysts are of dermoid type, these cysts have long pedicles which are particularly liable to twist. Dermoid cysts account for some 50% of torsions in young women.

#### Clinical features

The patient complains of severe cramping lower abdominal pain. A smooth round mobile mass may be palpable in the abdomen, and is often higher than would be expected from an ovarian mass. There may be tenderness and guarding over the mass, particularly if there is

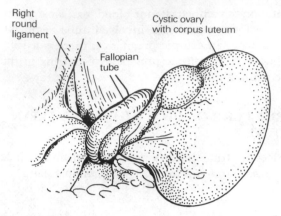

**Fig. 16.9** Torsion of an ovarian cyst

leakage from the cyst. Rupture results in diffuse peritonism.

The fallopian tube or a pedunculated uterine fibroid may also undergo torsion and present with a similar clinical picture.

### Treatment

Laparotomy is performed. The twisted pedicle is transfixed and ligated and the cyst is removed. Care should be taken to avoid rupture of the cyst as should it be malignant, cells may disseminate throughout the peritoneal cavity. The histology must be carefully reviewed. If malignant, a subsequent radical operation will be required.

## ACUTE SALPINGITIS

Acute salpingitis is most often due to gonococcal infection but streptococci and *M. tuberculosis* may also be responsible. Urethritis, cervicitis and a vaginal discharge occur 3–6 days following infection. At this stage, tubal involvement is unusual but following a menstrual period organisms spread to the lining of the uterus and tube. Both tubes are commonly involved and adhesions may seal the fimbriated end, leading to the formation of a pyosalpinx.

### Clinical features

Bilateral pain is felt low in the abdomen, often just above the inguinal ligament. This may be associated with increased frequency of micturi-

tion. The menstrual history is often irregular and there is pyrexia (39–40°C) and leucocytosis.

On vaginal examination there is unusual vaginal warmth, the cervix is tender and there is a purulent discharge. On inspection, the cervix is red and inflamed and a swab reveals the causal organism. If the tube is sealed and distended with pus (pyosalpinx) the vaginal findings may be less marked.

### Treatment

Treatment consists initially of antibiotic therapy. Laparotomy is undertaken only if acute appendicitis and ectopic pregnancy cannot be excluded or if a tubal abscess is suspected. In acute salpingitis, the tubes are red and on milking them gently there is a purulent discharge from which a swab is obtained. The abdomen is closed without drainage. The appendix is removed only if the infection is mild.

## NON-SURGICAL CAUSES OF THE ACUTE ABDOMEN

Acute abdominal pain can be produced by a number of conditions for which operation is contra-indicated. However, even when a non-surgical cause is suspected, it may not be possible to exclude serious abdominal disease and laparotomy may be required.

### NON-SPECIFIC ABDOMINAL PAIN

Approximately one-half of all patients sent to hospital with acute abdominal pain have no demonstrable cause, or are found to have a minor urinary tract infection of doubtful significance.

Non-specific abdominal pain is commonest in the young. Mesenteric adenitis, low grade urinary tract infection, mild gastroenteritis, the irritable bowel syndrome, cyclical ovarian problems and emotional upsets are possible causes. Tenderness is often present in the right iliac fossa and acute appendicitis most frequently suspected.

In such cases a period of careful observation is essential. Lapaorotomy is undertaken if pain and tenderness persist or if systemic indications of an inflammatory condition develop.

## ACUTE MESENTERIC ADENITIS

At one time acute mesenteric adenitis was believed to be viral in origin. It is now known that the majority of cases are caused by *Yersinia entercolitica* or *Y.pseudotuberculosis*. Most patients are between 5 and 15 years of age and present with a history of central or right sided abdominal pain, anorexia, nausea and vomiting. There may have been previous attacks of pain or a recent upper respiratory tract infection.

The patient is frequently flushed and pyrexial with an inflamed throat and cervical lymphadenopathy. Abdominal tenderness is usually higher in the abdomen and more diffuse than in appendicitis and may vary in its position on repeated examination or when the patient moves. Guarding and rebound tenderness are unusual.

Laparotomy is performed if appendicitis cannot be excluded. The lymph nodes in the mesentery of the terminal ileum are fleshy and enlarged and this may be associated with a red and thickened ileum (terminal ileitis). The appendix is normal but should be removed to avoid confusion in the future.

The diagnosis can be confirmed by culture of the responsible organisms from the stool or lymph nodes or by serological testing. However, as the condition is self-limiting and the patient usually recovers without event, this is not normally required. Histology of the lymph nodes or appendix reveals no specific changes.

## DIABETES MELLITUS

Acute abdominal pain and tenderness occur in 25% of patients with diabetic metabolic problems. The mechanism is uncertain but pancreatitis, stretching of the liver capsule, gastric distension and dehydration are possible explanations. Hyperamylasaemia is present in two-thirds of patients with diabetic keto-acidosis but it is unlikely that pancreatitis is responsible.

There is a history of thirst and polyuria, drowsiness and, in some instances, failure to maintain adequate insulin therapy. The patient appears dehydrated and ill, there is acetone in the breath and he/she may become comatose. The urine contains large amounts of sugar and acetone and there is hyperglycaemia and metabolic acidosis.

If the abdominal pain is due solely to diabetes, it should disappear rapidly with treatment. Persistence of pain and tenderness suggests an underlying surgical cause. In this regard, it should be remembered that a primary surgical problem, e.g. appendicitis, can cause secondary derangements of diabetic control.

If surgery is to be undertaken in these circumstances, vigorous treatment of keto-acidosis is required pre-operatively.

## ACUTE INTERMITTENT PORPHYRIA

An attack of acute porphyria is a rare cause of abdominal pain, the nature of which resembles small bowel colic. Vomiting is common but abdominal signs are seldom prominent. There may be a history of barbiturate ingestion which in a susceptible person can initiate an acute attack.

The diagnosis is suggested by the finding of porphyrins in the urine. Freshly passed urine is normal in appearance but becomes red on standing or on the addition of Ehrlich's aldehyde reagent. This test must be carried out on all patients with a familial trait of porphyria who are admitted with abdominal pain. Most now carry identification discs.

Porphyria and acute abdominal disease can coincide. Should it be considered advisable to operate the anaesthetist must be informed that the patient is porphyric so that barbiturates and other sensitising drugs can be avoided.

## HAEMOCHROMATOSIS

Abdominal pain occurs in one-third of patients with haemochromatosis. The pain is usually dull and boring in nature but can become severe and simulate acute cholecystitis or acute appendicitis.

## LEAD POISONING

The clinical picture of lead poisoning resembles that of porphyria. The diagnosis is suggested by a history of exposure to lead or by associated clinical findings of muscle palsy, a blue line on the gums or punctate basophilia on examination of the blood. Severe constipation is typical.

## DISEASE OF THE BLOOD AND BLOOD VESSELS

### Hereditary spherocytosis

Attacks of abdominal pain, nausea and vomiting associated with abdominal tenderness and icterus can coincide with episodes of haemolysis, probably as a result of minor intra-abdominal haemorrhage. Emergency laparotomy is seldom indicated. Cholelithiasis is common and cholecystitis should always be considered as a cause of abdominal pain in patients with this disease.

### Haemophilia

Abdominal pain in haemophiliacs is more often due to haemorrhage than to surgical pathology. Extraperitoneal bleeding is common and haemorrhage into the psoas sheath can simulate appendicitis. Haematoma formation in the gut wall can cause intussusception.

Despite this, a haemophiliac is not immune to surgical problems. If serious intra-abdominal pathology is suspected and operation advised, a haematologist must be consulted so that suitable precautions can be undertaken (Chapter 5).

### Anaphylactoid purpura (Henoch-Schonlein Purpura)

This is a rare cause of abdominal pain in children. It is usually associated with a streptococcal sore throat, abdominal colic, vomiting, bloody diarrhoea or intussusception preceding the development of skin purpura.

### Sickle-cell disease

This hereditary disease is virtually confined to negroes, particularly those from West Africa. There is an abnormal form of haemoglobin-S which crystallises when oxygen tension is reduced and results in increased osmotic fragility of the red cells and haemolytic attacks. These may be associated with abdominal pain, tenderness, guarding and icterus. The abdominal pain is most commonly due to splenic infarcts.

The correct diagnosis is suggested by associated chronic anaemia, bone and joint pain and leg ulcers. Examination of a blood film reveals characteristic appearances of the red cells. Gallstones occur in one-third of patients with sickle-cell disease. Cholecystitis must always be considered as a cause of abdominal pain.

### Polycythaemia vera

In this condition spontaneous thrombosis can cause splenic and mesenteric infarcts with acute abdominal pain.

### Polyarteritis nodosa

Nausea, vomiting, abdominal pain and diarrhoea affect 50% of patients with this disease. Occasionally severe protracted pain with fever, leucocytosis and abdominal tenderness suggests focal infarction within the abdomen. Pancreatitis, bleeding, perforation and obstruction are also reported as complications of this disease. Steroid therapy is indicated unless perforation or infarction of the intestine is suspected, when operation must not be delayed

# 17. Skin, Connective and Soft Tissues

*= Histiocytoma in dermis*

## COMPOSITION OF SKIN AND SUBCUTANEOUS TISSUES

### Skin (Fig. 17.1)

**The** *skin* of an adult has a surface area of some 1–1.8 sq metres. It is thinnest on the glans penis and eyelids and thickest on the palms, soles and back. Skin consists of two elements. The dermis is composed of collagen, elastic fibres and fat which support blood vessels, lymphatics, nerves and the epidermal appendages. The epidermis is avascular and consists of several layers of keratin-producing cells at different stages of differentiation and degeneration. The junction between epidermis and dermis is undulating. Projections of dermis push upwards into the epidermis to form 'dermal papillae' which carry capillaries and lymphatic channels which nourish the epidermis and permit fluid exchange. The dermal papillae are separated by ridges of epidermis, the 'rete pegs'.

The deepest layer of epidermal cells contains the basal germinal cells which produce the keratin producing cells or *keratinocytes*. The basal layer also contains pigment cells or melanocytes which donate melanin to the developing keratinocytes and are probably neuro-epidermal in origin. As the epidermal cells migrate to the surface they become increasingly keratinised and are eventually shed, the whole process taking around 28 days. Production of new epidermal cells (prickle cells) equals the rate of loss of fully keratinised cells, so that the thickness of the skin normally remains constant.

It is estimated that there are 2000 million melanocytes in the human skin. They secrete melanin which is synthesised from tyrosine and phenylalanine by cytoplasmic enzymes. They can

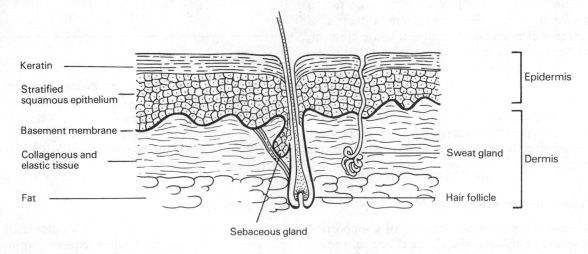

Keratin
Stratified squamous epithelium
Basement membrane
Collagenous and elastic tissue
Fat
Epidermis
Sweat gland
Dermis
Hair follicle
Sebaceous gland

**Fig. 17.1** Anatomy of skin

be recognised histopathologically by the dopa reaction, a histochemical staining reaction which depends on the presence of an oxidative enzyme which converts deoxyphenylalanine to melanin.

The pigment granules formed in the cytoplasm of melanocytes which can be demonstrated by silver stains, pass along dendritic processes to enter neighbouring epithelial cells. As the cells migrate towards the surface their contained melanin protects the germ cells of the basal epidermis and the melanocytes from the effects of ultraviolet light.

The skin appendages (hair follicles, sebaceous glands, and sweat glands) arise from the epidermis and grow down into the dermis and in some sites to the subcutaneous tissues. *The hair follicle* is a downgrowth of epidermal cells. At its end a papilla contains vessels and nerves to nourish and sensitise the hairs. The colour of the hair is due to pigment, which is produced by melanocytes which have colonised the hair follicle.

The *sebaceous glands* secrete sebum into the hair follicles. Sebum contains fatty acids and hydrocarbons and lubricates the skin and hairs.

*Sweat glands* are simple coiled tubular glands lying in the dermis and opening onto the surface. They are two types. *Eccrine* glands secrete salt and water over the entire surface of the skin; *apocrine* glands (which are present in the axilla, breast and genital regions) secrete a musty-smelling fluid into hair follicles.

The *nails* are flat horny structures composed of keratin which are implanted by a root into a groove of skin. They arise from a matrix of germinal cells which are seen as a white crescent, the lunula, at its base. On avulsion of the nail a new nail will grow from this germinal layer. The rate of a growth is about 3 mm per month.

The *nail bed* is composed of dermis with a thin layer of epidermal cells. If the matrix of a nail is destroyed, so that regeneration cannot occur these epidermal cells form a thick keratinised protective layer.

## Subcutaneous tissue

Subcutaneous tissue is composed of a supporting structure of collagen and elastic tissue containing fat, blood vessels, nerves and lymphatics. It is interposed between skin and the underlying muscles and is enclosed by the superficial fascia.

## DIAGNOSIS OF SKIN SWELLINGS

Three questions should be asked when confronted with a patient with a swelling which is visible on the surface.

1. *Is it in the skin or subcutaneous tissues?*. This is determined by 'pinching up' the skin over the swelling and attempting to move it from side to side. If the swelling is in the skin the two cannot be moved independently.

2. *Is it epidermal or dermal?* The stretched normal epithelium overlying a dermal swelling may look glossy but it remains smooth and ulcerates from pressure necrosis only when the swelling is large. An epithelial lesion causes roughening of the skin surface, papilliform growth or ulceration, even while the lesion is still small.

3. *Is the lesion pigmented?* Melanin produces black to brown pigmentation while haemosiderin produces brown to yellow pigmentation. In general melanin pigmentation is characteristic of melanocytic activity but certain other skin lesions (e.g. basal cell carcinoma or seborrhoeic keratosis) may show melanin pigmentation within constituent epidermal cells. Any warty growth is prone to bleeding and accumulation of blood may lead to red brown or yellowish pigmentation. Such pigmentation is a feature of vascular malformations (haemangiomas).

## CYSTS

Two main types of cyst occur in the skin and subcutaneous tissues (Fig. 17.2). The *sebaceous* or *epidermoid* cyst lies *within* the skin and is a dermal swelling covered by normal epidermis. The *dermoid cyst* lies in the subcutaneous tissues and is covered by normal skin.

## Sebaceous cysts

A *sebaceous cyst* has a thin wall of flattened epidermal cells and contains cheesy white material composed of epithelial debris and sebum

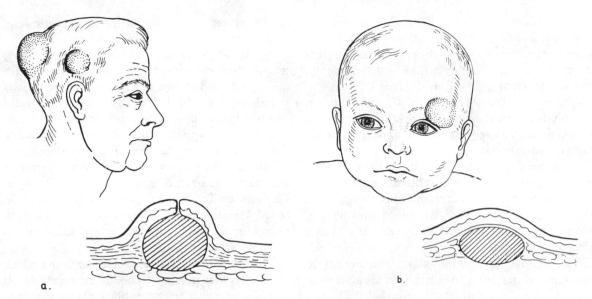

**Fig. 17.2** (a) Sebaceous and (b) dermoid cysts

with a characteristic sweet musty smell. Originally believed to be a retention cyst of a sebaceous gland, it is now believed to arise from a hair follicle. Common on hair bearing areas i.e. scalp, face, ears, neck, back and scrotum, a sebaceous cyst forms a hemispherical smooth soft swelling which lies within the skin. The skin *cannot* be moved over it. The overlying epithelium is normal but a small punctum marking the site of the involved hair follicle is common.

A sebaceous cyst may become infected. Then the overlying epidermis is hot, red and glazed. An infected cyst may discharge spontaneously.

*Treatment* of an uninfected sebaceous cyst consists of excision. Following infiltration of the skin and surrounding tissues with local anaesthetic, a small ellipse of skin is incised over the cyst. This allows traction to be applied so that the cyst can be dissected from the surrounding dermis and subcutaneous tissue without rupture (Fig. 17.3).

An *infected cyst* is incised. Excision is delayed until the inflammation has completely resolved.

## Dermoid cyst

This subcutaneous cyst arises from a nest of epidermal cells in the subcutaneous tissues. These originate either as an embryological anomaly, or by implanation of epidermal cells from the

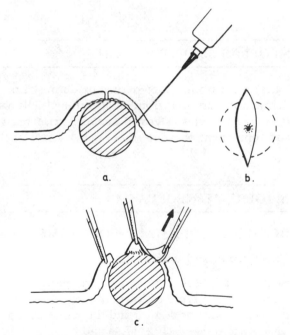

**Fig. 17.3** Removal of sebaceous syst. (a) Infiltration of local anaesthetic. (b) Ellipse of skin excised around punctum. (c) Cyst excised attached to skin ellipse.

skin by puncture. Congenital cysts are found at sites of embryonic fusion and are most common on the face around the forehead, base of nose and occiput; implantation dermoids occur at sites of minor injury such as the plantar surfaces of the fingers and hands.

A dermoid cyst is lined by squamous epithelium and contains sebum, degenerate cells and sometimes hair. A soft rubbery swelling forms deep to the skin. The cyst may be fixed deeply, particular when situated on the face.

*Treatment* consists of excision. Implantation dermoids can be removed under local anaesthesia. Congenital cysts require formal dissection under general anaesthesia.

*External angular dermoid* This is the commonest congenital dermoid. It is situated at the junction between the outer and upper margins of the orbit at the line of fusion of maxilla and frontal bones. Diagnosed in infancy the cyst is best removed when the child is a few years old. The cyst may be an hour-glass extension of an intracranial dermoid, the operation may prove to be extensive, and should be preceded by a skull X-ray and a CT brain scan.

## NEOPLASMS OF THE SKIN

These arise from the epidermis or dermis. Epidermal tumours arise from basal germinal cells or from melanocytes. Dermal tumours arise from any component of the dermis.

## EPIDERMAL NEOPLASMS

### BENIGN EPIDERMAL NEOPLASMS

#### Papillomas and warts

Benign warts (or papillomas) are particularly common. Two types of wart are seen; the infective (viral) wart or *verruca* and the senile wart or *seborrhoeic keratosis* (Fig. 17.4a and b).

*Infective warts* are found most commonly on the hands and fingers of young children and adults (*verruca vulgaris*). They are greyish brown, round or oval, elevated lesions with a filiform surface and keratinised projections. The warts may be studded with spots of blood pigment. These warts spread by direct inoculation and are commonly multiple. The natural history is one of spontaneous regression but if troublesome they

can be treated by caustics or freezing (acetic acid, liquid nitrogen or $CO_2$ snow).

Plantar warts (*verruca plantaris*) are particularly troublesome and are spread by contagion in swimming pools and showers. These warts are usually found under the heel or heads of the metatarsals. Flush with the surface they are covered by a thickened layer of epithelium and are intensely painful. They are treated by curettage or by liquid nitrogen.

Infective warts may also occur in the *perineum* and on the *penis* and may be of venereal origin. Cauliflower-like bulky papillomatous growths (condylomata acuminata) may occur in the perineum in syphilis, lymphogranuloma and in immuno-suppressed patients.

The *senile wart* is a basal cell papilloma which occurs in older persons (seborrhoeic keratosis). It forms a yellowish brown or black plaque greasy to touch and has a cracked surface which falls off in pieces. It has been likened to the end of a dirty paint brush. Senile warts are often multiple, particularly on the upper back and trunk, and are best treated by curettage.

*Pedunculated papilloma.* Simple non-infective papillomas can occur at any site. They form flesh coloured spherical warty masses which hang on a stalk of surrounding normal epithelium (Fig. 17.4c). If small they can be removed by snipping the pedicle with scissors or induced to necrose and drop off by tying a thread around it. If large, the papilloma and its pedicle is removed with an ellipse of normal skin.

### Kerato-acanthoma (molluscum sebaceum)

This lesion is important because of the likelihood of confusion with a squamous cancer. It forms a rounded hemispherical nodule which occurs most commonly on the face and has a mushroom like friable red centre core crusted with keratin (Fig. 17.5). Infective in origin it occurs in those over 50 years of age and has an alarmingly rapid growth. It is self limiting and heals following shedding of its central core. It can be cured readily by curettage.

### Benign melanoma (see below)

### Pre-malignant keratoses

Actinic or solar keratosis denotes the occurrence of small single or multiple firm warty spots on the face, back of the neck or hands of older, fair-

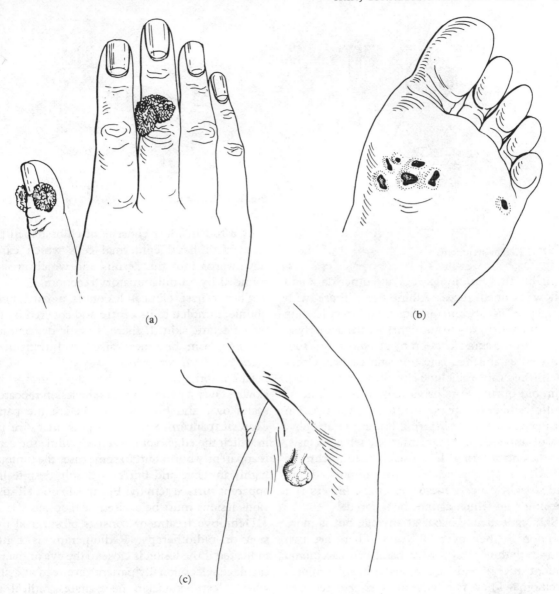

(a)

(b)

(c)

**Fig. 17.4** Some types of warts and papillomas. a. verruca vulgaris, b. plantar warts, c. pedunculated papilloma.

skinned persons who have been exposed excessively to sunlight. The scaly lesions drop off leaving a shallow premalignant ulcer. They should be removed surgically.

## INTRA EPIDERMAL CANCER (Carcinoma *in situ*, Bowen's disease)

This inactive form of cancer is non-invasive. It forms a discrete and often solitary raised brown or red fissured plaque which is keratinised. Histologi-

cally, the lesion consists of hyperplastic epithelial cells which have atypical forms but remain in situ.

When on the skin, the condition may be referred to as Bowen's disease; in-situ cancer of the glans penis, which is rare, is also known as 'erythroplasia of Queyret'.

## EPIDERMOID CANCER

Skin cancer occurs primarily on exposed areas and in those with poor natural protection against

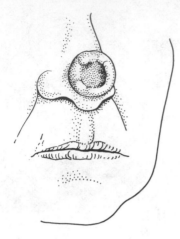

**Fig. 17.5** Kerato-acanthoma

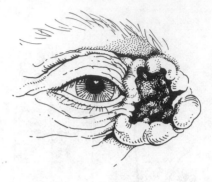

**Fig. 17.6** Rodent ulcer

sunlight. It is rare in negroes and other dark and yellow skinned races. Albinos and those with *xeroderma pigmentosa*, (a congenital defect leading to undue sensitivity to sunlight) are particularly at risk. Chronic skin irritation by arsenic, tar or soot is a well established cause of skin cancer. Other established causes include chronic ulceration (e.g. from old burns, scars or varicose ulcers). Therapeutic radiation causes an intense skin reaction with erythema and blistering leading to atrophy, loss of appendages, pigmentation, telangiectasis, fibrosis and scarring. In those exposed to chronic radiation such changes may pass unnoticed and lead to skin cancer. Fissuring of the fingers is a warning sign which cannot be ignored.

Skin cancer may occur at any age but is more common in men over 50 years. There are two distinct pathological forms: basal cell carcinoma (rodent ulcer) and squamous (or epidermoid) carcinoma. These two types of cancer behave very differently. A rodent ulcer is very slow growing, is only locally malignant, and seldom metastasises; a squamous carcinoma grows more rapidly and metastasises early to regional lymph nodes.

## Basal cell cancer (rodent ulcer)

Almost all rodent ulcers arise on the mid-portion of the face, typically on the nose, inner canthus of the eye, forehead and eyelids (Fig. 17.6). Rodent ulcers are rare in other sites; they never occur on the palms or soles of the feet. They occur at an earlier age than squamous cancers. Microscopi-

cally a rodent ulcer consists of club-shaped projections of basal epidermal cells which extend downwards into the dermis and which are surrounded by an inflammatory reaction.

The earliest clinical lesion is a hard pearly nodule, dimpled in its centre and covered by thin telangiectatic skin. If there is cystic degeneration the neoplasm becomes raised and translucent, *cystic basal cell carcinoma*.

Characteristically a rodent ulcer grows very slowly. Over a period of years the lesion repeatedly scales over and breaks down before the patient expresses concern. Spread may be of 'field-fire' type in which the edges spread actively while the centre is apparently burnt out. In some cases the tumour is highly invasive and burrows deeply despite little apparent surface activity. For this reason all suspicious lesions must be excised or biopsied.

Definitive treatment consists of surgical excision or radiotherapy. Radiotherapy is contraindicated if the lesion is close to the eye or overlies cartilage. Occasionally patients are seen at a stage where deep extension necessitates radical and complex reconstuctive surgery.

## Squamous cell cancer

This tumour occurs anywhere on the surface but is particularly common on the exposed parts i.e. ears, cheeks, lower lips, back of hands. All cancers arising from stratified squamous epithelium are also of this type. Chronic skin changes induced by chemical irritation, irradiation or ulceration are a predisposing factor and squamous cell carcinomas usually develops in a pre-existing area of epithelial hyperplasia or keratosis. In the mucosa e.g. of

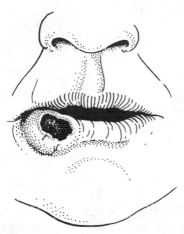

**Fig. 17.7** Squamous cancer

the lips the analogous change is leukoplakia (see Chapter 25). Malignant transformation forms a hard erythematous nodule which proliferates to form a cauliflower-like excrescence or ulcerates to form a malignant ulcer with a raised fixed hard edge (Fig. 17.7). Squamous cell cancer grows more rapidly than a rodent ulcer but not as rapidly as a kerato-acanthoma (see above). Metastases to regional lymph nodes occur early in the disease. The nodes become enlarged, hard and fixed. Histologically a squamous cell carcinoma consists of atypical squamous cells which infiltrate the underlying dermis to form concentric 'pearls' or 'nests'. Keratinisation is an obvious feature and epithelial bridges and prickle cells are numerous.

Treatment consists of wide excision or irradiation according to the size of the tumour, its site and aggressiveness, and whether lymph nodes are involved. Palpable lymph nodes should be excised by block dissection unless they are fixed, in which case palliative radiotherapy offers the only hope of control. In extensive tumours treatment with high-energy (fast) neutrons has proved superior to orthodox radiotherapy. Bleomycin and other chemotherapeutic agents are of limited value but occasionally affect worthwhile remission of advanced disease.

## DERMAL NEOPLASMS

Neoplasms arising from the connective tissue of the dermis rarely occur. Dermal fibroma, lipomas and neurofibromas form nodules in the skin covered by normal epidermis. Sweat gland tumours are also rare (see below).

### Dermatofibroma

This is hard dermal nodule, sometimes pigmented, and most commonly found on the lower leg in women. It is smooth and hemispherical in shape, being covered by normal epithelium. Histologically it consists of whorls of collagen fibres intermingling with fibroblasts and histiocytes containing haemosiderin. Previously known as a sclerosing haemangioma, it should be removed.

## MELANOCYTE TUMOURS

## BENIGN PIGMENTED MOLES

The pigment producing cells, *melanocytes*, lie in the basal layer of the epidermis. The number of melanocytes is fixed (approximately 2000 million), irrespective of the colour of the person, but the amount of pigment produced by them varies in individuals. As a developmental abnormality, conglomerates of melanocytes may migrate to the dermis or epidermis forming a mole (shapeless mass) or naevus. Such abnormal melanocytes are termed naevus cells and according to their site and activity they cause a variety of pigmented spots and swellings or 'naevi'.

### Common moles

Histopathologically moles are classified by the site of the clumps of naevus cells and their activity. Initially this takes place at the junction of epidermis and dermis; so-called *junctional change*. Moles showing active junctional change are common in childhood; all moles on the palms of the hands and soles of feet are of this type. Migration of the sheets or packets of naevus cells to the dermis produces an intradermal naevus; migration to dermis and epidermis produces a compound naevus (Fig. 17.8).

The common mole is a flat or slightly raised brown black lesion covered by normal epidermis.

It has a period of active growth during childhood due to junctional activity but usually becomes quiescent at puberty and may later atrophy. With migration of the naevus cells to the dermis the lesion becomes firm and raised, often associated with aberrant growth of hair. As the epidermis is not involved the surface of the lesion is smooth. Alternatively pigmented moles may be soft and rough - the *fleshy hairy mole* corresponding histologically to the compound naevus.

As only 1 in 100 000 moles become malignant, they need not normally be removed other than for cosmetic reasons. Active growth during childhood need not cause concern; but growth after puberty demands removal. Increase in pigmentation, scaliness, itching and bleeding also indicate excision. In brief any mole which has such characteristics suggesting malignancy or which has reached 0.7 cm in diameter should be removed with at least 1 cm of surrounding normal skin.

## Giant hairy mole

Unlike the common mole this congenital lesion is present at birth. It occupies a wide area which may correspond to a dermatome. Typical sites are the bathing trunk area and face (Fig. 17.9).

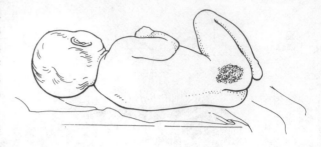

**Fig. 17.9** Diagram of giant hairy mole

Although the risk of malignant change is not great the lesion must be kept under observation. Removal with coverage of the large defect by skin grafting is often necessary for cosmetic reasons.

Histopathologically, the lesion is highly cellular. The cells contain abundant pigment and are confined to the dermis. Neurological elements may be present. These moles are often associated with neurofibromas and other congenital abnormalities.

## Blue naevus

This is a deep intradermal naevus, in which strap-shaped cells laden with melanin are scattered in

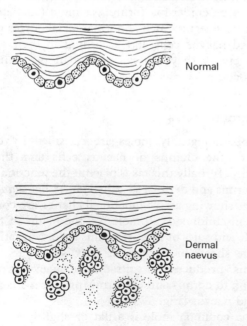

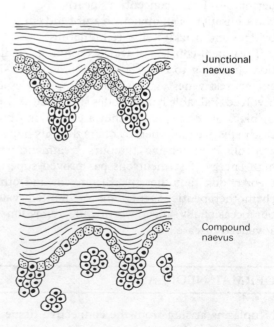

**Fig. 17.8** Histopathological types of benign mole

the deeper layers of the dermis. The cells may be of mesenchymal origin or may result from faulty migration. The blue colouration of the naevus is due to the optical effect caused by the depth of the lesions.

A blue naevus may develop at any time from birth to middle life and may form a blue-black papule (beauty spot) on the face or arms, or ribbon-like areas on the wrist, ankle or buttocks. The Mongolian spot of dark-skinned races is an example. It is a poorly defined brownish area in the skin overlying the sacrum and although present at birth, it later disappears.

### Halo naevus

This pigmented naevus is surrounded by a white circle of depigmentation associated with lympho-cytic infiltration. This phenomenon is believed to be of immune origin.

## MALIGNANT MELANOMA

Malignant melanomas predominantly affect the fair-skinned. They are rare in negroes except on depigmented areas such as the palms, soles and mucosa. Exposure to sunlight is a precipitating factor. In Scotland the disease incidence is 2.3 persons per 100 000 per annum compared with 17 in Queensland. Malignant melanomas are commoner in females than males, this due to an increased incidence on the lower leg.

About half of all malignant melanomas are believed to arise in pre-existing naevi. As the average person has 14 naevi the risk of any one becoming malignant is very small.

The essential feature of a malignant melanoma is invasion of the dermis by proliferating melano-cytes which have large nuclei, prominent nucleoli and frequent mitoses. Three distinct clinical pathological types are described.

### Melanotic freckle (lentigo maligna)

One in 10 malignant melanomas arise in a melan-otic or senile freckle (Fig. 17.10). This occurs most commonly on the face of elderly women affecting particularly the lower eyelids, cheek, side of nose, forehead or neck. The lesion begins

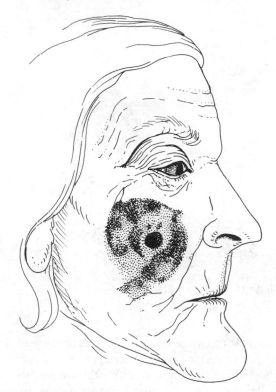

**Fig. 17.10** Lentigo maligna

as a brownish-red patch, grows slowly and centri-fugally, and advances and recedes over many years. The edge of the lesion is serrated and 'map-like' but the margin with normal skin is abrupt. Kaleidoscopic pigmentation of the surface is typi-cal.

During this pre-malignant phase, which may last for 10–15 years, there are conglomerates of large round melanocytes which extend laterally in the basal epidermis. The first clinical sign of malignancy is development of a brownish-red papule eccentrically within the freckle. This in-dicates vertical invasion. Microscopically abnor-mal melanocytes extend into the superficial der-mis.

### Superfical spreading melanoma

This is the commonest type of malignant mela-noma (Fig. 17.11). It occurs predominantly on the trunk but is also found on exposed parts. It is most common in the middle-aged.

During a pre-invasive phase which lasts at most

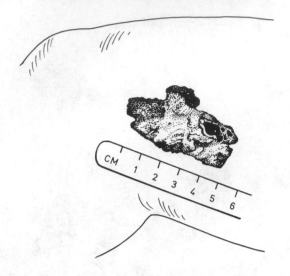

**Fig. 17.11** Superficial spreading melanoma

for a year or two, a wave of malignancy spreads in all direction from the basal region of the epidermis. Unlike the melanotic freckle the surface of the lesion is slightly raised and its outline indistinct. Pigmentation is again patchy and there is a profuse range of colours.

Vertical invasion of the dermis occurs while the lesion is still relatively small, and produces an indurated nodule which soon ulcerates or bleeds. A few longish white hairs may appear at the site of dermal invasion.

## Nodular melanoma

Nodular melanomas occur at any site or at any age (Fig.17.12). In females they are particularly common on the lower leg. Unlike the above two types, a nodular melanoma is vertically invasive and malignant from its onset. There is no preceding intra-epidermal lateral spread and therefore no surrounding pigmented macule. The total width of the lesion rarely exceeds that of 2 or 3 rete pegs.

A nodular melanoma starts as an elevated deeply pigmented nodule. It may occur at the site of a pre-existing benign naevus. The nodule steadily enlarges both on the surface and by centrifugal extension. This expansion is first detected by destruction of the normal skin lines on the surface of the pigmented lesion. It progressively darkens and the surface over the area of active growth becomes jet black and glossy. Bleeding results from trivial injury and is noted as a 'spotting' of blood on dressing or clothes. Crusting, scab formation and ulceration are typical. Itching and irritation are common.

In neglected tumours, satellite nodules may appear in the surrounding skin.

## Other types of malignant melanoma

An *acrolentigerous* melanoma has recently been described which suggests it occurs on the volar

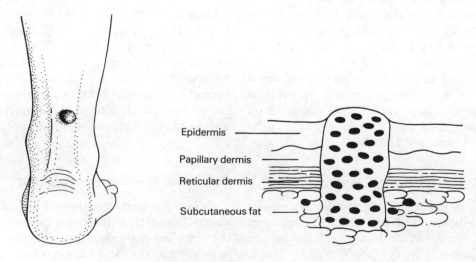

**Fig. 17.12** Nodular melanoma

surfaces of hands and feet and is of malignant lentigo type.

Not all malignant melanomas are deeply pigmented. *Amelanotic melanomas* do occur, and are pale pink in colour. They are usually associated with rapid growth, and in pure form are very rare.

A *subungual melanoma* occurs in middle age and elderly patients and most commonly affects the thumb or great toe. It is a cause of chronic inflammation below the nail, the *melanotic whitlow*, which is commonly misdiagnosed as a paronychia or ingrowing toenail. Pigmentation is not usually visible in the early stages, but a band of pigment may form later around the inflamed area.

## Spread

Malignant melanomas (particularly the nodular type) spread readily by lymphatic and blood streams. 'In transit' metastases may develop in the subcutaneous or intracutaneous lymphatics and form small painless discoloured nodules in the line of the lymphatics between primary lesion and regional lymph nodes. Lymph node metastases present as a firm enlargement of a single node which remains unattached and mobile. The lesion spreads then to the central lymph nodes. Blood borne metastases may occur at any site but are found most commonly in the liver, abdominal cavity, lungs, brain, skin and subcutaneous tissues. Extensive metastatic growth may be associated with excretion of melanin, or its enzymatic precursor 5S cystine-L-dopa in the urine. Some 5% of malignant melanomas present as metastases without a recognisable primary site.

## Prognosis

The most reliable prognostic indicator is the depth of the lesion (Fig. 17.13). The more superficial a tumour the better its prognosis. Depth can be measured either be reference to the normal layers of the skin (Clark) or by a micrometer gauge (Breslow). As normal skin layers are distorted by the tumour, reference points are difficult to define and the Breslow system is preferred.

Patients with tumours less than 0.7 mm in depth have a normal life expectancy after treat-

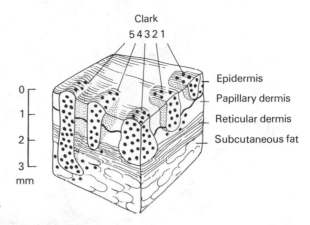

**Fig. 17.13** Methods of grading the depth of invasion of malignant melanoma

ment; 5-year survival rates in those with lesions 0.7–1.5 mm in depth average 70%; for those with lesions greater than 1.5 mm the 5-year survival rate is 30%.

The mitotic activity of the tumour also affects prognosis, and tumours may be graded according to the number of mitotic figures in a microscopic field.

As the melanotic freckle and a superficial spreading melanoma tend to remain superficial they are associated with a better prognosis than that found with melanomas of the nodular type.

## Treatment

The first essential step is to reach a diagnosis; if this is in doubt excision biopsy is performed. Frozen-section examination is reliable in 90% of cases, and one may proceed with definitive treatment if malignancy is confirmed.

*Curative excision.* Tumours of low malignancy e.g. lentigo malignum, are excised with a skin margin of 1.0 cm. If there is obvious invasive growth the margin should be wider (Fig. 17.14). On the limbs, removal of at least 5 cm of normal surrounding skin is advised; on the trunk some advocate removal of at least 10 cm. The tumour and surrounding skin are excised down to, but not including, the deep fascia so that the whole depth of subcutaneous fat is removed.

The defect is covered with a split skin graft. This is cut before the tumour is excised. In the case of limb melanomas the graft must be taken from the opposite arm or leg. If taken from the

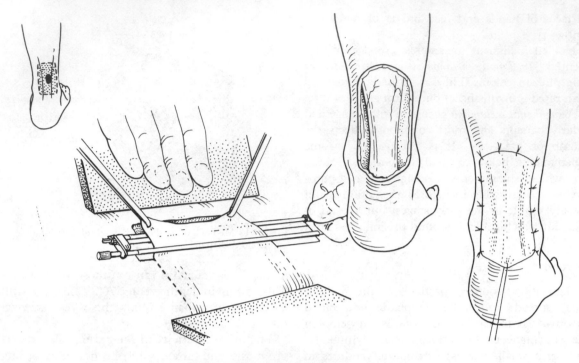

**Fig. 17.14** Excision of malignant melanoma

same limb there is a risk that seedling deposits of tumour may develop at the donor site.

*Lymph nodes.* Block dissection of regional lymph nodes is considered if the primary tumour is in the immediate vicinity of regional nodes, if there is microscopic evidence of deep dermal invasion, if dermal lymphatics are invaded or if the nodes are palpable. In doubtful cases, preliminary lymphangiography may define the state of the nodes.

An alternative method of treating lymph nodes is by endolymphatic infusion of radioactive gold or lipiodol which is trapped in the nodes and irradiates them.

In other cases i.e. when there is no evidence of node involvement, prophylactic node dissection or endolymphatic infusion has no advantage.

*Metastatic disease.* The management of metastatic melanoma is unsatisfactory. Occasional short-lived remissions have been reported with chemotherapy using DTIC (dimethyl triazeno imidazole carboxamide), BCNU (a nitroso-urea) and vindesine (a derivative of vincristine). Immune stimulation with BCG (Bacille Calmette-Guerin), C-parvum or vaccinia virus, or injection

of irradiated melanoma cells has also been used but without proven effect. Systemic therapy has been used as adjuvant treatment for primary disease but there is no evidence that it is beneficial.

## VASCULAR NEOPLASMS (haemangiomas)

The histological classification of haemangiomas is complex. They are best differentiated by their clinical behaviour i.e. whether they regress (involute) or persist.

### Involuting haemangiomas

These are true tumours arising from endothelial cells. They appear at or within a few weeks of birth, predominantly affecting the head and neck. If superficial an involuting haemangioma forms a bright red raised mass with an irregular bosselated surface, the so-called *strawberry naevus.* If deeply situated it forms a blue-black soft tumour which is covered by normal skin.

Active growth takes place for about 6 months. The tumour then remains static until the child is 2–3 years of age when it shrinks, and loses its colour. It usually disappears before the child is 7 years of age. They should be left severely alone.

## Non-involuting haemangiomas

These are hamartomas due to abnormal formations of blood vessels. There are two main types.

*Port-wine stain.* This is a red patchy lesion, often occupying the distribution of a peripheral nerve. Microscopically there are enlarged capillaries in the dermis lined by active looking endothelial cells. However the lesion neither grows nor involutes. It is treated by removal if small or by tattooing with a skin-coloured pigment if large. Treatment with the neodymium laser is under trial.

*Cavernous haemangioma.* This forms a bluish-purple elevated mass which empties on pressure and slowly refills. Unlike the strawberry naevus, a cavernous haemangioma does not appear until early childhood. Histologically it consists of mature venous-like structures which lie in a fibrous stroma and are lined by flat endothelial cells. It is treated by excision.

*Cirsoid aneurysm.* This is a variant of a cavernous haemangioma in which the mass of venous-like structures are fed directly by arterial blood and become tortuous, dilated and pulsating.

A common site is on the scalp. Pressure from the pulsating vascular mass erodes the skull. Penetrating channels may connect the superficial lesion with a similar malformation in the extra-dural space (Fig. 17.15).

The most effective treatment of a cirsoid aneurysm is complete excision following ligation of all its feeding vessels. As serious haemorrhage may complicate the operation, a preliminary angiogram is essential to show the distribution of the lesion and the anatomy of its arterial supply. Preliminary embolisation by injecting clot or metal beads into the feeding vessels may prove helpful.

*Granuloma pyogenicum.* This acquired condition is due to formation of a capillary haemangioma in a traumatised or infected area. There is a localised superficial polypoidal mass which is devoid of epithelium and resembles granulation tissue. The surface is fragile and bleeds easily. The differential diagnosis is from malignant melanoma or vascular metastases from a renal cancer. Demonstration of a pedicle is a good diagnostic guide. The condition is self-limiting in most cases. Excision of the lesion is performed if the diagnosis is in doubt.

## TUMOURS OF NERVES

### Neurilemmoma

This is an encapsulated solitary benign tumour which originates from the Schwann cells of a nerve sheath and forms a swelling in the course of the nerve. On clinical examination it is laterally mobile but fixed in the direction of the nerve (Fig. 17.16). It may cause radiating pain in the distribution of the involved nerve. Most *neurilemmomas* occur superficially in the neck or limbs. They grow slowly, have no malignant potential, and are readily treated by excision.

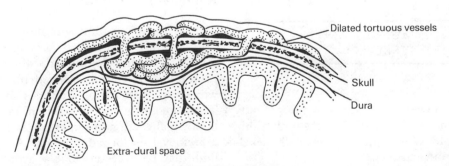

Fig. 17.15 Cirsoid aneurysm

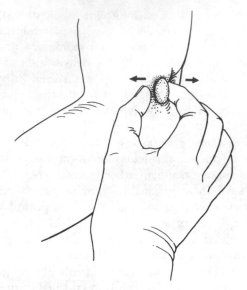

**Fig. 17.16** Neurilemmoma: lateral mobility

## Neurofibroma

This is regarded as a hamartoma of nerve tissue. The lesion may be solitary but more commonly they are multiple and associated with von Recklinghausen's disease. This is a genetically dominant condition present at birth or in early childhood. Multiple dermal and subcutaneous nodules arise from peripheral nerves and are associated with patches of dermal pigmentation forming *café-au-lait* spots. The tumours cause bony deformities particularly of the spine. It is important that this syndrome is recognised as the tumours are potentially malignant. Increase in size of existing swellings or appearance of new swellings suggests malignant change.

## TUMOURS OF MUSCLE AND CONNECTIVE TISSUES

### Lipoma

A lipoma is a slow growing benign tumour of fatty tissue. It forms a lobulated soft mass with a thin fibrous capsule. When large it occasionally develops sarcomatous change.

Although a lipoma can occur in the dermis most lipomas are subcutaneous and arise from the fatty tissue between the skin and deep fascia. Typical features are their soft fluctuant feel, their lobulation and the free mobility of overlying skin.

Lipomas also may arise from fat in the intermuscular septa when they form a diffuse firm swelling under the deep fascia which is more prominent when the related muscle is contracted. They may cause discomfort.

As a lipoma is radiolucent soft tissue X-rays can be diagnostic, but are only indicated when the diagnosis is uncertain and removal may pose problems. Unless small and symptomless they should be removed.

### Liposarcoma

A liposarcoma is the commonest sarcoma of middle age. It may occur in any fatty tissue but is most frequent in the retroperitoneum and legs. Wide surgical excision is the best initial treatment. This is difficult for retroperitoneal tumours and post-operative radiotherapy and chemotherapy are advised.

As the growth rate of a liposarcoma is slow, recurrence may be long delayed.

### Fibrosarcoma

This tumour arises from fibrous tissue at any site, but is most common in the lower limbs or buttock. It forms a large deep firm mass. Wide excision is the initial treatment of choice; radiation therapy may be required for recurrence.

### Rhabdomyosarcoma

This is a greyish-pink soft fleshy lobulated or well circumscribed tumour arising from striated muscle. The histological appearance resembles primitive (embryonal) striated muscle. A large variety of histological subtypes are described. The tumour is more common in children, is highly malignant and requires treatment by radical removal and/or radiotherapy. Amputation of a limb may be necessary but is avoided wherever possible.

## DISORDERS OF SWEAT GLANDS

### Hidradenitis suppurativa

This is a chronic infection of the apocrine glands in the axilla, perineum or groin. It most commonly affects the axilla of women and is precipitated by shaving, poor hygiene or the use of chemical deodorants. There are multiple intradermal abscesses which lead to sinus formation, fibrosis and a painful diffuse chronic infection of the skin.

As the apocrine glands discharge into the hair follicles, the condition is resistant to local antiseptics. Treatment by long-term tetracycline therapy may be successful. If not, surgical excision of the axillary skin with skin grafting is required.

### Hyperhidrosis

This is a disorder of the eccrine sweat glands which most commonly affects the axillae of young women. If severe, the eccrine glands can be scraped away from the undersurface of the skin by inserting a sharp curette through a small incision.

Excessive sweating of the hands or of the feet can cause social and economic difficulties. Sympathectomy may occasionally be indicated.

### Sweat gland tumours

A variety of adenomas of sweat glands are described which may give rise to dermal tumours. These are rare.

## GANGLION

This is a common cystic swelling arising from the fibrous capsule of a joint or fibrous tendon sheath. It contains mucoid material within a fibrous capsule and was once considered to be due to herniation of the synovial membrane of a tendon sheath or joint. A ganglion is now considered to result from degeneration of collagen.

A ganglion most commonly forms a smooth

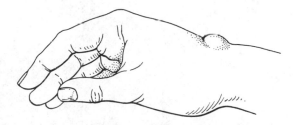

**Fig. 17.17** Ganglion in a typical site

tense hemispherical subcutaneous swelling on the dorsum of the wrist or foot (Fig. 17.17). Other sites include the palm of the hand, the palmar surface of a finger over the distal inter-phalangeal joint and the lateral side of the knee over the superior tibio-fibular joint. Those on the dorsum of the foot are bluish in colour due to the thin overlying skin. So-called *mucous cysts* arising from the small joints of the hand in older persons are also believed to be of similar origin. A ganglion should be differentiated from a bursa which is a fluid-filled fibrous swelling which overlies a bony exostosis.

A ganglion may be aspirated through a wide-bore needle or dispersed by firm pressure into the surrounding tissues. Recurrence after both procedures is common and excision under general or regional anaesthesia is preferred. A tourniquet is applied so that the operating field is bloodless, allowing careful and complete removal of the swelling.

## AFFECTIONS OF THE NAILS

### Onychogryphosis (hooked nail)

This is an overgrowth of a nail which resembles an ox or goat horn. The big toenail is most commonly affected (Fig. 17.18). Simple avulsion of the nail does not prevent recurrence of the deformity and excision of the nail bed is required. A flap of skin is reflected from the base of the nail and the germinal layer removed. Care must be taken to excise the edges of this layer completely or troublesome spikes of nail continue to grow. An alternative to excision of the nail bed is to cauterise it with phenol.

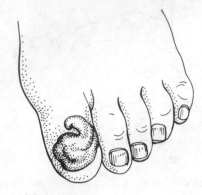

**Fig. 17.18** Onychogryphosis

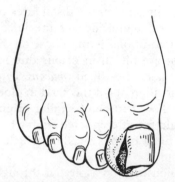

**Fig. 17.19** Ingrowing toenail

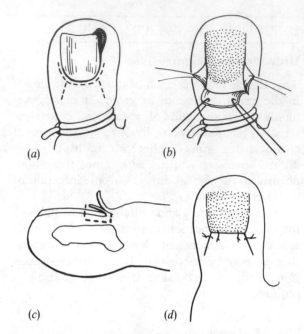

**Fig. 17.20** Operation for ablation of nail bed. (a) Skin incisions. (b) Nail avulsed and skin flaps raised. (c) Excision of nail bed. (d) Skin flaps sutured.

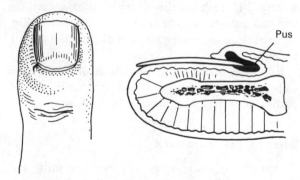

**Fig. 17.21** Paronychia — transverse section shows relation of pus to nail base

## Ingrowing toenail

This condition is due to the sharp edges of the nail impinging on the surrounding skin folds (Fig. 17.19). The skin is split and infection follows. The condition is painful and made worse by misguided attempts to cut away the nail.

The patient usually comes for help after infection has occurred. An attempt is made to 'lift out' the ingrowing portion of the nail by a pledget of gauze soaked in antiseptic. Then the patient is instructed to cut the nail square or shorter in the centre than at the edges, and to avoid wearing narrow shoes.

Once the infection has spread under the nail, or the nail has become deeply embedded, it is best to avulse the nail under general anaesthesia. Antiseptic footbaths then allow the infection to resolve rapidly. The patient is instructed on the correct way to cut the new nail. Should the condition recur, the nailbed must be ablated either surgically or with phenol (Fig. 17.20). Wedge excision of the lateral portion of the nail and underlying nailbed is no longer advised.

## Nail fold infections (paronychia)

Pain, redness and swelling develop at the side and base of a nail. This may extend around the nail and when fully developed produces a horseshoe swelling of the nail fold. Extension under the nail and into the underlying pulp space may occur (Fig. 17.21).

A minor paronychia will usually resolve but if

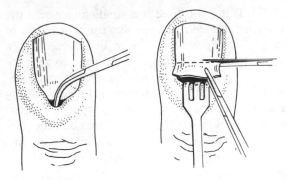

**Fig. 17.22** Operation for paronychia

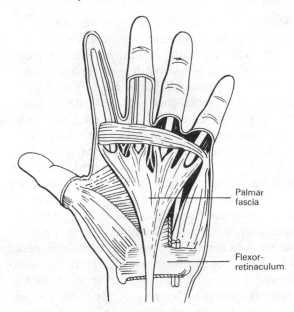

**Fig. 17.23** Flexor retinaculum and palmar fascia

the infection is extending an antibiotic (penicillin) should be given. Should the development of a tense shiny swelling indicate suppuration surgical drainage is required. A single unilateral incision may suffice but if the infection extends under the nail, a flap of skin should be reflected from the nailbase which is then excised to allow free drainage (Fig. 17.22). A simple vaseline gauze dressing is applied.

An acute paronychia may fail to resolve leading to chronic thickening of the nail fold. Fungal infection is a common cause of chronic paronychia and nail scrapings are essential for diagnosis. The possibility of a subungual melanoma must always be kept in mind.

tren's contracture. A similar condition affects the plantar fascia of the sole of the foot but because of constant stretching of the plantar fascia by weight-bearing, it often goes unrecognised.

The aetiology of Dupuytren's contracture is obscure. Some cases are familial, others are asso-

## FIBROSING AND CONSTRICTING CONDITIONS OF THE HAND

Contraction of fibrous tissue occurs in many parts of the body. Symptoms result from secondary constriction, and in the hand this may restrict free movement.

### Dupuytren's contracture

The palmar aponeurosis is a triangular fibrous structure which covers the tendons in the palm of the hand and prevents their forward dislocation (Fig. 17.23). It originates from the tendon of palmaris longus or flexor retinaculum and is inserted by fibrous bands into the proximal and middle phalanges of the fingers. Thickening and contracture of this aponeurosis is called Dupuy-

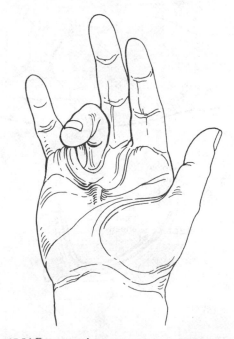

**Fig. 17.24** Dupuytren's contracture

ciated with alcoholism, epilepsy or chronic ill health, e.g. from pulmonary tuberculosis.

The first sign of the condition is the development of a small fibrous nodule or cord just distal to the distal palmar crease in the line of the 4th finger. The medial half of the palmar fascia becomes contracted so that the ring and little fingers become flexed and drawn onto the palm of the hand (Fig. 17.24). This causes a hooklike deformity and an object once grasped cannot be released. Other fingers progressively become involved. The skin of the palm either becomes raised, rock-hard and fused with the underlying fascia or puckered and indrawn. Vessels, nerves and tendons remain free from the fibrotic process.

If the patient is seen at an early stage, he is advised to keep stretching the aponeurosis by passively extending his fingers. Once the disease has given rise to contracture this is no longer helpful. If it is localised to a single finger, and the overlying skin remains mobile, the taut bands of the palmar aponeurosis may be divided by a subcutaneous fasciotomy. If multiple fingers are involved, complete excision of the palmar aponeurosis is required. In severe and long standing cases the capsules of the metacarpo-phalangeal and proximal inter-phalangeal joints become permanently contracted. A capsulotomy is then also necessary. Amputation of a single finger is sometimes necessary.

**Stenosing tenosynovitis**

This condition is due to the development of a fibrous stricture in a tendon sheath, usually at the site of a 'pulley' through which the tendons change direction. The tendons predominantly affected are those of the thumb at the level of the

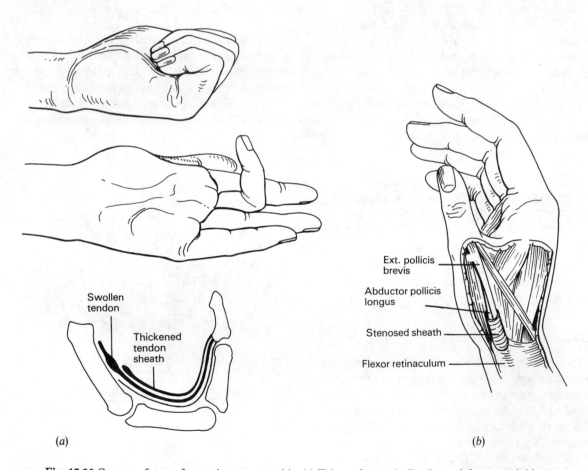

Swollen tendon

Thickened tendon sheath

Ext. pollicis brevis

Abductor pollicis longus

Stenosed sheath

Flexor retinaculum

(a)

(b)

**Fig. 17.25** Common forms of stenosing tenosynovitis. (a) Trigger finger. (b) De Quervain's tenovaginitis.

radial styloid and those of the finger in the distal part of the palm (Fig. 17.25).

*De Quervain's synovitis.* This is the name applied to stenosing tenosynovitis affecting the fibrous sheath of the tendons of the thumb, the abductor pollicis longus and extensor pollicis brevis, as they run through the tunnel at the tip of the radial styloid process. There is pain and tenderness over these tendons which is exaggerated by active or passive stretching of the tendons. Such simple domestic movements as wringing clothes or lifting a teapot may cause severe pain.

*Trigger finger.* This is the more common of the two conditions and is due to thickening of the fibrous flexor tendon sheath at the level of the metacarpo-phalangeal joint. Pain and tenderness at this site occur on active or passive movements of the affected finger. As the tendon is drawn through the narrowed portion of the sheath it develops a fibrous bulge which may prevent its ready return and 'lock' the finger in flexion. Attempts to extend the finger may require passive assistance when the tendon 'snaps' through the strictured area.

In infants and young children the thumb is mainly affected. As a child does not learn to extend the thumb passively, it remains flexed and maybe mistaken for a congenital anomaly. A palpable nodule at the base of the thumb is the clue to the true diagnosis.

These conditions can be corrected permanently by surgical decompression of the fibrous tendon sheath so that the thickened tendon is no longer obstructed.

### Nerve-compression syndromes

Nerves, being soft structures, are prone to compression when they run within fibrous or rigid compartments. Examples are compression of the median nerve as it passes under the pronator teres in the forearm; the ulnar nerve as it runs in the groove of the medial condyle of the humerus at the elbow or around the hook of the hamate in the hand; the lateral cutaneous nerve as it enters the thigh.

The commonest form of nerve compression is the carpal tunnel syndrome affecting the median

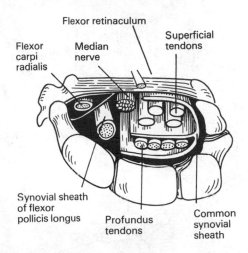

**Fig. 17.26** Anatomy of the carpal tunnel

nerve as it runs below the flexor retinaculum at the wrist (Fig. 17.26). This condition most commonly affects middle aged women, is a known complication of pregnancy or myxoedema, or may be precipitated by local oedema leading to increased tension under the retinaculum. Symptoms include pain particularly at night in the thumb and lateral three fingers, disturbance of sensation and wasting of those muscles supplied by the median nerve (first two lumbricals, abductor and flexor pollicis brevis, opponens pollicis).

Splinting of the wrist at night relieves the pain and is a useful diagnostic test. Relief may also follow the injection of hydrocortisone succinate under the retinaculum in the line of the nerve. Surgical decompression of the nerve is required if there is muscle wasting or when nerve conduction studies demonstrate a nerve block at the site of the retinacular tunnel. This simple operation can be performed through a small incision using a tenotome (Fig. 17.27).

## INFECTIONS OF THE HAND

The hand is prone to minor injury. Even the most trivial puncture wound must be treated with respect otherwise infections of the anatomical spaces within the hand or lymphangitis and lymphadenitis may rapidly develop.

In general a serious hand infection is managed

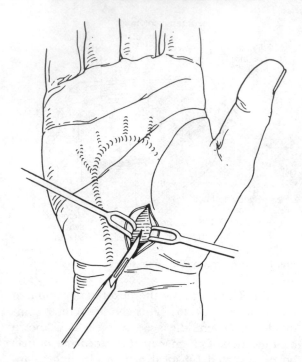

**Fig. 17.27** Relief of carpal tunnel syndrome

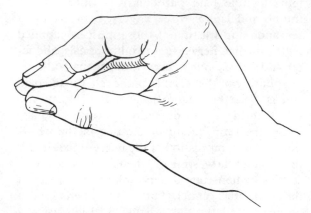

**Fig. 17.28** Position of function of the hand

by systemic antibiotics, elevation of the limb and immobilisation of the hand in the position of function i.e. with the thumb and fingers semi-flexed (Fig. 17.28). If rapid resolution does not occur, the infection must be drained.

### Collar-stud abscess

When a blister becomes infected a sub-epithelial abscess forms. If there is overlying callosity of the skin, this points through the dermis into the sub-dermal fat forming a collar-stud abscess with subepithelial and subdermal components. Such abscesses may track deeply into the anatomical spaces of the finger and hand. Early surgical treatment by deroofing the superficial compartment and dilating the dermal tract to allow free drainage of underlying pus is advised.

### Pulp space infection

The pulp space lies anterior to the distal phalanx and is divided into loculi containing fat and fatty tissue by septa running from the front of the phalanx to the skin (Fig. 17.29). Infection within the unyielding loculi rapidly builds up tension, causes pain and interrupts the blood supply to the distal phalanx, predisposing to septic necrosis of the bone.

For this reason surgical decompression is performed as soon as an abscess is suspected i.e. if the pulp is tense, swollen or red, or if the patient complains of throbbing pain. As it is important not to damage digital nerves and vessels, it is now recommended that incisions are placed longitudinally over the point at which the abscess points, or in the mid-line anteriorly. Such incisions must not cross the flexor crease over the distal inter-phalangeal joint for fear of entering the flexor tendon sheath, or joint capsule. The spaces over the middle and proximal phalanges may also be infected directly, but this is less common.

### Web space infections

The web spaces contain loose areolar tissue and form a path of least resistance for pus tracking from an infected blister situated distally in the palm or from the lumbrical canals to the fingers. The skin anterior to the web becomes thickened,

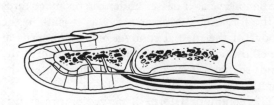

**Fig. 17.29** Pulp space

red and glazed but swelling is mainly dorsal. If there is collar-stud abscess in the distal palm the space is decompressed through this. Otherwise it is best opened through a small dorsal incision.

## Mid-palmar and thenar space infection

These potential spaces lie in the palm of the hand between the anterior surface of the metacarpals and interossei (mid-palmar space) or the adductor pollicis and the flexor tendons (thenar space). They may become infected by spread from a web space or tendon sheath, or by direct puncture.

Because the palmar aponeurosis restricts swelling anteriorly, swelling of the hand is disproportionately great on the dorsum which becomes grossly ballooned. Maximum tenderness is situated anteriorly over those parts of the spaces which are least covered by overlying tissues (Fig. 17.30).

These spaces are surgically decompressed by incisions placed over the site at which the infection points. Damage to vital structures is avoided

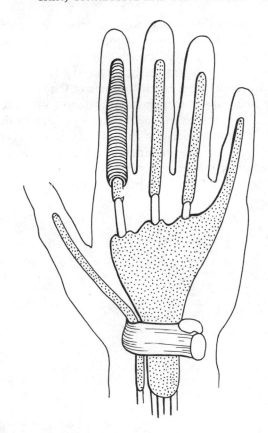

Fig. 17.31 Anatomy of flexor tendon sheaths

by blunt dissection through the deeper tissues. If there is no obvious site of pointing the spaces may be opened either from the medial or lateral sides of the hands.

## Acute tenosynovitis

To allow free and frictionless movement in all positions of the hand, the flexor tendons are enclosed in two layers of synovium separated by fluid and surrounded by a fibrous sheath (Fig. 17.31). Infection may gain access to these synovial spaces either by spread of contiguous infection or by direct puncture, and spreads rapidly within their anatomical confines.

Most commonly acute tenosynovitis affects the flexor sheath of a finger, which becomes grossly swollen and semiflexed. Any attempt to move the tendon either actively or passively causes severe pain. Such passive movements must be tested gently. Tenderness is maximal just proximal to the

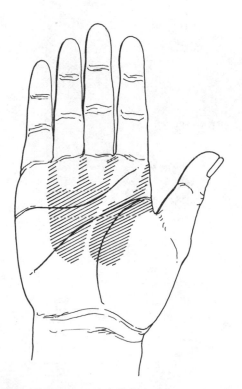

Fig. 17.30 Midpalmar and thenar spaces

crease over the metacarpo-phalangeal joint where the digital tendon sheath projects into the palm.

Infection of the flexor sheath of the thumb spreads into the 'radial bursa' on the lateral side of the palm of the hand. Infection of the sheath of the little finger may involve the common flexor sheath. In this event there is gross oedema of the whole hand, especially the dorsum. The fingers are held in the semiflexed position and any attempt at movement or stretching of the flexor tendons is painful. There is diffuse tenderness over the palm which is maximal on the medial side and may also be elicited in the forearm above the flexor retinaculum.

If there is no immediate response to intensive conservative therapy, surgical decompression of the affected sheath should be carried out. Otherwise necrosis of the tendon may occur. Normally a sheath is decompressed through two small incisions through which pus can be evacuated and soft catheters inserted to allow irrigation and instillation of an appropriate antibiotic.

# 18. The Breast

## ANATOMY AND PHYSIOLOGY

The breast is an appendage of skin and is a modified sweat gland. It contains some six to eight segments of glandular tissue, each drained by a duct opening onto the nipple. The primary secretory unit is a group of saccular alveoli draining into a ductule, the 'terminal duct-lobular unit'. In the resting state this secretes watery fluid which is believed to be re-absorbed through the walls of larger ducts (Fig.18.1)

The alveoli and ducts are lined by a single layer of epithelial cells, the last centimetre of the main ducts by stratified squamous epithelium. Myo-epithelial cells surround the ducts (but not the lobules). Being contractile, they move secretions along the duct system.

The shape of the female breast is due to fat contained within fibrous septa. In adolescents and young adults the breast is firm and prominent; with age the glandular and fibrous elements atrophy, the skin stretches and the breast sags.

The breast lies between the skin and pectoral fascia to which it is loosely attached. It extends from the second to sixth ribs and from the lateral border at the sternum to the mid-axillary line. A prolongation of parenchymatous tissue, the axillary tail runs upwards between pectoralis major and latissimus dorsi to blend with the fat of the axilla. The breast has an excellent blood supply. Laterally this comes from branches of the lateral thoracic artery and perforating branches of the intercostal vessels; medially from perforating branches of the internal mammary artery. Its veins follow the same course. The lymphatics are profuse and run within the substance of the breast

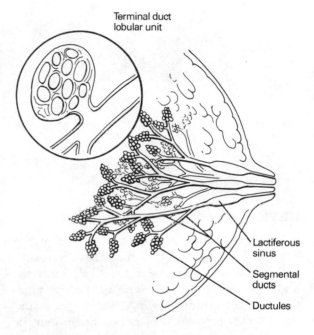

**Fig. 18.1** Structure of the breast and its secreting unit

medially to the internal mammary nodes (which lie under the medial ends of the ribs close to the internal mammary artery) and laterally to nodes along the lateral thoracic vessels (pectoral group) and subscapular vessels (subscapular group). From these nodes lymph passes up through the central and apical axillary nodes to the subclavian trunk. A few lymphatics pierce the pectoral fascia and enter the chest with the perforating vessels, some draining into occasional nodes lying between the pectoral muscles. Although lymph from the medial part of the breast may drain medially, lymph from all parts of the breast may drain laterally through the axillary lymph nodes,

205

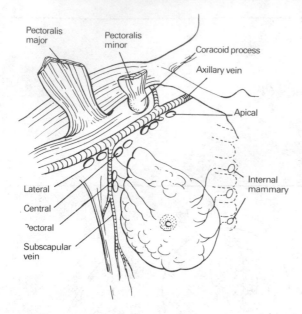

**Fig. 18.2** Axillary and internal mammary nodes draining the breast

which are generally regarded as the main route of spread of malignant disease (Fig. 18.2).

## DEVELOPMENT OF THE BREAST

Early in uterine life two 'milk ridges' form on a line from mid-clavicle to groin. These consist of differentiated ectodermal cells which form the buds of mammary glands. The number and position of these glands vary in different species but small 'accessory' buds of breast tissue may lie anywhere along the milk lines. In women there are two pectoral buds. Solid cords or cells extend into the subcutaneous tissues to develop into the alveoli and ducts of the adult breast.

Apart from a transient burst of activity in the new-born due to circulating hormones of maternal origin, the breast remains dormant until puberty. Then the onset of cyclical hormonal activity stimulates growth, branching of ducts, and formation of ductules and primitive terminal duct lobular units. The size and shape of the post-pubertal breast is not determined by the amount of glandular tissue but by fat.

Although in the resting state terminal duct lobular units can be recognised microscopically, lobular development is only marked during pregnancy. Secretions can be obtained by suction

from the nipple of some 75% of young women. After the menopause lobules normally disappear and secretions become sparse.

## HORMONES AND BREAST DEVELOPMENT

Breast development depends on the endocrine system. Studies in rodents suggest that oestrogen, adrenocortical steroids and growth hormone promote development of ducts, that prolactin is essential for alveolar formation and that full lobulo-alveolar development such as that found in late pregnancy requires a growth tetrad of oestrogen, progesterone, prolactin and growth hormone. During pregnancy the placenta is an important source of these hormones.

In pregnant females the high levels of ovarian and placental steroids inhibit lactation. Following delivery, reduction of oestrogens increases sensitivity of the mammary epithelium to the lactational complex (prolactin, growth hormone and cortisol). Suckling stimulates release of prolactin and oxytocin, the latter stimulating the myo-epithelial cells to eject milk into the terminal ducts. These effects are reversed with weaning.

## NORMAL AND ABNORMAL GROWTH

Enlargement of one or both breasts may be observed in the new-born. This may be associated with secretion of a colostrum-like fluid, 'witches' milk, from the nipple. These changes are due to stimulation by hormones of maternal origin and are temporary.

As puberty approaches the breast enlarges again, initially as a firm 'button' of breast tissue beneath the nipple. At first, this may be unilateral and a cyst or fibro-adenoma may be suspected. One should never interfere surgically with developing breasts lest inadvertent mastectomy be performed. The only exception to this rule is unequivocal evidence of malignancy, which in this age group is exceedingly rare. Early skin fixation and ulceration is characteristic.

During the menstrual years the breast undergoes cyclical changes, which can cause heaviness, discomfort and increasing nodularity during the latter part of the menstrual cycle.

Excessive growth of connective tissue and fat in one or both breasts may occur following puberty (virginal hypertrophy) and can cause discomfort and embarrassment. Reduction mammoplasty may be required but should not be advised until fully mature.

Small breasts also can cause embarrassment. Various methods of enlarging the breast have been tried. These include massage with hormonal creams, and injection of paraffin wax or silicone (see p. 212). Safe augmentation can be achieved by inserting a silicone rubber prosthesis behind the breast tissue or under the pectoral muscles.

Complete failure of development of both breasts at puberty may be due to ovarian agenesis. In Turner's syndrome this is associated with infantilism, short stature, web-neck and cubitis valgus. Failure of breast development may be accompanied by absence of the pectoral muscle or can result from inappropriate surgery before or during puberty. The ease of reconstruction depends on the availability of tissues and the size of the opposite breast. In its simplest form it requires only the insertion of a silicone rubber prosthesis.

---

## EXAMINATION OF THE BREAST (Fig.18.3)

### CLINICAL EXAMINATION

#### History

The patient should be asked if she has any symptoms referrable to the breast, and in particular whether she has noted any discrete abnormality or other areas of texture different from normal. Premenstrual discomfort, nipple discharge, recent retraction or distortion of the nipple are enquired about.

It is important to determine whether the patient has had any previous breast complaint, has attended a breast clinic, had a mammogram or biopsy or whether there is a family history of breast cancer. Routine enquiries include number of children and whether breast-fed, the patient's age at first pregnancy, her menstrual status and date of last menstrual period.

### Physical examination

It is important to have a strict routine for examination of the breast. The patient is undressed to the waist and sits facing the examiner. The breast is inspected from in front while the patient's arms are placed by her side, raised above her head, and finally placed upon her hips. The examiner looks for asymmetry, visible lumps, flattening, skin tethering, abnormal fixation of the breast or retraction and altered axis of the nipples. The patient is then asked to place her hands on the examiner's shoulders and to lean forward. The breasts are again inspected and gently palpated. The fingers are slid behind the outer border of the pectoralis major to seek enlarged pectoral lymph nodes.

Further palpation of the breast is best carried out with the patient lying down and with each shoulder supported in turn by a small pillow. If the arm is raised and the hand tucked behind the patient's head the breast 'flows' over the chest wall. The patient should be asked to point to any abnormality she is aware of and this area examined first. Thereafter each quadrant of each breast is examined in turn by careful palpation between the fingers and underlying chest wall.

Palpation is repeated with the patient's arms at her side. The axillary, central apical and subscapular axillary lymph nodes are then palpated, the arm being supported to relax the axillary muscles. Supraclavicular nodes are best palpated from behind.

Should a lump be palpated its position, size (measured by a calliper), consistency and discreteness must be carefully recorded. It is particularly important to decide whether a lump is smooth, roughened, nodular or whether it is separate from surrounding breast tissue or integrated within it. Fixity to skin is sought by pinching up the skin overlying the mass, fixity to the pectoral muscle by assessing the mobility of the mass first with the pectoral muscles relaxed then with them contracted. This is achieved by asking the patient to place her hands on her hips and press.

If the patient complains of discharge from the nipple an attempt should be made to reproduce this, to determine whether it arises from one or several ducts and to test it for blood. Pressure is applied to the alveolar margin with the finger

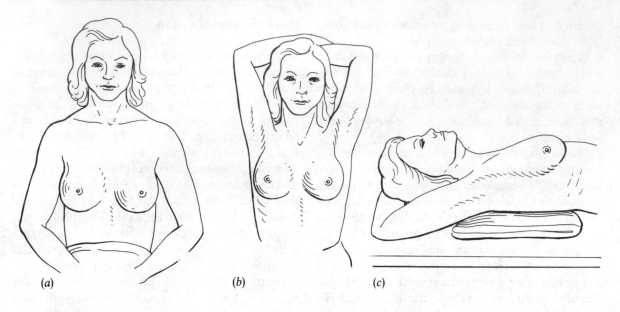

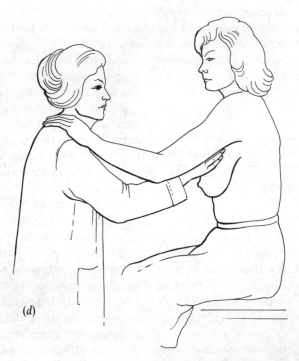

**Fig. 18.3** Examination of the breast. (a) + (b) Inspection. (c) Position for palpation. (d) Palpation of axillae.

'around the clock', palpating for a dilated duct or nodule and observing if the discharge can be produced (Fig. 18.4). If unsuccessful the breast tissue immediately under the nipple is picked up and gently compressed.

The discharge is tested for blood and a smear made for cytological examination. If it arises from one duct, note should be made of the position of that duct and whether its orifice is dilated.

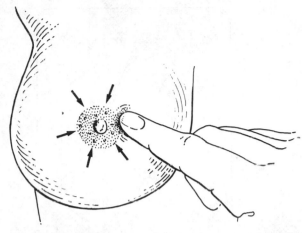

**Fig. 18.4** Method of differential 'round the clock' palpation to induce discharge

## ANCILLARY METHODS

### Needle aspiration

Needle aspiration of a breast lump is carried out in the clinic using a 20 ml syringe and a 19 gauge needle (Fig. 18.5). A special handle is available to apply constant suction but is not necessary.

The mass is steadied between the finger and thumb and the needle inserted into it through the overlying skin. The 'consistency' of the mass gives useful information; the sudden relief of resistance on entering a cyst, the tough rubbery feel of fibrocystic breast tissue, and the grittiness of a cancer are typical.

A cyst is emptied of fluid (see below). If the lesion is solid an aspiration biopsy is taken by applying suction at constant pressure and advancing and withdrawing the needle several times through the centre of the tumour. The pressure on the syringe is released, the needle and syringe removed and contents of the needle expressed onto a slide and smears prepared.

### Mammography

Mammography (soft tissue radiology of the breast) uses high resolution fine grain film, high intensity screens and X-rays of low penetrating power. With modern systems the dose of radiation is small (0.1 rad per film).

Xeromammograms (see Chapter 1) are particularly useful for examining the breast as they highlight changes of density by a 'brush' effect, show calcifications clearly, and can be read in reflected light. As the dose of radiation is larger that with mammography (at least 1 rad per film), xeroradiography is reserved for postmenopausal women.

With both systems, the lateral and craniocaudal films are standard. Recently a single oblique view has been developed which shows the whole breast. This is taken from upper medial to lower lateral aspects of the breast and is particularly suitable for 'screening' well women for breast cancer (Fig. 18.6).

### Thermography

Once popular for examining the breast, thermography has limited diagnostic value and is seldom used (see Chapter 1).

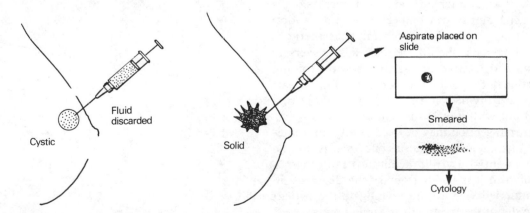

**Fig. 18.5** Needle aspiration of a breast mass

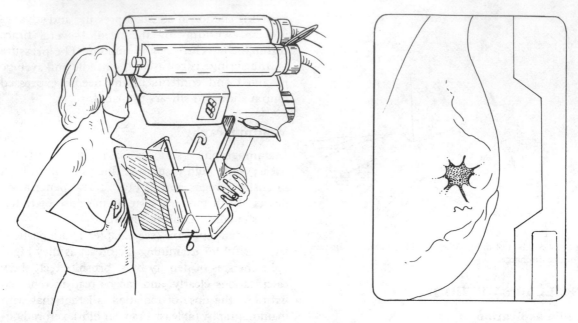

**Fig. 18.6** Single oblique mammography

## Histology

Traditionally the histology of breast lesions is obtained by excision biopsy, often combined with frozen section examination. Closed biopsy methods are now standard in specialist breast clinics. The simplest device is a Trucut needle by which a core of tissue is removed under local anaesthesia (see Chapter 1).

## BREAST BIOPSY

Surgical removal of a benign lesion from the breast is a common operation. If the lesion is superficial biopsy can be performed under local anaesthesia, otherwise a general anaesthetic is used. Incisions should be placed transversely following the curve of the breast and avoiding distortion of the breast contour. The breast tissues are divided and the lesion carefully dissected out with a little surrounding tissue.

A frozen section may be used to give an immediate histological diagnosis but this is by no means essential. Even if the diagnosis of cancer is unequivocal it is better to make the diagnosis in an unhurried way and to investigate the patient before definitive treatment is carried out.

Removal of mammographically visible but im-

palpable lesions poses particular problems. Some surgeons simply perform wide local or segmental resection of the area concerned but it is better to localise the lesion radiologically before operation using a hooked stylet needle. Following excision the specimen must be X-rayed to confirm that the lesion has been removed (Fig. 18.7).

Frozen section examination of small mammographic lesions is not advised. Considerable experience and expertise are required for their pathological assessment.

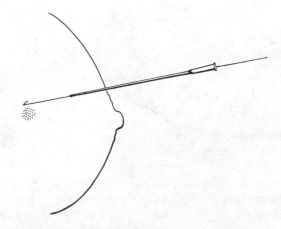

**Fig. 18.7** Localisation of non-palpable mammographic lesion to facilitate excision

## INFLAMMATION

### ACUTE AND CHRONIC MASTITIS

Inflammation of the breast may accompany systemic infection. Acute mastitis can complicate mumps, while causes of chronic mastitis include tuberculosis, hydatid disease, syphilis and actinomycosis. These are rare. The common form of acute mastitis is staphylococcal infection of local origin and occurs most frequently during the puerperium. Infection gains access from a cracked nipple and good hygiene has done much to reduce its incidence.

Acute mastitis starts as a localised area of inflammation which is painful, red, indurated and tender. It may resolve spontaneously or spread through the breast which becomes swollen, hot and oedematous. Fever and toxicity occur. Necrosis and pus formation forms a multilobular abscess. Fluctuation may be elicited but only if the abscess is superficial. The involved skin is then glazed and thin. If the abscess lies deeply within or behind the breast fluctuation is absent.

Antibiotic therapy can prevent the full development of acute mastitis but it must be given early in the disease and in adequate doses. The choice is based on the likely sensitivity of the organisms. For domiciliary practice a combination of penicillin and cloxacillin may prove satisfactory; when in hospital a cephalosporin or erythromycin are preferable. Cessation of breast feeding is normally advised. Firm support may be all that is needed. Alternatively a synthetic oestrogen (quinestrol 4 mg) or bromocriptine (2.5 mg twice daily) may be given.

An abscess should be drained surgically. Indications for drainage are a fluctuant mass, glazed red oedematous skin or persistence of local signs of infection for more than five days, or of severe systemic upset for more than 48 hours after full antibiotic treatment.

At operation, loculi are broken down to form a single cavity which is drained. A curved transverse incision is made, the abscess opened and a finger inserted to break down the septa. A biopsy is taken from the abscess wall and a tube drain brought out through the wound or at the most dependent part of the breast (Fig. 18.8).

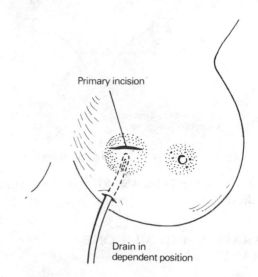

Primary incision

Drain in dependent position

**Fig. 18.8** Drainage of a breast abscess

Pus is sent to the laboratory for identification of the organism and its sensitivity. Antibiotic therapy is continued for a few days and the drainage tube removed when drainage ceases. If it is small, some surgeons prefer to excise an abscess under antibiotic cover rather than to drain it.

Inadequate antibiotic therapy alters the natural history of the disease. Necrosis and pus formation are retarded, fibrosis is increased and the breast becomes chronically thickened and honeycombed with pus. The resemblance to an inflammatory cancer can be startling. Treatment is by multiple incisions and drainage. Biopsy of several areas of breast tissue is mandatory.

### MAMMILLARY FISTULA

This condition of young women is due to blockage by a keratin plug of a lactiferous sinus in the nipple. The sinus becomes dilated, its epithelium undergoes squamous metaplasia and infection leads to a subareolar abscess. This either bursts spontaneously or is incised, to form a fistula opening at the areolar margin (Fig. 18.9)

Recurrent attacks of acute inflammation and intermittent discharge of pus through the 'mammillary fistula' follow. Treatment is by surgical exploration with excision of the wall of the lactiferous sinus, its related cavity and in some cases a segment of breast tissue. Alternatively, as in operation for fistula-in-ano, the lactiferous sinus

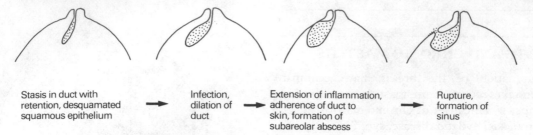

Stasis in duct with retention, desquamated squamous epithelium → Infection, dilation of duct → Extension of inflammation, adherence of duct to skin, formation of subareolar abscess → Rupture, formation of sinus

**Fig. 18.9** Stages in the formation of a mammillary fistula

between the fistula and the orifice of the duct may be de-roofed and the lining excised.

## PARAFFIN AND SILICONE GRANULOMAS

The current desire for large breasts has led women with small breasts to seek augmentation. Initially liquid paraffin was injected into the sub-mammary space. Unfortunately, paraffin migrated into the breast tissues causing an intense low grade inflammatory reaction, and formation of abscesses and chronic sinuses. Organic polymers of silica (silicones) of glue-like consistency were then developed and these also were injected into the sub-mammary space. Pure silicones are inert but the use of inferior grades to which irritants were added to prevent migration resulted in inflammatory reactions. Multiple painful lumps, 'silicone granulomas', developed through the breast; the overlying skin became inflamed and often broke down to form multiple sinuses. Systemic reactions such as granulomatous hepatitis also occurred from absorption of the chemical. Mastectomy is the only possible treatment.

It is now recognised that even 'medical grade' silicone should not be injected. If mammary augmentation is indicated it should be performed by the insertion of a prosthesis consisting of silicone gel enclosed in a silicone rubber envelope.

## BENIGN EPITHELIAL TUMOURS

### FIBROADENOMA

A fibroadenoma is the commonest breast mass of young women. It is a well-defined, small, painless, smooth firm swelling which is clearly demar-

cated from the surrounding breast tissue and is characteristically mobile: 'the breast mouse'. Frequently fibroadenomas are multiple. Mammography may reveal a round ovoid density with a radiolucent halo from compression of surrounding fat. However its density may be similar to that of breast tissue and it may not be detectable. In later life it may form a dense, coarsely calcified mass.

On gross examination a fibroadenoma is clearly demarcated from surrounding breast tissue, which suggests encapsulation. Its cut surface is granular, whitish-brown, glistening and bulges outward. Interweaving clefts form dark lines.

Microscopically there are two components: proliferation of fine connective tissue 'fibro' and an abnormal multiplication of ducts and acini, 'adenoma'. These two components are present in varying degrees and produce a wide range of histological appearances.

A typical fibroadenoma is slow-growing and self-limiting. It takes some 6 to 12 months to double in size and usually stops growing when some 3 cm in diameter. If untreated it may undergo hyalinisation and merge with surrounding tissue or may form a hard calcified mass. Nevertheless it is wise to excise a fibroadenoma as in a young patient a carcinoma may be indistinguishable. A fibroadenoma may grow during pregnancy and there is always a slight risk of later malignant change.

*Soft fibroadenoma.* A variant of fibroadenoma with more rapid growth is found in older women. This is softer in consistency than the typical lesion of the young patient but is still quite benign and is cured by excision.

A *giant fibroadenoma* is a distinct entity in young adolescent females. It is rare in Britain but common in some African countries, appearing a few years after puberty and growing rapidly to a very large size. The girl usually complains that one breast has become larger than the other. On examination the involved breast is distended asymmetrically by a large softish lobular tumour in which clefts can be palpated. The skin is thin with distended veins yet the tumour is not fixed to skin or to deeper tissues. Mammography demonstrates a large well-defined opacity within the breast.

These tumours are quite benign and cured by local excision, provided this is complete.

## CYSTOSARCOMA PHYLLODES

This tumour is so called because of the leaf-like masses of tumour tissue which project into cystic cavities and the 'sarcomatous' appearance of the connective tissue stroma. It is fibro-epithelial in origin, the typical deep elongated clefts being lined by epithelial cells. Some believe that it originates in a fibroadenoma. Myxomatous degeneration and metaplastic formation of fibrous and fatty elements are common. If the stroma becomes frankly malignant (3–12%) metastases may occur. These are of sarcomatous (blood-borne) type.

Clinically a cystosarcoma forms a rapidly growing unilateral tumour in women of 40–50 years. Typical are its irregular 'bosselated' surface, palpable deep clefts and the shiny stretched thin skin containing grossly dilated veins (Fig 18.10). Lymph node enlargement is rare.

Treatment consists of total mastectomy combined with axillary node sampling. As local recurrence is the main problem wide removal of tissue is advised with replacement by a musculo-cutaneous flap. Radiotherapy is of no value.

## CYSTIC DISEASE AND EPITHELIAL HYPERPLASIA

### Definitions

*Cystic disease* is regarded as a disease of the breast lobules. Dilatation of the duct system is known as duct ectasia, although the two conditions may coincide. Inspissated secretions may exude from dilated ducts during operations for cystic disease.

Cystic disease is a condition of late premeno-

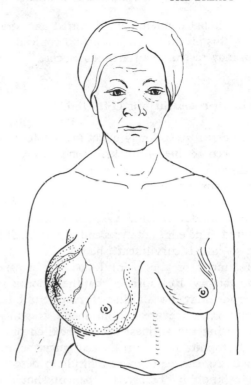

**Fig. 18.10** Clinical appearances of Cystosarcoma phyllodes

pausal and menopausal women. Unlike cancer its incidence does not increase with age and it is rare in postmenopausal women. It is probably a disorder of involution. Several small cysts develop by dilatation of acini within the lobule, these being separated by fine connective tissue of intralobular type. These small cysts coalesce to form large cysts lined by epithelium, which may show metaplastic transformation to apocrine (sweat gland) type. If the outflow tract becomes obstructed a large tension cyst forms which is filled with clear yellow, green or brownish fluid.

*Benign epithelial hyperplasia* is commonly associated with cystic disease and may consist of adenosis or epitheliosis. Adenosis is non-neoplastic glandular hyperplasia in which all epithelial units within a lobule are hypertrophied and lie within fine connective tissue stroma. Epitheliosis is solid epithelial hyperplasia occurring within small ducts, ductules and even acini. When extensive this forms finger-like projections of epithelium which some call papillomatosis. If adenosis is accompanied by marked proliferation of fibrous tissue the condition is called 'sclerosing adenosis'.

The epithelial elements are distorted and strangled by this proliferation, and microscopically the lesion may resemble a scirrhous cancer.

## Clinical presentations (Fig. 18.11)

*Diffuse cystic disease* may affect the whole breast which becomes heavy, thickened and lumpy. Pain and discomfort are common, particularly in the premenstrual phase of the cycle.

On mammography the breast parenchyma is dense and ductal and vascular shadows are obscured. The edges of cysts and fibrotic nodules form so-called 'curvilinear' shadows.

Treatment of the painful nodular breast is unsatisfactory. Reassurance that the lesion is not cancerous may be all that is required, but if discomfort is severe, antihormone treatment, either using the antioestrogen tamoxifen or the gonadotrophin inhibitor danazol may be prescribed. As cancer is more difficult to detect in such a 'knobbly' breast, the patient should be kept under review.

*Localised thickening*. This is caused either by a conglomeration of small cysts or by fibrosis. The patient notices that a segment of one breast differs in texture from the rest. This area may have become particularly prominent towards the end of a menstrual cycle, but unlike the rest of the breast does not resolve and soften after the period finishes.

On clinical examination the area feels rubbery, thickened and nodular. It is more readily palpated by the fingers than with the flat of the hand. Mammography is essential and any suggestion of discrete opacity or microcalcifications indicates the need for biopsy. Provided the mammograms do not show such change the patient may be kept under review. Clinical suspicion of a discrete nodule within the area makes biopsy mandatory regardless of the mammographic findings.

Sclerosing adenosis gives rise to a firm mobile nodular mass, which may suggest malignant disease. On needle aspiration it feels tough and rubbery, rather than hard and gritty. Biopsy is the only safe course of action. Because the microscopic appearances can resemble scirrhous cancer, careful examination of the gross specimen (a greyish-white nodular mass) and of multiple paraffin sections is desirable to avoid inappropriate mastectomy.

*Tension cyst*. A cyst forms a firm or hard mass in the breast. This may be well-demarcated, smooth and mobile, or integrated into an area of fibrocystic disease when its surface feels irregular. The clinical differentiation of a cyst from a cancer is not always easy; absence of fixation to the skin is a helpful guide.

The diagnosis can readily be confirmed by fine-needle aspiration. The needle traverses the wall of the cyst to enter the fluid-filled cavity, from which typical yellow, green or brown cyst fluid is aspirated. Usually a cyst contains 5–15 ml; but much larger amounts can occur.

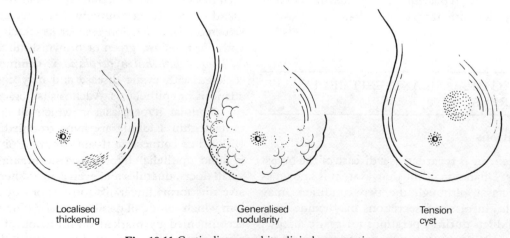

Localised thickening        Generalised nodularity        Tension cyst

**Fig. 18.11** Cystic disease and its clinical presentation

Needle aspiration is a safe method of treating a breast cyst, provided certain precautions are taken:

1. The breast must be palpated carefully after aspiration. A hollow may be felt at the site of the cyst so that the surrounding breast tissue is more clearly palpable. There should be no residual discrete mass.

2. The cyst fluid should be examined for blood. Cytological examination of the cyst fluid is unhelpful.

3. Mammograms should be requested. These may show additional cysts in one or other breast but no signs of cancer.

4. The patient should be re-examined in 3 to 4 weeks' time to determine whether the cyst has remained empty. If it has re-filled, one further aspiration may be done. Re-filling thereafter is a definite indication for removal.

Indications for excision biopsy are: a residual mass after aspiration, significant blood in the cyst fluid, a suspicious mammogram, and repeated re-filling of the cyst.

## Risk of malignancy

The risk of developing cancer in women with cystic disease is reported to be 2–3 times higher than normal. Such reports are retrospective studies. There are no good prospective studies in which women with cystic disease have been matched with normal controls, both being meticulously followed over a long period of time. As epithelial elements are believed to be at risk attempts have been made to classify atypical appearances of ductal and lobular epithelium. These are difficult to interpret and require detailed study. A breast must never be removed on a frozen section report of epithelial atypia.

## DISEASES OF DUCTS

### DUCT ECTASIA (Fig. 18.12)

This is an inflammatory disease of breast ducts. It is characterised by dilatation of the major ducts, which fill with inspissated pultaceous creamy secretion and is associated with periductal inflam-

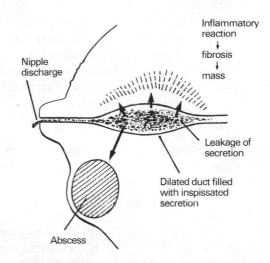

**Fig. 18.12** Duct ectasia and its clinical presentation

matory reaction in which round cell infiltration predominates. It is not known whether the dilatation of the ducts occurs first and is followed by leakage of secretions which initiate the periductal reaction, or conversely whether periductal reaction occurs first, destroying elastica and allowing duct dilatation.

The disease occurs most commonly in women over the age of 50 years and may produce one or more of the following clinical signs:

1. Discharge from the nipple — bloody, serous or creamy — arising from one or more ducts

2. Retraction or inversion of the nipple due to shortening of the ducts

3. An episode of acute inflammation with a hot, tender swelling involving a segment of the breast usually close to the areola with red overlying skin. An acute abscess may form and require drainage. This may lead to the development of a mammillary fistula. Anaerobic organisms may be present and antibiotic therapy is under trial.

4. Chronic inflammation affecting a localised area or segment of the breast (plasma-cell mastitis). This forms a hard craggy area within the breast which may be associated with tethering and dimpling of overlying skin and nipple retraction. Its similarity to cancer has led to inappropriate mastectomies.

The treatment of duct ectasia is excision of the involved ducts and surrounding breast tissue. When there is discharge or nipple inversion, a circumareolar incision is made, the nipple reflected and a cone of tissue including the main ducts excised from the centre area of the breast. If the disease affects a single segmental duct, that duct and its associated segment of breast tissue is removed.

## DUCT PAPILLOMA

Benign papillomatous growths can form from the epithelial linings of the main ducts. They may be pedunculated or sessile, and are situated within 1 cm of the nipple. Bleeding from the nipple is characteristic and originates from a single duct, the orifice of which is dilated and slit-like. The papilloma may be felt as a small nodule at the areolar margin. Pressure at that point reproduces the discharge (Fig.18.13).

Mammography shows a dilated duct and/or a small round opacity close to the nipple and on ductography a filling defect is demonstrated. Treatment is by surgical excision of the involved duct.

## THE PAINFUL BREAST

Pain, discomfort and heaviness in the breasts are common symptoms which if severe can interfere

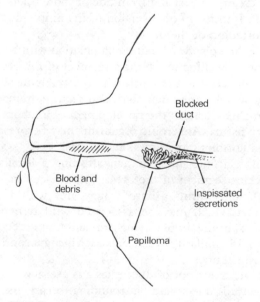

Fig. 18.13 Duct papilloma

with the normal sex-life of a woman and cause irritability and depression. Breast pain may be cyclical, occurring predominantly in the premenstrual phase, or non-cyclical, when its occurrence has no relationship to the menstrual cycle. The former frequently is associated with tender nodularity and fullness of the breast most pronounced in its upper outer quadrant and is generally assumed to be of hormonal origin. Non-cyclical pain may be associated with inflammatory disease of the breast, duct ectasia, or as a symptom of neurosis.

The breasts should be carefully examined, including, in women over 35 years, a mammogram. Most patients have no local disease, but if cysts are present they should be aspirated and tender fibrous nodules may require excision.

Many patients with breast pain are helped by reassurance that there is no serious disease present. If cyclical symptoms are severe the anti-prolactin bromocryptine, the anti-oestrogen tamoxifen, the anti-gonadotrophin danazol or evening primrose oil are reported to give some relief.

## MISCELLANEOUS TUMOURS

### CONNECTIVE TISSUE TUMOURS

*Benign* connective tissue tumours, lipomas, angiomas, leiomyomas, neurofibromas, etc. are rare. A lipoma of the breast forms a soft lobulated mass which on mammography is radiolucent. Its importance lies in its confusion with the 'pseudo-lipoma', the soft fatty mass which can surround a small scirrhous carcinoma and is caused by indrawing of surrounding fat by fibrous spicules.

Fibrosarcoma, lymphosarcoma, rhabdomyosarcoma, angiosarcoma and osteogenic sarcoma are all rare. Unlike the cystosarcoma (see above) there are no epithelial elements in these tumours. A sarcoma presents as a rapidly enlarging breast mass. Spread occurs predominantly by the bloodstream and gives rise to metastases in lungs and other viscera. Treatment is by radical local surgery. They are radioresistant.

*Lymphoma*. The breast may be the site of a

lymphomatous deposit. This forms a smooth, discrete and firm mass resembling a fibro-adenoma. Axillary lymph nodes are typically rubbery and discrete.

*Secondary tumours.* Metastases can occur within the breast and form a well-defined discrete mass which mammographically is usually well-defined. Primary sites are most commonly bronchus, thyroid and malignant melanoma and, should it have been involved by cancer, the other breast.

## SCREENING FOR BREAST CANCER

Recognition that breast cancer presents frequently at an incurable stage has led to interest in the earlier detection of the disease. Programmes of education and 'self-palpation' have been instituted, in which women are encouraged to seek advice for the smallest abnormality. With the development of mammography, it soon became apparent that small cancers of less than 1 cm in diameter could be visible radiologically before they became clinically obvious. Small discrete opacities, areas of disturbed breast architecture and clusters of irregular spicules of calcification may point to a cancer months or even years before it is clinically obvious. Programmes of routine breast examination, clinical examination and mammography or mammography alone have now been instituted in many countries. One, in Sweden, relies on a single oblique mammogram of each breast as the initial screening procedure; this considerably reduces the cost of screening programmes.

As screening is expensive it is important to know that it reduces the mortality of the disease. The only evidence that this is so comes from a study carried out in New York, in which 60 000 women of age 40–64 were randomly allocated for annual screening by clinical examination and mammography or for routine medical care. The number of cancers detected in these two groups over a 5-year period was the same; but the fatality rates of those in the screened population were one third less than the controls.

Good surgical back-up services are essential to an efficient screening programme. They are particularly important when dealing with small mammographic lesions which may be completely impalpable even on careful re-examination of the breast. Pre-operative radiological localisation by the insertion of a small hooked metal marker and postoperative radiographs of the specimen to ensure that the lesion has been removed are essential aids (see p. 210).

Considerable experience and expertise are required for the histopathological examination of these mini-lesions. Rapid diagnosis by frozen section has no place; the pathologist must define the site of the lesion by slicing the specimen and if necessary X-raying the slices. He will also wish to examine relevant areas of normal as well as diseased breast tissue by microscopy.

Radiation can induce breast cancer. It has been calculated that for each rad of radiation received by the breast there will be six extra cancers per million women, starting after a latent period of 10 years. Radiation dose must therefore be kept low. With modern systems of sensitive films vacuum-packed with highly intensifying screens, a complete two-view examination of the breast can be performed with a dose to the breast of a fraction of a rad. In Britain mammography for screening is not advised in women under the age of 45 years.

## CANCER OF THE BREAST

Cancer of the breast is an adenocarcinoma arising from epithelium lining the ducts and acini. Some believe that all cancers arise in the terminal duct lobular unit but traditionally such tumours are divided into ductal and lobular types. Both duct and lobular cancers may be invasive (infiltrating) or non-invasive (non-infiltrating) or *in situ*. Only invasive cancers metastasise.

### TYPES OF INVASIVE CANCER

*Duct cancers.* 80% of invasive cancer of the breast is of ductal type of 'nondescript histological pattern'. However duct cancers with specific histological features do occur. Those of greatest importance are:

*Medullary cancer.* This is a well-delineated tumour accounting for 5% of cancers. Microscopically it is sharply and completely circumscribed. It consists of syncytial sheets of large neoplastic cells with a substantial diffuse infiltrate of mononuclear lymphoid cells. Its prognosis is better than that of a typical duct cancer.

*Tubular cancer.* This is a well-differentiated tumour which accounts for some 10% of invasive breast cancers and is typified by proliferation of small tubular duct-like structures which are haphazardly arranged in a loose cellular stroma. It is this type of cancer which may be confused with sclerosing adenosis. Its prognosis is better than average.

*Mucoid cancer.* Like medullary cancer this is well circumscribed. It is a rare tumour, characterised by a copious matrix of mucinous tissue. It also has a relatively good prognosis.

*Lobular cancer.* Lobular invasive cancer accounts for 5–10% of breast cancers. It is typified by the bland homogeneous nature of its small cells. As with duct carcinoma various histopathological types are described, including cribriform, solid and tubular types. The differentiation between lobular and duct cancers is not easy and there is no single criterion by which they can be identified.

## IN-SITU CANCER

Non-invasive cancers of the breast are confined to the ducts and acini and have not penetrated the basement membrane of the epithelial cell layer. Lobular carcinoma *in situ* is usually an incidental finding in biopsy specimens of post-menopausal women. There is total involvement of one or more lobules with small neoplastic round cells. Intraduct carcinoma is usually detected as microcalcifications on mammography. The epithelial cells of otherwise normal ducts and lobules undergo malignant change and either cling to the duct wall or form papillary masses within the ducts. Both lobular and intraduct carcinoma in situ have a long natural history and a good prognosis. This is further considered below.

## BIOLOGY AND NATURAL HISTORY

### Spread of breast cancer

Invasive breast cancer spreads by lymphatics and blood stream and direct invasion (skin, chest wall)

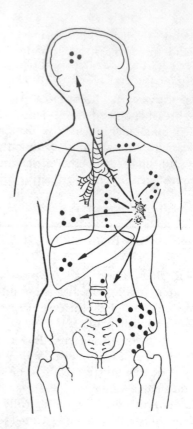

**Fig. 18.14** Spread of breast cancer to regional nodes, liver, bones, lung and brain

(Fig. 18.14). The regional lymph nodes most commonly involved lie in the axilla, in relation to the lateral thoracic (pectoral group) and sub-scapular vessels (sub-scapular group). From these disease spreads to the glands lying along the axillary vein (central group) up to the level of the first rib (apical group) (Fig. 18.2). Supraclavicular nodes may also be affected.

Although tumours in all parts of the breast can give rise to axillary node metastases, those in the medial half may also spread to the internal mammary group of nodes lying along the internal mammary vessels within the mediastinum. This is most common when the axillary lymph nodes are also involved and only occasionally are the internal mammary nodes the sole route of spread. Internal mammary node involvement is a bad prognostic feature and usually indicates spread to mediastinal nodes and pleural cavities.

The orthodox view was that the phenomenon of spread of breast cancer has 'two steps', initial spread to the regional lymph nodes and only then to distant organs. It is now known that tumour cells can bypass the node 'filter' and that spread by both lymphatic and bloodstream occurs contemporaneously. Systemic spread can occur to any site but metastases are particularly common in the skeleton, lungs, liver, brain, the ovaries and peritoneal cavity.

## Aetiology

Breast cancer is the commonest cancer affecting the female population of Western countries; 7% of women develop the disease. In Japan, Africa and South America its incidence is one sixth of that in Europe, Scandinavia or North America. This difference affects mainly postmenopausal women and is not explained by any known risk factors. There is a positive correlation between crude fat intake and breast cancer incidence and some believe that dietary factors are important in aetiology.

Certain other factors which increase the risk of developing the disease are recognised. Early age at menarche, late age at first pregnancy, nulliparity, late age at menopause, upper social class, a previous history of benign breast disease and a family history of breast cancer are all associated with an increased incidence. Some of these risk factors have been examined alone or in combination in populations of women undergoing breast screening to see whether women at increased risk can be selected for intensive examination. However the factors are not sufficiently sensitive for this purpose.

Only women who have already been treated for breast cancer (whose opposite breast is at risk) and those with a mother or sister who has been treated for the disease justify special surveillance.

The relationship between atypical changes in the breast epithelium and later development of breast cancer is obscure. At present only frank in situ cancer is a proven antecedent of invasive disease.

## Natural history

The incidence of breast cancer increases with age, but is most common in women of 55–60 years. There is a fall-off in incidence during the meno-

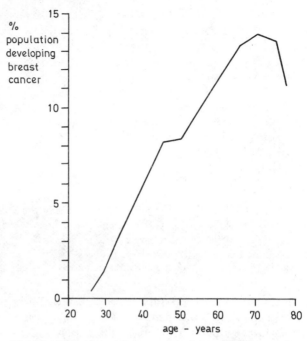

**Fig. 18.15** Prevalence of cancer of the breast related to age

pause which has led some to believe that there are two distinct types of breast cancer affecting respectively premenopausal and postmenopausal women (Fig. 18.15). Different aetiological factors may then be concerned.

Breast cancer is a slow-growing disease and metastases may develop many years after apparently successful local treatment. Recurrence-free interval and survival time are affected by the extent of the disease at the time it presents. The larger a tumour and the more extensive the local spread the worse its prognosis. Lymph node involvement affects survival adversely, the larger the number of lymph nodes involved the worse the prognosis. Only 30% of women with four or more invaded axillary lymph nodes will survive for 5 years.

Biological factors also affect the aggressiveness of the disease. These include the type of tumour and tumour-host relationship. The histological grade of differentiation (based on degree of tubule formation and regularity of nuclear size and shape), tumour contour, degree of lymphocytic infiltration and reactive changes in the regional lymph nodes all affect prognosis. Thus tumours which are well-differentiated, have a smooth con-

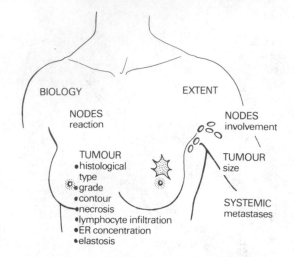

Fig. 18.16 Biological factors influencing prognosis

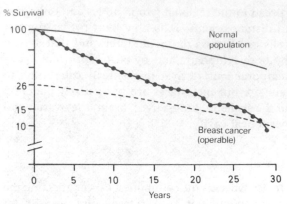

**Fig. 18.17** Survival curve of women with breast cancer (----
is parallel to normal survival) (source as Fig. 15.8)

tour, exhibit marked lymphocytic infiltration and
evoke reactive enlargement of regional lymph
nodes have a better prognosis than poorly differentiated lesions with a spiculated contour and no
lymphocytic infiltration or reaction in regional
nodes (Fig. 18.16).

Recently it has been found that tumours with
oestrogen receptor activity (see p. 227) and
extensive focal periductal elastosis also have a
better prognosis. These features may also reflect
tumour differentiation.

## Curability

There are now several reports of the long-term
follow-up of women with breast cancer treated
only by local means. As a result it is now recognised that 'cure' (as defined by survival for a
normal life-span free from disease) is achieved in
less than 30% of 'operable' patients. If all cases
are considered including those inoperable when
first seen, the 'cure rate' is less than 20% (Fig.
18.17).

It is also now evident that even when a patient
has attained her normal life-span, she has still a
high probability of dying from metastatic breast
cancer. Metastases and local recurrence may
develop even as long as 40 years after primary
treatment. Calculation of absolute cure rates in
terms of eradication of disease is therefore virtually impracticable.

## DIAGNOSIS

### History

### Clinical examination of breast

Breast cancer usually presents as a lump which is
painless or at most associated with a tingling
discomfort. It most commonly occurs in the upper
outer quadrant of the breast and may have caused
recent nipple retraction. Visible signs of fixation
are carefully sought. These include asymmetry of
the breast, flattening of its contour, dimpling or
puckering of the overlying skin and retraction or
altered axis of the nipple. These signs are more
evident when the patient is sitting with her hands
raised above her head or when with her hands on
her hips, she pushes out her chest.

The mass is usually readily palpable and classically it is hard with an irregular surface merging
with surrounding breast tissue. Cancer in a fatty
breast may be deceptively soft due to 'packaging'
of surrounding fat by the contraction of the
fibrous framework of the breast. This may even
be mistaken for a lipoma.

It is important to appreciate that any discrete
lump, no matter how small or mobile, can be a
cancer. This is particularly important in the
young woman with a glandular breast in whom
cancer cannot be distinguished clinically from a
small fibroadenoma.

Some patients present with advanced local
disease and exhibit skin ulceration, infiltration or
oedema or fixity and obvious contraction of the
whole breast to the chest wall. In such cases the
diagnosis should not be in any doubt.

The regional lymph nodes in the axilla and supraclavicular fossa are carefully palpated and the findings recorded. It should be noted whether nodes are palpable and if so whether they are soft, hard, mobile, matted or fixed to surrounding structures.

## Needle aspiration

The main differentiation is between cancer and a cyst and aspiration with a fine (19 gauge) needle is performed. If no fluid is obtained an aspirate should be examined cytologically.

Fine needle aspiration cytology is performed by repeatedly advancing the needle through the tumour while suction is applied. On withdrawal, the tissue aspirated into the needle is expressed onto a slide, fixed and stained.

## Radiology

In expert hands this has an accuracy of diagnosis of 95%. Radiology or xeromammography is ordered. A cancer forms a dense opacity containing small clustered microcalcifications and with an indefinite outline from which irregular spicules or spikes penetrate straight out into the surrounding breast. Secondary signs of tumour include thickening of the overlying skin, distorted duct and vascular pattern, and dilated veins (Fig. 18.18). Mammography is of less diagnostic value in the young women in whom the density of the lesion differs little from that of the parenchymatous tissue. Mammography is important for the full examination of the contralateral breast.

## Tru-cut

The final diagnosis of cancer rests on histopathology. A tissue sample can be obtained by Tru-cut needle biopsy under local anaesthesia. Not only does this avoid frozen section, it also allows further assessment of the patient before operation. Fine needle aspiration cytology, if expertly carried out, can provide sufficient evidence of malignancy to proceed.

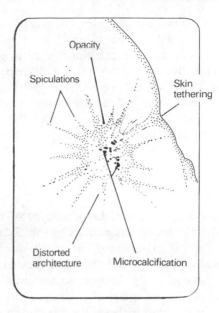

**Fig. 18.18** Mammographic signs of cancer

## STAGING

The international TNM system of classifying breast cancer (UICC) allows grouping into clinical stages which traditionally have determined curability by local treatment. It was considered that if the growth was confined to the breast and regional (axillary) lymph nodes every tumour cell could be eradicated by mastectomy and axillary clearance or by combinations of surgery and radiotherapy. This is no longer accepted. Nevertheless careful clinical staging allows the comparison of patients and defines patients with local disease suitable for surgical treatment. Clinical staging has two main drawbacks:

1. Palpability of axillary lymph nodes is not synonymous with tumour involvement

2. Clinical methods are insufficiently sensitive to detect small 'micrometastases' in viscera and bones. The first drawback has been resolved by acceptance of the need for histological staging of nodes. Removal of some or all of the axillary nodes for histopathological examination is now a mandatory part of breast cancer surgery.

It was hoped that development of more sensitive methods of detecting occult metastatic disease would resolve the second problem. However the use of radionuclide, ultrasonic and CT scans and of sophisticated tests of organ function have not proved of great value.

At present routine examination of a patient with early breast cancer for occult metastatic disease should include only X-rays of chest and pelvis, haematological examination and liver function tests.

The current system of staging is shown in Table 18.1.

## TREATMENT

Until recently the orthodox treatment of cancer limited to the breast and axillary lymph nodes was either 'radical mastectomy' in which the breast was totally removed and the axilla cleared of all lymph nodes, or by 'simple mastectomy' when the breast only was surgically removed but radiotherapy was given to 'sterilise' the lymph nodes and skin of the chest wall. Realisation that these procedures resulted in long-standing cure in only a minority of patients led to reappraisal of the objectives of treatment and to introduction of systemic as well as local methods of control as well as more conservative forms of local treatment.

### Local therapy

*Stages I and II.* For tumours of 5 cm or less in size with no skin involvement or chest wall fixation (T1, T2, a or b) mastectomy is still considered by many to be the treatment of choice. Provided the axillary lymph nodes are not fixed to each other or to surrounding structures (N0, N1) the axilla may either be surgically cleared of all nodes or alternatively node sampling may be performed. Sampling entails removal of the pectoral or lower axillary nodes for histological examination.

There is no need for postoperative radiotherapy if the axilla has been cleared even if node histology is positive. However, if sampled nodes are involved by tumour, radiotherapy is advised to control presumed residual disease in the unremoved nodes. This selective policy has the advantage that high surgical dissection of the axilla or radiotherapy are avoided in node-negative patients.

**Table 18.1** Summary of TNM classification of breast cancer.

*Primary tumour*

| | | |
|---|---|---|
| Tis | Pre-invasive carcinoma | |
| | Paget's disease (no tumour) | |
| T0 | No evidence of primary tumour | |
| T1 | tumour $\leqslant 2$ cm | a. no fixation to underlying pectoral fascia and/or muscle |
| T2 | tumour 2–5 cm | |
| | | b. fixation to underlying pectoral fascia and/or muscle |
| T3 | tumour $>5$ cm | |
| T4 | Any size with direct extension to chest wall or skin | |
| | T4a: fixation to chest wall | |
| | T4b: oedema, infiltration, ulceration skin or satellite nodes | |
| | T4c: both of above | |

*Regional lymph nodes*

| | |
|---|---|
| N0 | No palpable homolateral axillary lymph nodes |
| N1 | Moveable homolateral axillary nodes |
| | N1a: not considered to contain growth |
| | N1b: considered to contain growth |
| N2 | Fixed homolateral axillary nodes |
| N3 | Homolateral supraclavicular or infraclavicular nodes or oedema of arm |

*Distant metastases*

| | |
|---|---|
| M0 | No evidence of distant metastases |
| M1 | Evidence of distant metastases |

Recently there has been a swing towards conservation of the breast and, for tumours of less than 2 cm in diameter, local excision of the mass with radiotherapy to the remaining breast and 'nodal regions' would appear to give control equal to that of a mastectomy.

*Stage III.* Provided there is no skin involvement or deep fixation tumours over 5 cm in size may still be suitable for mastectomy but this should be followed by radiotherapy. If there is skin involvement or deep fixation (T4) surgery is contraindicated but local control can be achieved by radiotherapy.

Clinical lymph node status affects the choice of local treatment only when nodes are fixed. In this event surgical treatment of the axilla is contraindicated.

When indicated, radiotherapy is planned to treat fields which include the breast, surrounding chest wall, axilla, supraclavicular and internal mammary lymph nodes. Using mega voltage equipment, tumour doses of 4500 rad can be delivered without severe reactions in the overlying skin. Irradiation of the tumour area can if necessary be 'boosted' either using accelerated electrons or by implants of radium. Alternatively plastic tubes can be implanted into which radiation sources e.g. of iridium can be 'after loaded'.

Following radiotherapy the skin must be kept dry during the erythematous reaction. The patient is advised not to wash and a light talc is applied. If moist desquamation occurs zinc and castor oil ointment is applied. The reaction to radiotherapy usually lasts 5–6 weeks. Patients must avoid direct sunlight on the area for several years or serious sunburn may result.

## Adjuvant systemic therapy

The objective of systemic therapy is to reduce the growth potential of micrometastases. The best indicator of the existence of such systemic spread is axillary node status.

Clinical trials suggest that chemotherapy given as a short course perioperatively or in the longer term delays recurrence and improves survival of premenopausal women with involved axillary nodes. The effect in postmenopausal women is less clear, and chemotherapy is not generally advised as a routine.

Although it is accepted that ovariectomy or ovarian irradiation performed at the time of mastectomy may delay recurrence in the young woman with involved nodes, it has little effect on ultimate survival. A recent report from Toronto suggests that addition of low-dose steroid therapy with prednisone 5 mg b.d. results in significant prolongation of life.

The role of hormone therapy in postmenopausal women is under study. Trials of anti-oestrogen therapy are currently being undertaken and are reported to indicate benefit. The value of oestrogen receptors in selecting appropriate therapy for patients with primary disease is uncertain.

There is at present no evidence that systemic treatment has any part to play in management of women with uninvolved axillary nodes. Although long-term survival statistics indicate that most of such women eventually die of their disease their duration of life may be long.

## COMPLICATIONS OF TREATMENT

### Lymphoedema of the arm

A troublesome complication of breast cancer is lymphoedema of the arm. This may be due to malignant infiltration of axillary lymphatics but more commonly it is a complication of surgery and radiotherapy. Radical removal of the lymph nodes in the axilla interrupts lymph drainage from the arm and this is made worse by postoperative irradiation. Lymphoedema is more common when infection has complicated surgery. Thrombotic occlusion of the axillary vein may also occur. Lymphatic and venous obstruction together cause massive arm swelling.

Oedema is first noted in the hand and spreads up the arm. If untreated the whole arm can gradually become swollen, brawny, hard, heavy and painful. Infection from minor injuries leads to attacks of cellulitis and lymphangitis which extend lymphatic obstruction. In rare cases small nodules of tumour appear in the skin; these have been described as angiosarcomatous but more frequently are metastatic from breast cancer.

Treatment is by intermittent compression with an inflatable arm cuff (Fig. 18.19) and a supportive arm stocking. The patient is warned to avoid minor trauma and should wear gloves when carrying out rough work or gardening. Rarely a forequarter amputation may be indicated for massive lymphoedema when the limb becomes an intolerable burden for the patient.

Recently micro-techniques have been developed for performing lymphatico-venous anastomoses. To be successful, these must be carried out at several sites in the limb as soon as lymphoedema is suspected.

## Psychological effects of mastectomy

Cancer of the breast induces great psychological stress. Following mastectomy one third of patients have moderate or severe anxiety and depression and are in need of psychiatric help. The effects include intolerance of body image, concern about its effect on husband and family and anxiety about relationships with other people. As a result a patient may withdraw from her normal social relationships, and radically alter her domestic and sexual activities.

While many of these problems are related to the mutilation of mastectomy, fear of the disease and uncertainty about the future play an important

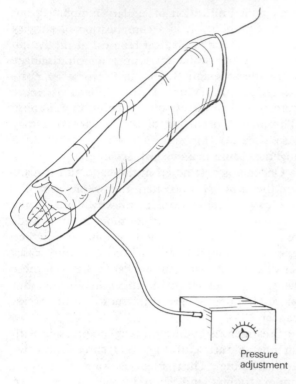

**Fig. 18.19** Pneumatic compression to treat lymphoedema of the arm

role. Good counselling helps; while in theory this is an important role of the surgeon, in practice it is difficult to achieve and in many specialist units nurse councillors are now employed. Not only are they responsible for keeping the patient informed of the nature of her disease and its treatment, but also to give advice on the best type of prosthetic support.

If a patient is completely intolerant of her mastectomy, breast reconstruction can be performed. In its simplest form this consists of insertion of a silicone gel prosthesis under the pectoral muscles. Where loss of tissue or post-radiation fibrosis is marked it may be necessary to advance a musculo-cutaneous flap of latissimus dorsi to form new skin covering for the false breast (Fig.18.20)

In some specialised centres these methods of reconstruction are now offered to patients requiring mastectomy as primary procedures. Alternatively, mastectomy can be avoided by local excision and radiotherapy (see above).

## ADVANCED BREAST CANCER

In its later stages breast cancer can cause distressing symptoms e.g. from ulcerating and fungating lesions on the chest wall, dyspnoea from lung and pleural involvement, or pain from bone metastases. At this stage the objective of treatment is to relieve symptoms and improve the quality of life; one must not prolong life at the expense of increasing misery. As control of the disease will only reduce symptoms, measures to effect tumour regression should normally be instituted as soon as overt metastatic disease is recognised. These include local treatment by surgery or radiotherapy and systemic treatment by endocrine means or by chemotherapy.

## ASSESSMENT OF THE PATIENT

When treating metastatic disease it is important to measure what one has achieved. Otherwise giving ineffective treatment may be prolonged; and this may cause more discomfort than that due to the untreated disease. Three parameters are relevant: the tumour, the symptoms caused by it, and morbidity of the treatment. These must be separately assessed.

Various criteria are used to measure tumour regression. These require serial measurements of tumour deposits either clinically or from X-rays. Responses are not clear-cut, and there is a 'grey area' within which it is difficult to be certain whether a tumour is regressing or becoming worse.

The measurement of symptomatic response is even more difficult. Various self-assessment scales are available by which the patient can record her own symptoms and from which it can be determined whether they are improving or getting worse. Typical symptoms are pain, breathlessness, fatigue etc. Activity ratings are also available, by which an objective estimate can be made of day-to-day activity expressed numerically.

The morbidity of treatment varies according to the methods used. Structured questionnaires can be used to determine side-effects and to assess their progress.

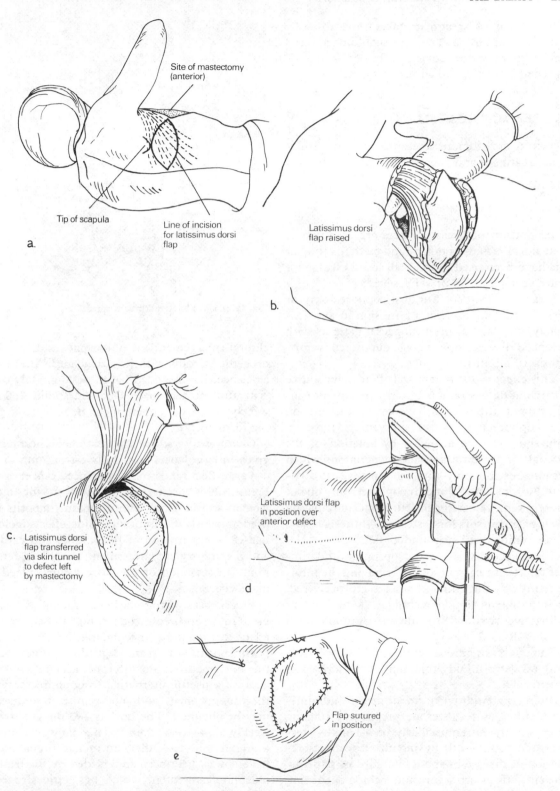

**Fig. 18.20** Latissimus dorsi flap reconstruction of the breast (a silicone prosthesis may be inserted under the latissimus flap)

Any form of treatment takes time to exert benefit. In general 2–3 months should be allowed before therapy for advanced breast cancer is regarded as ineffective and is changed.

## SYSTEMIC TREATMENT

Systemic anti-tumour measures include endocrine treatment and chemotherapy.

### Endocrine therapy

A proportion of breast cancers are sensitive to their hormone environment and methods to alter this have been used to treat advanced disease for many years (Fig. 18.21). These are:

*Endocrine ablation.* Surgical oophorectomy or ovarian irradiation effect a remission in approximately one third of premenopausal patients with advanced disease. The average duration of remission is 18 months.

This effect is due to removal of the main source of circulating oestradiol. In older (postmenopausal) women the ovaries have ceased to function and oophorectomy is of no value. However, remissions can be achieved by ablation of the adrenals or the pituitary gland, operations which became possible only with the synthesis of cortisone. Adrenalectomy and hypophysectomy do not directly remove oestrogen, but reduce circulating levels of precursors for oestrogen synthesis by the breast tumour and surrounding fat.

Adrenalectomy is a major operation and simpler microsurgical methods of removing the pituitary through the ethmoid sinuses are preferred. An alternative simple technique is to implant radioactive yttrium($^{90}$Y) into the pituitary fossa transnasally.

The effects of adrenalectomy and hypophysectomy on general body functions are described in Chapter 39.

*Androgens.* Additive hormone therapy administered either as testosterone propionate 100 mg twice weekly intramuscularly or as methyl-testosterone 5 mg t.i.d. by mouth also effects remission of disease in about one third of patients. The side effects are severe and include deepening of the voice, coarsening of the skin, hirsutism,

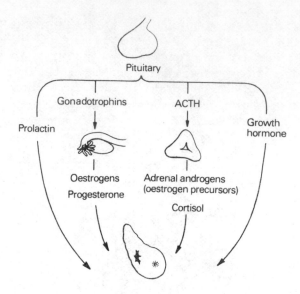

**Fig. 18.21** Hormones and breast cancer

clitoral enlargement and abnormal sex drive. Androgenic steroids with less virilising effects have since been developed. That most commonly used is nandrolene decanoate (Deca-durabolin) 100 mg weekly. If there is benefit it can be reduced to 100 mg fortnightly.

*Oestrogens.* Paradoxically, oestrogenic hormones, given in large doses (e.g. stilboestrol 5 mg t.i.d.) can also effect remission of advanced cancer of the breast. This occurs particularly in the older woman and in those whose tumour deposits are predominantly in soft tissues. Side-effects include nausea, pigmentation of the nipple, and cardiac and respiratory embarrassment from fluid retention. On cessation of the drug vaginal bleeding may occur.

*Progestogens.* Progestational agents are also used to treat breast cancer but these are less effective than other agents, particularly in the postmenopausal woman. High-dose progesterone therapy (medroxyprogesterone acetate — Provera) is a useful alternative to oophorectomy in the young woman, and good remission of disease may be obtained. The dose is 400 mg i.m. twice weekly for 4 weeks; then 100 mg daily per mouth.

*Antioestrogens.* Other hormonal preparations have now largely been superseded by the triphenylamine tamoxifen, which has antioestrogenic effects. It acts by preventing the binding of oestradiol and remission rates are equal to those of other agents. It has the great advantage of few side-effects and easy administration. Occasional thrombocytopenia, jaundice and vaginal bleeding are described. One tablet 10 mg twice or three times daily is recommended.

*Aminoglutethamide.* In the past suppressing doses of glucocorticoids (prednisolone 10 mg t.i.d. were used alone or combined with oophorectomy as a form of 'medical adrenalectomy'. The anti-convulsant aminoglutethamide specifically inhibits the conversion of cholesterol to pregnenolone in the adrenal cortex and blocks the synthesis of all adrenocortical steroids. It also affects the conversion of C 19 steroids to oestrogen in peripheral tissues e.g. fat. Given in a dose of l g daily it is used as an alternative to adrenalectomy in patients with breast cancer. Maintenance steroid therapy is also required. As this must also suppress the 'feed-back' secretion of ACTH the dose of 40 mg cortisol (hydrocortisone) acetate daily is recommended.

*Prolactin inhibitors.* Levo-dopa and bromo-ergocriptine have been used in the management of advanced breast cancer. There is no convincing evidence of benefit.

## Chemotherapy

Single-agent chemotherapy is relatively ineffective in breast cancer. Combinations of cell cycle dependent and independent drugs are now preferred. These include alkylating agents (cyclophosphamide) and antimetabolites (methotrexate and 5-fluorouracil). Doxorubicin (Adriamycin) is the most effective of the drugs, and most courses of treatment for advanced disease now include this agent. Its total dose is limited by its cardiotoxic effects.

Cyclical combination chemotherapy will cause remission in 60% of patients. The duration of remission is relatively short, averaging 6 months. Typical regimes are given in Table 18.2.

## Selection of therapy

The availability of oestrogen receptor assays has rationalised anti-tumour therapy in breast cancer. Oestrogen receptors are specific cytoplasmic proteins which have a high affinity for the binding of oestradiol, and which translocate with oestradiol into the nucleus to activate its growth-promoting effect (Fig. 18.22). Oestrogen binding is a specific property of all oestrogen target tissues (e.g. uterus, vagina, breast) and is present in 60% of breast cancers.

The presence or absence of cytoplasmic oestrogen receptor is now recognised to be a valuable guide to the likely hormone responsiveness of the tumour. Those tumours which do not possess this activity are refractory to endocrine treatment;

**Table 18.2** Some regimes of chemotherapy used in the treatment of advanced breast cancer.

| | |
|---|---|
| *CMF* | |
| Cyclophosphamide | 750 mg/m² ⎫ |
| Methotrexate | 50 mg/m² ⎬ I.V. q. 3-weekly |
| 5-fluorouracil | 600 mg/mS ⎭ |
| *VAP* | |
| Vincristine | 1.4 mg/m² (max. 2 mg) I.V. ⎫ |
| Adriamycin | 50 mg/m² I.V. ⎬ q. 3-weekly |
| Prednisolone | 10 mg qds × 5 days P.O. ⎭ |
| *Mitoxanthrone* | |
| Remains *experimental*, possible substitute for adriamycin with potentially less cardiotoxicity. Alopecia, nausea and vomiting are not a major problem. | |
| | 14 mg/m² I.V. as 45 min. infusion in 5% dextrose. |
| | q. 3-weekly |
| *CHOP* | |
| Cyclophosphamide | 750 mg/m² I.V. ⎫ |
| Hydroxy-adriamycin | 50 mg/m² I.V. ⎬ q. 3-weekly |
| Oncovin (vincristine) | 1.4 mg/m² I.V. ⎭ |
| Prednisolone | 10 mg qds × 5 days P.O. |

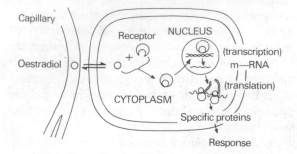

Fig. 18.22 Oestrogen receptors

those with it have a 50% chance of response. Patients with advanced receptor-negative tumours should be treated with chemotherapy, those with receptor-positive tumours by endocrine therapy.

In the premenopausal woman with a receptor-positive tumour removal of functioning ovaries should precede other forms of endocrine treatment. Not only does this offer the most effective method of reducing oestrogenic influences, but patients who respond beneficially to this are likely to gain further response from adrenalectomy or hypophysectomy when their tumour subsequently relapses.

In the postmenopausal patient a trial of tamoxifen therapy (10 mg t.i.d. for 2–3 months) is usual, irrespective of receptor status. If there is a good response the drug should be continued. On relapse, or if there is no response, further treatment will depend on the fitness of the patient and the oestrogen receptor status of the tumour. A trial of aminoglutethamide is worthwhile: if this is successful a hypophysectomy or adrenalectomy may be considered. Otherwise the only useful alternative is chemotherapy.

## GENERAL

The support of the patient with advanced breast cancer includes more than the control of the tumour. Palliation includes control of symptoms; and this is particularly important in those who fail to respond to endocrine treatment or chemotherapy. The methods which are available have been outlined in Chapter 15.

## SPECIAL PROBLEMS

Certain types of metastatic disease require special methods for their control.

*Pleural metastases*. Pleural effusions in those with a history of breast cancer are regarded as malignant until proven otherwise. Symptoms of severe dyspnoea demand aspiration: this is best carried out by tube thoracostomy, a small chest drain being inserted through the 8th and 9th space in the midaxillary line and connected to water seal drainage to which suction is applied (25 cm water). Fluid should be sent for cytology (Fig. 18.23).

Pleural effusions usually respond well to systemic therapy. If not, the local instillation of a cytotoxin may be required, bleomycin being the preferred agent. Following tube thoracostomy 60–120 mg is injected in 100 ml saline: the tube is clamped while the patient lies supine, prone and on either side, after 24 hours the clamp is removed and the tube reconnected to an underwater seal with suction to empty the chest completely.

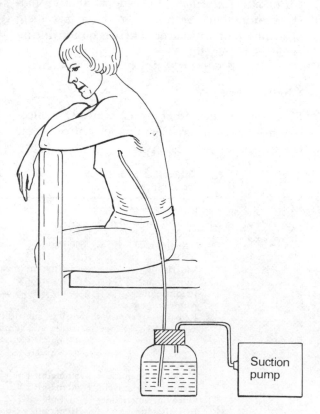

Fig. 18.23 Pleural aspiration

*Lung metastases.* Discrete lung metastases do not cause severe symptoms. Lymphangitis carcinomatosa, in which the pulmonary lymphatics are infiltrated by cords of tumour, causes bronchospasm and severe dyspnoea. This may be helped by steroid therapy (prednisone 30 mg daily) and bronchodilators (salbutamol). Chemotherapy is the preferred treatment.

*Hypercalcaemia.* Transient elevations of serum calcium are seen in 40% of patients with bone metastases. More severe hypercalcaemia (over 3 mmol/l) associated with gastro-intestinal, renal and neuromuscular symptoms occurs in 10% and may be rapidly induced by hormone or diuretic therapy. Most prominent symptoms are nausea, constipation, thirst and polyuria, personality change and muscle weakness, these usually being associated with increasing bone pain.

Persistent levels over 3 mmol/l must be reversed. Infusions of sodium chloride correct dehydration and promote excretion of calcium; diuretics are given to maintain a urine output of 3–5 l daily and steroids (prednisone 60 mg daily) to reduce bone resorption and hypercalcaemia. Oral and intravenous phosphate will predictably lower serum calcium according to the dose. This sequesters calcium and precipitation in kidneys, blood vessels and soft tissues is a long-term problem. Oral phosphate 1–3 g daily is usually given but can cause diarrhoea.

Mithramycin 25 mg/kg rapidly reduces serum calcium by interfering with osteoclastic function but is toxic. Effective anti-tumour therapy is an essential part of management.

*Bone metastases.* These are usually of osteolytic type. The majority of patients with widespread bone metastases have pain and are disabled. Systemic therapy is essential but local radiotherapy (2000 rad over 5–7 days) can relieve pain and promote healing. Radiotherapy to an osteolytic lesion is particularly valuable in weight-bearing bones and may prevent pathological fracture. It also may prevent vertebral collapse and paraplegia. If fracture occurs orthopaedic reinforcement may be required. This can include total hip replacement.

*Spinal cord compression.* Compression of spinal cord by extradural tumour is common in breast cancer. The condition must be recognised early and treatment instituted promptly. Patients with back pain who develop neurological symptoms are treated as surgical emergencies. A myelogram is performed to determine the site and extent of compression. The spinal column is surgically decompressed and postoperative irradiation arranged. The duration of symptoms prior to treatment is the most important guide to recovery and delay must be avoided.

*Brain metastases.* Rising intracranial pressure and neurological dysfunction associated with intracerebral metastases cause severe problems. As soon as cerebral secondaries are suspected high-dose steroid therapy (dexamethasone 10 mg i.v. then 4 mg i.m. 6 hourly) should be given and a CT scan arranged. Oral dexamethasone 2 mg t.i.d. may be continued.

Whole head irradiation (3000 rad over 3 weeks), although accompanied by loss of hair, is worthwhile. Neurosurgical excision is rarely indicated unless an apparently single lesion is demonstrated on CT-scan. Then its removal may give striking palliation.

*Liver metastases.* Progressive liver failure and jaundice result from infiltration of the liver by metastatic disease. Occasionally endocrine treatment can induce dramatic shrinkage but this is rare and liver metastases generally are regarded as rapidly fatal. Steroid therapy may improve well-being.

## MALE BREAST

### GYNAECOMASTIA (Fig. 18.24)

Enlargement of the male breast is becoming increasingly common. Histologically it consists of duct and fibro-epithelial elements; alveolar formation is rare. Although clinically it is usually unilateral, mammograms will normally show hypertrophy of breast tissue of both sides. Irritation and tenderness of the nipple may be a feature.

Gynaecomastia must be differentiated from cancer. Helpful guides are its concentricity, its firmness and the lack of skin fixation or ulceration. A cancer is eccentric in relation to the nipple, stony hard and fixed.

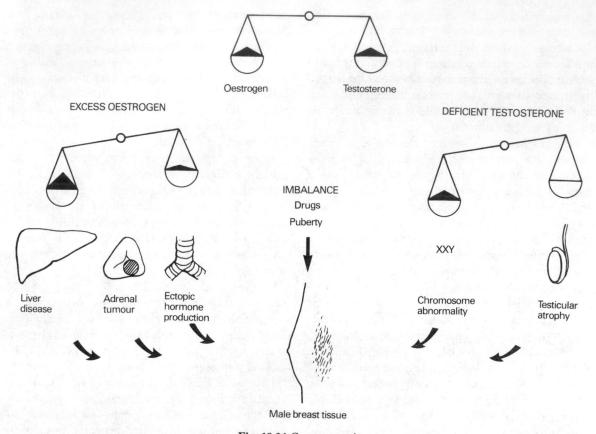

Oestrogen          Testosterone

EXCESS OESTROGEN                                                DEFICIENT TESTOSTERONE

IMBALANCE
Drugs
Puberty

Liver        Adrenal     Ectopic                XXY
disease      tumour      hormone                Chromosome              Testicular
                         production             abnormality             atrophy

Male breast tissue

**Fig. 18.24** Gynaecomastia

Gynaecomastia results from excessive hormonal drive. It is a physiological event at puberty and at the 'male menopause'. In older men it may be associated with testicular atrophy, low testosterone and high gonadotrophin levels.

Drugs are an important cause of gynaecomastia (Table 18.3). Digitalis, spironolactone, phenthiazines and cimetidine are most common. As spontaneous resolution may occur there is no need to stop the treatment unless pain and tenderness are severe, or the patient unduly disturbed by his enlarged breast.

Increased levels of circulating oestrogens are an obvious cause of gynaecomastia. This may be due to the administration of oestrogens for therapeutic purposes e.g. in the treatment of cancer of the prostate, or to their excess production e.g. in testicular feminisation, or as a result of an oestrogen-secreting tumour of the adrenal gland. Ectopic hormone production by a bronchial carcinoma and other tumours can also cause the condition.

**Table 18.3** Some common drugs associated with gynaecomastia.

| | |
|---|---|
| Amphetamines | Oestrogens |
| Andrenocorticosteroids | Oxerutins |
| Androgens | Radioactive iodine |
| Bendrofluazide | Reserpine |
| Cimetidine | Salbutamol |
| Digoxin | Spironolactone |
| Marihuana | |

Failure to metabolise steroid hormones e.g. in chronic liver disease may also result in gynaecomastia. When due to excess hormonal stimulation gynaecomastia is usually bilateral. Provided there is no endocrine cause, a gynaecomastic breast can be removed by a simple operation preserving the nipple and overlying skin.

## CANCER

Cancer of the male breast is rare. Because of the lack of breast tissue it rapidly becomes fixed to the skin and chest wall and readily ulcerates. Treatment is similar to that for the female but, because of shortage of skin, skin grafting or replacement by a musculo-cutaneous flap is likely to be required. Metastatic cancer in the male follows a similar pattern to that in women but is frequently hormonal-sensitive. Excellent regressions of disease have been noted with stilboestrol therapy, and with orchidectomy, adrenalectomy and hypophysectomy. If acceptable to the patient orchidectomy is the best initial therapy for metastatic disease.

# 19. Surgery of Cardiac Disease

Surgical treatment of heart disease is relatively new. With the development of safe techniques for cardiopulmonary bypass since the mid 1950s, surgery now offers a prospect of effective treatment for many forms of heart disease. In view of the high prevalence of heart disease, cardiac surgery is now a major speciality-indeed surgery for coronary artery disease is presently one of the commonest forms of surgery undertaken in the United States.

Results of cardiac surgery continue to improve. Though further changes and modification of techniques are to be expected, the principles involved are common to other fields of surgery.

## The cardiac surgical unit

Cardiac surgery makes a demand on a number of specialities and requires a specialised staff. Several surgeons, anaesthetists, theatre staff and perfusion and monitoring staff are required for the average cardiac operation. Patients are usually in theatre for 3 or 4 hours, and require intensive postoperative care for at least the first postoperative day. The cost of cardiopulmonary bypass equipment, prosthetic valves and surgical equipment, as well as the demands on blood transfusion, biochemical and haematological services make the provision of a cardiac surgical service a major undertaking. Such a service can only function in association with a cardiological service with full investigative facilities.

## PRINCIPLES OF SURGICAL TREATMENT

Rational application of surgical treatment for heart disease requires:

1. Accurate assessment of the patient
2. Knowledge of the natural history of the condition
3. Knowledge of therapeutic possibilities, including techniques and results of surgery.

## ASSESSMENT OF THE PATIENT

Patients considered for cardiac surgery are usually referred to a cardiologist for assessment. Referral may be because of symptoms, such as chest pain or dyspnoea, or because of the findings on routine examination of an abnormality, usually a cardiac murmur.

The *history, physical examination,* findings of *electrocardiography* and *chest radiography,* and at times *echocardiography,* enable the cardiologist to diagnose the lesion in most cases. It is important to assess the severity of the lesion and the pathological effects it may be having on the heart itself, the lungs, or other organs.

*Cardiac catheterisation* and *angiocardiography* are usually undertaken where surgical treatment is contemplated, and are used at times to aid diagnosis or assess results of surgery.

*Cardiac catheterisation* provides data about pressures and oxygen saturation in the major vessels and cardiac chambers. This will allow assessment of severity of obstruction at a stenotic valve or calculation of amount of shunting through abnormal communications (Fig. 19.1). *Angiocardiography* or *selective coronary angiography* where radio-opaque contrast medium is injected into a cardiac chamber or coronary artery during cineradiography gives the surgeon clear visualisation of the morphology of the abnormality present (Figs. 19.2, 19.3).

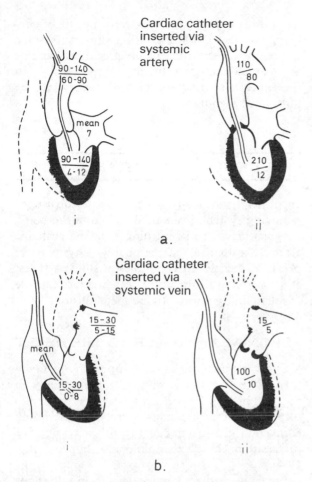

Cardiac catheter inserted via systemic artery

90-140 / 60-90    mean 7    90-140 / 4-12

110 / 80    210 / 12

a.

Cardiac catheter inserted via systemic vein

mean 4    15-30 / 5-15    15-30 / 0-8

15 / 5    100 / 10

b.

**Fig. 19.1** Cardiac catheterisation. (a) Cardiac catheter inserted via systemic artery showing: (i) Normal left heart pressures; (ii) Pressure in aortic stenosis. (b) Cardiac catheter inserted via systemic vein showing: (i) Normal right heart pressures; (ii) Pressure in pulmonary stenosis.

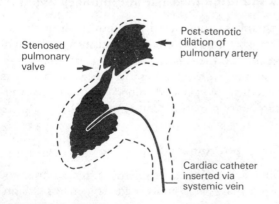

Stenosed pulmonary valve

Post-stenotic dilation of pulmonary artery

Cardiac catheter inserted via systemic vein

**Fig. 19.2** Angiographic appearance of pulmonary valve stenosis

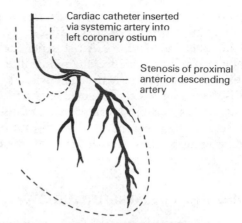

Cardiac catheter inserted via systemic artery into left coronary ostium

Stenosis of proximal anterior descending artery

**Fig. 19.3** Selective left coronary angiogram

In addition to having accurate knowledge of the cardiac defect the surgeon requires a *general assessment* of the patient.

*General physical examination* may reveal conditions requiring specific investigation and management. Dental sepsis should be treated. A specific assessment of lung function, renal function, hepatic function and coagulation function is required.

Lung function is commonly compromised in the elderly by chronic bronchitis, patients on long-term diuretic treatment may have elevated blood urea levels, and those in long-standing cardiac failure may have secondary liver impairment. Patients with coronary artery disease may have evidence of important vascular disease elsewhere, such as carotid bruits, which merits further investigation.

Patients requiring valve replacement may have a contra-indication to long-term anticoagulation — e.g. peptic ulceration, which will influence the choice of valve prosthesis.

With current techniques of anaesthesia, operative and post-operative care, only major abnormalities of other systems jeopardise surgical results sufficiently to contra-indicate surgery.

## NATURAL HISTORY

Knowledge of the natural history of any condition influences the timing and urgency of surgical treatment. For example, it is known that symptomatic aortic stenosis carries a poor prognosis and early surgery is advised. Ventricular septal defects may close spontaneously in childhood and so the decision regarding surgery can be deferred provided pulmonary vascular disease is not thought likely to develop. Atrial septal defects usually cause heart failure in middle life and elective surgical closure is usually advised.

It is becoming widely accepted that left main coronary artery disease has a poor prognosis and that isolated right coronary artery disease has a good prognosis. This knowledge may influence choice of medical or surgical treatment.

## THERAPEUTIC POSSIBILITIES

The surgeon must be aware of medical measures available to the cardiologist and must understand the effects of drugs. For example, beta-blocking drugs are commonly used for angina and may modify the response of the heart to drugs used postoperatively.

The hazard of any particular surgical procedure also influences decisions about surgery. Closure of atrial septal defects carries a very low risk while the risk of mitral valvotomy makes this operation advisable relatively early in the natural history of mitral stenosis. On the other hand, the greater risk of valve replacement and continuing problems with prosthetic valves mean that this operation is less lightly advised.

In general terms, surgical treatment of heart disease is undertaken for:

1. *Relief of symptoms* by improving cardiac function. Examples are the treatment of exertional dyspnoea due to mixed mitral valve disease by replacement of the mitral valve, or treatment of angina pectoris by aorta-coronary bypass grafting.

Mild symptoms well managed by medical measures usually do not warrant surgery; severe symptoms or poor response to medical measures usually require surgery.

2. *Alteration of natural history of the disease.* Examples are resection of aortic coarctation to avoid complications of hypertension, or treatment of Fallot's tetralogy to avoid thrombotic complications of polycythaemia or death in cyanotic spells, or treatment of severe aortic stenosis to prevent myocardial damage or death.

The decision to advise surgery for this reason is not always easy. It requires knowledge of the natural history and the long-term results of surgery, and also implies advising surgery in some symptom-free patients. In practice most patients are operated on for treatment of symptoms and in the expectation that the natural history will be influenced favourably.

## CARDIOPULMONARY BYPASS

In principle, *cardiopulmonary bypass* consists of removing systemic venous blood from the body, oxygenating it, and returning it to the systemic arterial system at a reasonably physiological pressure, devoid of gas bubbles or solid particles, at a controlled temperature, and at a rate capable of maintaining normal tissue metabolism.

## SURGICAL APPROACH TO THE HEART

Vertical sternotomy is the approach generally used. The sternum is divided longitudinally in the midline and the pericardial cavity is opened to display the heart and major vessels, the ascending aorta and right atrium being readily accessible for preparation for cardiopulmonary bypass (Fig. 19.4).

Previous cardiac surgery results in adhesions between the heart and pericardial cavity or back of sternum, increasing the difficulty of a second operation.

### Cannulation for cardiopulmonary bypass

Systemic venous blood is removed through two plastic cannulae inserted via incisions in the right atrium into the superior and inferior venae cavae. A cannula is inserted high in the ascending aorta to return oxygenated blood from the cardiopulmonary bypass circuit (Fig. 19.5).

### Cardiopulmonary bypass circuit (Fig. 19.6)

The major technical problems with cardiopulmonary bypass have concerned oxygenator design. Most centres use one of a number of commercially produced, disposable, bubble oxygenators

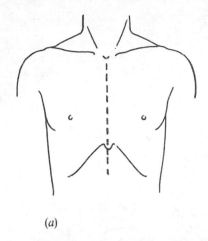

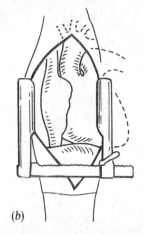

(a)                                    (b)

**Fig. 19.4** Surgical approach to the heart. (a) Vertical sternotomy incision;
(b) right atrium and ascending aorta.

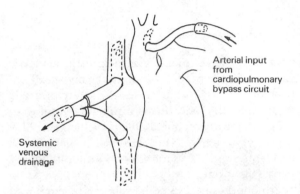

**Fig. 19.5** Cannulation for cardio-pulmonary bypass

which incorporate a heat exchanger. Oxygen is bubbled through a column of blood on its way through the oxygenator, allowing removal of carbon dioxide and oxygenation of the blood. Defoaming sponge then removes gas bubbles before the blood runs into a reservoir to be pumped back to the body by a simple roller pump. This results in an even arterial perfusion pressure of between 50 and 100 mmHg. The absence of a physiological pulse pressure for several hours does not appear unduly deleterious, but newer pumps can provide a pulsatile flow.

Cooling is inevitable during extracorporeal transit. A heat exchanger is usually incorporated in the oxygenator, and the temperature of the circulating water is adjusted to warm the blood back to 37°C, or to induce (and finally correct) systemic hypothermia during cardiopul-

monary bypass. The circuit is filled with an isotonic fluid (e.g. Ringer's solution) and air is meticulously excluded from the arterial side of the circuit.

Blood accumulating in the operating field during cardiopulmonary bypass is removed by suction and returned to the circuit. A system for venting or removing blood from the left side of the heart is often used to prevent cardiac distension or lung congestion when the heart is unable to eject blood.

### Heparin

Before inserting the cannulae for cardiopulmonary bypass heparin is given into the circulation to prevent blood from clotting in the extracorporeal circuit. Additional heparin is given during long procedures and is neutralised with protamine after discontinuing cardiopulmonary bypass.

### Hazard of emboli

Care is taken to avoid introduction of air into the systemic arterial system and to remove air from the heart chambers before allowing ejection into the aorta. Intracardiac thrombosis and calcium from calcific heart valves can act as emboli. The most profound effects follow cerebral emboli in that severe cerebral damage can result.

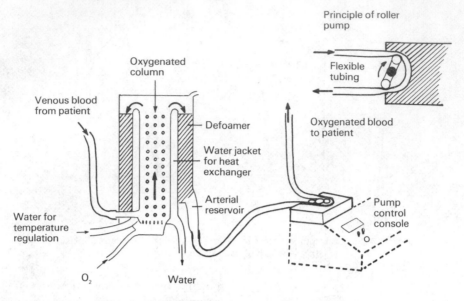

**Fig. 19.6** Diagram of cardio-pulmonary bypass circuit

## Sterility

All parts of the extracorporeal circuit with which blood comes into contact must be sterile. The commercially produced oxygenators are pre-sterilised. It is usual practice to give a broad-spectrum antibiotic over the operation period to reduce the risk of bacteraemia.

## Myocardial protection

During many cardiac operations the ascending aorta is cross-clamped once cardiopulmonary bypass has been established. This interrupts flow into the coronary arteries and renders the myocardium ischaemic. Aortic cross-clamping is essential prior to opening the aortic root for access to the aortic valve. It is also of great help in providing a bloodless, immobile, relaxed heart for most cardiac procedures.

Interruption of coronary flow is followed by ischaemic cardiac arrest within a few minutes, changes in mitochondria within 15 minutes, and increasing myocardial damage after about 30–45 minutes. Where cross-clamping of the aorta beyond about 30 minutes is required (as for valve replacement) some form of myocardial protection is necessary. This may be achieved by directly cannulating and perfusing the coronary arteries

with oxygenated blood via their ostia at aortic valve replacement, or by cooling the myocardium. Cooling to 28–30°C increases the safety of aortic cross-clamping, and this is frequently employed, using the extracorporeal heat exchanger. This degree of systemic hypothermia also allows helpful temporary reductions of cardiopulmonary bypass flow rate.

Profound topical hypothermia can be employed to increase the safety of myocardial ischaemia. It is achieved by irrigating the heart after aortic cross-clamping with large volumes of cold saline at about 4°C. Infusion of cold potassium-containing solutions into the coronary arteries to induce cardioplegia is currently widely used, often in combination with moderate systemic and profound topical hypothermia, to allow two hours or more of safe ischaemia. Myocardial rewarming, and activity, occurs rapidly once coronary blood flow is restored.

Ventricular fibrillation is common after rewarming and is sometimes induced deliberately to prevent ejection from the heart while air is removed. Direct application of defibrillating paddles to the ventricles restores an effective beat.

Incisions in ventricular muscle impair contractility and are kept to a minimum. Right ventriculotomy is used for repair of Fallot's tetralogy. Incisions are closed with continuous non-absorbable sutures (Fig. 19.7).

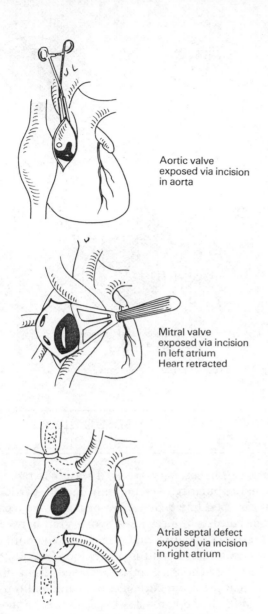

Aortic valve
exposed via incision
in aorta

Mitral valve
exposed via incision
in left atrium
Heart retracted

Atrial septal defect
exposed via incision
in right atrium

**Fig. 19.7** Surgical exploration of intracardiac structures with cardio-pulmonary bypass

# SURGERY FOR VALVULAR HEART DISEASE

## TYPES OF VALVULAR DISEASE

*Mitral valve disease* is usually due to rheumatic fever, although a history of rheumatic fever is not always obtained. The valve may become regurgitant due to annular dilatation during the acute episode and is associated with pancarditis. Surgery is usually required for the late results of chronic inflammation which may cause predominant *mitral stenosis* due to commissural fusion and leaflet thickening, predominant *mitral regurgitation* due to annular dilatation and retraction of leaflet tissue, or a *mixed* lesion due to combination of commissural fusion, leaflet thickening and chordal shortening. Valve calcification is common after long-standing inflammation.

Less commonly, mitral regurgitation is due to chordal rupture, leaflet degeneration, infarction or rupture of papillary muscle due to ischaemic heart disease, or to left ventricular dilatation in severe cardiac failure.

*Infective endocarditis* may affect any diseased heart valve and cause rapid deterioration in valve function.

*Aortic valve disease* may be due to rheumatic fever with predominant stenosis, predominant regurgitation, or a 'mixed' lesion. Calcification occurs in long-standing disease. A congenitally bicuspid aortic valve may be stenotic early in life, but stenosis is more commonly a late manifestation of valve calcification.

Syphilitic and dissecting aortic aneurysm are less common causes of aortic regurgitation.

*Tricuspid valve disease* may be due to rheumatic involvement or to 'functional' annular dilatation in patients with mitral valve disease complicated by severe pulmonary hypertension. The tricuspid valve may also be congenitally abnormal.

*Pulmonary valve disease* is usually congenital stenosis with varying degrees of commissural fusion or hypoplasia of the valve annulus.

## CONSERVATIVE MEASURES FOR ABNORMAL VALVES

Reasonably satisfactory haemodynamic function in the patient's own valve is preferable to a prosthetic valve. Conservation of valves is always preferred if feasible.

The stenosed mitral valve may be opened by *mitral valvotomy*. This is applicable to a mobile valve with commissural fusion as the main abnormality (evidenced by loud first sound and opening snap, with absence of radiological calcification). With a finger inserted through a small incision in the left atrial appendage a dilator is inserted through the left ventricular apex and guided into the stenosed mitral orifice. Rapid opening of the dilator breaks down commisural fusion. The operation does not severely impede cardiac action and does not require cardiopulmonary bypass.

*Pulmonary* and *aortic valvotomy* are performed using cardiopulmonary bypass, visualisation of the valve, and division of the fused commissures.

*Regurgitant valves* are less easy to conserve. Aortic and pulmonary valves are not commonly repaired. Mitral or tricuspid regurgitation due primarily to dilatation of the annulus may be dealt with by reduction in the size of the annulus to restore competence (annuloplasty).

## VALVE REPLACEMENT

Cardiopulmonary bypass is required with exposure of the valve. A diseased valve which cannot be conserved is excised leaving a rim of valve tissue to facilitate suturing in a replacement. It is often necessary to remove calcium from the valve annulus.

The surgeon has a choice of a large variety of valve prostheses for valve replacement. This reflects the continuing problems with prosthetic valves, although many earlier problems have been largely overcome (Fig. 19.8). In general there are two categories of prosthetic valve:

1. *Artificial valves*. These are made of non-biological materials and do not mimic natural valves. Of the large number available, the Starr-Edwards caged ball valve, and the Bjork-Shiley tilting disc valve are perhaps best known. All artificial valves are subject to thrombosis on the valve, with resultant embolism or valve failure. Indefinite oral anticoagulation (Warfarin) is used to reduce this hazard, and is started as soon as postoperative blood loss ceases.

2. *Biological valves*. The currently favoured biological valve is a glutaraldehyde-prepared porcine aortic valve mounted on a frame for insertion. Its advantage is the absence of thrombo-embolism without the need for anticoagulation. Long-term durability is as yet unproven.

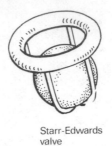
Starr-Edwards valve

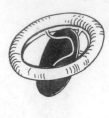
Bjork-Shiley valve

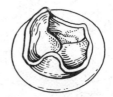
Glutaraldehyde prepared porcine valve

**Fig. 19.8** Types of artificial heart valve

## SURGERY FOR ISCHAEMIC HEART DISEASE

Surgery for coronary artery disease has rapidly gained popularity over the past decade, particularly in the United States. In principle the technique consists of inserting a bypass graft between the ascending aorta and the relatively normal coronary artery beyond an obstruction (Fig. 19.9).

The saphenous vein is removed from the patient at the commencement of operation for use as a graft. Cardiopulmonary bypass is used to allow ischaemic arrest for a quiet bloodless operative field. The coronary vessels are opened beyond known obstructions which have been angiographically demonstrated prior to surgery. Fine instruments and sutures are used to insert the bypass graft between aorta and coronary artery.

*Endarterectomy* or removal of an atheromatous core will often disobliterate a blocked vessel allowing insertion of a graft. Revascularisation for poorly functioning myocardium due to ischaemic fibrosis is unrewarding. Thus, surgery is applicable to patients with angina pectoris in whom coronary angiography demonstrates severe

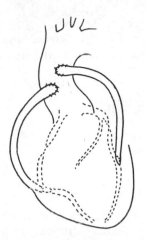

**Fig. 19.9** Bypass grafts for right and left anterior descending coronary obstruction

obstruction (loss of 70% or more of coronary lumen) in a major coronary vessel, and in whom left ventriculography demonstrates reasonably good left ventricular function. Precise indications are not agreed. Severe angina or poor response to medical treatment are the usual indications.

The risk of surgery is low and relief of angina is often complete. The effect on natural history is not yet agreed; longer follow-up is required.

## SURGERY FOR COMPLICATIONS OF CORONARY ARTERY DISEASE

Myocardial infarction is the usual complication of coronary artery disease and is not generally amenable to surgical help.

Ventricular aneurysm is a complication of infarction which is amenable to surgery. Healing of transmural infarction may leave a large weak fibrous scar which bulges to form the aneurysm, thus compromising left ventricular function and leading to cardiac failure. The aneurysm can be resected using cardiopulmonary bypass, taking care to avoid dissemination of underlying mural thrombus. The resultant defect is closed with strong non-absorbable sutures buttressed with Teflon felt.

Less commonly, where acute myocardial infarction involves the interventricular septum or a papillary muscle of the mitral valve, muscle rupture results in a ventricular septal defect or mitral regurgitation, causing a major, and often rapidly fatal, haemodynamic load on an already compromised heart. Urgent surgery is occasionally successful.

## SURGERY FOR CONGENITAL HEART DISEASE

Congenital heart disease occurs in about 6 to 8 per 1000 live births. There are many varieties and only the common defects are discussed here. Although effects may become apparent only late in life (e.g. congenital bicuspid aortic valve) the problem usually presents in childhood. The severe lesions which present in the first few months of life have a lower surgical success rate, although cardiopulmonary bypass is feasible in the newborn.

### Palliative surgery

Palliative surgery most frequently involves construction of a systemic-pulmonary shunt to increase pulmonary blood flow in conditions which result in poor pulmonary blood flow and cyanosis. The usual application is in Fallot's tetralogy where anastomosis of the subclavian artery to pulmonary artery (Blalock-Taussig shunt) is a relatively simple operation giving good palliation and allowing definitive repair to be deferred for 2 or 3 years. Palliative surgery may be the only course open for severe anomalies. Improving techniques mean that definitive repair is now undertaken in younger children and palliative surgery is avoided if possible.

### Patent ductus arteriosus

The ductus arteriosus allows pulmonary artery blood to bypass the airless lungs during intra-uterine life. Failure of normal closure results in left-to-right shunting of systemic blood into the pulmonary circulation as pulmonary vascular resistance falls after birth. This may produce cardiac failure in infancy, requiring urgent surgery. More commonly, the shunt is well tolerated, and the characteristic 'machinery' murmur in the second left interspace is the reason for referral. Cardiac failure occurs in middle life if the condition is not remedied.

Surgery carries little risk and is always advised. The duct is either divided and sutured between vascular clamps, or ligated with thick, non-absorbable suture material.

### Coarctation of the aorta

Narrowing of the aorta usually occurs just beyond the left subclavian artery. The diagnosis is suggested if the femoral pulses are absent or delayed, and radiological rib notching is often evident in older patients. The untreated patient is at risk from complications of proximal hypertension and operation is advised. The aorta is mobilised above and below the coarctation which is then excised with re-anastomosis of the aorta using non-absorbable suture material. An intervening graft is occasionally required.

### Atrial septal defect

Atrial septal defects result in left-to-right shunting of blood because of greater distensibility of the right ventricle and higher left atrial pressure. This causes increased pulmonary blood flow, a delayed pulmonary second sound and the radiological finding of pulmonary plethora. If untreated, the defect causes cardiac failure in middle life.

Surgical repair is advised when the diagnosis is made and carries little risk. Cardiopulmonary bypass is used and the defect is closed through the right atrium. It it usually possible to approximate the edges of the defect but a patch of pericardium or Dacron is occasionally required.

### Ventricular septal defect

Defects in the ventricular septum result in left-to-right shunting because of the higher left ventricular pressure. Surgery may be required in infancy for cardiac failure refractory to medical treatment, but is usually advised before school age for defects of significant size. Evidence of raised pulmonary vascular resistance in childhood is an indication for early surgery. Severe pulmonary vascular disease contra-indicates surgery.

Cardiopulmonary bypass is used. The ventricular septal defect is exposed via a right ventriculotomy or through the right atrium and tricuspid valve. A patch of Dacron is sutured into the defect. Tricuspid valve tissue and conducting tissue are closely related to the defect and injury must be avoided.

### Tetralogy of Fallot

This condition consists of obstruction to right ventricular outflow-either from pulmonary valve stenosis, muscle hypertrophy, or hypoplastic pulmonary artery-and a large ventricular septal defect. Right ventricular pressure is at systemic level and right-to-left shunting causes cyanosis.

Palliative systemic-pulmonary shunting may be undertaken in the first year or two if severe cyanosis with polycythaemia or cyanotic spells are present. Total correction is usually advised before school age. Cardiopulmonary bypass is required. If a palliative shunt is present it is closed. The outflow obstruction is removed and the ventricular septal defect is closed. The operation carries a fairly low risk and results are usually good in that cyanosis is abolished and full activity is possible.

## SURGERY FOR PERICARDIAL DISEASE

*Chronic constrictive pericarditis* has many causes. The commonest is tuberculous pericarditis, which is usually inactive when the disease is seen by the surgeon. Systemic venous congestion occurs because the heart cannot expand fully in diastole to accept normal venous return.

Resection of the dense constrictive fibrous tissue can be achieved through a vertical sternotomy with careful dissection on the beating heart, although some surgeons prefer to use cardiopulmonary bypass.

## SURGERY FOR CARDIAC TRAUMA

Cardiac injuries are not commonly seen by the surgeon. Stab wounds of the heart usually cause rapidly increasing tamponade. Urgent thoracotomy on the side of the stab wound with opening of the pericardium immediately relieves tamponade, allowing time for blood transfusion and suture of the cardiac injury.

# POSTOPERATIVE CARDIAC SURGICAL CARE

Before closure of the chest after any cardiac operation tubes are placed for drainage of blood and connected to under-water seal bottles. These tubes prevent tamponade by escape of blood from around the heart, and allow measurement of postoperative blood loss. Postoperative observation in an intensive care area is essential for the first 24 to 48 hours.

## CARDIAC OUTPUT

Adequate cardiac output is evidenced by normal tissue perfusion as assessed by peripheral skin temperature (palpation or skin temperature probe), mental responsiveness, adequate urine flow (measured from bladder catheter — 0·5 ml/kg/hour is adequate) and maintenance of normal acid/base balance.

Continuous assessment is made of *pulse rate* (from oscilloscope display of electrocardiogram), *blood pressure* (recorded from peripheral arterial cannula used for per-operative monitoring) and atrial pressure (usually right atrial or central venous, but left atrial if the pulmonary vascular bed is abnormal). *Low cardiac output*, evidenced by fall in peripheral skin temperature, mental unresponsiveness, oliguria and developing metabolic acidosis, may be due to:

1. *Oligaemia* caused by inadequate replacement of blood loss, or vasodilatation in a patient previously vasoconstricted due to systemic hypothermia. There is tachycardia, hypotension and low atrial pressure. Treatment is rapid blood transfusion to restore normal parameters.

2. *Heart failure* due to surgical trauma, ischaemia, complicating myocardial infarction or dysrhythmia. There may be normal or rapid pulse rate, hypotension and high atrial pressure. Treatment consists of administration of inotropic drugs such as isoprenaline, adrenaline or dopamine, and correction of any electrolyte or acid/base abnormalities.

3. *Cardiac tamponade* is due to accumulation of blood around the heart and is usually due to clot blocking the drainage tubes. There is tachycardia, hypotension and high atrial pressure. Tamponade can be difficult to distinguish from heart failure. Sudden onset of these signs, particularly if blood loss has been heavy, makes tamponade the likely diagnosis. When suspected the treatment is immediate re-opening of the chest for evacuation of clot and control of bleeding.

## BLOOD LOSS

Blood loss in excess of 200 ml/hour in an adult requires that the chest be re-opened. An active bleeding site may be found but often there is generalised oozing. Haematological studies may reveal the cause (e.g. free heparin or low platelet count) and suggest specific therapy.

## VENTILATION

It is common practice for patients to remain on a ventilator for several hours after cardiopulmonary bypass to ensure adequate ventilation and allow bronchial suction until stable cardiovascular function is confirmed.

## COMPLICATIONS OF CARDIAC SURGERY

The commonest complications are *excessive bleeding* and *low cardiac output* in the early postoperative period. *Systemic embolism* is manifested by signs of cerebral injury.

*Cardiac arrest* may be due to ventricular fibrillation consequent on myocardial irritability due to falling serum potassium level. Treatment consists of prompt external cardiac massage, maintenance of ventilation, defibrillation, correction of any abnormality of serum potassium and acid/base balance, and inotropic support if required.

*Renal failure* is an occasional complication requiring peritoneal dialysis.

Patients with poor pre-operative lung function may require prolonged ventilation with gradual weaning from the ventilator, regular removal of retained bronchial secretions and treatment of pulmonary infection.

# 20. Chest and Mediastinum

The respiratory system comprises those organs which bring atmospheric gases into proximity with the blood to permit exchange of oxygen and carbon dioxide, fundamental to continuing tissue metabolism. It includes the airways, the lungs and the thoracic cage.

## THE AIRWAYS

The passages which conduct air into the lungs are traditionally described as the *upper respiratory tract* (nose, pharynx, larynx) and *lower respiratory tract* (trachea, bronchi and their subdivisions). This arbitrary descriptive separation is reinforced by the fact that the upper respiratory tract is a concern of ear, nose and throat surgery and the lower respiratory tract a concern of thoracic surgery.

The *upper respiratory tract* has the functions of conducting, filtering, warming and humidifying air, and maintaining separation of air from alimentary contents. The nasal passages are lined by mucous membrane with large surface area and rich vascular supply. This ensures warming of inspired air to body temperature and complete humidification before the air reaches the lower respiratory tract. The nasal hairs, the ciliated epithelium, and the mucus from submucosal glands in the nasal cavity filter and trap particulate matter.

During ventilation via endotracheal tube (as during anaesthesia, or in managing crush injuries of the chest) or via tracheostomy it is important to supply filtered, warmed and humidified air. Failure to do so results in drying and injury of epithelium of the lower respiratory tract, thickening of lower respiratory tract secretions and likelihood of infection (tracheobronchitis).

Topical laryngeal anaesthesia (as sometimes used for bronchoscopy) may impair separation of saliva and air and result in inhalation of saliva into the trachea. Eating and drinking should be avoided until such local anaesthesia has worn off.

The anatomy of the *lower respiratory tract* is of considerable importance in thoracic surgery.

The *trachea* is a tube made up of incomplete cartilage rings joined by fibrous tissue; the cartilage rings are deficient posteriorly. Ciliated mucous membrane lines the trachea. The trachea extends from the cricoid cartilage down to the *main carina*, the bifurcation into left and right main bronchi. In the adult the trachea is about 10 cm long.

In the neck the trachea is a midline structure unless deviated by pressure from a mass or mediastinal movement affecting its lower end.

The trachea divides at the main carina into left and right *main bronchi* — the right, being a more direct continuation of the trachea, is more commonly entered by inhaled foreign bodies. The lobes of the lungs are supplied by *lobar bronchi* which divide into *segmental bronchi*. Their anatomical arrangement is fairly constant, and is readily demonstrable by the investigations of bronchography and bronchoscopy. Figure 20.1 shows the arrangement and nomenclature of the lobar and segmental bronchi. The bronchi continue to subdivide, the cartilage plates in their walls become less prominent, until after 15 to 25 divisions the resultant small air passages are devoid of cartilage in their walls and are known as *terminal bronchioles*.

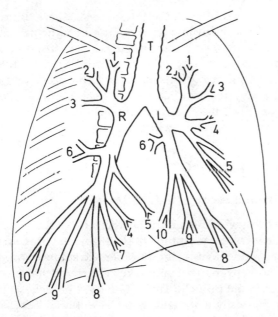

**Fig. 20.1** Diagram of bronchial tree as seen on left oblique bronchogram

T — Trachea
R — Right main bronchus
L — Left main bronchus

| Right Lung | | | Left Lung | | |
|---|---|---|---|---|---|
| 1 Apical | } | upper lobe | 1 Apical | | |
| 2 Posterior | | | 2 Posterior | | |
| 3 Anterior | | | 3 Anterior | } | upper lobe |
| 4 Lateral | } | middle lobe | 4 Superior Lingular | | |
| 5 Medial | | | 5 Inferior Lingular | | |
| 6 Apical | | | 6 Apical | | |
| 7 Medial basal | | | | | |
| 8 Anterior basal | } | lower lobe | 8 Anterior basal | } | lower lobe |
| 9 Lateral basal | | | 9 Lateral basal | | |
| 10 Posterior basal | | | 10 Posterior basal | | |

The bronchi and bronchioles are surrounded by smooth muscle which is capable of constricting the lumen (as occurs in asthma). The tracheobronchial tree is lined by pseudostratified ciliated epithelium three or four layers deep in the trachea, but decreasing in height peripherally until it is a single layer of ciliated cuboidal epithelium in the bronchioles. Goblet cells in the mucosa and submucosal mucous glands produce a film of surface mucus which is constantly moved up to the larynx by the cilia to clear inhaled dust particles. Interference with this cilial clearing action occurs when dry air is allowed into the trachea or when a bronchus is blocked. The result is a likelihood of infection.

A further protective mechanism for removal of intrabronchial material is the *cough reflex*. The explosive blast of air which clears inhaled foreign material or excessive bronchial secretions requires the ability both to close the glottis and to build up sufficient intra-bronchial pressure. Thus an endotracheal tube or tracheostomy or chest wall muscle weakness (as may occur with postthoracotomy pain) will interfere with this cough mechanism and predispose to intra-bronchial infection.

## MANAGEMENT OF THE AIRWAYS

Maintenance of unobstructed airways and control of ventilation are important in anaesthesia and surgery for most thoracic surgical conditions. The interruption of the pumping action of the thoracic cage which occurs with thoracotomy, major chest injury or skeletal muscle relaxation in general anaesthesia necessitates *mechanical ventilation*. There are many different models of mechanical ventilator available which deliver air, or mixtures of air and oxygen, to the patient at predetermined rate, pressure or volume. Warming of the ventilating gas, with adequate humidification, is essential to avoid drying and injury of the bronchial mucosa. The ventilating gas must be delivered to the airways under pressure to produce movement of gas into the lungs with lung expansion simulating the normal lung expansion achieved by the normal thoracic cage pumping action. This requires an effective seal between the delivering tube and the airways — in practice usually achieved by use of a *cuffed endotracheal tube* (Fig. 20.2).

The cuff near the end of the tube is inflated with air sufficient to produce a leak-proof seal

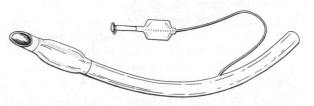

**Fig. 20.2** Endotracheal tube

between the cuff and the trachea. A danger of the cuff is the possibility of pressure on the tracheal mucosa producing ischaemic necrosis, ulceration, and subsequent infection or late stricture formation. Prolonged pressure on the cords from the endotracheal tube is another hazard. As the cough mechanism is impaired by the presence of an endotracheal tube regular aspiration of bronchial secretions is required. This requires gentle suction down the tube with a sterile catheter to avoid mucosal injury or infection.

If prolonged mechanical ventilation is necessary for more than about 5 days, as may occur with crush chest injury, the airway is better managed by *tracheostomy* with insertion of a cuffed tracheostomy tube for mechanical ventilation. This can be changed for a non-cuffed tracheostomy tube once mechanical ventilation is no longer required. Such a tube allows access to the tracheobronchial tree for aspiration of secretions and helps to achieve adequate ventilation by reducing airways dead-space.

### Tracheostomy

Bypassing of the upper airways carries the disadvantages of losing the warming and humidifying functions of the upper airways, the risk of introducing infection into the lower respiratory tract and the abolition of an effective cough.

Careful aseptic technique in bronchial aspiration is essential in management. Nevertheless, tracheostomy is valuable when prolonged mechanical ventilation is required — the initial airways control by cuffed endotracheal tube usually being maintained for about 5 days.

Tracheostomy should be undertaken with airways control by endotracheal tube, general anaesthesia and careful aseptic technique. The operation now rarely requires to be undertaken as a life-saving urgent procedure as was often the case in the past with life-threatening upper airways obstruction due to diphtheria.

A transverse incision is made in the neck between the suprasternal notch and the cricoid cartilage. The incision is deepened in the midline between the strap muscles. The isthmus of the thyroid may require upward retraction. The trachea is exposed and an opening is made. An inverted U-flap in the anterior wall (Bjork flap) or a vertical midline incision through the second, third and fourth tracheal rings allows insertion of the tracheostomy tube as the endotracheal tube is withdrawn. This ensures that access to the airways for ventilation and aspiration is never lost. The tracheostomy tube should be securely anchored to the neck to avoid displacement.

## EXAMINATION OF THE AIRWAYS

### Bronchoscopy (Fig. 20.3)

Direct viewing of the airways from the larynx down to the beginning of the segmental bronchi is a routine investigation in thoracic surgery. Bronchoscopy may be undertaken either with a rigid or a flexible bronchoscope. The rigid bronchoscope is basically a straight metal tube with a bevelled smooth end for safer insertion between the vocal cords. The instrument carries a light source near its tip, and a small tube fastened to the other end enables a high pressure jet of oxygen to be blown intermittently down the bronchoscope. This entrains air and will readily maintain ventilation on the anaesthetised and paralysed patient. General anaesthesia is preferable, although the procedure can be undertaken with local anaesthesia. The neck is extended to allow insertion of the bronchoscope between the cords into the trachea. Care is required to avoid damage to teeth by levering the bronchoscope on them. Gentle positioning of the head allows the bronchoscope to be advanced into the main bronchi. A right-angled telescope can be used to look into bronchi arising from the side walls of main bronchi. Bronchoscopy enables the investigator to examine the major airways. Bronchial tumours may be recognisable and can be biopsied with forceps. Secretions aspirated at bronchoscopy can be examined cytologically for malignant cells, and a fine sponge may be inserted into a selected bronchus to abrade cells for biopsy (brush biopsy). Further diagnostic information can be obtained by seeing compression or distortion of bronchi — as for example the widening of the main carina with loss of its normal sharp dividing ridge indicating involvement of carinal lymph nodes by tumour — a sign of inoperability in lung cancer.

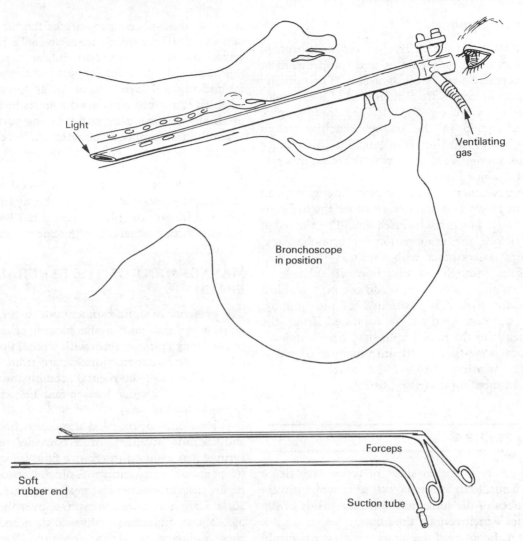

**Fig. 20.3** Bronchoscopy

## Foreign bodies

Sudden onset of coughing, dyspnoea and stridor, especially in children, is suggestive of the presence of an inhaled foreign body. Stridor is the main physical finding. Radiologically there may be no obvious abnormality, or there may be obstructive emphysema on the affected side, or later there may be lobar or whole lung shrinkage. Occasionally the foreign body is radio-opaque. Bronchoscopy is usually required with a degree of urgency. The foreign body is extracted through the broncho-scope with forceps. Occasionally, especially if long-impacted, bronchoscopic removal is impossible and thoracotomy is required to open the bronchus (bronchotomy) for removal of the foreign body. Where a foreign body has been present for a long time infective damage in the obstructed bronchial segments may be so severe as to necessitate resection of the affected lung tissue.

Bronchoscopy is also used for the aspiration of blood or inspissated secretions after thoracic operations, or for removal of secretions or pus in postoperative patients who fail to clear their own secretions and develop tracheobronchial infection. This may be due to pain or weakness impairing coughing; physiotherapy is of great value in avoiding this complication.

## Bronchography

It is possible to see the trachea and main bronchi on plain chest radiography, and compression or displacement may be recognisable. Tomography will give more precise visualisation of these major airways. However, for detailed radiographic demonstration of the tracheobronchial tree a radio-opaque medium is injected into the trachea and radiographs are made with the medium coating the major bronchi.

The commonest use for bronchography is in the diagnosis and assessment of extent of bronchiectasis. The bronchial tree should be cleared of pus before the examination by bronchoscopy. General anaesthesia with injection of contrast medium through an endotracheal tube gives predictable results. Ventilation can be controlled while the patient is positioned for radiography. The contrast medium is aspirated from the trachea after the radiographs have been obtained.

Local anaesthesia with introduction of radio-opaque medium through the larynx or cricothyroid membrane is also possible.

## THE PLEURA

The pleura is a thin sheet of connective tissue with a surface mesothelial cell layer which covers the lobes of the lungs and lines the inside of the cavities which contain the lungs.

Over the lobes of the lungs this pleura is firmly adhered to underlying parenchyma and is known as visceral pleura. It has a blood supply from the bronchial arteries and is not sensitive to painful stimuli.

The visceral pleural layer is continuous at the lung hilum with the *parietal* pleura, which lines the interior of the thoracic cage and covers the mediastinum and diaphragm. The parietal pleura is sensitive to pain and has the same blood supply as the related underlying structures. The parietal pleura can be fairly readily stripped from the mediastinum and chest wall.

*The pleural space.* The parietal and visceral layers of pleura are normally in contact, the lungs being fully expanded to fill the hemithoraces. Normally the pressure between the pleural layers is below atmospheric pressure as the lungs contain elastic tissue which tends to make the lung retract and shrink toward the hilum.

The pleural space only appears when the parietal and visceral layers separate, as for example when air is allowed between the layers by rupture of an air-containing cyst at the lung surface, or when fluid accumulates between the layers as in the case of pleural effusion due to underlying inflammation in the lung.

Inflammation of the pleura or blood between the pleural layers may result in fibrous adhesions which obliterate the pleural space; the lung then becomes firmly adherent to the chest wall.

## MANAGEMENT OF THE PLEURAL SPACE

The presence of significant amounts of air, blood, effusion or pus within the pleural space compresses lung and interferes with its function. This requires intervention quite apart from dealing with the cause of the pleural accumulation.

Drainage of a pleural space may be performed in the following ways:

*1. Aspiration of the pleural space.* A fine trocar and cannula attached via a two-way tap to a syringe may be used to remove fluid for diagnostic purposes or to empty a pleural space when rapid reaccumulation is not anticipated (Fig. 20.4). Care is required to aspirate over the site of pleural accumulation — physical signs and recent chest radiographs dictate the site. Skin preparation, aseptic technique and adequate local anaesthesia of the selected intercostal space are important.

*2. Insertion of an intercostal tube.* Continuous drainage via an intercostal tube is preferable to repeated aspirations. A wide bore tube is more successful than an aspirating needle in removing thick blood or pus.

Aspiration at the selected site confirms the correct choice of site. A trocar and cannula are inserted through the intercostal space (Fig. 20.5). The trocar is removed and a clamped intercostal tube is threaded through the cannula. The cannula is removed; the intercostal tube is connected to an underwater seal bottle and unclamped, and the tube is secured to the chest wall. The under-

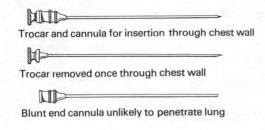

Trocar and cannula for insertion through chest wall

Trocar removed once through chest wall

Blunt end cannula unlikely to penetrate lung

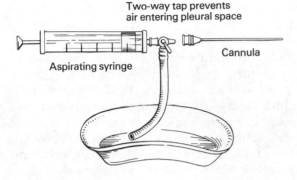

Two-way tap prevents
air entering pleural space

Cannula

Aspirating syringe

Fig. 20.4 Equipment for aspiration of the pleural space

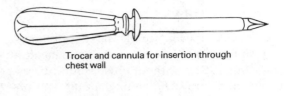

Trocar and cannula for insertion through
chest wall

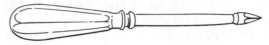

Trocar removed once through chest wall

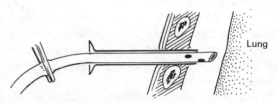

Lung

Clamped intercostal tube passed through cannula

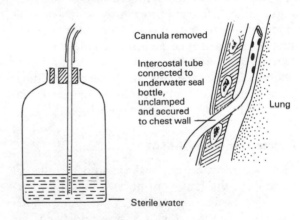

Cannula removed

Intercostal tube
connected to
underwater seal
bottle,
unclamped
and secured
to chest wall

Lung

Sterile water

Fig. 20.5 Pleural intubation

water seal allows fluid or air to drain but prevents return into the chest. The gentle negative pressure it creates in the pleural space assists lung expansion.

Once drainage has ceased, usually after a day or two, the tube is removed briskly and a previously placed suture may be tied to obliterate the tube tract and a sterile dressing applied.

*3. Open drainage by rib-resection.* Long-standing accumulation of pus in the pleural space leads to formation of adhesions of lung to chest wall around the pleural accumulation. More efficient drainage is obtained by resecting several centimetres of rib over the lower extent of the pleural space and inserting a wide-bore tube which drains into a bottle or dressing. The tube and dressings are changed frequently until healing occurs. The site for rib resection is judged by chest radiography following insertion of radio-opaque medium into the pleural space.

*4. Thoracotomy and clearance of the pleural space.* The pleural space may not drain by aspiration or intercostal tube drainage if considerable quantities of blood clot are present. This may require thoracotomy for its removal. The presence of constricting fibrous tissue over the lung

may prevent its re-expansion. This may complicate undrained haemothorax or empyema and requires thoracotomy for decortication of the lung. The fibrous layers over the lung and chest wall are dissected off to allow re-expansion.

*Pleural space management after thoracotomy.* Drainage of the pleural space by insertion of one or more intercostal tubes connected to underwater seal drainage is performed after many thoracic operations. The tubes are inserted during the operation to prevent accumulation of blood from an oozing operative field, or air from a leaking lung surface (as for example after pulmonary lobectomy where blood and air often leak from the interlobar surface for a day or two).

# PNEUMOTHORAX

The presence of air in the pleural space is known as pneumothorax. This may arise spontaneously, usually in a patient without obvious lung disease. The patients are usually young and fit, and present with sudden onset of chest pain and dyspnoea. There is hyperresonance to percussion and absence of breath sounds over the affected side of the chest. Chest radiographs show absence of lung markings — usually with the shrunken lung readily visible at the hilum. Smaller degrees of pneumothorax may be less obvious — the lung edge may be discernible away from the chest wall. In about a third of cases spontaneous pneumothorax recurs.

Less commonly spontaneous pneumothorax is associated with lung disease such as emphysema, lung abscess, pneumonia, tuberculosis or occasionally carcinoma. Pneumothorax may occur as a result of injury — penetrating chest wounds resulting in lung laceration or open communication between the pleural space and atmosphere, or blunt injury resulting in fractured ribs which lacerate the lung. Usually blood and air accumulate in the pleural space in this case — *haemopneumothorax.*

## Tension pneumothorax

This occurs where air leakage into the pleural space from the lung continues to increase intrapleural pressure — usually by coughing which increases intrabronchial pressure and hence air leakage. This causes complete lung compression and mediastinal displacement to the non-affected side with severe dyspnoea. Urgent treatment is required — a needle inserted through the chest wall relieves tension while preparation is made for pleural intubation.

## Recurrent spontaneous pneumothorax

This requires additional measures. When the same side has been affected three times or more it is recommended that permanent fusion of the lung to chest wall is produced. This may be performed most reliably by the operation of *pleurectomy.* Through a short thoracotomy the parietal pleura is stripped from the chest wall and removed. The chest is closed with intercostal underwater seal drainage. Fusion of the lung to the raw chest wall is permanent. A similar effect can be achieved by instillation of an irritant such as iodised talc which induces a pleurisy and a likelihood of permanent obliteration of the pleural space (*pleurodesis*).

# HAEMOTHORAX

The presence of blood in the pleural space (haemothorax) may result from injury, from leakage of an aortic aneurysm or dissection, or occasionally as a spontaneous event with no demonstrable cause. Penetrating injury may result in haemothorax due to bleeding from intercostal vessels, lung, or injury to heart or major vessels. Blunt injury or crush injury usually causes haemothorax as a result of rib fractures which cause bleeding from the fracture sites, or are associated with bleeding from torn intercostal vessels or lacerated lung. Severe deceleration injury may cause shearing of the descending aorta with mediastinal haematoma around the ruptured aorta — leakage from this haematoma presents as haemothorax.

Small collections of blood in the pleural space will resolve satisfactorily. Aspiration of larger collections is advisable — and this may be the only treatment required for haemothorax following injury. Where considerable bleeding has occurred blood transfusion will be required to treat oligaemic shock and aspiration may require to be repeated. In this case insertion of an intercostal tube connected to underwater seal drainage allows more accurate assessment of the rate of blood loss. Continued or excessive bleeding may require thoracotomy for control of the bleeding. Thoracotomy is occasionally required for evacuation of haemothorax where clotting prevents satisfactory intercostal tube drainage.

When haemothorax is caused by leakage from aortic aneurysm it indicates the likelihood of imminent disruption of the aorta and requires urgent surgical treatment.

# EMPYEMA

The presence of pus in the pleural space is known as empyema. This usually arises as a result of spread of infection from infected lung conditions such as pneumonia, lung abscess or infection distal to bronchial carcinoma or from pulmonary tuberculosis. Unresolved haemothorax consequent on thoracic injury carries a risk of infection with empyema formation. Leakage from the oesophagus, which may complicate oesophageal carcinoma or oesophageal instrumentation or surgery, results in empyema. Less commonly empyema may be due to amoebiasis where spread is from an hepatic focus, or due to fungal infection. In infants staphyloccal lung infection may cause empyema, usually with associated pneumothorax.

The diagnosis of empyema is dependent on the detection of signs of pleural effusion (dullness to percussion, absent breath sounds, radiological appearance of pleural opacity), with signs of infection. Confirmation is obtained by aspiration of the pleural space and culture and sensitivity testing of the aspirated pus.

The surgical management of empyema is dependent on the duration of the condition, the state of the pleural cavity, the causative organism and the underlying pathological cause.

Empyema of recent onset is usually characterised by thin pus (infected effusion) and there is little thickening of the pleura and no fusion of the pleural layers. At this stage resolution may occur, and antibiotic treatment may aid this resolution.

If repeated aspiration is required an intercostal tube with underwater seal drainage may be more convenient. However in more long-standing empyema thick pus and fibrin will often fail to drain in this way and rib resection will be required (see p.253). Physiotherapy and physical activity speed resolution.

When encountered at a late stage the pleural thickening due to fibrin deposition may have resulted in fibrosis which results in permanent constriction of the underlying lung and restriction of chest wall movement. At this stage thoracotomy is required to allow dissection of the chronic empyema cortex from the lung and the interior of the chest wall (decortication).

## THE LUNGS

Each lung is contained within its hemithorax and is attached at the *hilum* to the mediastinum. The main bronchus, pulmonary artery and pulmonary veins are the major structures in the hilum; lymphatics and lymph nodes, bronchial arteries and nerves are also present.

The left lung is divided by an oblique fissure into upper and lower lobes; the right lung has an oblique fissure from which a transverse fissure runs forward resulting in an upper, a middle and a lower lobe. The depth of the fissure varies; lobes may be well separated or nearly totally fused. Lobar bronchial obstruction causes infection in the affected lobe, with fluid accumulation in the lobe, or shrinkage due to air absorption. This consolidation or shrinkage can be recognised and the affected lobe identified radiologically.

The lung lobes are divided by fibrous tissue septa, which radiate out from the hilum, into bronchopulmonary segments each supplied by a segmental bronchus (Fig. 20.1). The branches of the pulmonary arteries are somewhat variable, but they accompany the branches of the bronchial tree and are important in supporting the lung tissue.

Each bronchopulmonary segment is divided into lobules each supplied with a bronchiole and a pulmonary ateriole. The bronchiole divides further within the lung lobule to form five to nine terminal bronchioles each ending in an *acinus*. The acinus consists of the terminal bronchiole which divides into respiratory bronchioles and finally alveolar ducts which have numerous confluent rounded pouches arising from them, known as alveoli. The acinus is supplied by an acinar arteriole which branches with the terminal bronchiole and ultimately gives rise to capillary loops on the outer surface of the alveoli. The capillary loops drain into veins in the interacinous tissue and these veins then run toward the lung hilum in the connective tissue between lobules.

Exchange of oxygen and carbon dioxide occurs between the alveolar gas and the blood in the capillary loops. The alveoli are lined by a thin layer of flattened epithelium lying on a basement membrane which is applied to the alveolar basement membrane. This constitutes the 'alveolocapillary membrane' or blood-air barrier across which gas exchange readily occurs.

## INFECTIVE LUNG CONDITIONS

### Lung abscess

Breakdown of tissue within an area of pneumonia to form an abscess is relatively uncommon with antibiotic therapy. Inhalation of foreign material during a period of loss of consciousness may be followed by infection in the obstructed bronchial segments with subsequent abscess formation. The patient is ill, pyrexial, producing large quantities of foul-smelling sputum. Chest radiography shows a rounded opacity with a fluid level. Bacteriological examination of the sputum aids choice of antibiotic. Postural drainage and physiotherapy help to resolve the abscess. Occasionally rupture into the pleural space results in empyema (pyopneumothorax) requiring pleural drainage.

A major problem commonly encountered is distinguishing an infective lung abscess from a cavitating carcinoma or occasionally a cavitating pulmonary infarct.

### Bronchiectasis

In bronchiectasis parts of the bronchial tree are dilated, with abnormal bronchial walls and associated infection in the bronchi and surrounding lung parenchyma. The condition may be congenital, but probably more commonly follows childhood infections, particularly tuberculosis, measles and whooping cough, in which transient bronchial obstruction is followed by bronchial wall destruction and permanent dilatation. The condition may be widespread but commonly affects the lower lobes, or the lingula or right middle lobe. Persistent cough, unpleasant sputum, haemoptysis, and liability to recurrent chest infections are the main features. Chest radiography may show little change; bronchography is required for diagnosis.

Postural drainage, physiotherapy and antibiotics for acute infective flare-ups are the main methods of treatment. If symptoms are sufficiently troublesome and bronchography demonstrates bronchiectasis confined to one or two lobes only, resection of the affected lobes or segments is often worthwhile.

## BENIGN LUNG TUMOURS

Benign tumours of lung are uncommon. The usual presentation is at routine chest radiography where a mass is shown within the lung. The diagnostic problem may then be considerable. Tuberculoma, pulmonary infarct and metastatic tumour must be considered. Previous chest radiographs, if available, may help as a mass which has been present unchanged for many years is likely to be benign. Sputum cytology may help in diagnosis of bronchial carcinoma. Provided that lung function is satisfactory the advisable course is resection of the mass because of the possibility of its being a bronchial carcinoma, or a tumour with borderline malignancy. Prolonged observation may result in an early carcinoma spreading to become inoperable.

### Bronchial carcinoid

Bronchial carcinoid or bronchial adenoma arises in the major bronchi and causes cough and haemoptysis. This tumour occasionally is associated with the carcinoid syndrome. It is usually non-invasive but occasionally metastasises. The red appearance of the tumour when seen bronchoscopically may suggest the diagnosis.

### Adenoid cystic carcinoma

Adenoid cystic carcinoma or cylindroma is even less common. This tumour arises in trachea or major bronchi and has a greater liability to malignant behaviour.

### Hamartoma

Hamartoma is a developmental abnormality resulting in a mass of tissue with cartilage, muscle and epithelium. It rarely causes symptoms, but may cause bronchial obstruction.

Other benign tumours in lung are rareties. They are almost invariably diagnosed after their resection. It is important not to remove lung tissue unnecessarily when resecting tumours thought to be benign. Palpation at surgery may aid in assessment and frozen section may be useful.

# LUNG CANCER

Lung cancer is a carcinoma arising from the bronchial tree. It is one of the commonest malignant tumours and has increased in frequency over the past 30–50 years. It usually presents in the age group of 50–60 years and is about 10 times more common in men than in women. Cigarette smoking is the major predisposing factor, but exposure to asbestos, chromates and urban life are factors which may be implicated.

Histologically the tumour may be squamous-celled (50%), anaplastic, oat-celled or undifferentiated (35%) or adenocarcinoma (15%). The exact incidence of each type varies in different series. Some areas of the same tumour may have metaplastic change of cell type.

The tumour may be situated 'centrally' — i.e. in the major bronchi where it is visible at bronchoscopy. 'Peripheral' tumours arise within the lung from smaller bronchi and are not visible at bronchoscopy. The tumour may produce symptoms of haemoptysis and cough (or more commonly in smokers a change in cough) due to ulceration and local irritation. If sufficient interference with cilial clearing occurs, or if the tumour blocks a bronchus, there is infection of the distal bronchial tree resulting in pneumonia. Failure of expected resolution of pneumonia in a patient over 40 years old should suggest the possibility of an underlying carcinoma.

Erosion of the growing tumour into a large blood vessel occasionally results in massive blood loss with life-threatening haemoptysis.

The tumour spreads in the lung by invading surrounding lung parenchyma and contiguous structures such as the pericardium, atrium, pleura, chest wall or oesophagus. Tumours arising in the upper lobe apex may invade the brachial plexus, sympathetic chain, and adjacent ribs causing severe pain and Horner's syndrome (Pancoast tumour).

Spread of the tumour by lymphatic spread to hilar and mediastinal lymph nodes results in mediastinal tumour masses which may compress or distort mediastinal structures (e.g. superior vena caval obstruction or widening of the main carinal angle may result). Further lymphatic spread into cervical nodes may produce cervical adenopathy which may be palpable and can be biopsied.

Blood-borne metastases may occur in most viscera; commonest sites are cerebral, skeletal, liver, skin and adrenal.

Uncommon manifestations of bronchial carcinoma are described which are not necessarily related to metastases. They include peripheral neuropathy, myasthenia, acanthosis nigricans, superficial thrombophlebitis, finger clubbing and hypertrophic pulmonary osteo-arthropathy and a variety of endocrine disturbances.

## Presentations

With the many methods of pathological spread it is not surprising that there are so many modes of presentation. The commonest complaints are of cough, haemoptysis, chest pain and shortness of breath. Headaches, back pain, skin nodules, hoarseness, general malaise and weight loss are other presentations. 'Unresolved' pneumonia in the older adult is an important presentation. The discovery of a pulmonary opacity on routine chest radiography is another mode of presentation.

## Investigation

Physical examination may show finger clubbing, evidence of weight loss, lymph node enlargement (particularly in the supraclavicular region), or skin nodules. There may be hoarseness of the voice, suggestive of recurrent laryngeal nerve invasion. Examination of the chest may show evidence of pulmonary consolidation or atelectasis due to bronchial obstruction.

*Chest radiography* almost always shows an abnormality — either due to the tumour mass or lymph node metastases at the hilum, or due to consolidation or atelectasis of lung in the area of an obstructed bronchus. Evidence of involvement of other structures can be obtained by chest radiography. Elevation of a hemidiaphragm due to phrenic nerve involvement indicates the likelihood of inoperability. Erosion of ribs or vertebral bodies also indicates the likelihood of inoperability.

*Bronchoscopy* will allow direct viewing of 'central' tumours which can then be biopsied for histological examination. 'Peripheral' tumours themselves will not be visible, but cytological examination of bronchial secretions aspirated at bronchoscopy or brush biopsy may give cytological confirmation of the diagnosis.

Bronchoscopy gives valuable evidence in assessing operability. Main carinal widening indicates subcarinal lymph node metastasis and inoperability. Tumour involving a main bronchus up to the main carina, or into the trachea, is generally inoperable.

*Lymph node biopsy.* Any palpable supraclavicular lymph nodes should be biopsied — tumour spread to these nodes indicates inoperability.

*Mediastinoscopy.* Biopsy of lymph nodes in the upper and anterior mediastinum through a short suprasternal or parasternal incision may similarly provide evidence of lymph spread but these techniques are not undertaken by all surgeons and their value remains disputed.

*Barium swallow.* Gross distortion of the barium-filled oesophagus on radiography may similarly indicate the presence of involved lymph nodes and the likelihood of inoperability, but the investigation is not uniformly performed.

### Assessment of pulmonary function

In contemplating surgical treatment for bronchial carcinoma the surgeon must consider not only the likelihood of the tumour being localised to lung tissue which can be removed totally, but also the likelihood of the remaining lung tissue being adequate to maintain satisfactory respiration. This latter judgement is not always simple; many complex tests of lung function are available and the pulmonary physician can help in assessment. In practice the surgeon is guided by the pre-operative activity of the patient (ability to climb a flight of stairs), results of ventilatory function tests (vital capacity and forced expiratory volume in 1 second), and the likely extent of surgery. Resection of an airless obstructed lobe clearly is less likely to impair subsequent lung function than is resection of a functioning lung with a small central tumour.

### Treatment

Evidence of inoperability is usually present in well over half of patients — as for example the presence of metastases or obvious unfitness for thoracotomy due to chronic bronchitis or emphysema. The outlook for these patients is bleak: the majority are dead within a year and any treatment is mainly symptomatic. For those in whom there is no evidence of spread, resection of the tumour offers the only prospect of cure, and even then 5-year survival is disappointing — being no more than 30% to 40%.

The principle of surgical treatment is the removal of the tumour within the affected lobe or lung together with the hilar lymph node drainage. If the tumour is confined to a lobe the operation of lobectomy is performed. When the tumour crosses a fissure to involve upper and lower lobe, or where a main bronchus is involved the operation of pneumonectomy is performed.

*Radiotherapy* is used to palliate bronchial carcinoma where severe pain is caused by skeletal involvement of Pancoast tumour, or where obstruction of superior vena cava or trachea causes severe distress. As an adjunct to surgical resection radiotherapy has been disappointing.

*Chemotherapy.* Cytotoxic drugs have had little success in palliation of bronchial carcinoma and are not commonly used.

Because of the disappointing results of resection for bronchial carcinoma and the likelihood of spread from the primary site leading to inoperability before symptoms arise it is advised that any unexplained pulmonary opacity discovered by routine chest radiography be resected.

## OPERATIONS TO THE LUNG

### Thoracotomy

Exposure of the lung for resection of a lobe (lobectomy) or the whole lung (pneumonectomy) is performed by thoracotomy. Opening the pleural space necessitates provision for inflating the lungs during operation. This requires insertion of a cuffed endotracheal tube to allow intermittent positive pressure ventilation during anaesthesia. General anaesthesia with skeletal muscle relaxation is used.

The patient is positioned in the lateral position on the operating table with a support under the loin to increase the prominence of the side of the chest uppermost. The skin is prepared and draped for surgery with sterile technique.

The skin incision curves from between the medial border of the scapula and the vertebral spines, below the scapular angle and into the inframammary crease. The incision is deepened through the subcutaneous fat and fascia. Diathermy is used to control bleeding points. The chest wall muscles that require division are latissimus dorsi and the lower digitations of serratus anterior. The chest is entered by stripping the periosteum from the border of the 5th or 6th rib and incising the periosteal rib bed and pleura. The opening is spread by moving the ribs at their ends — the costal cartilages and costo-vertebral joints. Thus a long incision is essential to ensure a wide opening — the *lateral thoracotomy*. For operations designed to approach the anterior chest (e.g. anterior mediastinum) or posterior chest (e.g. thoracic aorta) the emphasis of the incision may be anterior or posterior (*antero-lateral thoracotomy* or *posterolateral thoracotomy*). However, in both cases it is necessary to strip periosteum from the rib over most of its length to allow spreading of the ribs.

Following operation a pleural drain may be inserted via the chest wall below the incision if leakage of air or blood is anticipated. Closure of the thoracotomy requires apposition of the ribs with heavy sutures and reconstitution of the muscle layers, fascia and skin.

## Pneumonectomy

Before commencing pneumonectomy for tumour the surgeon gently palpates the tumour to confirm that it does not invade chest wall or mediastinum. The pulmonary veins and main pulmonary artery are ligated and divided. The main bronchus is resected close to the main carina avoiding a residual stump. The bronchus remaining should not be crushed, and contamination of the operative field from endobronchial secretions must be avoided. Non-absorbable bronchial sutures or staples are used. Leakage (bronchopleural fistula) is a serious complication which is less common with careful technique. Hilar and mediastinal lymph nodes are removed as far as possible in continuity with the resected lung.

The pneumonectomy space is commonly not drained, unless excessive oozing is anticipated. Gradual filling of the space by serum and blood over the next few weeks is followed by gradual fibrosis, movement of the mediastinum to the pneumonectomy side, and elevation of the diaphragm and crowding of the ribs.

## Lobectomy

If the appropriate operation is lobectomy (tumour or other pathology localised to a lobe) the fissure is deepened toward the hilum. The lobar bronchus is divided, and the lobar arteries and vein are divided and ligated. Small air leaks from the lobe surface require insertion of pleural drains.

The remaining lobe or lobes expand to fill the space left in the hemithorax. Crowding of ribs, elevation of the hemidiaphragm and movement of the mediastinum contribute to making the hemithorax smaller on the lobectomy side. As a result usually there is no pleural space left by a week after lobectomy.

## THE THORACIC CAGE

The driving force for the movement of air into the lungs via the airways is provided by muscular contraction. The diaphragm is the major muscle involved in normal resting breathing. As it has a dome-like shape shutting off the lower end of the thoracic cage, contraction results in flattening of the diaphragm and an increase in intrathoracic volume. This results in lowering of intrathoracic pressure, which is transmitted to the airways, and air flows into the lungs. Additional respiratory drive comes from elevation of the ribs by the intercostal muscles. Because the ribs slope downward and forward from their pivot axis on the vertebrae their elevation increases the anteroposterior and to a lesser extent the transverse measurement of the thorax.

Expiration is largely a passive phase. The lungs contain elastic tissues causing a natural recoil toward the lung hilum; once chest expansion is relaxed the airways pressure increases and air flows out.

With greater respiratory effort, as with active exercise or where there is airways obstruction (as in asthma) additional ventilatory effort is made by using 'accessory muscles of respiration' — the scalenes, pectorals and sternomastoids; and for forced expiration (or coughing) the abdominal wall muscles are contracted. The bony framework of the thoracic cage provides the necessary element of rigidity for creating this pumping mechanism.

If the thoracic cage is affected by disease or surgery there may be severe impairment of ventilation. The most striking and obvious example is the total failure of ventilation following skeletal muscle paralysis during anaesthesia. Muscle weakness or spasm due to pain is a common cause of inadequate ventilation following thoracic or upper abdominal operations. The thoracic cage may be restricted in its movement by ankylosing spondylitis or by fibrous tissue within the thoracic cage following organisation of a haemothorax. Impairment of ventilation may also occur if the negative pressure generated by thoracic cage expansion is not transmitted to the airways. This occurs when the pleural space around the lung is in communication with the atmosphere (either via the chest wall or via the lung — pneumothorax) or where part of the lung framework is unstable as a result of multiple fractures creating a 'flail' segment.

## CHEST WALL DEFORMITIES

### Pectus excavatum

This is a deformity of the thoracic cage in which the sternum is posteriorly displaced. This results in a depression in the precordial area and displacement of the heart toward the left. Systolic murmurs are often present but cardio-respiratory function is not usually unduly impaired. The main problem is the distress caused by the cosmetic deformity and this is the justification for surgery. Surgery involves resecting costal cartilages on either side of the sternum to allow the sternum to be pulled forward. Malleable metal strips are then placed across the front of the ribs and behind the sternum to hold it forward until stability results from regeneration of costal carti-

lages in the normal position. The metal strips may be removed several months later.

### Pectus carinatum

This is a similar type of deformity but the sternum is anteriorly displaced. The principle of surgery is similar to that for pectus excavatum.

## THORACIC INJURY

Thoracic injury is common following major traffic accidents and military injuries. It is commonly associated with major injury to other parts of the body — in particular the head, the abdomen and the skeletal system.

Although head injury, abdominal injury or major orthopaedic injury may require urgent treatment, thoracic injuries frequently lead most rapidly to death, and relatively simple intervention, if prompt, may be life-saving.

### Airway obstruction

Crush injury or blunt injury to the chest commonly results in lung contusion and bleeding into the bronchial tree. When the integrity of the chest wall is lost, as with multiple rib fractures causing flail chest, or if coughing is suppresed by unconsciousness, blood in the bronchial tree, or inhaled pharyngeal blood or secretions or vomited gastric contents may rapidly produce fatal suffocation. The provision of an *unobstructed airway* is therefore an urgent priority. This may be achieved in the unconscious patient by a *pharyngeal airway*, or by inserting an *endotracheal tube*, which has the advantage of allowing tracheobronchial suction for clearing of the airway.

### Fractured ribs

Direct blows to the chest wall may result in fracture of one or more ribs. Pain, exacerbated by breathing or coughing, is the main problem. This tends to inhibit ventilatory movement of the related lung. In the elderly or the bronchitic this may be followed by serious bronchopneumonia. For this reason attempts to immobilise the frac-

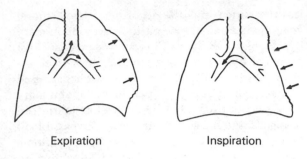

Expiration                    Inspiration

**Fig. 20.6** Effect of flail segment on the chest wall

ture area by strapping are best avoided. Analgesia, if necessary with local anaesthesia, is required.

## Flail chest

Loss of chest wall integrity due to a flail segment occurs when a number of ribs are fractured in such a way as to produce paradoxical movement of a segment of the thoracic cage. Inspiratory efforts then result in indrawing of the 'flail' segment and expiratory efforts result in bulging of the flail segment (Fig. 20.6). The effect on ventilatory movement of airways gas is catastrophic — effective ventilation is severely compromised by air moving into and out of lung on the affected side instead of moving through the trachea.

This condition is rapidly reversed by inserting a cuffed endotracheal tube and using mechanical positive pressure ventilation. This will usually be required for several weeks. Once urgent treatment has been undertaken, tracheostomy can be performed. This allows prolonged positive pressure ventilation, tracheal aspiration and earlier weaning from ventilation, due to dead space reduction. As the chest wall fractures begin to heal a degree of rigidity returns. This reduces the tendency for paradoxical movement of the flail segment and unassisted ventilation usually becomes possible after 2 to 3 weeks.

If thoracotomy is required (as for example for continued bleeding) it is often feasible to immobilise at least some of the rib fractures at the same time by wiring or pinning. This may sufficiently reduce subsequent paradoxical ventilation to avoid the need for prolonged ventilation and the risks of tracheostomy.

## Pneumothorax and surgical emphysema

Sharp penetrating injuries which lacerate lung result in pneumothorax or haemopneumothorax. This may require pleural drainage. Occasionally blunt injury results in fracture of a major bronchus or trachea. Air leakage is rapid and requires suture of the leak. Surgical emphysema is caused by air in the tissue planes. It gains access from airways or lung when they are injured and may spread widely over chest, abdomen, neck and face giving a distressing bloated appearance and crackling of the air-filled tissues. The condition subsides spontaneously over several days.

## Haemothorax

Sharp penetrating injuries, such as stab wounds, bullet wounds, or fractured ends of ribs from crush injuries may all result in bleeding from laceration of intercostal vessels, chest wall muscle, lung tissue or heart and major vessels. Blood accumulates within the pleural space — *haemothorax*. The effects of this blood loss are those of oligaemic shock as well as impaired lung function due to compression of lung on the side of the injury. In addition, if lung is injured, bleeding may occur into the airways, adding airways obstruction to the problems of the injured patient. Air leaking from lacerated lung further compresses that lung by pneumothorax (traumatic haemo-pneumothorax). Urgent chest X-ray is required. The principles of management are:

1. The provision of unobstructed airway;
2. Drainage of the pleural space by insertion of a pleural tube connected to underwater seal drainage, and
3. Replacement of blood.

The rate of blood loss from the pleural drain is a guide to further treatment. Usually bleeding slows and finally ceases spontaneously, blood replacement and continual pleural drainage being all that is required. If blood loss is excessive and continued, thoracotomy is required to control bleeding sites. The loss of 200 ml/hour or more in an adult usually requires thoracotomy. Similarly, failure of pleural drainage to clear the pleural space requires thoracotomy. The usual cause is blood clot obstructing the pleural tube. If left alone a large clotted haemothorax may undergo organisation and fibrosis, severely compromising lung movement. At thoracotomy the commonest bleeding site is from lacerated intercostal vessels which can be undersewn or diathermied. Bleeding from lung is accompanied by air leak, and smaller lacerations can be repaired with absorbable sutures. Occasionally gross laceration of lung requires lobectomy for control of haemorrhage.

Bleeding from major vessels or heart usually produces rapidly fatal haemorrhage. Stab injuries of the heart, however, commonly cause death by pericardial tamponade. Recognition of hypotension, tachycardia and systemic venous engorgement with a stab wound near the heart (anterior chest or epigastrium) requires urgent thoracotomy and opening of the pericardium. Release of pericardial clot results in dramatic improvement and allows time for insertion of sutures into the cardiac laceration.

## Aortic rupture

Rapid deceleration injury, such as seen in traffic accidents, or in falls from a height, may result in shearing of the aorta at a point 2 or 3 cm beyond the left subclavian artery in the descending aorta. The tear is frequently circumferential and the aortic ends retract apart. Massive exsanguination may result immediately, but it is possible for aortic adventitia, mediastinal connective tissue and pleura to contain the blood as a false aneurysm. Ultimate rupture usually occurs within days, occasionally much later.

Clinically, the condition is suspected when chest radiography shows mediastinal widening in a patient who has sustained deceleration injury. Other sources of bleeding, such as sternal fracture, cause mediastinal haematoma and the diagnosis requires confirmation by aortography as an urgent procedure. Irregularity of the aorta just beyond the left subclavian artery with extravasation of opaque medium confirms the diagnosis. Repair of the aortic rupture should be undertaken urgently.

Left thoracotomy reveals extensive haematoma over the mediastinum. If bleeding elsewhere in the body (e.g. liver, spleen, brain) is not a prob-

lem the patient may be heparinised and femoral vein to femoral artery partial cardiopulmonary bypass may be used. This allows avoidance of proximal hypertension when the aorta is cross-clamped and also allows return of lost heparinised blood to the patient. If partial cariopulmonary bypass is not used a special tube (Gott shunt) can be placed into the ascending aorta to bypass blood into descending aorta or femoral artery. Some surgeons do not use either method, but rely on speed in operating. Spinal cord ischaemic injury is a hazard of all methods. The proximal aorta is surrounded with a tape and a distal aortic tape is placed beyond the anticipated rupture. Dissection at the site of rupture should not commence until the aorta has been clamped proximally between common carotid and left subclavian arteries, and distally to the descending aorta. The ruptured aorta is readily identified. The gap caused by aortic retraction is repaired by sewing in a length of woven dacron graft.

## THE MEDIASTINUM

The mediastinum is that region of the thorax between the lungs. It includes the heart and great vessels, the trachea and main bronchi, oesophagus and nerve and lymphatic tissue (Fig. 20.7).

An arbitrary descriptive division of the mediastinum aids discussion of diagnostic problems.

*Superior mediastinum* is that area superior to an imaginary line between the sternal angle and the lower border of the 4th thoracic vertebra.

*Anterior mediastinum* is that area between the heart and the back of the sternum — normally only a potential space.

*Posterior mediastinum* is that area between the heart and the vertebral column and posterior chest wall.

*Middle mediastinum* is occupied by the heart, the structures of the lung hila and major vessels.

## MEDIASTINAL MASSES

These are of a large variety. They may be *infective* (e.g. mediastinal abscess from oesophageal perforation, or tuberculous abscess from a thoracic

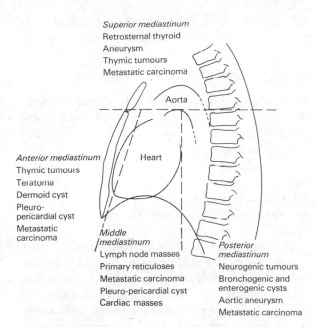

Superior mediastinum
Retrosternal thyroid
Aneurysm
Thymic tumours
Metastatic carcinoma

Aorta

Anterior mediastinum          Heart
Thymic tumours
Teratoma
Dermoid cyst
Pleuro-
pericardial cyst
Metastatic
carcinoma

Middle
mediastinum                          Posterior
Lymph node masses                mediastinum
Primary reticuloses              Neurogenic tumours
Metastatic carcinoma             Bronchogenic and
Pleuro-pericardial cyst          enterogenic cysts
Cardiac masses                   Aortic aneurysm
                                 Metastatic carcinoma

**Fig. 20.7** Diagram of the mediastinum as seen on lateral chest X-ray

vertebral body), *benign tumours* (e.g. neuro-fibroma), *malignant tumours* (e.g. lymphosarcoma or secondary lymph node metastasis from bronchial carcinoma), *developmental abnormalities* (e.g. enterogenous cyst) or *aneurysms* (atherosclerotic, syphilitic, dissecting or traumatic).

The presentation is commonly that of a symptom-free mass detected on routine radiography, or that of mediastinal pressure symptoms due to compression of mediastinal structures. *Tracheal compression* causes stridor and breathing difficulty, *superior caval* compression causes a feeling of distension in the head and neck with venous engorgement. Compression or distortion of the *oesophagus* produces dysphagia. Pressure on the heart may cause dysrhythmias or even heart failure.

In practice the radiological appearances are not always easy to assess. A lung mass adjacent to the mediastinum may be indistinguishable from a mediastinal mass. Aortic aneurysm of the ascending aorta, arch or descending aorta should always be considered. Radiologically aortic aneurysms may not be obviously pulsatile on screening; and many other masses pulsate due to transmitted pulsation. Aortography is required if this diagnostic possibility is raised.

## Superior mediastinum

1. Retrosternal *thyroid* enlargement due to any cause may cause tracheal compression, with dyspnoea and stridor. Most retrosternal goitres connect with the thyroid in the neck. Radio-isotope scanning may aid in diagnosis. Surgical removal is usually possible from the neck — rarely is it necessary to split the sternum.

2. *Aneurysm* of the aortic arch, innominate artery or origin of carotid arteries may produce a mass which compresses trachea or oesophagus and requires arch aortography for delineation. Resection of these aneurysms usually requires cardiopulmonary bypass with systemic hypothermia for cerebral protection during any brief periods of interruption of cerebral blood flow, and a means of artificial cerebral perfusion from the arterial side of the the cardiopulmonary bypass circuit.

3. There is an association between *thymic tumours* and myaesthenia gravis which is not clear. A number of patients with myaesthenia gravis have thymic tumours. Resection of the thymus (whether or not it contains a tumour) is frequently followed by cure or amelioration of myaesthenia. Surgery is recommended if there is a radiologically visible thymic tumour, or if medical therapy with neostigmine is unsatisfactory.

Neostigmine is given in the pre- and postoperative period. Vertical sternotomy gives best access to the thymus which is dissected free and removed after controlling its vascular connections.

## Anterior mediastinum

1. *Thymic tumours* may occur in the anterior mediastinum.

2. *Teratoma*: this tumour usually contains endodermal, mesodermal and ectodermal tissue. Malignant change may occur in any element. The most common site for teratoma is the ovary, followed by the anterior mediastinum.

The dermoid cyst is a benign variety in which ectodermal elements including skin, hair or teeth predominate. Pressure symptoms or routine radiology draw attention to the condition.

## Posterior mediastinum

*1. Neurogenic tumours. Neurofibroma* arises on an intercostal nerve. Occasionally it entends into the vertebral canal through an intervertebral foramen where it may cause cord compression. Malignant change is rare.

*Ganglioneuroma* arises on the sympathetic chain. Malignant change may occur.

*Neuroblastoma* occurs in children: it is usually malignant.

*2. Bronchogenic and enterogenous cysts.* Foregut tissue in the posterior mediastinum may give rise to cysts which contain bronchial or gastric epithelium.

*3. Masses arising from oesophagus.* Oesophageal carcinoma or rhabdomyoma (or rhabdomyosarcoma), or the dilated oesophagus of oesophageal achalasia, or a hiatus hernia occasionally cause diagnostic difficulty, but their presentation is usually distinctive.

## Middle mediastinum

*1. Pleuro-pericardial cysts.* These are thin-walled cysts containing clear fluid which arise from the pericardium. They are benign and rarely produce pressure symptoms.

*2. Lymph node masses.* Hilar and mediastinal lymph node enlargement due to any cause may present as a mediastinal mass. The commonest cause for this is lymph node metastasis from bronchial carcinoma, although many other primary sites may metastasise to mediastinal nodes.

Hodgkins' disease may present because of mediastinal lymph node enlargement; tuberculous lymph node enlargement as part of a primary tuberculous infection is a very common cause of mediastinal mass in countries where tuberculosis is common. Sarcoidosis is another cause for lymph node enlargement.

*3. Cardiac aneurysm or tumour.* Left ventricular aneurysm is usually fairly easy to diagnose – it follows myocardial infarction and electrocardiographic and radiological findings are usually helpful. Cardiac tumours are rare; their diagnosis is not often apparent until exploratory thoracotomy.

## General principles of management

Careful attention to history and physical examination may be helpful e.g. the presence of cervical lymphadenopathy, hepatomegaly or splenomegaly may suggest reticulosis.

The radiological picture may be helpful, but is not often diagnostic. The commoner causes and sites of mediastinal masses have been mentioned but rarer conditions or unusual sites are encountered.

Because of the risk of development of pressure effects, or risk of malignant change in a benign lesion, or spread of an early malignant lesion, it is advised tht asymptomatic mediastinal masses be removed. Every effort should be made to establish the diagnosis beforehand — particularly to avoid encountering an aortic aneurysm without forewarning and to avoid unnecessary surgery for disseminated disease (as for example Hodgkins' disease).

Where symptoms of compression are present the common explanation is malignant tumour (primary or secondary). If this can be confirmed, radiotherapy or cytotoxic therapy may be appropriate (e.g. bronchial carcinoma with spread causing superior vena caval obstruction). Care must be taken to avoid the assumption that malignancy is the cause of pressure symptoms, or that it is inoperable (e.g. retrosternal goitre may be wrongly diagnosed as a malignant tumour). Where there is doubt exploratory surgery is required. The usual approach is by lateral thoracotomy on the side on which the mediastinal mass is most obvious. For thymic tumours vertical sternotomy provides excellent exposure. Retrosternal goitre is usually accessible from the neck.

## DISEASES OF THE OESOPHAGUS

These are considered in Chapter 26.

# 21. Peripheral Vascular Disease

## ATHEROSCLEROSIS AND OCCLUSIVE ARTERIAL DISEASE

Occlusive arterial disease is now the commonest cause of death in the Western World. It is most frequently due to atherosclerosis, the underlying cause of which remains obscure. The complications are readily understood and are due to partial or complete occlusion of an involved vessel, potentiated by secondary thrombosis. In the limbs, this leads to the development of ischaemic pain on exercise (claudication), ischaemic rest pain and, eventually, gangrene. Local haemodynamic factors such as movement of arteries across joints, turbulence at orifices and bifurcations, sucking effects on the intima, and trauma may influence the distribution of the disease and the risk of thrombosis. So also may such general factors as obesity, hypercholesterolaemia, diabetes mellitus and diet. Cigarette smoking and hypertension adversely affect the outcome of occlusive arterial disease; exercise may confer some protection.

*Thrombosis* starts where a vessel wall is irregular, ulcerated, narrowed or widened and progresses to partial or complete occlusion. Collateral vessels dilate to compensate for the reduced flow of blood in the main vessel and may eventually serve as an efficient, if temporary, bypass.

As the origins of the collaterals are themselves frequently diseased, the degree of compensation is variable. When this bypass mechanism fails, symptoms return or become more severe.

During the period of partial occlusion, *thrombus* may become dislodged to form an *embolus* which lodges distally, often at sites of bifurcation.

This may be a single or recurrent event. Recurrent emboli may greatly compromise the 'run-off' through distal vessels.

The majority of arterial emboli do not originate from vessels but from the heart, usually when there is atrial fibrillation or a mural thrombus following myocardial infarction. Occasional causes of embolisation include vegetations on valves and prosthetic heart valves.

With increasing age, arteries tend to lengthen, widen and lose the elasticity of the media, features which facilitate *aneurysm* formation. Aneurysms may also form beyond an area of stenosis due to increased turbulence (post-stenotic dilatation).

*Dissection* of the arterial wall most frequently follows medial degeneration, especially when complicated by hypertension. An intimal tear allows blood to enter the vessel wall and so create two lumens. In most cases the outer adventitial layer also ruptures eventually but rarely the dissection re-enters the true lumen through the intima further down the vessel (Fig. 21.1).

Drug therapy does not affect the course of atherosclerosis. Neither anticoagulants nor clofibrate have been proven to limit the disease or prevent its complications. Antiplatelet drugs which prevent thrombosis offer future promise. Vasodilators are generally useless.

## OCCLUSIVE ARTERIAL DISEASE OF THE LOWER LIMB

### AORTO-ILIAC OCCLUSION

The aorto-iliac segment includes the abdominal aorta and iliac vessels (Fig. 21.2). Though less

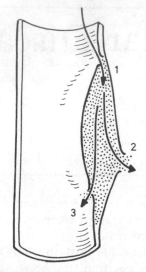

**Fig. 21.1** A diagram of a dissecting aneurysm of aorta showing: (1) initial intimal tear, (2) adventitial rupture, (3) intimal rupture.

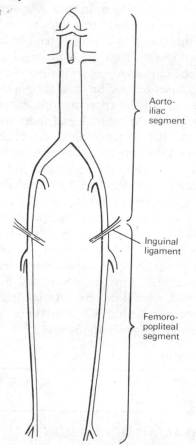

**Fig. 21.2** Anatomy of aorto-iliac and femoro-popliteal segments

frequently affected by atherosclerosis than the femoro-popliteal segment, its occlusion is a common cause of vascular insufficiency in the lower limbs. The disease may affect only the bifurcation of the aorta or extend to involve the common iliac vessels.

Extension of thrombosis is slower than in the femoro-popliteal region, and the external iliac artery may remain free of disease for a considerable time. As the collateral circulation is greater than in the femoro-popliteal segment, the progress of symptoms is slower.

### Clinical features

Buttock and thigh claudication are classical features which may be associated with impotence in males. However, many patients present with calf claudication or rest pain. The femoral pulses are reduced or absent, and auscultation may reveal a bruit in the upper femoral region or over the aortic bifurcation. The distal pulses may or may not be palpable. Signs of ischaemia in the lower limb are usually minimal.

## FEMORO-POPLITEAL OCCLUSION

In the lower limb atherosclerosis most frequently affects the femoro-popliteal segment of the arterial tree (Fig. 21.2). This includes the common femoral, profunda femoris, superficial femoral and popliteal arteries.

The initial lesion is only partially occlusive and affects a short segment of the artery. It is frequently situated close to the termination of the superficial femoral artery at the adductor hiatus. Generally there are no symptoms or, at most, calf claudication may be present. The ankle pulses are intact, the only clinical sign being a bruit in the region of the adductor hiatus.

Secondary thrombosis with occlusion inevitably develops. Initially, the collateral circulation compensates adequately so that symptoms are limited to periods of exercise. This stable state of affairs may last for many years.

If thrombosis extends to involve the femoral and popliteal arteries in continuity, the collateral circulation begins to fail. Decompensation leads to a dramatic worsening of peripheral ischaemia.

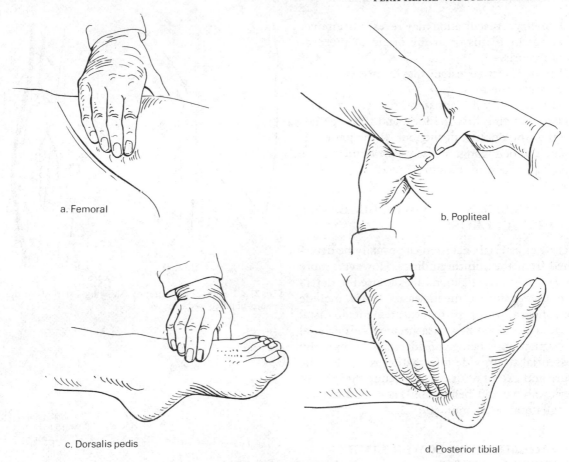

a. Femoral

b. Popliteal

c. Dorsalis pedis

d. Posterior tibial

**Fig. 21.3** The palpation of pulses

Stenosis at the origin of profunda femoris or at the popliteal bifurcation, or occlusion of the tibial or peroneal vessels hastens decompensation.

## Clinical features

*Symptoms.* The commonest presenting feature of femoro-popliteal occlusion is *intermittent claudication* affecting the calf. Initially the patient can 'walk through' the pain, but later he must stop and rest for several minutes before continuing. With progressive circulatory impairment, the claudication distance shortens until finally the patient is crippled. Often the claudication distance remains unchanged over long periods of time or may even improve as the collateral circulation develops.

*Rest pain* in the toes and foot occurs most commonly at night and indicates extensive occlusion. It is hot and burning in nature and may be relieved by the patient uncovering his foot, hanging his leg out of the bed or elevating it on pillows. Paraesthesia, numbness and tingling also occur. During this phase, minor trauma may lead to infection and precipitate gangrene.

*Signs.* The skin of the leg is white and shiny. There is loss of hair and the nails become opaque and brittle. Elevation of the leg results in immediate increase in pallor which is exaggerated when the patient exercises his calf muscles by dorsiflexion and plantar flexion of the foot. When the leg is brought back to the horizontal, the appearance of reactive hyperaemia is delayed and the venous filling time is prolonged relative to the normal limb.

The femoral and sometimes the popliteal pulse are palpable but the dorsalis pedis and the posterior tibial pulses are invariably absent (Fig. 21.3). These findings can be confirmed by oscillometry. Auscultation may reveal a bruit over the adductor hiatus or at the origin of the profunda femoris.

Chronic infective lesions may be present, notably between the toes.

Gangrene may be apparent. It usually starts distally, affecting first the toes, and then spreading on to the dorsum of the foot. If the patient is confined to bed, gangrene may start at the heel as a result of pressure (decubitus ulcer).

## INVESTIGATION OF LOWER LIMB ATHEROSCLEROSIS

The *site* of arterial occlusion can usually be determined from the clinical findings. However, more sophisticated investigations are required to determine the *extent* of the disease. These include ultrasonography, pressure measurements in distal arteries, and blood flow measurements. If arterial reconstruction is being considered, arteriography is essential to provide information regarding the nature and extent of disease, to define the state of arteries above and below the lesion, and display the collateral circulation (Fig. 21.4).

## MANAGEMENT OF LOWER LIMB ATHEROSCLEROSIS

Restoration of blood flow to the ischaemic part relieves pain, promotes healing of gangrenous areas, and improves function. Failed surgical reconstruction may leave the patient worse off than before, and careful and critical preoperative evaluation is necessary. For this reason most patients are treated initially by conservative measures which include general care and care of the limb.

### Conservative measures (Fig. 21.5)

*General care.* Cardiac failure, diabetes and hypertension are controlled. Anaemia is corrected and, as nicotine is a vaso-constrictor, patients should stop smoking. Hyperlipidaemic states are corrected as far as possible.

Malnourished patients are given a high protein diet and vitamin supplements.

Analgesics may be required to relieve pain. Narcotics are avoided for fear of addiction.

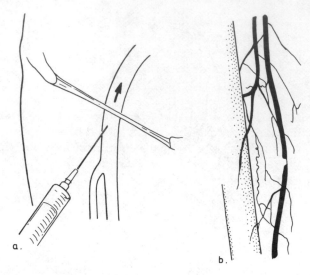

**Fig. 21.4** Femoral arteriography (showing a stenosis of the femoro-popliteal segment

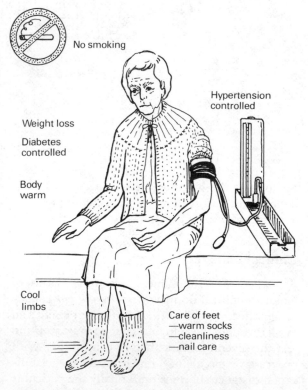

**Fig. 21.5** Conservative measures in arterial disease

Aspirin is a useful analgesic with antiplatelet properties but stronger analgesics are often necessary. Anticoagulants and vasodilators are of doubtful value.

*Care of the limb.* It is essential to avoid precipitating gangrene. The patient is warned to avoid extremes of heat (which increases metabolism) or cold (which causes vaso-constriction). The feet must be protected from trauma and kept clean and free from infection. The nails are trimmed regularly, preferably by a chiropodist so that skin trauma can be avoided. Socks should be soft (but not tight), should not have elasticated tops, and should be kept clean and well fitting. Constricting clothes or garters of any type are avoided.

There are no drugs which reliably increase blood flow to limbs affected by occlusive vascular disease. Buerger's exercises consist of intermittent elevation and dependency of the limb to increase blood flow and are still prescribed by some.

Should gangrene occur, the limb is kept cool and exposed. Moist dressings are avoided. Infection is treated promptly by antibiotics. The leg is supported so that the heel is not submitted to pressure. Reflex heating, by placing a warm pad over the abdomen to induce peripheral vasodilatation is still practised, though its value is doubtful.

## Sympathectomy

In a normal limb sympathectomy results in dilatation of skin vessels so that the limb becomes warm, pink and dry. It does not increase muscle blood flow or benefit claudication, and lumbar sympathectomy has an uncertain role when major vessels are affected by occlusive vascular disease.

In many centres, sympathectomy is performed only if there is evidence of skin ischaemia or rest pain and to enhance the effects of an arterial reconstruction. Destruction of the lumbar sympathetic chain by para-vertebral injection of phenol (chemical sympathectomy) has recently been brought back into use (Fig. 21.6). Not only does this avoid a major operation (and it can be performed on a trial basis), but it can be repeated if sympathetic function returns. Its likely effect can be determined by a preceding test injection of local anaesthetic.

## Arterial reconstruction

All patients with severe intermittent claudication, rest pain, or threatened or established gangrene should be considered for arterial reconstruction. Techniques available include 'patch grafting' to widen a stenotic vessel, removal of atherosclerotic plaques and thrombus, and bypass of occluded vessels. For a good result, the small distal vessels must be patent, i.e. there must be adequate 'run-off'. Amputation will be required if reconstruction fails. Also the sequence of events may be delayed by sympathectomy.

*Aorto-iliac segment.* Significant aorto-iliac disease must be corrected before distal recon-

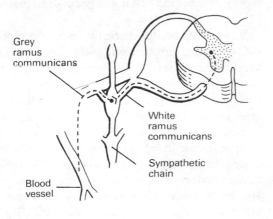
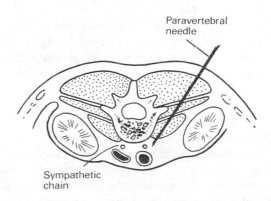

a.                                       b.

**Fig. 21.6** Sympathectomy showing (a) the vascular sympathetic supply, and (b) the direction of insertion of a paravertebral needle for phenol block

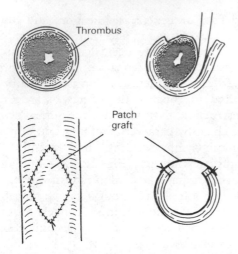

Fig. 21.7 Thromboendarterectomy and patch grafting

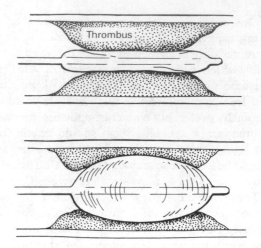

**Fig. 21.8** Balloon angioplasty

struction is considered. Stenotic lesions of the aorto-iliac system require surgical treatment as occlusion is inevitable. Patches with vein or synthetic material can be used to widen the stenotic area and local thrombo-endarterectomy may also be necessary (Fig. 21.7). Isolated stenotic lesions can be dilated by transluminal angioplasty using a special balloon catheter which is inserted under local anaesthesia and guided with image intensification (Fig. 21.8).

When there are multiple stenoses or occlusions, the choice of treatment rests between thrombo-endarterectomy and aorto-femoral profunda bypass grafts. Synthetic grafts (Dacron) are favoured, and patency rates of 90% at 5 years have been reported.

Graft infection, pseudo-aneurysm formation or thrombosis are rare complications. An infected suture line may rupture requiring ligation of the vessel and removal of the graft. In this event flow to the limb can be restored by a long bypass graft from the axillary artery to the femoral artery, or less frequently, from the opposite femoral artery ('cross-over graft'). The results are less satisfactory than those of direct aorto-iliac reconstruction.

*Femoro-popliteal segment.* An isolated stenotic lesion may be treated by a 'patch graft' of vein. This can prevent secondary thrombosis for many years and does not compromise future major arterial reconstruction. Vein patch grafting has particular value in disease affecting the profunda

femoris, the main collateral channel to the lower limb. Atherosclerosis commonly affects only its origin while the main stem of the profunda femoris remains remarkably disease-free. If thrombosis is more extensive, the patch graft (profundoplasty) may be combined with a thrombo endarterectomy, which removes thrombus and sclerosed intima from the stenosed segment (Fig. 21.8). Reconstruction of the profunda femoris almost always improves the distal circulation, can abolish rest pain, and occasionally heals gangrenous lesions.

Thrombosis of a short segment of the femoro-popliteal artery can usually be left untreated; in most instances the collateral circulation maintains peripheral blood flow.

When advanced atherosclerosis compromises the collateral circulation, major reconstructive surgery is required. This involves a bypass procedure between femoral and popliteal, tibial or peroneal vessels (Fig. 21.9). An autogenous vein graft is preferred and the long saphenous vein is suitable in 70% of cases. The cephalic vein can be used although in 50% of patients it is too small. Stripping of the long saphenous vein for varicosities should be avoided in patients at risk from arterial occlusive disease. If no vein is available, synthetic materials such as Dacron, PTFE (Gortex) or Dardik biograft (specially treated human umbilical vein) can be used. These are expensive and give less satisfactory long-term results than autogenous vein when used below the groin.

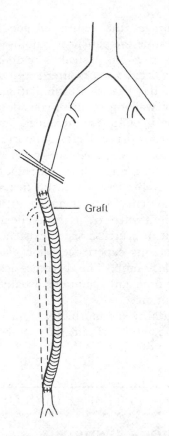

**Fig. 21.9** Bypass procedure showing a synthetic graft or autogenous vein bypassing an occluded femoro-popliteal segment

When synthetic grafts are used, prophylactic antibiotic therapy is advised.

Cross-clamping of vessels is necessary to allow an anastomosis to be made. As this carries a risk of thrombosis, heparin (5000 units) is injected intravenously before the clamps are applied.

## DIABETES AND ARTERIAL DISEASE

Up to 10% of patients with peripheral arterial disease suffer from diabetes mellitus. Of patients with *severe* ischaemia of the distal lower limb, 30–50% are diabetics.

Diabetic arteritis (or angiopathy) is predominantly a disease of vessels of arteriolar size. However, the majority of diabetics with peripheral arterial disease also have larger vessels involved with atherosclerosis indistinguishable from that of non-diabetic patients. In about 30% of diabetics, the large vessels appear healthy and normal pulses are present. When large and small vessel disease co-exist the prognosis for limb salvage is worse than in non-diabetic patients with equivalent degrees of large vessel occlusion.

The progress of arterial disease in diabetics is affected adversely by two further factors:

1. Infection in the ischaemic part, facilitated by the high sugar content of the tissue which favours bacterial growth.

2. Diabetic neuropathy with loss of sensation so that the patient may be unaware of minor trauma with its risks of infection.

Many diabetic patients have a degree of autonomic neuropathy, so that sympathetic function is lost. The foot is warm and dry, particularly when large vessel disease is not present.

Control of the diabetes and eradication of infection are essential for successful treatment. In patients with large vessel disease and severe ischaemia, arterial reconstruction is indicated. Although the results are poorer than in non-diabetic patients, the line of eventual amputation may be moved distally. If sympathetic function is preserved, sympathectomy may also allow distal amputation.

In patients with small vessel disease and neuropathy, but with healthy large vessels, infection leads only to local gangrene. Local removal of gangrenous tissue and adequate drainage of pus usually leads to healing, though this may be slow.

## AMPUTATION

Amputation is performed for extensive atherosclerosis when limb salvage by reconstruction has failed or is not feasible. The level of amputation was once dictated by 'sites of election' for the fitting of the prostheses, but with modern prostheses carrying total contact plastic sockets, this is no longer necessary. The major determinant of the level of amputation is skin viability.

Long stumps have disadvantages if insufficient room is left for an artificial joint. However, they permit greater surface area for contact with the prosthesis and limb control is improved.

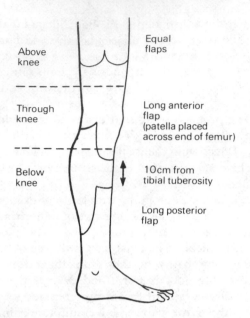

Fig. 21.10 Site of amputation

One-third of all leg amputations are carried out above the knee. The remainder are performed through or below the knee (Fig. 21.10). The site depends on the level of the principal arterial lesion, the extent of ischaemic damage, the presence or absence of infection, and the general state of the patient. As indicated above, skin viability is now the most important determinant of site and thermography can be used to define this.

In an elective amputation the skin is closed by primary suture. Drainage is the rule and prevents haematoma formation and wound breakdown. The main nerves are divided proximal to the site of amputation. A 'neuroma' always develops on the end of the nerve and if this is trapped in the scar, pain can be severe.

If there is infection or severe trauma, the amputation wound is left open. Delayed primary suture is performed some days later.

Antibiotic cover with penicillin to prevent anaerobic infection is advisable in all cases.

For an above knee amputation, a non-rigid dressing is used. Firm bandaging helps to mould the stump and controls post-operative oedema. In through-knee or below knee amputations, a rigid dressing of light plaster is preferred.

Intensive post-operative physiotherapy prevents flexion contracture of the hip and/or knee and encourages the return of good function. Where possible the patient is mobilised immediately after operation. Usually a temporary artificial limb is fitted 3 weeks after amputation when the wound has healed. Rehabilitation to ensure satisfactory walking requires considerable effort on the part of physiotherapists, nurses and doctors. Strong psychological support is essential. The above-knee amputee faces greater problems than those with more distal amputations. Myocardial or cerebral vascular insufficiency may prevent the patient from using an artificial limb satisfactorily, when resort must be made to a wheel-chair or crutch-assisted existence.

Most patients experience some *phantom pain* from the lost limb. This becomes less troublesome with time and symptoms usually disappear with reassurance.

The mortality and morbidity of major amputation is substantial. Pulmonary embolism is a major cause of death.

# CAROTID-VERTEBRAL OCCLUSION

## THE STROKE SYNDROME

Blood flow to the brain depends as much on the state of the extracerebral vessels as of those within the brain. Stenosis or occlusion of extracranial arteries, particularly the internal carotid, is an important cause of stroke (see Chapter 22). Occlusive disease of the carotid and vertebral systems causes two distinct ischaemic syndromes; the carotid syndrome (with associated hemiplegic effects) and the vertebro-basilar syndrome (with symptoms referable to the hind-brain).

### Carotid syndrome

Ischaemic attacks due to carotid insufficiency are typically transient. There is contralateral motor and sensory disturbance associated with ipsilateral monocular visual disorders (amaurosis fugax). The attacks may last for minutes or for hours.

Initially there is no residual neurological defect but the attacks become more frequent, last longer and lead to neurological deficits. Early recognition and treatment of the syndrome is vital as the interval between the onset of transient ischaemic attacks (TIA) and a full-blown hemiplegic stroke is often short.

## Vertebro-basilar syndrome

This is associated with attacks of vertigo and diplopia with unilateral or bilateral sensory and/or motor impairment. Different sides may be involved in different attacks. Residual neurological defects are rare.

## Examination and investigation

Other causes of transient cerebral ischaemia, particularly vasculitis and cardiac arrhythmias must be ruled out. Examination of the neck reveals that the carotid pulse is diminished or absent on one or other side. A bruit is audible over the involved carotid or vertebral artery and a thrill may be felt. Pulsation in the retinal vessels may be decreased unilaterally.

Non-invasive screening of the carotid artery by Doppler ultrasound oculoplethysmography and carotid phono-angiography may be useful but arteriography is the most reliable investigation. An arch aortogram to visualise the carotid and vertebral arteries is performed by retrograde catheterisation through a catheter introduced into a femoral artery. Digital subtraction angiography (DSA) is currently being evaluated and offers much promise for the future.

## Treatment

*Carotid syndrome.* The objective of treatment of symptomatic disease is early removal of the source of athero-emboli so that cerebral blood flow is increased and transient ischaemic attacks and major strokes are prevented. The artery is occluded proximally and distally and incised through the stenosed area. The atheromatous lesion is removed (endarterectomy) and the artery closed with or without a patch graft. The cerebral circulation is protected by an indwelling internal shunt during the procedure (Fig. 21.11).

The indications for surgical treatment in patients with asymptomatic bruits are not well defined.

Once a significant neurological deficit has occurred, the risks of the operation may outweigh its possible advantages. In selected cases in which the patient has occlusion of the internal carotid and symptoms referable to the ipsilateral hemisphere, blood flow can be increased by extra- to intra-cranial bypass involving anastomosis of the superficial temporal artery to a branch of

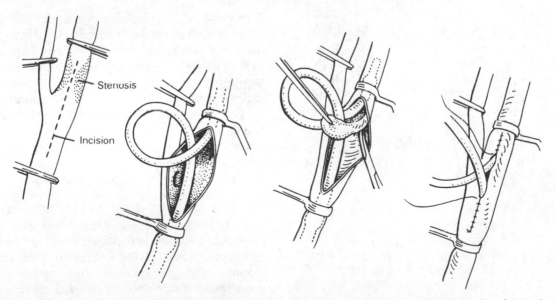

**Fig. 21.11** Cartoid endarterectomy showing the use of an internal Javid shunt inserted to bypass the site of operation

the middle cerebral artery. An operating microscope is used.

*Vertebral syndrome.* Surgery on the vertebral artery is performed less frequently, and usually comprises local endarterectomy of its origin with patch angioplasty.

## SUBCLAVIAN ARTERY OCCLUSION

Atherosclerosis causes ischaemia of the upper limb much less frequently than in the lower limb. The collateral circulation is better, the muscle mass is smaller, and intermittent usage of the arms makes claudication less likely.

Occlusion of the subclavian or axillary artery occasionally produces an ischaemic limb. Brachial arterial pressure is reduced in comparison with the other side, and a bruit may be heard over the site of the occlusion. If the subclavian artery is occluded proximal to the origin of the vertebral artery, the 'subclavian steal' syndrome may result. Reversal of flow in the vertebro-basilar artery provides a collateral circulation to the affected arm at the expense of the basilar circulation (Fig. 21.12). Symptoms of vertebro-basilar insufficiency occur when the arm is exercised, and ischaemic changes may sometimes occur in the

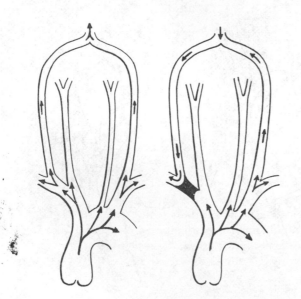

**Fig. 21.12** Subclavian steal syndrome

contralateral limb. The diagnosis is confirmed by arch aortography.

Subclavian artery occlusion is treated by insertion of a bypass graft of autogenous vein or synthetic material. This runs between the common carotid artery and the subclavian or axillary artery beyond the occlusion.

## AORTIC ARCH SYNDROME

This condition was first described in young women and is due to arteritis affecting the main branches of the aorta. There is cerebral vascular insufficiency with syncopal attacks and ischaemia of the upper limbs. Pulses are absent in the neck and/or upper limbs, hence the name 'pulseless disease'.

The arteritis may have an auto-immune basis and steroid therapy benefits some patients. Surgical treatment, by endarterectomy or bypass grafting gives disappointing results and there is a tendency for occlusion to occur at anastomotic sites.

## RENAL ARTERY STENOSIS

Narrowing of the renal artery reduces perfusion of the juxta-glomerular apparatus, with increased release of renin and angiotensin, and hypertension (Fig. 21.13). Atherosclerosis accounts for two-thirds of cases and occurs principally in males. Narrowing of the renal artery as a result of fibromuscular hyperplasia predominantly affects young females.

The onset of hypertension due to renal artery stenosis is often sudden and the patients are usually younger (< 35 years) or older (> 60 years) than those with essential hypertension. The diagnosis is suspected if a bruit is heard over the renal area or epigastrium. Deficient renal perfusion can be demonstrated by an isotope renogram using radio-iodinated para-amino hippuric acid. An excretion (intravenous) urogram shows diminished or delayed excretion of dye on the affected side. Differential renal func-

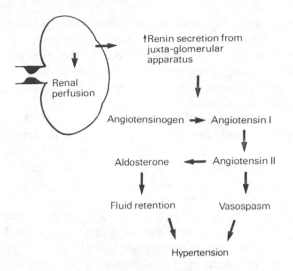

**Fig. 21.13** The effects of renal artery stenosis

tion studies may be performed by catheterising both ureters; sodium concentration is reduced in urine from the affected kidney. Arteriography confirms the diagnosis.

Surgical reconstruction by disobliteration, patch grafting or an aorto-renal bypass graft restores flow satisfactorily in 80% of patients. One-third of patients become normotensive, one-third have some reduction in blood pressure, and one-third are not improved. Balloon dilatation (transluminal angioplasty) offers an alternative form of treatment which can be repeated. A balloon catheter is inserted through a femoral arterial puncture, guided radiologically to the point of stenosis, and then inflated.

## BUERGER'S DISEASE (THROMBOANGIITIS OBLITERANS)

This is an uncommon form of obliterative arterial disease which affects young males who are heavy smokers. At one time there was an erroneous belief that it was more common in Jews. The disease affects medium-sized vessels which show lymphocytic infiltration of the arterial wall, thrombosis and peri-arterial fibrosis. Neighbouring veins are often thrombosed and the thrombophlebitis may be migratory.

Though the upper limb may be affected, the disease most commonly involves the lower limb. As the proximal large vessels are free from disease, claudication is not a prominent feature, except in the foot. Severe rest pain, ischaemic changes and progressive ulceration and gangrene are typical features. Examination often reveals intact pedal pulses with swelling and redness of the digits, a fungal infection in the web spaces or chronic paronychia.

Arteriography shows healthy main vessels, narrowing of the small arteries and, in the early stages, an absence of collateral circulation. With time, a profuse collateral circulation may develop.

### Management

Excellent remissions of disease follow cessation of smoking if this can be achieved but the disease progression is usually slow and relentless. Low molecular weight Dextran given intravenously may aid management during an exacerbation. Pain relief can be difficult, and addiction to narcotics may occur. Sympathectomy, either by chemical or surgical means, may delay the need for amputation. Sepsis is controlled by appropriate measures.

## ARTERIAL EMBOLISM

Arterial embolism is a less frequent cause of limb ischaemia than atherosclerosis. It tends to occur in older patients and is most commonly associated with ischaemic cardiac disease, particularly with atrial fibrillation (present in 50% of cases) or cardiac failure. Cardioversion may precipitate embolisation. One third of patients have had a proven myocardial infarction; one quarter have a history of previous embolism. Sub-acute bacterial endocarditis and prosthetic heart valves can produce multiple emboli, which may be infected. Emboli may also originate from mural thrombi associated with atherosclerosis in proximal main arteries. Trauma to a vessel, for example, during arterial catheterisation may lead to thrombus formation and embolisation.

Most frequently an embolus consists of organised clot and lodges at the bifurcation of an artery. Occlusion is aggravated by thrombosis spreading proximally and distally from the embolus, and occlusion of collaterals can lead to gangrene.

## Clinical features

The leg is most commonly affected by an embolus lodging at the femoral bifurcation. Classical features include pain, pallor, coldness, paraesthesia, loss of sensation, and loss of power with varying degrees of paralysis. There is poor venous filling and the limb becomes mottled with cyanotic patches. Peripheral pulses are usually absent.

Emboli may occur during sleep, when some of these features are not noticed, or they may be completely silent. The degree of ischaemia depends on the site and duration of the obstruction and the extent to which the collateral circulation can compensate.

The differential diagnosis includes acute arterial thrombosis, dissecting aneurysm, deep vein thrombosis, venous gangrene and arterial trauma. A careful history and clinical examination supported by electrocardiography and chest X-ray will usually differentiate between these diagnoses. Limb blood flow should be assessed by Doppler ultrasound. Arteriography is necessary only if there is doubt as to whether the occlusion is embolic or thrombotic, i.e. when there is acute-on-chronic ischaemia. Full blood count, blood sugar, urea and electrolytes are estimated routinely.

## Management

Ischaemia can be reversed completely if embolus is diagnosed and treated promptly. The first priority is to preserve life and supportive measures to correct cardiac decompensation include digitalis, diuretics and anti-arrhythmic agents. Blood pressure must be maintained.

Systemic heparinisation is started immediately to prevent or minimise propagation of thrombus and reduce the risk of deep vein thrombosis. Early surgery is indicated; the artery is opened under local anaesthesia to allow removal of the embolus with a Fogarty balloon catheter. Early

operation has dramatically improved the limb salvage rate but mortality remains at around 25%. Embolectomy is contraindicated in the presence of massive gangrene and amputation will be needed unless the patients's general condition precludes surgery.

The degree of limb ischaemia on presentation gives a good indication of the likely outcome. Lack of motor activity with a 'wooden' feel to the muscles suggests that amputation is likely to follow. Restoration of blood flow in the face of advanced ischaemia may cause cardiac or renal complications (arrhythmias, hypotension and oliguria) due to release of breakdown products of myoglobin and haemoglobin.

Where surgery is contraindicated, systemic heparinisation (2000–4000 units hourly) may allow limb survival. Thrombolytic agents such as streptokinase are of little value.

## Some technical considerations

*Femoral embolus.* The common femoral, profunda and superficial femoral arteries are approached by a vertical incision in the groin. After controlling these vessels by vascular clamps, the common femoral artery is incised longitudinally and a Fogarty catheter passed distally as far as possible down the superficial femoral artery. The balloon is inflated and the catheter withdrawn slowly, maintaining inflation of the balloon (Fig. 21.14).

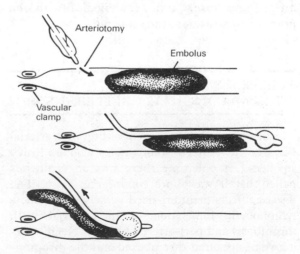

**Fig. 21.14** Femoral embolectomy by means of the Fogarty balloon catheter

Several passages may be necessary to remove all propagated thrombus. The procedure is repeated down the profunda femoris and up the common femoral artery. Operative arteriography is then performed to ensure that the distal arterial tree is patent; back-bleeding through the arteriotomy wound is not a reliable sign. Heparin therapy is continued post-operatively for 2–3 days and the patient is prescribed oral anticoagulants for 6 months.

*Saddle embolus of the aorta* is dealt with by removal of thrombus through bilateral groin incisions. Operative angiography is necessary to determine that proximal and distal arterial trees are patent.

*Embolism of the upper limb* is less common. Emboli may lodge with equal frequency in the subclavian, axillary and brachial arteries. Though the collateral supply in the upper limb is better than the lower limb, embolectomy should be performed in the majority of cases. An arteriotomy in the axillary artery under local anaesthesia allows adequate proximal and distal access. Operative angiography is used to confirm patency of the arterial tree. Limb viability is assured if the radial or ulnar artery is patent.

### Post-operative care

A close check must be kept on the pulses to detect further embolisation. Following restoration of circulation, ischaemic muscle swells and the increased tissue pressure in osteo-fascial 'compartments' (e.g. anterior or posterior tibial compartments) may compromise blood flow to the muscle or to distal parts of the limb. Urgent decompression of the affected compartment is achieved by extensive incision of the overlying fascia (*fasciotomy*).

## ANEURYSM

An aneurysm is an abnormal dilatation of an artery (or occasionally a heart chamber), which may be congenital or more commonly, acquired. Arterial aneurysms are 'true' or 'false' (Fig. 21.15).

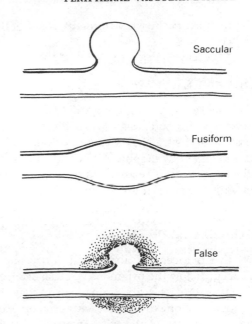

**Fig. 21.15** Types of aneurysm

## TRUE ANEURYSMS

A *true* aneurysm is enclosed by all three layers of the arterial wall.

*Acquired* aneurysms result from degeneration of the media and elastic lamina, due to atherosclerosis or syphilis with expansion of the affected part of the vessel. Though not strictly speaking an aneurysm, *dissection* of the arterial wall is usually considered in conjunction with aneurysmal dilatation. It may result from insertion of an arterial catheter into a peripheral artery, but more commonly affects the aorta as a consequence of destruction of the media (containing the elastic fibres) in atherosclerosis.

In subacute bacterial endocarditis, septic emboli may lodge within the vasa vasorum and form an intramural abscess. This may give rise to an *infective* or (as it is often wrongly termed) a *mycotic* aneurysm.

Turbulence of the blood stream within an aneurysm leads to the laying down of thrombus and its progressive enlargement with erosion of neighbouring structures and eventual rupture. The wall of an aneurysm frequently becomes calcified and can be seen on a radiograph.

*Congenital* aneurysms occur in the cerebral arteries and are saccular or fusiform, depending on whether part or the whole circumference of the wall is weakened.

## FALSE ANEURYSMS

A *false* aneurysm may follow a traumatic tear of the vessel wall. Blood escapes through the intima and media and stretches the adventitia, which forms a sac lined by organised clot and supported by adjacent tissues. The sac remains in communication with the arterial lumen and is pulsatile.

## ABDOMINAL AORTIC ANEURYSM

Ninety-five per cent of abdominal aortic aneurysms occur below the origin of the renal arteries. An aneurysm of the abdominal aorta may be continuous with one of the thoracic aorta, or more commonly it is associated with aneurysmal dilatation of the iliac, femoral or popliteal arteries. Most patients are elderly and have ischaemic heart disease or peripheral vascular disease. Rupture of the aneurysm is the most common hazard. Without operation 50% of patients will die within 2 years and all but a few will die within 5 years.

### Clinical features

An abdominal aortic aneurysm may present in the following ways:

1. An *asymptomatic* pulsating mass is found on routine clinical examination of the abdomen.

2. *Abdominal pain* may develop centrally or in the lumbar region. It may be referred to the flank and simulate renal colic.

3. *Leakage or rupture* may cause severe abdominal or back pain and hypovolaemic shock. An episode of relatively minor pain often precedes the onset of catastrophic rupture by an interval of days or even weeks. This pain is due to a small leak of blood — the *herald bleed*.

A pulsatile abdominal mass is present in 90% of cases and is associated with guarding and distension if leakage on rupture has occurred. If its upper limit lies below the level of the renal arteries, the mass is separated by an interval from the costal margin. The femoral pulses may be diminished in volume.

A straight abdominal X-ray will show calcification of the aneurysmal wall, particularly on a lateral view. Ultrasound is a useful investigation to determine the size of the aneurysm and the urgency of operation. If leakage has occurred, ultrasound will demonstrate the presence of an extravascular haematoma. In this circumstance impending rupture demands immediate operation.

Arteriography is seldom indicated in an unruptured aneurysm. It is contraindicated when rupture is suspected as any delay in treatment is unacceptable.

### Management

The treatment of choice is resection of the aneurysm and replacement of the aorta with a Dacron graft. A single tube graft is used unless the aortic bifurcation or iliac vessels are involved when a bifurcated (trouser) graft is needed. The limbs of the bifurcated graft are anastomosed either to the common or external iliac arteries, or to the common, superficial or deep femoral arteries (Fig. 21.16).

All aneurysms over 5 cm should be operated on electively unless there are general contraindications. In that event the progress of the aneurysm is monitored by ultrasonic screening. A leaking or ruptured aneurysm requires immediate operation. The mortality is 50% compared to 2–3% for

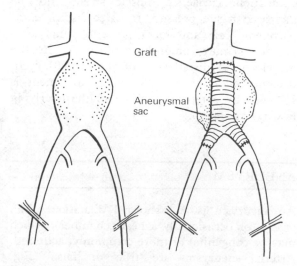

Fig. 21.16 Resection of an aortic aneurysm

elective cases. Myocardial infarction and renal failure are the two main post-operative complications of aneurysm surgery. Operative mortality depends on the experience of the surgeon and his team, and transfer to a specialist centre is recommended. Such transfer is rendered safer if the patient wears a 'G-suit' to maintain external pressure on the abdomen, so containing the aneurysm and any extravascular haematoma. The G-suit is removed in the operating theatre when the surgical team is ready to start the operation.

## DISSECTION OF THE AORTA

Aortic dissection is a relatively common condition with a high mortality. The dissection normally starts in the ascending aorta or proximal descending aorta, and spreads distally. The patients are usually hypertensive, but dissection may also occur in pregnancy or as a result of trauma. Patients with Marfan's syndrome are particularly prone to dissection.

The onset of aortic dissection is accompanied by *excruciating* chest pain which spreads to the back and abdomen. If the ascending aorta is involved the signs are of upper limb ischaemia; dissections of the descending aorta affect the lower limbs. Severe chest pain associated with diminution of arm or leg pulses should always raise the suspicion of dissection. Involvement of spinal arteries may cause paraplegia, and that of the renal arteries acute renal failure. Pulmonary oedema is often present. External rupture of the dissection leads to severe hypovolaemic shock.

### Treatment

Urgent treatment consists of anti-hypertensive treatment (e.g. with sodium nitroprusside), stabilisation of the circulation and pain control. Aortography is undertaken to confirm the diagnosis.

Dissection of the ascending aorta is treated by resection of the affected part of the vessel and insertion of a graft. Aortic valve replacement may also be necessary. Uncomplicated dissection of the descending aorta is usually managed conservatively with anti-hypertensive therapy, but grafting is indicated if pain is uncontrolled, if the circulation cannot be stabilised, or if external rupture occurs.

Fifty per cent of untreated patients die within 48 hours. Sixty per cent of treated patients survive 5 years.

## PERIPHERAL ANEURYSMS

Aneurysms affecting peripheral vessels form pulsating swellings in the line of the vessel. Symptoms arise from compression of adjacent structures, and venous thrombosis and neurological compression are particularly common.

Arteriography defines the site and extent of the aneurysm and the state of the distal arteries. Treatment consists of resection of the aneurysm with insertion of an autogenous vein graft or synthetic graft.

## ARTERIOVENOUS FISTULA

An arteriovenous fistula is an anomalous communication between an artery and vein; it may be congenital or acquired (traumatic).

*Congenital* fistulas result from persistence of fetal arteriovenous communications and are usually multiple. They occur most frequently in the lower limb but may be found in the abdominal viscera. Congenital fistulas are usually detected in childhood. The affected limb is longer, thicker and warmer than the other. There is marked varicosity of the long saphenous system, and venous insufficiency may cause skin ulceration (Fig. 21.17).

A *cirsoid aneurysm* is a form of congenital arteriovenous fistula with multiple communications between arterial and venous systems.

*Traumatic* fistulas are usually single. The communication may be direct (*aneurysmal varix*) or involve a communicating false aneurysm (*varicose aneurysm*) (Fig. 21.18). Blood is shunted at high pressure into the vein causing it to dilate so that its wall becomes thickened and arterialised.

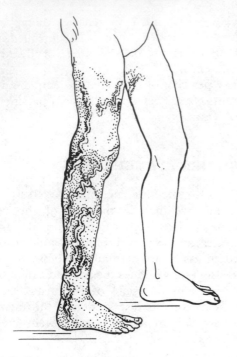

**Fig. 21.17** Congenital A-V fistula

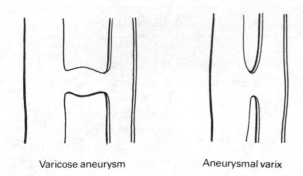

Varicose aneurysm          Aneurysmal varix

**Fig. 21.18** The two types of traumatic A-V fistula

Shunting of large volumes of blood leads to distal ischaemia. There may be a compensatory increase in cardiac output and systolic pressure, a fall in peripheral resistance and diastolic blood pressure, and widening of pulse pressure. Cardiac failure and pulmonary oedema may lead to death if the fistula is not treated.

A palpable pulsatile mass with a thrill or bruit may be present. Occlusion of the fistula by pressure leads to slowing of the heart. Arteriography is used to confirm the diagnosis and localise the lesion before surgery.

## Management

*Congenital fistula.* Surgical excision of multiple congenital fistulas is hazardous and simple support with an elastic stocking is usually advised. Rarely amputation is required for gangrene or haemodynamic effects. Localised congenital fistulas can be treated effectively by excision of the dilated veins and ligation of the feeding arterial supply. In certain cases, selective catheter thrombosis carried out by a radiologist skilled in such procedures is highly effective.

*Traumatic fistulas.* Traumatic fistulas rarely close spontaneously and surgical repair is usually necessary.

## VASOSPASTIC CONDITIONS

Vasospastic conditions are initially reversible but irreversible changes follow secondary thrombosis.

## RAYNAUD'S SYNDROME

### Primary Raynaud's phenomenon

This disease affects young women most commonly and is an abnormal reaction of the peripheral vessels to cold. The hands are usually affected, though in some patients the feet are also involved. A positive family history is often present.

The changes are bilateral and symmetrical. Paroxysms of pallor, acrocyanosis, coldness and numbness of the fingers occur on exposure to cold. On rewarming, the fingers become bright red and there is an associated burning sensation which may amount to severe pain. The colour change fades gradually and normal sensation returns.

Progressive nutritional changes occur with atrophy of the skin and pulps of the fingers, chronic infections (e.g. paronychia), and ulceration. Digital gangrene may supervene eventually despite persistence of peripheral pulses (Fig. 21.19).

The diagnosis is made by precipitating an attack by immersing the hands in cold water (15°C) for several minutes. Arteriography may

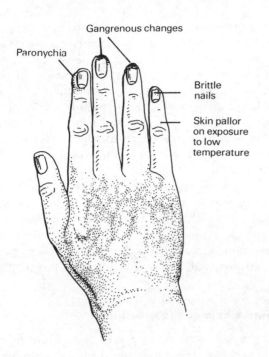

Paronychia

Gangrenous changes

Brittle
nails

Skin pallor
on exposure
to low
temperature

**Fig. 21.19** The clinical appearances in Raynaud's syndrome

show occlusion of digital arteries. Secondary Raynaud's phenomenon must be ruled out (see below).

The patient is advised to avoid cold, wear protective, loose fitting gloves and avoid minor trauma and other causes of infection. Smoking should be banned. Alpha-adrenergic blocking agents can prove useful. Sympathectomy to release vasomotor tone may be helpful in severe cases. Amputation of digits may be required.

### Secondary Raynaud's phenomenon

Intermittent attacks of Raynaud's phenomenon may be precipitated by frostbite, by the use of vibrating tools and by collagen disease. Unlike the primary form there is no sex preponderance and the feet are more commonly affected. The management is similar to that of primary Raynaud's disease with avoidance or appropriate treatment of the precipitating cause.

### Acrocyanosis

This abnormal reaction to cold also affects young females and is difficult, if not impossible, to distinguish from primary Raynaud's phenomenon. Arteriolar constriction and sluggish capillary flow cause abnormal coldness and cyanosis of the extremities. In the skin over the calf the cyanosis assumes a reticulate pattern. On exposure to warmth the small arteries dilate so that the capillary flow increases and the skin becomes red.

The management is similar to that of primary Raynaud's disease. Sympathectomy is valuable in severe cases.

## FROSTBITE

Exposure of the extremities to extremes of low temperature causes variable skin loss affecting the fingers, toes and ears.

Treatment consists of rapid rewarming, heparinisation and infusion of low molecular weight dextran. Sympathectomy may limit necrosis but amputation of digits may be necessary.

## ARTERITIS (OTHER FORMS)

There are a group of diseases affecting connective tissues which lead to degeneration of arterial walls with fragmentation of elastica and fibrinoid necrosis of the intima and media. Raynaud's phenomenon, haemorrhage or purpura can occur. The underlying condition is treated, usually with steroids, and anti-coagulants may be required. Sympathectomy is of value in a few patients but amputation is sometimes necessary.

## VASCULAR TRAUMA

Direct arterial damage may occur as a result of blunt or penetrating trauma. Iatrogenic damage during arteriography is increasingly common, and inadvertent intra-arterial injection of pentothal or narcotics can cause arterial injury. Compression of an artery may follow swelling of tissues within an osteo-fascial compartment or rigid dressings, or the vessel can be occluded by direct pressure from splints or plasters.

Secondary thrombosis at the site of injury occludes the vessel. The degree of distal ischaemia depends on the state of the collateral circula-

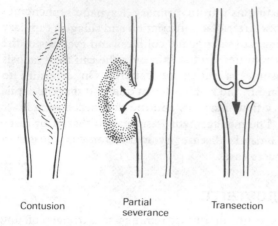

| Contusion | Partial severance | Transection |

**Fig. 21.20** Types of arterial injury

tion, and whether distal extension of thrombus occludes entry points from collaterals. While arterial spasm at or beyond the site of injury contributes to distal ischaemia, its importance has been overemphasized. Occlusion by thrombosis is the significant factor.

Arterial injuries may be divided into three categories (Fig. 21.20):

## Complete severance

The vessel is completely divided, for example, by a knife or bullet. The ends of the vessel retract and constrict. Thrombosis occurs rapidly at the cut ends and compression by local tissues further limits blood loss, which may be surprisingly small. In patients with severe atherosclerosis, the artery has less capacity to retract and constrict and serious haemorrhage is more likely.

Distal pulses in the limbs are lost immediately. Pallor, paraesthesia, paralysis, pain and poikilothermia (coldness), the 5 Ps of acute ischaemia, develop subsequently.

## Incomplete severance

Partial division of an artery results from penetrating injury (including those from surgical knives, drills or needles) or from closed injury when the vessel is lacerated by a fragment of a fractured bone.

Partial continuity of the vessel prevents retraction, and contraction of circular muscle at the site of injury tends to hold the laceration open. Haemorrhage is severe and if the overlying tissues are intact, a pulsating haematoma develops. If the laceration is open to the exterior, exsanguinating haemorrhage may follow. Diminution of distal pulses and signs of distal ischaemia are less pronounced than after complete severance of a vessel. If an accompanying vein is damaged at the time of injury an arteriovenous fistula is likely to develop (see p. 273).

Failure to diagnose the injury may lead to the slowly surrounding haematoma being misdiagnosed as an abscess. The results of incision and drainage of such an 'abscess' require little description. Occasionally the haematoma remains relatively small and a *false aneurysm* forms.

## Non-severance (contusion)

Contusion of an artery results from blunt injury or excessive stretching, and is not uncommon in fractures. Contusions may result from penetrating injury, for example, when a high velocity bullet passes close to an artery, or from a needle or catheter damaging the intima without significantly damaging the outer coats of the vessel. The injury produced by direct intra-arterial injection of irritants also falls into this category.

Intimal damage leads to the development of thrombus or elevation of an intimal flap which occludes the vessel. If damage to the vessel wall is more extensive, an intramural haematoma may further compromise the lumen.

External bleeding is absent or minimal. Pulses are minimally affected at first but signs of ischaemia develop over the next few hours. If the injury is unrecognised, a true aneurysm may later occur.

## Management

In closed injuries clinical suspicion is of prime importance if limbs and lives are to be saved. Even then some arterial injuries are not apparent immediately but become obvious when complications arise.

Control of haemorrhage has precedence. The limb is elevated (to control venous haemorrhage) and direct pressure is applied over the wound. A tourniquet is rarely necessary. Blood volume is restored by transfusion.

If the peripheral circulation remains impaired despite adequate replacement, surgery is needed urgently. Arteriography may help to define the site and extent of injury, but should not delay definitive surgical treatment.

*Surgical treatment*. Early reconstruction is advised for injuries of larger arteries but minor arteries may be ligated. End-to-end suture may be possible but any gap should be bridged by graft. Autogenous vein graft is preferred, as insertion of a synthetic graft may be complicated by infection, thrombosis and secondary haemorrhage. Incomplete lacerations may be repaired by a vein patch graft. Contusions are treated by resection of the damaged segment of vessel, with end-to-end suture or insertion of a vein graft.

Associated fractures are immobilised, if necessary by internal fixation. Heparin or dextran therapy helps to preserve patency of the reconstructed vessel in the initial stages. Antibiotic cover is advisable.

Intra-arterial injection of irritant materials is managed more conservatively if possible. The artery is flushed with heparinised saline and irrigated with reserpine. Full systemic doses of heparin, opiates and antibiotics are given.

---

## DISORDERS OF THE VEINS

### VENOUS DRAINAGE OF LOWER LIMB

The *superficial veins* of the lower limb are the long and short saphenous veins and their tributaries. The vessels lie outwith the deep fascia and carry only 10% of the venous return from the limb. The long saphenous vein runs from in front of the medial malleolus of the ankle, up the medial side of the leg. It penetrates the deep fascia (cribriform fascia) at the saphenous opening (4 cm below and lateral to the pubic tubercle) to enter the femoral vein. The short saphenous passes up the lateral side of the lower leg from behind the lateral malleolus of the ankle and ends in the popliteal vein.

The *deep venous system* consists of intermuscular and intramuscular veins. These accompany the arteries and carry 90% of the venous return from the limb.

Communicating veins connect the superficial and deep venous systems and perforate the deep fascia at variable points (perforating veins). The greatest numbers are situated just behind the posterior edge of the tibia above the ankle, but they also occur below and above the knee.

Venous return from the leg is an active process. Muscle action compresses the deep veins, and flow is directed upwards by numerous 'one-way' valves. With relaxation of the 'muscle pump', blood is sucked in from the superficial system. Reflux from deep to superficial systems is prevented by valves in the perforating veins (Fig. 21.21). The venous pressure at the ankle is approximately 100 cm water (zero at Rt atrium), but during exercise this is reduced to 30–40 cm. It is because of this relatively high pressure that

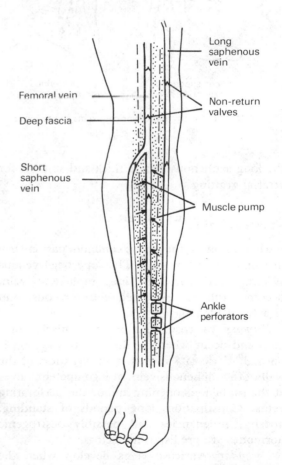

**Fig. 21.21** Mechanism of venous return from lower limb

Long saphenous vein

Femoral vein

Non-return valves

Deep fascia

Short saphenous vein

Muscle pump

Ankle perforators

* Ensure that deep veins are patent before avulsion of superficial veins.

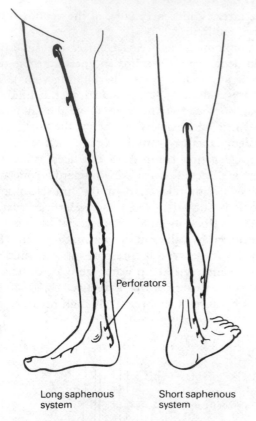

**Fig. 21.22** The distribution of varicose veins in the lower leg

the long saphenous vein is thick and suitable for arterial grafting.

## Varicose veins

Varicose veins of the leg are common, particularly in women (F:M = 5:1). The superficial venous system, particularly the long saphenous vein, becomes dilated, elongated and tortuous, and clearly visible (Fig. 21.22).

*Primary* varicose veins are particularly common and occur when the deep venous system is normal. Varicosity results from weakness of the wall of the saphenous vein, or incompetent valves at the saphenous opening and/or the perforating veins. Constipation, long periods of standing, obesity, pregnancies and possibly oestrogenic hormones are predisposing factors.

*Secondary* varicose veins develop when the deep venous system is thrombosed or has been thrombosed and become recanalised with destruction of its valves. The muscle pump now functions so that its full pressure is transmitted to the superficial system. Other causes of 'secondary' varices include arteriovenous fistulas (see p. 273) and an abdominal tumour.

## Clinical features

Varicose veins cause few symptoms but are unsightly. Aching in the limbs may be troublesome when the patient stands for long periods and is sometimes associated with ankle swelling. Skin changes include itching, dryness and scaling. Accumulation of haemosiderin (from rupture of small venules) leads to hyper-pigmentation of the skin which also becomes atrophic and thin. Varicose eczema may precede ulceration. Secondary varices are usually more prominent and because superficial venous pressure is so high, secondary complications are common.

Sudden *rupture* of a varix can lead to profuse and frightening haemorrhage. It is readily controlled by elevation of the limb and pressure on the bleeding site.

## Examination

Examination is designed to detect incompetence of the communicating system. A cough impulse over the long saphenous vein indicates free communication with the inferior vena cava and sapheno-femoral incompetence can be confirmed by the *Trendelenberg test* (Fig. 21.23). The limb is elevated to empty the saphenous system and a tourniquet is applied to the thigh just below the saphenous opening. Rapid filling of the varicose saphenous vein when the patient stands indicates incompetence of perforating veins distal to the tourniquet. Rapid filling from above when the tourniquet is removed indicates sapheno-femoral incompetence.

Incompetent perforating veins below the sapheno-femoral junction can be defined accurately by applying multiple tourniquets to isolate segments of the limb. Distension of superficial veins within a segment indicates incompetence.

In all patients with varicose veins the abdomen must be examined to exclude an abdominal or

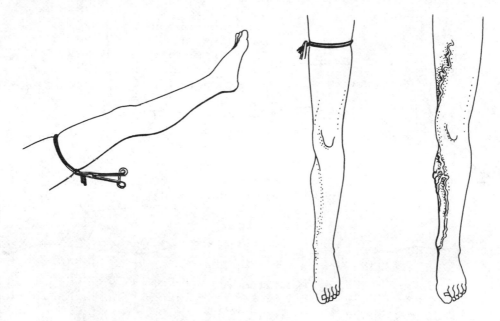

Fig. 21.23 The Trendelenberg test demonstrating sapheno-femoral incompetence

pelvic mass. A rectal examination is also performed. If it is suspected that the varicose veins are secondary (e.g. if there is a history of deep vein thrombosis, or skin changes are marked), phlebography is essential. Severe varicose veins in children or young adults should raise the suspicion of a congenital arteriovenous fistula.

## Management

*Conservative*. Mild cases are treated conservatively with elastic support, regular exercise, weight reduction where necessary and avoidance of constricting garments.

*Sclerotherapy*. For small localised varices due to incompetent perforating veins in the lower leg or recurrent varices after operation, sclerotherapy is the treatment of choice. The sites of incompetence are defined while the patient stands. The patient then lies down and the leg is elevated to empty the veins. Sodium tetradecyl sulphate (0.5 ml of 3% solution) is injected into the vein at the site of each incompetent perforator (Fig. 21.24). The superficial vein is occluded with the fingers above and below the injection site to direct sclerosant into the perforating vein. Each injection site is compressed with a bevelled sorbo pad and a crepe bandage is firmly applied. An elastic stocking holds the bandage in place. Compression is maintained for 6 weeks during which time the patient is instructed to walk for several miles daily.

*Surgery*. Sclerotherapy is unsuitable for incompetent perforating veins above or around the knee and when there is demonstrable sapheno-femoral incompetence. The sapheno-femoral junction is displayed at operation under local or general anaesthesia and *all* tributaries running into the upper 2–3 inches of saphenous vein are ligated and divided (Fig. 21.25). The saphenous vein is ligated flush with the femoral vein, divided and the upper few inches of the vein removed. Incompetent perforators at lower levels are exposed through small incisions, ligated and divided.

At one time 'stripping' was advised to remove the saphenous vein after division at the saphenofemoral junction. It is now considered important to preserve the upper portion of the vein (which seldom is varicosed) to provide a graft for arterial reconstruction should this ever be required.

## VENOUS ULCERATION

Venous or gravitational ulceration was once regarded as a common complication of varicose

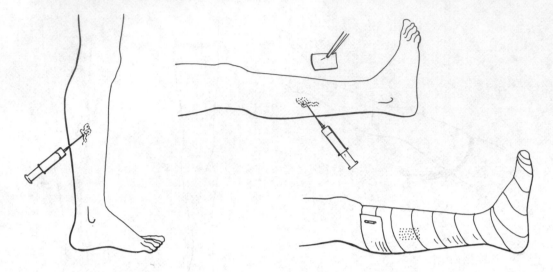

**Fig. 21.24** Sclerotherapy

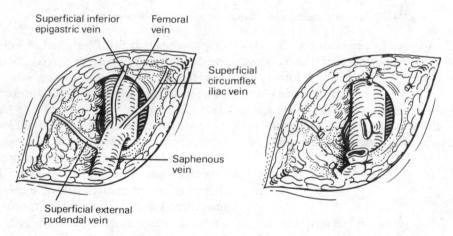

**Fig. 21.25** Femoro-saphenous disconnection with ligation of the tributaries of the long saphenous vein

veins. It is now a recognised part of the syndrome of chronic venous insufficiency following thrombosis of the deep veins. After recanalisation the valves are destroyed, subjecting the superficial system to high pressure. Severe and long standing varices result.

A venous ulcer occurs typically on the medial side of the lower half of the leg. This is the site of multiple perforating vessels and of a localised increase in venous pressure. Disturbed capillary haemodynamics lead to localised ischaemia and tissue necrosis.

## Clinical features

The ulcer is usually large and shallow with sloping edges and a base of unhealthy granulation tissue. The surrounding skin is hyperpigmented and eczematous. Fibrosis from haemosiderin deposition may involve the whole circumference of the leg and lead to a 'gaiter-like' constriction. A venous ulcer is painful and readily becomes infected. Repeated episodes of infection further contribute to fibrosis. Very rarely a long standing varicose ulcer is complicated by the development of a squamous carcinoma.

## Management

The patient must be fully investigated for systemic conditions which may predispose to venous thrombosis or to ulceration. Phlebography is essential to determine the state of the deep veins and must precede any operation.

Ulcer healing can be achieved by relieving venous hypertension by bed rest and high elevation of the limb. A mild antiseptic dressing is applied to combat infection. Alternatively, a compressing bandage is used to supply a firm support against which muscle action can increase venous return. The bandage must be applied meticulously from below with even pressure and must be worn at all times when out of bed. Exercise is essential if the ulcer is managed by a compressing bandage.

Once the ulcer has healed, venous hypertension must be relieved if recurrence is to be prevented. Superficial varices are dealt with and perforating vessels in the lower leg are ligated. This is best done by incising the skin and deep fascia vertically and ligating the perforating vessels in the subfascial compartment.

---

## DEEP VEIN THROMBOSIS AND PULMONARY EMBOLISM

---

### SUPERFICIAL THROMBOPHLEBITIS

This inflammation of the superficial veins is commonly associated with trauma or irritation after injections, or infusions. It may occur spontaneously, particularly in women taking oral contraceptives. The affected vein is tender and indurated, and the overlying skin is red and warm. The changes usually remain localised but may involve the length of the vein and can extend through communicating channels to involve the deep veins. Resolution occurs in a few days leaving a linear patch of brown pigmentation and a fibrosed cord-like vein.

Treatment consists of analgesics, support stockings and active exercise. Should suppuration occur, incision and antibiotics may be required. Rapidly spreading thrombophlebitis may require

ligation of the vein to prevent proximal spread.

A migrating type of superficial thrombophlebitis is seen occasionally in association with malignant disease.

### DEEP VEIN THROMBOSIS (DVT)

Deep vein thrombosis is a common complication of a surgical operation and 30–50% of patients dying in hospital have thrombi in the deep veins of the leg.

The veins first affected are those of the calf muscles (the soleal sinuses) in which a platelet thrombus leads to venous occlusion and formation of a clot of red blood cells enmeshed in fibrin. This clot may extend to involve the popliteal and femoral veins. Thrombosis may also occur in pelvic veins, involving the ilio-femoral segment.

Pulmonary embolism is a serious complication of deep venous thrombosis (Fig. 21.26). Significant embolisation rarely occurs from calf veins, but is a real risk when the ilio-femoral segment is involved (see p.283). A DVT may develop without symptoms, and the first evidence of its occurrence may be a fatal pulmonary embolus.

### Aetiology

Three factors are traditionally associated with venous thrombosis: venous stasis, intimal damage, and hypercoagulability of the blood. All three are aggravated by surgical operation.

*Venous stasis.* Lack of active muscle movement during anaesthesia allows blood to stagnate in the

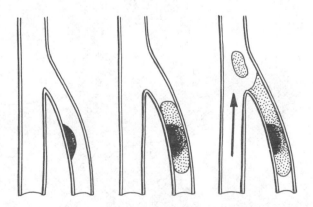

**Fig. 21.26** The propagation of deep vein thrombosis

intermuscular venous sinuses. Venous stasis by itself does not cause thrombosis; other factors must also be present.

*Intimal damage.* Platelet deposition follows injury to the delicate intimal lining. Injury may be caused by pressure on the calves by the operating table, insertion of venous catheters, or external compression.

*Hypercoagulability.* The coagulability of the blood depends upon the balance between clotting factors and thrombolytic mechanisms. Following an operation there is increased adhesiveness of platelets, increased blood viscosity and decreased fibrinolysis. Oral contraceptive agents and parturition both decrease thrombolysis and increase the risk of DVT.

### Associated factors

Factors predisposing to DVT before, during and after operation include obesity, age (over 45 years), prolonged bed rest, malignant disease, varicose veins, a previous history of venous thrombosis, polycythaemia, operations of the hip and pelvis, and the administration of oestrogens.

### TYPES OF THROMBOSIS

#### Distal (calf vein) thrombosis

This is the most common site for the first development of DVT. Clinical signs include aching or heaviness in the calf, tenderness over the deep veins, and minimal oedema. However, these signs are present in only 50% of cases, and DVT should always be suspected in a person who develops slight pyrexia and tachycardia while confined to bed. Equally, all patients who complain of calf pain may not have developed DVT.

The inaccuracy of clinical diagnosis of DVT has led to the use of $^{125}$I-fibrinogen scanning to detect the development of calf vein thrombosis and of venography to confirm the diagnosis.

*Fibrinogen uptake.* Potassium iodide (100 mg) is given 48 hours preoperatively to block thyroid uptake. An intravenous injection of 100 $\mu$c $^{125}$I fibrinogen is given the day before operation. Radioactivity at defined points along the length of both legs is monitored daily. A sustained rise of radioactivity over the calf suggests that fibrinogen has accumulated as a result of thrombosis (Fig. 21.27).

*Phlebography.* Suspicion of calf vein thrombosis is an indication for bilateral ascending venography (Fig. 21.28). Occluding cuffs are placed above the ankle and in the mid thigh and 30-40 ml of 45% sodium diatrozoate injected into a vein on the dorsum of the foot. Serial X-rays are taken. Filling defects, abrupt obstruction to flow, nonfilling of deep channels, and diversion of flow indicate thrombosis.

On release of the thigh tourniquet the femoral veins and the ilio-femoral segment are seen, although they may not fill completely with this technique. Streaming of dye may wrongly suggest a filling defect. Femoral phlebography with direct injection into the femoral veins may be needed if thrombosis in the ilio-femoral segment is still suspected.

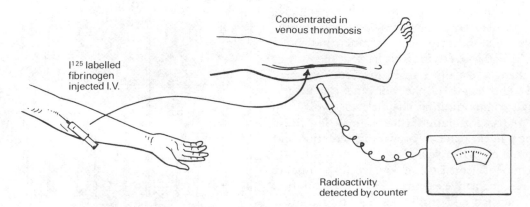

Concentrated in venous thrombosis

I$^{125}$ labelled fibrinogen injected I.V.

Radioactivity detected by counter

**Fig. 21.27** Fibrinogen scan

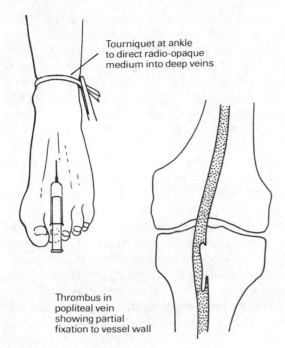

Tourniquet at ankle to direct radio-opaque medium into deep veins

Thrombus in popliteal vein showing partial fixation to vessel wall

**Fig. 21.28** Venography

*Management.* Thrombosis limited to the calf veins is treated by elevation of the legs, active movement, and early ambulation with supporting stockings. Progress is monitored daily and heparinisation (see below) may be needed if there is evidence of extension of thrombus.

## Proximal (ilio-femoral) thrombosis

Involvement of the ilio-femoral segment by non-occlusive thrombus may cause pain and tenderness over the common femoral vein or remain asymptomatic. *Occlusion* leads to oedema of the limb, and gross swelling may result if both common femoral and iliac veins are involved.

The limb is often white due to associated arterial spasm (*phlegmasia alba dolens*). Alternatively, if there is total obstruction of *all* venous outflow from the limb, cyanosis is marked (*phlegmasia caerulea dolens*) and venous gangrene is imminent. $^{125}$I-fibrinogen scans are of little or no value in detection of ilio-femoral thrombosis. The proximity of the femoral artery and abdominal wounds frequently introduce error. A Doppler ultrasonic scan indicates whether venous flow is impaired. Squeezing the calf normally increases flow in the femoral vein if the intervening veins are patent; this augmented flow does not occur in iliac vein thrombosis and changes in flow during respiration are abolished (Fig. 21.29). More sophisticated methods of detecting altered venous flow (e.g. impedance plethysmography to monitor the total blood content of the limb and its movement) are available in specialised centres.

*Management.* If ilio-femoral thrombosis is suspected, femoral phlebography must be carried out

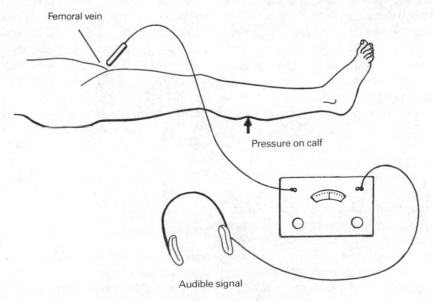

Femoral vein

Pressure on calf

Audible signal

**Fig. 21.29** Ultrasonic examination

urgently. If the diagnosis is confirmed an intravenous bolus of heparin is given (10 000 units or 100 units/kg) and a constant infusion pump used to deliver 1000 units an hour. The thrombin time is estimated at 6 hours and should be 3 times normal. The dose of heparin is adjusted accordingly. Heparin is continued for 10 days. Oral anticoagulants (phenindione 75–100 mg daily) are started 2 days before heparin is discontinued and are used to maintain the prothrombin time at 2.0–2.5 times normal. The optimal duration of oral anticoagulant therapy is controversial; some surgeons discontinue therapy after 6 weeks while others prescribe it for 6 months.

An alternative regime involves use of a thrombolytic agent such as streptokinase to lyse the clot. The initial dose is 300 000 units given over 30 minutes either directly into the femoral vein or into a peripheral vein, followed by 1 million units over 6 hours. Bleeding, pyrexia and allergic reactions are complications and this form of therapy is not used widely.

Surgical removal of the clot (thrombectomy) is no longer popular and it is indicated only for phlegmasia caerulea dolens which might lead to venous gangrene.

## Care of limb

In major vein thromboses the limb is elevated and the patient kept in bed for 7–10 days to allow adherence of clot. A firm elastic supporting bandage is then applied and active exercises and ambulation are started. Support is maintained for 3–6 months so that venous flow is promoted and recanalization encouraged.

## Prophylaxis

Various methods of prophylaxis can be used during and after operation, and are particularly important in high-risk patients.

*Care of the limbs.* In many units graded compression stockings are worn by all patients having an operation. In the operating theatre care is taken to avoid compressing the calf and the ankles are supported on rubber blocks. Alternative methods of stimulating venous return include pneumatic leggings into which air is regularly cycled and electrical stimulation of the calf muscles. Early post-operative ambulation is encouraged.

*Altered blood coagulability.* Many surgeons employ low-dose subcutaneous calcium heparin 5000 units 8 or 12 hourly, commencing with premedication and given until the patient is fully ambulant or at most for 5–7 days. The incidence of DVT and the risk of pulmonary embolus are reduced with minimal risk of inducing bleeding.

Dextran 70 also reduces the incidence of DVT and can be used as an alternative to heparin. A 500 ml infusion is commenced pre-operatively and continued during the operation. Further infusions of 500 ml are given daily for 4 days. Circulatory overload, bleeding and anaphylaxis are uncommon but recognised complications. Antiplatelet drugs (e.g. aspirin or prostacyclin) may be of value, but are still under assessment.

All of these prophylactic measures are less effective in patients having hip surgery, in whom oral anticoagulation with phenindione is advised by some surgeons.

## PULMONARY EMBOLUS

Prior to the introduction of prophylaxis against DVT, one in 400 surgical patients died from pulmonary embolus post-operatively. Although the incidence of DVT can now be reduced, not all surgeons employ prophylaxis routinely and pulmonary embolus remains a problem in hospitalised patients, particularly in those with associated factors known to increase the risk of DVT.

Embolism results from detachment of a thrombus from a vein, most commonly in the lower limb (70%) or pelvis (20%). Five per cent of emboli originate in the right atrium. Although DVT precedes pulmonary embolus in almost all cases, it is apparent clinically in only 20% of cases before embolisation occurs.

Two types of pulmonary embolism are described:

### Major embolism

Massive embolus with occlusion of two-thirds or more of pulmonary artery flow results in acute chest pain, followed by severe dyspnoea, cyanosis, hypotension and collapse.

A systolic murmur is audible over the pulmonary artery.

As two-thirds of all fatal pulmonary emboli cause death within 30 mins of onset, the immediate aim is to maintain cardio-respiratory and neurological function with active resuscitation and monitoring of vital signs.

The sternum is thumped with a fist in an attempt to fragment the embolus in the pulmonary artery. The diagnosis of embolus is confirmed by urgent pulmonary angiography and heparin (bolus dose of 20 000 units) is given intravenously. Full heparinisation should be maintained to keep the clotting (thrombin) time 2–3 times normal. An alternative is thrombolytic therapy. One million units of streptokinase are given with 100 mg hydrocortisone sodium succinate (to prevent anaphylaxis) intravenously. A further 1 million units are given by intravenous infusion over the next 8 hours, during which the patient's vital signs are continuously monitored. Hydrocortisone 50 mg 6-hourly is continued for 24 hours after cessation of streptokinase therapy. Should the patient recover consolidation and a pleural effusion will be noted on chest X-ray.

Pulmonary embolectomy using cardio-pulmonary bypass has been used successfully, though the overall results are not superior to anti-coagulant or thrombolytic therapy. Nevertheless, if facilities are available, embolectomy is indicated if the patient's condition does not improve over the first 2 hours. This must be preceded by pulmonary angiography.

## Minor embolism

Smaller emboli result in peripheral pulmonary infarcts of varying size, most frequently in the lower lobes. Sudden dyspnoea is common, often followed by pleuritic chest pain, tachycardia and pyrexia as infarction develops. Haemoptysis is relatively uncommon. Clinical signs of pulmonary infarction may follow and include decreased air entry, moist rales and a friction rub.

An electrocardiograph shows right axis deviation with prolonged PR interval, depressed ST segment in leads I and II, and an inverted T wave in leads II and III. A chest X-ray may show decreased markings with increased translucency in the peripheral lung fields, a prominent pulmonary artery, and enlarged cardiac shadow. Linear atelectasis may be noted. Later there may be a wedge-shaped area of consolidation, and/or a pleural effusion.

A ventilation-perfusion lung scan (V-Q scan) is a more sensitive investigation. Gamma scintigraphy following the intravenous injection of 99m-technetium labelled macroaggregates of albumin is used to delineate the pulmonary vasculature (perfusion scan). As atelectasis may also be associated with a perfusion defect a ventilation scan with $^{133}$Xenon is used to confirm that the ventilatory spaces are normal. Pulmonary angiography can be used to define the state of the pulmonary artery but is generally required only if operation is contemplated.

Recurrent minor pulmonary emboli lead to pulmonary hypertension.

## Management

The main objective in the care of the patient with minor emboli is prevention of further embolisation. One third of fatal emboli are preceded by a minor 'herald' episode and residual life-threatening thrombus in the leg veins must be excluded by bilateral venography.

Systemic heparinisation is started at once and is followed by oral anti-coagulation. If venography reveals a loosely attached thrombus in the ilio-femoral segment, further major embolisation is likely. It can be prevented by inserting a filter in the inferior vena cava below the renal veins (Fig. 21.30). The filter can be introduced through the internal jugular vein and positioned under radio-

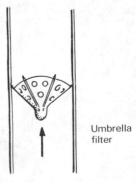

Umbrella filter

**Fig. 21.30** IVC filter

logical control. Direct surgical removal of the thrombus (thrombectomy) is associated with a high incidence of re-thrombosis and is seldom indicated.

Oral anti-coagulation should be continued for 6 months to prevent permanent occlusion of pulmonary vessels and pulmonary hypertension.

## OTHER FORMS OF VENOUS THROMBOSIS

### Inferior vena cava thrombosis

Inferior vena cava thrombosis results from extension of an ilio-femoral thrombosis, but more commonly complicates abdominal malignant disease. There is bilateral leg and scrotal oedema, distended collateral veins are obvious in the abdominal wall, and ascites may develop.

Management is symptomatic with diuretics and support stockings for the legs. Anticoagulation is indicated in non-malignant cases.

### Superior vena cava thrombosis

Mediastinal tumours or enlarged nodes (e.g. from breast or bronchial carcinoma) may obstruct the superior vena cava and induce thrombosis. Central venous catheters, for pressure measurement or to administer total parenteral nutrition, may also cause thrombosis of the SVC as of subclavian and axillary veins. There is marked oedema and cyanosis of the head and neck with distention of neck veins. The site of obstruction is defined by venography. Radiotherapy or systemic therapy may relieve symptoms by inducing remission of the obstructing disease. Anticoagulation is indicated.

### Subclavian and axillary vein thrombosis

This may complicate malignant disease in the axilla, or follow surgery or irradiation of axillary lymph nodes. Spontaneous axillary vein thrombosis sometimes occurs in young healthy adults. It usually results from excessive muscular excercise, and compression of the vein as it crosses the first rib may be involved. Insertion of a catheter, particularly when used for parenteral nutrition, is an occasional cause of thrombosis.

Axillary or subclavian vein thrombosis leads to a dull ache and feeling of fullness in the limb, which becomes swollen. Venous collaterals develop over the front of the shoulder and anterior chest wall. Total venous obstruction may lead to venous gangrene.

Ten per cent of patients develop a pulmonary embolus, and two-thirds develop persisting fatigue of the arm. Treatment consists of heparinisation, elevation of the arm, and elastic support. In young patients venous thrombectomy should be considered and is claimed to improve exercise tolerance.

# 22. Principles of Neurosurgery

## INTRODUCTION

Although there is evidence that so-called primitive man trepanned skulls, and that in medieval times crude attempts at trepannation, tumour removal and nerve section were made, surgical neurology is a relatively new specialty. Its modern development began in the late 18th century and owes more to the rapid increase in understanding of neurological anatomy, physiology and pathology than to improvements in surgical technique. Although the general principles of surgery are just as important as in other surgical fields, special techniques peculiar to neurosurgery have been developed. As new techniques became available an increasing number of conditions previously considered inoperable acquired surgical importance.

Conditions affecting the central nervous system which may require surgical intervention may be classified as:

1. congenital disorders
2. degenerative disorders
3. infection
4. vascular disorders
5. neoplasia
6. trauma (Ch. 11)
7. miscellaneous disorders

These disorders may affect the central nervous tissue itself, the coverings of the nervous tissue (meninges, etc.) or the bony compartments containing the nervous system (skull and vertebrae). The signs and symptoms produced may either be *generalised* (e.g. headache, vomiting, alterations in conscious level) due to increase in intracranial pressure, or *localised* (e.g. paralysis, sensory defect), resulting from damage in a specific area, which may be caused by trauma, local pressure, ischaemia or haemorrhage.

## INCREASED INTRACRANIAL PRESSURE

Because the nervous system is enclosed in a rigid bony framework, increase in the mass content produced by tumour, haemorrhage, oedema, or failure to reabsorb cerebrospinal fluid, results in an increase in pressure within the framework, particularly within the cranium. In the child, the ununited cranium permits expansion of intracranial contents with smaller increases in intracranial pressure than in the adult; in certain situations hydrocephalus results (p.294).

Intracranial pressure normally fluctuates throughout the day, and may increase during coughing, defaecation, or other circumstances producing an increase in the intrathoracic pressure. Such transient rises do no harm, only sustained increases producing disorder.

Increases in intracranial pressure lower perfusion pressure (intracerebral arterial pressure minus intracranial pressure) but initially, autoregulatory processes maintain an effective perfusion pressure of > 40 mmHg. Vasodilatation of intracranial vessels occurs along with an increase in extracranial blood pressure, resulting in increased cerebral flow. If raised intracranial pressure is unrelieved, bradycardia, hypertension and respiratory abnormalities (e.g. apnoea) develop. Unrelieved increased intracranial pressure progresses to irreversible oedema, vasoparalysis and death.

Pressure may not increase uniformly throughout the intracranial and spinal cavities, producing distortion of vessels and local ischaemia. Marked displacement of intracranial structures may occur and there are three major types:

1. *Transfalcine herniation.* The cingulate gyrus herniates beneath the free edge of the falx. The anterior cerebral artery may be compressed sufficiently to produce medial hemisphere infarction, but otherwise there are no obvious clinical signs other than deterioration in conscious level.

2. *Transtentorial herniation.* The medial part of the temporal lobe is pushed downwards through the tentorial notch to wedge between the tentorial edge and the midbrain (Fig. 22.1). The opposite cerebral peduncle is pushed against the sharp tentorial edge, and the midbrain and uncus become wedged at the tentorium. The aqueduct is compressed, obstructing flow of cerebrospinal fluid, and venous obstruction produces midbrain haemorrhage. The condition of the patient rapidly deteriorates. Epidural haematomas, or tumours or contusions of the temporal lobe are the usual causes.

Upward herniation is less common, but sometimes occurs with posterior fossa tumours. The pons and superior cerebellum become impacted at the tentorium.

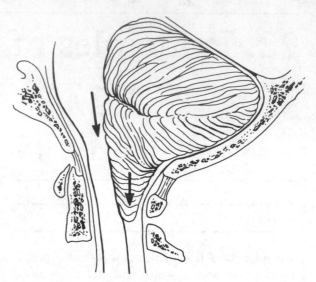

**Fig. 22.2** Foraminal herniation

3. *Foraminal herniation.* The cerebellar tonsils and medulla are displaced downwards through the foramen magnum, and cerebellar impaction occurs (Fig. 22.2). This may follow lumbar puncture and removal of cerebrospinal fluid in patients with raised intracranial pressure. Deterioration with loss of consciousness and decerebration is rapid. Thus, lumbar puncture should *not* be performed in patients suspected of having increased intracranial pressure.

### Signs and symptoms of increased intracranial pressure

The principal symptoms are headache, vomiting and visual disturbance (Hippocratic triad) and papilloedema may be detected. Clinical suspicion should be aroused by any one of these signs or symptoms.

*Headache* is common in patients with tumour, but may be absent. It is usually generalised, dull and aching, exacerbated by straining, coughing or defaecation, and classically worse in the morning when it may be accompanied by vomiting.

*Nausea or vomiting* is more common in posterior fossa tumours than supratentorial lesions and may be due more to medullary displacement than to generalised increase in pressure.

*Visual disturbance and papilloedema.* Transient *amblyopia* or blurred vision may occur in one or

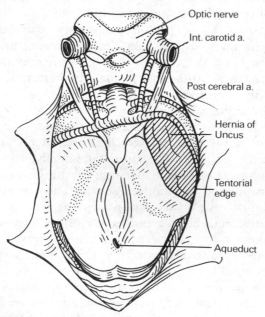

Optic nerve

Int. carotid a.

Post cerebral a.

Hernia of Uncus

Tentorial edge

Aqueduct

**Fig. 22.1** Transtentorial herniation

both eyes, particularly during straining or stooping. In the early stages of *papilloedema*, the retinal veins appear full and may show nipping and there is blurring of the nasal margin of the optic disc. Later, the disc becomes reddened and congested, with haemorrhagic streaks radiating from its edges, and filmy exudates form. Papilloedema is often present or more marked in one eye, but this is usually of no localising significance.

*Weight loss and anorexia* may be present and usually indicate tumour.

*Bradycardia and mild hypertension* are common in the later stages. *Intellectual deterioration and disorders of consciousness* occur as intracranial pressure rises progressively.

## DISORDERS OF CONSCIOUSNESS

Swelling, ischaemia or displacement of brain stem structures produce dysfunction of the reticular activating system in the brain stem which is concerned with consciousness. Continuing brain stem compression leads to deterioration of consciousness, coma and death.

Assessment of conscious level is invaluable in the observation of patients with a variety of neurological disorders, where even minor changes in conscious level may indicate the need for urgent treatment. The following system for classification of disordered consciousness has general acceptance:

*Grade 1*
*Alert and orientated* (AO): responds readily and accurately to question and command. Orientated in time, place and person.
*Grade 2*
*Disorientated or confused* (D): disorientated in time, place and person.
*Grade 3*
*Drowsy — vocal response to stimuli* (VRS): patient can be roused briefly by strong stimuli to respond vocally.
*Grade 4*
*Stuporous — purposeful response to stimuli* (PRS): patient can be roused briefly by strong stimuli to respond purposefully but not vocally.
*Grade 5*
*Coma — absent or abnormal response to pain*

**Table 22.1** Glasgow coma scale.

| Eyes | Open | spontaneously | 4 |
|---|---|---|---|
| | | to verbal command | 3 |
| | | to pain | 2 |
| | No response | | 1 |
| Best motor response | To verbal command | obeys | 6 |
| | To painful stimulus | localises pain | 5 |
| | | flexion withdrawal | 4 |
| | | flexion abnormal (decorticate rigidity) | 3 |
| | | extension (decerebrate rigidity) | 2 |
| | | no response | 1 |
| Best verbal response | | oriented and converses | 5 |
| | | disoriented and converses | 4 |
| | | inappropriate words | 3 |
| | | incomprehensible sounds | 2 |
| | | no response | 1 |
| Total | | | 3–15 |

(ARP): the patient does not respond vocally or purposefully. There is diminished or absent corneal reflex, depressed or absent cough or swallowing reflexes, sluggish or fixed pupils. Superficial reflexes are absent. Deep reflexes are diminished and the response to painful stimulation, particularly midline sternal pressure, is decorticate or decerebrate.

A large number of coma classifications have been prepared and the most useful are those which record patients' responses to stimulation by vocal responses, motor or pupillary reaction. Some of these are well-established systems and of especial value in research (Table 22.1).

## FOCAL SIGNS OF INTRACRANIAL LESIONS

Compression or destruction of different parts of the brain often produces subtle signs and symptoms long before there is evidence of increased intracranial pressure. The following signs are general pointers to the site of the pathology but are not specific. Displacement and resulting ischaemia frequently produce symptoms from parts of the brain distant from the causative lesion.

*Frontal lobe.* Intellectual and emotional change. Expressive dysphasia (dominant lobe lesions).

Contralateral faciobrachial weakness in convexity lesions and contralateral lower limb weakness in medial lesions. Focal epilepsy. Lateral gaze paralysis with the eyes deviated to the side of a destructive lesion; lateral gaze fixation with the eyes deviated away from the side of an irritating lesion. Urinary and faecal incontinence. Anosmia.

*Parietal lobe.* Contralateral faciobrachial sensory loss in convexity lesions and lower limb loss in medial lesions. Astereognosis. Sensory epilepsy. Receptive or global aphasia (dominant lobe).

*Occipital lobe.* Dyslexia (dominant lobe). Hemianopia.

*Temporal lobe.* Emotional changes. Temporal lobe epilepsy. Memory loss. Receptive auditory disorder.

*Cerebellum.* Ipsilateral weakness. Hypotonia. Ataxia. Dysmetria. Nystagmus.

*Brain stem.* Cranial nerve palsies. Long tract motor and sensory signs.

*Cerebello-pontine angle.* Functional disturbance in all or some of the 5th to 12th cranial nerves. Weakness of the contralateral arm and/or leg. Ipsilateral ataxia.

*Basal tumours.* Anosmia (unilateral or bilateral). Optic atrophy. Paresis of eye movement.

*Pituitary or parapituitary tumours.* Visual disturbance. Endocrine abnormalities.

## REACTION OF CENTRAL NERVOUS SYSTEM TO INJURY OR INFECTION

The central nervous system reacts to injury in a way similar to that of other tissues. Oedema is however more prominent due to damage to the blood-brain barrier allowing albumin, $Na^+$ and water to pass into the extracellular fluid. Oedema may be exacerbated by a number of factors, including a rise in $Pa_{CO_2}$. The injured area becomes surrounded by increased numbers of glial cells which act as phagocytes to remove dead neurones and other material, and which tend to localise infection. Fibrosis (gliosis) or scarring is the final outcome.

Oedema may result in loss of function of involved neural cells, with recovery of function as the oedema resolves. Irritation of cells may also result from oedema, or from their involvement in the scar process, leading to epilepsy or pain if pain fibres are involved. Replacement of destroyed neurones by regeneration is not possible in the central nervous system.

## INVESTIGATION OF NEUROLOGICAL DISORDERS

Though many sophisticated investigations are available, a detailed history and careful examination are essential to utilise investigations rationally.

*Full blood counts* should be done in all patients. Severe anaemia should arouse the suspicion of metastatic disease, while polycythaemia in a patient with posterior fossa symptoms suggests cerebellar haemangioblastoma. A raised white count suggests infection.

*Lumbar puncture and CSF examination* may assist or confirm a provisional diagnosis of meningitis, subarachnoid haemorrhage, or neoplasm. The investigations should not be carried out if raised intracranial pressure is suspected, because of the risk of foraminal herniation and cerebellar coning.

### Plain radiography

X-rays of the *skull* or *spine* should be routine. Metastatic disease of the spine or skull is often clearly seen; a narrowed intervertebral disc space will confirm a provisional diagnosis of prolapsed intervertebral disc. Congenital disorders may be revealed by the abnormal shape of the skull. Raised intracranial pressure in children produces expansion of the sutures, while in adults the posterior clinoid processes are thinned. Enlargement of the sella turcica or internal auditory meatus may occur in patients with pituitary or acoustic tumours respectively, while the vascular markings of the skull may be enlarged in the region of a vascular tumour such as a meningioma. Bony erosion or overgrowth (hyperostosis) are other features of meningioma. Calcification of the pineal gland or choroid plexus may reveal displacement of these structures, while abnormal calcification may develop within certain cysts or tumours (Fig. 22.3).

A *chest X-ray* should always be taken. 25% of

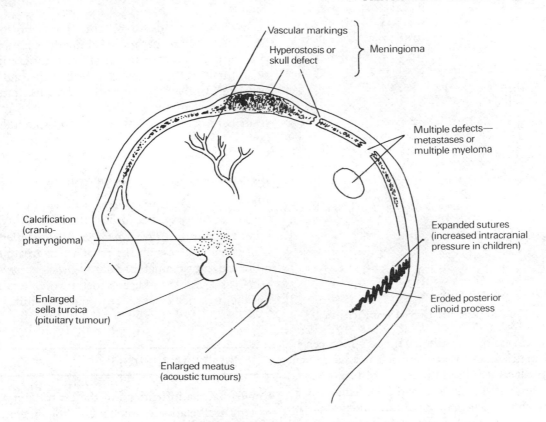

Fig. 22.3 Pathological changes in skull X-ray

cerebral tumours are secondary deposits from lung cancer; the chest X-ray may also reveal metastases from other primary sites.

## Contrast radiology

Dye may be injected to outline the spinal cord and nerve roots (*myelography or radiculography*) or the cerebral ventricles (*ventriculography*) (Figs. 22.4 and 22.5). The ventricles and basal systems may also be filled with air injected via lumbar puncture (*pneumo-encephalography*), though this technique is contra-indicated if raised intracranial pressure is suspected. *Angiography* may reveal lesions such as aneurysms and arteriovenous malformations, and display the relationship of important arteries to tumours.

Though angiography and ventriculography have been to a large extent superseded by computerised axial tomography, they still hold an important place in investigation.

*Computerised axial tomography* is a non-inva-

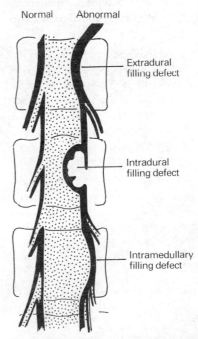

Fig. 22.4 Contrast radiology. Normal (left) and abnormal (right) myelogram.

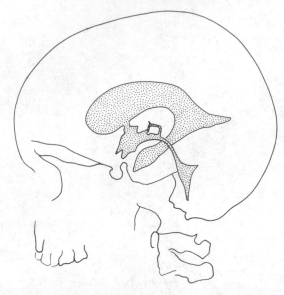

**Fig. 22.5** Contrast radiology. Normal ventriculogram.

sive, accurate diagnostic technique which can be performed without risk. Ventricular enlargement and displacement, and the extent of tumours and abscesses with their associated oedema can be clearly shown. Haemorrhages and clots show up as dense areas, and the presence of even small haemorrhages and associated oedema may indicate the arterial system involved in subarachnoid haemorrhage.

*Cerebral isotope scans.* Technetium-99 is usually used (Fig. 22.6). Vascular tumours such as meningiomas, metastases and some gliomas are readily revealed, though the vascularity of the

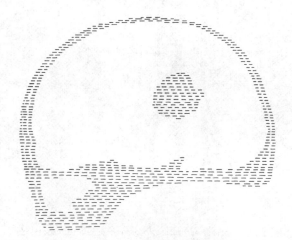

**Fig. 22.6** Cerebral isotope scan. Tumour uptake.

neck muscles tends to obscure posterior fossa tumours. Though isotope scanning does not provide as good anatomical detail as computerised axial tomography, it is a valuable method of assessing tumour vascularity following radiotherapy or chemotherapy, and may also be used to study cerebral blood flow and cerebrospinal fluid flow.

### Electrophysiological measurements

*Electroencephalography* is less used than formerly, except in epilepsy, because of the availability of other techniques. *Intracranial pressure monitoring* is of value in assessing the response to treatment of raised intracranial pressure. *Echo-encephalography* is a simple and useful method of determining the presence or absence of midline shift.

## CONGENITAL LESIONS

Congenital malformations of the central nervous system are relatively frequent. Though genetic counselling and advances in intra-uterine diagnosis are beginning to reduce the number of babies born with severe defects, minor defects will undoubtedly continue to occur. The causative role of viral infection and ingestion of certain drugs and toxic substances during pregnancy is well established, and prophylactic measures may now be taken. Children with mild defects who are likely to live independent lives should be offered immediate surgical treatment, but surgery may not enable children with major defects to live independent lives. Such children may therefore be denied surgery, but unfortunately a proportion survive with much greater defects than had surgery been undertaken. Currently, therefore, simple corrective surgery is offered to all, except those with severe defects associated with bladder abnormalities.

### SPINAL DISORDERS

These are common. *Dysrhaphism* is due to defective closure of the neural tube, and includes such conditions as spina-bifida occulta, simple meningocoele and meningomyelocoele. Closure of the neural tube begins in the mid-dorsal region and extends cranially and caudally. Thus thoracic defects are rare, cervical defects are uncommon, while lumbar and lumbo-sacral defects are common.

## Spina bifida occulta

This common condition is not usually associated with neurological defect. The overlying skin may be hairy, dimpled, or have an associated fat pad. Occasionally a fibrous band tethers the cord, producing increasing symptoms as the vertebral column grows and the spinal cord 'ascends' the vertebral canal. The onset of paraesthesia or sphincter disorders is usually due to an associated lesion such as a cord lipoma, or *diastemyelia* where the cord is split by a projection from the posterior surface of a vertebral body. A sinus may connect the skin and spinal canal in a few cases, and is a rare cause of meningitis in children. Plain X-rays may reveal an abnormality of the lamina, or failure of fusion of the laminar arches.

Patients with neurological disorders require surgical treatment. Paraesthesia, backache and sphincter disorder due to tethering by a fibrous band are dramatically relieved by division of the band. Splitting of the cord by a bony spur can be dealt with by careful removal of the spur. Intraspinal lipomas are often diffuse; though removal has been facilitated by microscopic techniques, severe neurological disturbances may result.

## Simple meningocoele

The defect is usually lumbar and results from failure of fusion of laminae (Fig. 22.7). The subarachnoid space is distended and protrudes through the defect. The arachnoid fuses with the skin forming a membrane to which nerve roots may be adherent. The cord, however, is normal and often there are no neurological abnormalities.

## Meningo-myelocoele

The condition occurs most commonly in the lumbar region (Fig. 22.8). Spinal nerve roots and the cord adhere to the membrane because of distension of the central canal and may be exposed

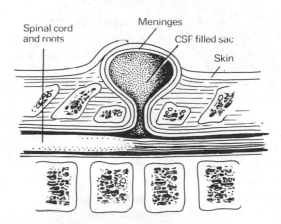

Fig. 22.7 Meningocoele

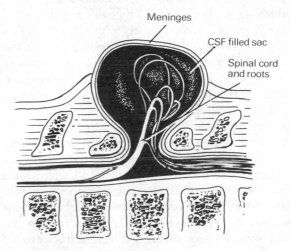

Fig. 22.8 Meningo-myelocoele

on the surface. Cranio-cerebral malformations such as hydrocephalus are commonly present.

There is usually serious motor and sensory loss affecting the lower limbs and sphincters due to involvement of the cauda equina. Bladder paralysis is of the lower motor neurone type with paralysis of the detrusor muscle and pelvic floor musculature.

These patients often require complex and lengthy corrective procedures, and urinary continence is difficult to achieve.

## Syringomyelia and syringobulbia

Distension of the central canal of the cord or a paraventricular extension of the fourth ventricle results respectively in syringomyelia or syringobulbia. Though the genesis of the condition is debated, most believe it to result from failure of closure of the connection between the fourth ventricle and the central canal coupled with failure of development of exit foramina in the membrane around the cerebellar tonsils.

Symptoms, which are steadily progressive, appear in the third decade and affect men more commonly than women. In the cord, distension of the central canal gradually compresses and destroys the decussating pain and temperature pathways producing 'dissociated sensory loss' (loss of pain and temperature sensation but not touch) over the upper part of the body, most often in the fingers. Trophic lesions develop on the hands and arms due to loss of pain sensation. The small muscles of the hand are often involved early with resulting deformity and wasting. Ultimately the long tracts become involved, producing paresis and sensory changes below the level of the lesion. Denervation arthritis (Charcot's joints) may occur.

The condition is treated by creating an opening in the membrane around the cerebellar tonsils, allowing drainage of cerebrospinal fluid. Occasionally a persisting communication with the central canal may be plugged. A posterior fossa approach is used. Isolated cysts of the cord may be drained by direct puncture either via laminectomy or percutaneously. Orthopaedic deformities may require correction e.g. arthrodesis of unstable joints.

## MALFORMATIONS OF THE SKULL

These are less common than spinal defects.

### Meningocoele and encephalocoele

Protrusions of meninges only (meningocoele) or meninges with brain (encephalocoele) through a skull defect occur most commonly in the occipital region, and are usually associated with other abnormalities such as hydrocephalus and mental retardation.

### Craniostenosis

Premature fusion (before 4 years of age) of skull sutures results in restriction of the growing brain and an increase in intracranial pressure. The shape of the skull is determined by which sutures fuse. Associated ophthalmic disorders such as exophthalmus are common. Severe cases are treated by excision of the involved sutures. The edges are then lined with dura or plastic material to retard re-union and allow the brain to expand.

### Orbital hypertelorism

This group of malformation is produced by overgrowth of anterior fossa structes resulting in widening of the intercanthal distance and persistence of clefts and fusion lines. The disorder is relatively common in a mild form, but in its most advanced form produces gross malformation, requiring treatment by excision of the central sutures and transposition of the lateral masses.

### Epidermoid cysts

These contain cheesy debris and arise from skin which has been engulfed by bone. They expand the bone and erode the skull, producing a scalloped lytic area.

### Miscellaneous malformations

Malformations associated with autosomal chromosomal abnormalities, such as Down's syndrome, micro-encephaly or macro-encephaly, and porencephaly, are not correctable. Tuberous sclerosis is a form of neuro-ectodermal dysplasia associated with mental retardation and epilepsy in which astrocytes form pale firm tubers in the cortex and subependyma, which occasionally become malignant. Angiomatous malformations of skin (usually in the distribution of the ophthalmic branch of the trigeminal nerve), or retina and meninges (Sturge-Weber syndrome) may be associated with epilepsy and mental retardation. The vessels rarely rupture, and symptoms are related to the epilepsy.

## HYDROCEPHALUS

Cerebrospinal fluid is produced by the intra-ventricular choroid plexus, passes from the lateral ventricles via the narrow foramen of Munro into the slit-like third ventricle and then through the aqueduct of the upper brain stem into the widening fourth ventricle. From here the fluid passes via 'exit foramina' in the lower part of the fourth ventricle into the cisterna magna, afterwards flowing over the surface of the brain and spinal cord to be absorbed by cerebral veins and arachnoid granulations. Hydrocephalus results when the production of cerebrospinal fluid exceeds absorption and is usually associated with increased intracranial pressure. Though a choroid plexus papilloma may produce hydrocephalus by oversecretion of CSF, much the commonest cause of hydrocephalus is obstruction to flow with consequent failure of CSF to reach sites of absorption (Fig. 22.9).

Obstruction may be truly congenital due to failure of communications between ventricles as in aqueduct stenosis, or acquired as a result of tumour or fibrosis (gliosis) following infection or haemorrhage. For the sake of simplicity the acquired types of hydrocephalus are also considered in this section. When the obstruction occurs within the ventricular system the condition is called *non-communicating* or *internal hydrocephalus*. *Communicating* or *external hydrocephalus* exists when the ventricular system is patent, but absorption by the arachnoid granulations is prevented by blood or fibrosis, or occasionally by their failure to develop.

Hydrocephalus usually presents at birth or in early infancy with characteristic enlargement of the head. Presentation in later childhood or in adult life is associated with the signs and symptoms of raised intracranial pressure.

If the cause of hydrocephalus can be removed (e.g. cysts, thin membranes, certain tumours), this should be done after preliminary drainage of the ventricles via a right frontal burrhole. Lumbar puncture should be avoided because of the risk of medullary 'coning'. If the cause cannot be removed, a ventricular shunt may be performed (Fig. 22.10). A catheter is inserted into a lateral ventricle and tunnelled subcutaneously into the neck where it is inserted into the internal jugular vein and passed into the superior vena cava or right atrium (ventriculo-atrial shunt). Alternatively, the catheter is tunnelled to the abdomen to be inserted into the peritoneal cavity (ventriculo-peritoneal shunt). The catheter incorporates a one-way valve to prevent reflux of blood, and a chamber which may be milked or compressed to prevent clotting and encourage flow. Despite this, blockage is frequent, especially in children, necessitating revision or replacement of the catheter.

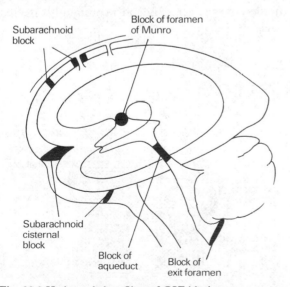

Fig. 22.9 Hydrocephalus. Sites of CSF block.

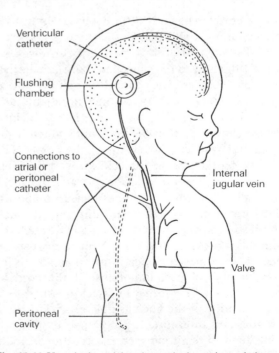

Fig. 22.10 Ventriculo-atrial and ventriculo-peritoneal shunts

## CEREBRAL PALSY

Cerebral palsy may result from agenesis, birth injury, or infection. There is often a history of neonatal distress, cyanosis and feeding difficulties. Though many patients have normal intelligence, mental subnormality is common and as the child grows it becomes evident that development is retarded. Spasticity and athetoid movements become marked and the abnormal movements may be so violent that the patient cannot sit up, and joint contractures develop. In milder cases, there is a characteristic 'scissors' gait with adduction of the legs and equina varus posture.

Treatment consists of physiotherapy, and special education in mild cases, but the major disability often progresses so that the patient becomes helpless and unable to dress or feed himself. Joint deformities may be relieved by tendon transposition or neurectomy. Stereotactic destruction of thalamic or cerebellar nuclei is often successful in relieving lower limb spasticity.

## DEGENERATIVE DISEASES OF THE VERTEBRAL COLUMN

Degenerative changes in the intervertebral discs are common at all levels in the spine. Intervertebral discs consist of three parts-the *cartilage endplates* adherent to the cancellous bone of adjacent vertebral bodies, the central semifluid *nucleus pulposus* which is relatively incompressible and inelastic, and which is surrounded and retained by the slightly elastic *annulus fibrosus* which regulates and restricts movement of the spine. The intervertebral disc is subject to severe and repeated compression, and degenerative changes may allow protrusion of the nucleus pulposus. This can occur in an upward direction through the cartilage endplate, or horizontally through the annulus fibrosus. Horizontal protrusion usually occurs in a postero-lateral direction and is of considerable clinical importance if the cord or nerve roots are subjected to direct pressure.

Herniation of the nucleus pulposus is usually a gradual and intermittent process, so that symptoms tend to remit between exacerbations. Acute herniation may however occur, usually in response to severe trauma with flexion injury. The annulus fibrosis ruptures allowing posterior (central) protrusion of the nucleus with sudden severe neurological deficit.

If the nucleus pulposus has lost substance by protrusion or desiccation (as occurs in advancing age) the relaxed fibres of the annulus fibrosis bulge outwards and the 'disc space' narrows. Strain on the apophyseal joints results in osteophyte formation and narrowing of the intervertebral foramina. Osteophyte formation also occurs around the disc margin. This condition is known as *spondylosis*. With continuing degeneration, osteophytes may protrude on to the cord or nerve roots (Fig. 22.11).

Spinal *osteoarthritis* is a disorder affecting the posterior apophyseal joints and produces back pain without distant radiation. It should be distinguished from spondylosis (which depends on disc degeneration) although the two frequently co-exist in older patients.

## CERVICAL SPINE

### Cervical spondylosis

Degenerative changes in the cervical spine are common and start in adolescence. Compression of a nerve root in an intervertebral foramen produces pain, usually in the neck but often radiating to the shoulder or arm, which is exacerbated by rotation of the neck. The most commonly affected level is C5–6.

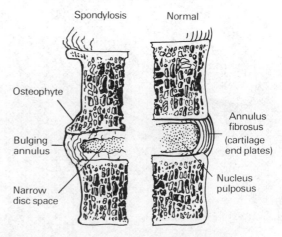

**Fig. 22.11** Intervertebral disc. Normal and abnormal.

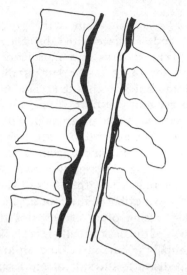

**Fig. 22.12** Cord compression by cervical spondylosis

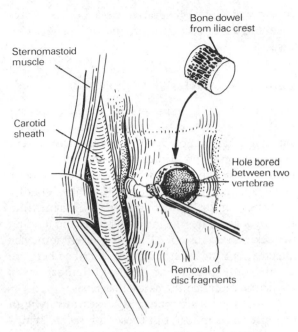

**Fig. 22.13** Anterior cervical decompression and fusion

Plain X-rays of the spine show narrowing of one or more disc spaces and foramina with osteophyte formation. Myelography may demonstrate nerve compression, and in severe cases compression of the cord (Fig. 22.12).

Treatment is initially conservative and comprises physiotherapy, neck traction and prescription of a supporting cervical collar. If there is more severe compression as evidenced by weakness and paraesthesia, such conservative therapy is not effective, and some form of decompression is required. Through an anterior approach a central core of disc and related vertebra is removed and the lateral portion of the disc is curetted away. A dowel of bone taken from the iliac crest is then hammered into the central core to stabilise the two vertebrae (Fig. 22.13).

### Acute cervical disc prolapse

Acute prolapse is uncommon and fortunately most protrusions are small. The patient presents with acute onset of neck pain which radiates down the arm in the area of the involved root or roots. Symptoms usually resolve following conservative management with analgesics, neck traction and use of a cervical collar. Persistence of symptoms is an indication for surgery, while patients with major prolapse and long tract signs (which may include quadriparesis) require urgent operation.

The disc fragments may be removed through a posterior approach or less commonly by anterior decompression which is usually accompanied by vertebral fusion.

### THORACIC SPINE

Thoracic disc degeneration with formation of osteophytes and foraminal narrowing is relatively common, though surgical treatment is seldom required.

Acute disc prolapse, though uncommon, requires urgent surgery because the narrow calibre of the vertebral canal in the thoracic region favours cord compression. Acute pain in the distribution of the segmental nerves may be accompanied by paraparesis or paraplegia depending on the degree of prolapse.

An anterolateral or posterolateral approach is used to avoid injuring the acutely compressed spinal cord.

### LUMBAR SPINE

Disorders of the lumbar spine are extremely common. Low backache (*lumbago*), with pain radiating down one or both legs (*sciatica*) may be caused by a variety of conditions. Metastases from lung, breast or prostatic cancer should always be considered, but degenerative disease of the vertebrae and discs accounts for the vast majority of cases.

## Lumbar spondylosis

As a result of bulging of the annulus fibrosis, osteophytes form at the disc margins. Posterior osteophyte formation reduces the diameter of the vertebral canal, while additional stress on the posterior joints results in hypertrophy of the joint bone and ligaments, reducing the canal laterally. There is thickening of the laminar arch, and the ligamentum flavum degenerates, losing its elasticity and tending to buckle on extension. All lumbar vertebrae may be affected, but the severe changes described here are usually only present at the lower lumbar level. Radiculography confirms the diagnosis.

Most patients are managed conservatively with exercise and support, but those with severe symptoms will require decompression by laminectomy.

## Acute lumbar disc prolapse

Acute disc prolapse is most common in the 4th and 5th decades of life and occurs more frequently in men than in women. It is frequently associated with degenerative spinal disease elsewhere. During torsion stresses on the disc (e.g. twisting when carrying heavy weights), the annulus fibrosis may be torn allowing protrusion of the nucleus pulposus.

If rupture occurs through the central portion of the annulus, the roots of the cauda equina are compressed and the patient has severe back pain without a predominant root involvement, urinary retention, and weakness below the knees. This is the *cauda equina syndrome*, and urgent surgical relief is necessary.

More commonly the prolapse occurs posterolaterally and compresses and angulates the nerve emerging at that level. The most common sites for prolapse are at the L4–5 and L5–S1 level, the roots affected being L5 and S1 respectively. Prolapse above L4–5 becomes less common as one ascends. The majority of patients recover on conservative management, though patients with symptoms which persist for more than six weeks should be offered surgical treatment.

*Signs and symptoms.* Pain is the predominant symptom, and is exacerbated by coughing or sneezing. Tendon jerks and muscle power are diminished according to the site of the lesion. *Straight leg raising* stretches the sciatic nerve and pulls on nerve roots, resulting in pain if the roots are stretched over a disc protrusion. The straight leg raising test is measured in degrees and reflects the amount of root compression. The limit of straight leg raising is normally between 80–90°, but it may be reduced on the affected side to less than 30°. Dorsiflexion of the foot at the limit of straight leg raising often exacerbates the pain. Examination of the back usually reveals flattening of the lumbar spinal curve and mild lumbar scoliosis, concave to the side of the lesion. This scoliosis is exaggerated when the patient is asked to bend forward.

*L5–S1 prolapse.* Involvement of the S1 root produces pain which radiates down the back of the thigh and lateral aspect of the leg onto the lateral border of the foot and the lateral three toes. Sensory changes may be detected in this distribution. The ankle jerk is diminished or absent, and plantar flexion of the foot is weak, so that the patient has difficulty in standing on his toes.

*L4–L5 prolapse.* The L5 root is compressed causing pain radiating from the back down the back of the thigh, and then passing medially from the lateral aspect of the leg to the dorsum of the foot and into the great toe. Sensory changes may similarly be detected in this distribution. The ankle jerk is normal, but dorsiflexion of the foot is weak.

*L3–L4 prolapse.* L4 root involvement produces pain and sensory disturbance down the front of the thigh and medial aspect of the leg on to the medial malleolus. The knee jerk is diminished or absent, and there is quadriceps weakness.

Full examination of the abdomen including rectal examination is imperative as retroperitoneal or pelvic pathology may also produce severe back pain with radiation if nerves become involved.

*Investigations.* The diagnosis is often apparent from the history and physical examination, though some difficulty may result when an adjacent root is involved in addition to the root at the level of the prolapse. PA and lateral X-rays of the lumbar spine are essential and often show narrowing of the involved disc space. Radiculography is indicated if the diagnosis remains in doubt.

*Treatment.* Immediate *strict* bed rest is mandatory. The patient should lie flat; though not permitted to sit for meals, he may be allowed up for toilet purposes. Most patients improve within two to three weeks and are allowed up after four weeks.

Patients with major protrusions are unlikely to respond satisfactorily and should be offered early surgery, and any patient not progressing satisfactorily after six weeks bed rest requires operation. The prolapsed disc material is removed through a posterior approach. The results of operation are good for those with acute disc prolapse, though pain may recur in those with generalised spinal disease.

### Spondylolisthesis

There is a bilateral defect in the pars interarticularis of the neural arch of the fifth lumbar vertebra (i.e. *spondylolysis*) which allows the anterior part of the vertebra, comprising the body, pedicles, transverse processes and superior articular facets, to slide forward upon the sacrum (i.e. *spondylolisthesis*).

Spondylolysis is probably not a congenital defect, although there is an inherited tendency in some patients, and signs and symptoms may appear in childhood, most often between 10 and 15 years of age. Vertical stresses on a weakened neural arch may be responsible for the slipping, while in adults it may follow stress fracture in mature bone, or facet deficiency due to degenerative joint disease.

In children, the condition is usually painless, though a prominent lumbar lordosis may be detected. The normal presenting symptom in adolescents or adults is backache exacerbated by exercise. Sciatica may develop as a result of S1 root pressure. The diagnosis is confirmed radiologically.

Symptomatic younger patients are treated by lumbosacral fusion, but as this is a major undertaking, older and less fit patients are usually managed with a spinal brace.

### Spinal stenosis

In this congenital condition there is generalised narrowing of the vertebral canal. Symptoms do not occur until middle life, and are associated with other degenerative changes such as spondylosis, which are more likely to produce symptoms as a result of the narrow canal. Several nerve roots are often affected.

Treatment is along the lines of that for spondylosis though operation (laminectomy with or without fusion) is more frequently necessary.

---

## VASCULAR DISORDERS

---

### INTRODUCTION

The metabolic demand of the brain is greater than any other organ, requiring a considerable blood supply. The cerebral blood flow of 800 ml per minute (16% of cardiac output) is provided by two systems; the carotid arteries supply the forebrain, and the vertebral arteries supply the hindbrain. The two systems communicate freely in the circle of Willis (Fig. 22.14).

The common carotid artery divides into the external carotid artery which supplies the soft tissues of the head and the dura, and the internal carotid artery which enters the skull to supply the brain. After passing through the carotid sinus, the

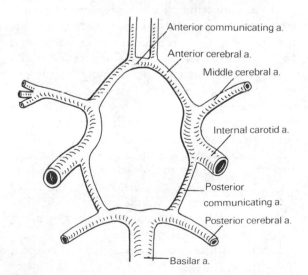

**Fig. 22.14** Circle of Willis

internal carotid artery divides into the anterior cerebral artery and the middle cerebral artery. The two vertebral arteries join within the skull to form the basilar artery which supplies the cerebellum and brain stem and then divides into the posterior cerebral arteries which pass through the tentorium to supply the occipital lobe and the posterior two-thirds of the medial aspect of the hemisphere.

As a result of the major communications occurring in the circle of Willis, occlusion of any of the major arteries may be compensated by collateral flow.

Disorders of the central nervous system resulting from vascular disease are due mainly to occlusion or to haemorrhage.

## OCCLUSIVE VASCULAR DISEASE (See also Ch. 21)

Symptoms most often result from occlusive disease affecting the *extracranial* vessels. The lumen of the carotid or vertebral vessels may be narrowed or occluded by arteriosclerotic changes in the arch of the aorta, in the neck (particularly at the carotid bifurcation), or at the level of entry into the skull. Though arteriosclerotic disease may be widespread in the cerebral vessels, *intracranial occlusion* is usually embolic.

### Transient ischaemic attacks (TIA)

Small thrombic and platelet aggregates attached to atheromatous plaques, and occasionally small portions of the plaques themselves may embolise from larger vessels to lodge in small intracranial vessels and produce sudden and alarming symptoms, which are often transient. Symptoms depend on which vessels are obstructed, but in carotid disease there is commonly unilateral blindness and contralateral weakness, with associated speech disorder if the dominant hemisphere is affected. Auscultation over the carotid bifurcation will detect a bruit in 70% of patients, and ophthalmo-dynometry may reveal lower pressure on the affected side. The extent of the lesion is revealed by angiography, though this is not without risk.

Embolectomy has been attempted on occasion, but 50% of patients with TIA will have a major stroke within five years if the primary lesion is not treated. Stenotic lesions in the neck arteries are relatively easy to relieve; those arising in the aortic arch are more difficult. Gentle handling of the carotid artery is essential to avoid dislodging thrombi, and if the pressure in the distal carotid artery is less than 50 mmHg a bypass procedure is used to lessen the risk of postoperative stroke.

Unfortunately many patients suffer from generalised arteriosclerotic disease, and a high proportion suffer fatal myocardial infarction within a few years of surgery.

### Cerebral thrombosis

Stenotic lesions may progress to complete occlusion with thrombus formation which extends up the carotid tree. If the collateral circulation via the circle of Willis is defective, cerebral infarction occurs (cerebral 'thrombosis'). In many cases a precarious circulation is maintained: in suitable patients if facilities exist this may be improved by anastomosing an extracranial vessel such as the superficial temporal or occipital artery to one of the intracranial vessels.

## HAEMORRHAGE

Intracranial haemorrhage may be intracerebral, subarachnoid, subdural or extradural. Extradural and subdural haemorrhage usually results from trauma and is considered separately in Chapter 11.

### Intracerebral haemorrhage

Intracerebral haemorrhage is relatively common in the middle-aged and elderly. The risk is particularly high in patients with hypertension and diabetes, and justifies the prophylactic therapy of hypertension. In hypertension the perforating arteries of the middle cerebral arteries develop microaneurysms which rupture and tear open the internal capsule. Intracerebral haemorrhage may also occur from rupture of 'berry' aneurysms located deep within the brain, from arteriovenous malformations, or from trauma producing brain lacerations.

The onset is abrupt and the majority of patients become comatose with stertorous respiration and flaccid hemiparesis. About 30% of patients die within three days, but some survive with partial recovery of function.

Emergency procedures to remove intracerebral haematomas are rarely successful since bleeding continues. If patients survive the initial haemorrhage, their recovery may be impeded by the presence of haematoma. In such cases, evacuation of the clot through a burr-hole may result in marked improvement.

## Subarachnoid haemorrhage

In more than 50% of patients the haemorrhage is due to rupture of an aneurysm, while in 15% arteriosclerotic disease is the cause. Arteriovenous malformations, trauma, and haemorrhage in association with tumour or infection account for the remainder.

Intimal proliferation and degeneration of the internal elastic lamina produces a weakness of arterial walls, particularly at sites of congenital weakness in the circle of Willis. Failure of the media to develop allows the intima to bulge and form an aneurysm. The majority of aneurysms occur in the anterior portion of the circle of Willis, only 15% being sited in the posterior portion.

Though 10% of patients present with symptoms due to local pressure effects of the aneurysm (e.g. 3rd cranial nerve palsy in posterior communicating artery aneurysm), or with signs suggesting tumour, the majority have no symptoms until the aneurysm ruptures. Sometimes the patient has pre-ictal symptoms of vague headache or neck pain, while the first haemorrhage (ictus) may be relatively mild and pass unrecognised.

Rupture of the aneurysm into the subarachnoid space produces sudden severe headache, neck stiffness and photophobia. Kernig's sign indicates meningism. The patient's conscious level is affected in varying degrees from mildest disorientation to deep coma, and sudden death may occur. These symptoms, apart from meningism, are mostly due to vasospasm. The focal signs depend on the vessels affected, but are commonly related to the aneurysm's parent vessel, for example middle cerebral artery aneurysm rupture commonly produces faciobrachial paresis. Associated rupture into brain substance is more serious than subarachnoid haemorrhage, and is the usual cause of sudden death.

*Diagnosis and assessment.* The diagnosis is confirmed by lumbar puncture. The fluid is evenly blood-stained, as opposed to a 'traumatic tap' which progressively clears. Oxyhaemoglobin appears within a few hours of haemorrhage, giving an orange colour to the supernatant fluid. By three days bilirubin (due to red cell breakdown) is present and gives the supernatant fluid a characteristic yellow colour (xanthochromia).

A special grading system (Botterell) is used to assess the patient:

*Group A*
Grade 1: Conscious, with or without signs of subarachnoid blood
Grade 2: Drowsy, without significant neurological deficit
*Group B*
Grade 3: Drowsy and confused or with mild neurological deficit
Grade 4: Major neurological deficit and generally deteriorating, possibly the result of intracerebral clot
Grade 5: Moribund or nearly so, with vegetative disturbance and extensor rigidity.

In practice group A patients are fit for angiography; group B patients are not. Patients in group A have a much better prognosis, and are fit for definitive surgery directed at the aneurysm. Patients in group B may sometimes be improved by removing intracerebral clot.

*Skull X-rays* usually show no abnormality, though a giant aneurysm may erode a clinoid process or have a calcified wall. CT *scan* may reveal a large aneurysm, but is more useful in detecting oedema or intracerebral haemorrhage. *Angiography* should be deferred until the patient is alert and has no evidence of vasospasm. Though the clinical picture may suggest the site of the aneurysm it is important to have a complete picture of the cerebral circulation, as aneurysms are commonly multiple (Fig. 22.15).

*Management and prognosis.* Mortality is high in the first week, but falls steadily after the second week. Without operation the mortality is 60% by two months. 50% of patients who survive the first haemorrhage die within 5 years without surgery. Thus, surgical treatment should always be con-

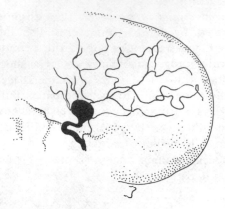

Fig. 22.15 Diagram of angiogram showing internal cartoid aneurysm

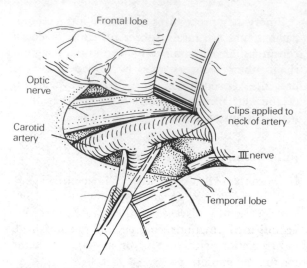

Fig. 22.16 Clipping of posterior communicating artery

sidered after the first bleed. Experience has shown that the optimum time to operate is during the second week following the first haemorrhage, providing the patient is in Botterell Grade 1 or 2.

While awaiting surgery the patient is confined to complete bed rest and given oxygen because of the vasospasm. Sedation may be required. If neurological signs are present, dexamethasone (10 mg stat. and 4 mg 6 hourly) is given. Hypertension is treated by hypotensive drugs, aiming to reduce the blood pressure by 10%. Antifibrinolytic therapy reduces the risk of re-bleeding by preventing lysis of the peri-aneurysmal clot. Epsilon-amino caprionic acid (EACA) is the most frequently used preparation and reduces the risk of re-bleeding to 10–15%.

*Operation.* Most aneurysms are now treated by a direct approach under induced hypotension. Using the operating microscope, the neck of the aneurysm is exposed and a special clip is then applied (Fig. 22.16). The aneurysm can be strengthened by coating it with plastic material or by wrapping it in gauze to cause a fibrous reaction. The mortality rate of operation (5%) is substantially less than non-operative treatment, but despite meticulous technique vasospasm may result in brain oedema requiring energetic treatment with steroids and other anti-oedema agents.

Common carotid artery ligation is the procedure of choice for aneurysms within the cavernous sinus or for giant aneurysms of the carotid system, provided angiography has revealed a satisfactory cross-circulation. The procedure is normally done under local anaesthesia, so that the patient's speech, behaviour, sensation and motor function can be monitored after clamping of the common carotid artery. If these parameters remain satisfactory for five minutes, the vessel is ligated and the clamp removed.

## ARTERIOVENOUS MALFORMATIONS

These congenital malformations may occur close to ventricular walls, in the substance of the brain, or on the cerebral cortex. Composed of a complex mass of abnormal arteriovenous connections, they vary in size from small lesions undetectable by conventional angiography to large masses occupying major portions of brain. The lesions frequently bleed, and are the commonest source of subarachnoid haemorrhage in the younger age groups, or they may cause epilepsy. Once bleeding has occurred the risk of re-bleeding is high; within 10 years 20% of patients die and a further 30% suffer severe disability from recurrent haemorrhage. If bleeding occurs in childhood, the chance of normal life expectancy is very small; the prognosis improves with increasing age at the first bleed.

Arteriovenous malformations are best demonstrated by angiography, though CT scans enhanced by contrast media will reveal moderate sized to large malformations. Calcification in some malformations will be shown on plain X-rays, and occasionally a bruit may be heard.

The malformation may be locally excised or removed by block resection (lobectomy). Pre-operative embolisation of contributing vessels with small plastic spheres may facilitate resection, and the recent introduction of the laser beam 'knife' has given promising results. Carefully directed cobalt radiotherapy is an alternative to resection, and excellent results have been claimed.

## Spinal arteriovenous malformations

These lie over the posterior surface of the cord and form loops of vessels which may involve cord substance. Thrombosis frequently occurs in the vessels, producing cord ischaemia. Symptoms are often progressive, with pain, weakness and ultimate paraplegia. Excision using the operating microscope is the only available treatment, but its long-term value is uncertain.

# INFECTION

Infection of the central nervous system and its coverings acquires surgical importance if it produces a mass (abscess or oedema), hydrocephalus, or osteomyelitis, or occurs as a result of a breach or absence of the coverings (Fig. 22.17).

## INTRACRANIAL INFECTION

### Osteomyelitis of the skull

Bone may become infected by penetrating wounds, during surgery, by local extension (from sinuses, the middle ear or mastoid), or by blood-borne infection. Pus may track into the subgaleal space or involve the overlying scalp to produce 'Pott's puffy tumour', and there is often an associated small extradural abscess. The infection is difficult to eradicate, and may require removal of large areas of calvarium, which may subsequently be replaced with an acrylic plate.

### Extradural abscess

Extradural abscess is usually secondary to osteomyelitis and most often occurs close to the middle

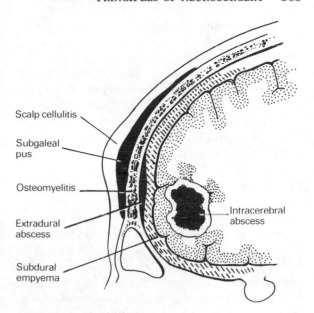

**Fig. 22.17** Types of cranial infection

Labels: Scalp cellulitis; Subgaleal pus; Osteomyelitis; Extradural abscess; Subdural empyema; Intracerebral abscess

ear, the mastoid air cells, or the paranasal sinuses. Trauma is another frequent cause. Pus may infiltrate into the pericranium to produce Pott's puffy tumour, and frequently breaks through the dura to produce meningitis, subdural empyema or cerebral abscess.

Systemic upset is usually severe. There is local tenderness, and focal neurological signs may result from thrombophlebitis of superficial cortical veins. Facial nerve paralysis is frequent when mastoiditis is the source.

Treatment involves the use of large doses of antibiotics, drainage, excision of any infected bone, and drainage of infected sinuses or mastoid air cells as appropriate.

### Subdural empyema

Subdural empyema (pus within the subdural space) is commoner than cerebral abscess in the western world. It may follow penetrating wounds or surgery, but is most commonly associated with paranasal or ear infection, which may spread to the subdural space along emissary veins or via dural sinuses.

Pus may spread over the whole hemisphere, beneath the falx to involve the opposite hemisphere, or beneath the tentorium. It may accumulate in multiple sites, making treatment difficult.

Although accumulation of pus exerts pressure on the brain, symptoms are largely the result of venous thrombosis. Patients may present with disordered consciousness, paresis and epilepsy and with signs of meningitis. Spread of infection is revealed by altering localising signs. Deterioration of consciousness in patients with a history of frontal sinusitis or ear infection should arouse suspicion of subdural empyema.

Plain X-ray of the skull may reveal opaque air sinuses, but the diagnosis is confirmed by angiography or CT scan. Immediate treatment is indicated. Multiple burrholes are made to drain the pus, and catheters are inserted through which antibiotics are instilled 4-hourly in addition to systemic administration. The common infecting organisms are staphylococcus and streptococcus, which determines the choice of antibiotic until bacteriological reports are available. Occasionally, removal of a large area of skull may be necessary to achieve adequate decompression. Anticonvulsant treatment is continued indefinitely. Despite these measures, the mortality is 20–35%, and residual paresis and epilepsy are common.

## Cerebral abscess

Though the brain is relatively resistant to infection, abscess formation may occur, particularly if there has been previous damage due to haemorrhage, trauma or anoxia. Initially there is a cerebritis (encephalitis) and at this stage antibiotics may prevent development of an abscess; usually however the brain tissue necroses to form pus around which a tough glial capsule develops which is resistant to passage of antibiotics.

Abscesses may develop, in descending order of frequency from:

1. Direct extension from the paranasal sinuses, mastoid or middle ear
2. Haematogenous spread, most commonly in patients with bronchiectasis or lung abscess, or patients with cyanotic heart disease with a right-to-left shunt
3. Direct penetrating trauma-now a much less common cause than formerly.

The presentation is often acute, with high fever, progressive disturbance of consciousness and evidence of increasing intracranial pressure. If the abscess is chronic and walled-off, systemic signs of infection may be minimal and the presentation is that of a slowly expanding localised mass.

Diagnosis requires a high degree of suspicion, and is confirmed by CT scan (Fig. 22.18) or pyography (Fig. 22.19). Echo-encephalography

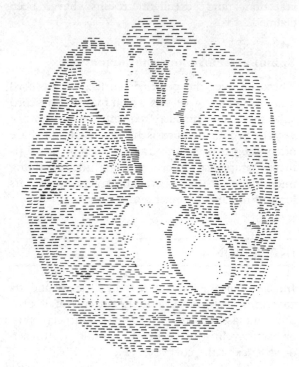

**Fig. 22.18** Right posterior fossa abscess. Diagram of CT scan.

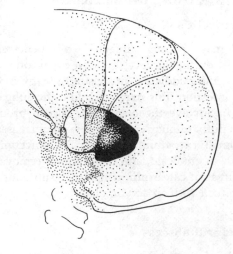

**Fig. 22.19** Temporal lobe abscess. Diagram of pyogram with air.

shows midline shift and electro-encephalography may show large delta waves.

*Treatment.* Urgent treatment is necessary. In the acute stage of encephalitis, systemic antibiotics in high doses and anti-oedema agents are administered, and may localise the infection. Once localisation has occurred, drainage through a burrhole is indicated, and a catheter inserted into the cavity so that antibiotics can be instilled regularly. Systemic antibiotics are continued for 10 days while the size of the cavity is monitored by CT scanning. Encapsulated abscesses and cerebellar abscesses are exciscd, while if a patient does not become rapidly more alert following drainage of an abscess, excision should be undertaken.

Nearly 50% of patients with cerebral abscess develop epilepsy, and anticonvulsant therapy should be continued indefinitely. With early diagnosis, the mortality is low, but the overall mortality rate of 30–50% reflects the failure to make an early diagnosis.

## INFECTIONS OF THE SPINE

### Tuberculosis

Tuberculosis of the spine is still relatively common in the 'developing' countries. The bovine form, from infected milk, is the usual agent and most commonly affects the thoracic spine.

Infection initially affects the anterior border of one or more vertebral bodies with development of caseous necrosis, and spreads through the disc space to affect the adjacent upper or lower vertebra. The disc space narrows because of loss of fluid. A paraspinal abscess develops which may compress the cord and nerve roots, and the disc may sequestrate into the abscess. Collapse of the anterior part of the vertebral body occurs if there is sufficient damage, producing angulation of the spine, and in severe forms a gibbus. Severe angulation may produce cord compression and paraplegia — Pott's paraplegia — in 10% of cases.

The paticnt prcsents with back pain, limitation of spinal movement, and systemic signs of infection. Cord compression produces neurological deficits. Spinal X-rays show narrowing and irregularity of the disc space with erosion of the vertebral body, while paravertebral abscess may

be seen as a soft tissue mass. Angulation is seen in later cases.

Early treatment carries a good prognosis, and even if cord compression has occurred from an epidural abscess, the prognosis is favourable. The late form of Pott's paraplegia is due to ischacmic changes in the cord and carries a poor prognosis for recovery. If tuberculosis is suspected, triple chemotherapy is instituted, and the patient nursed in bed in a plaster cast. When adequate chemotherapy has been given, the diagnosis is confirmed by biopsy, infected material removed, and if necessary the spine is stabilised by bone grafting. The presence of pus or signs of compression are indications for urgent drainage. All necrotic material is removed, and bone grafts (from resected rib or iliac crest) are inserted to stabilise the spine.

### Osteomyelitis of the spine

The usual infecting organism is *Staphylococcus aureus*. The infection arises most often as a result of haematogenous spread from boils, dental root infections, tonsillitis or otitis media, but may follow local trauma or operation.

The infection is most common in adolescence and early adulthood, and is much more common in males than females. In contrast with spinal tuberculosis, the lumbar region is most often infected, the illness is usually more acute and severe, and the development of large paravertebral abscess or vertebral collapse is uncommon. Radiological signs are absent in the first 10–14 days after which some signs of bone erosion and regeneration and loss of disc space appear.

Treatment consists of immobilisation in a plaster cast, and administration of large doses of the appropriate antibiotic as determined from culture of material from the primary site or from blood culture. An associated abscess should be drained by an anterolateral approach and the area debrided, with or without bone grafting.

### Epidural abscess

Epidural abscess may arise from haematogenous spread from an infected skin lesion, from the urinary tract, or from local spread of a vertebral infection. The patient develops severe pain and the signs of cord compression, with retention of urine. Plain X-rays are usually normal in the absence of an established bone infection, but myelography confirms the compression.

Antibiotics and urgent evacuation of the pus are indicated. In the absence of local bone infection a laminectomy approach is used, but an anterolateral approach is used if the abscess is secondary to vertebral infection.

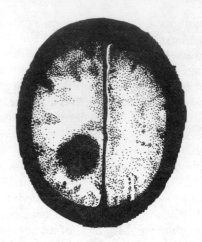

Fig. 22.20 Meningioma. Diagram of CT scan.

## NEOPLASMS

## INTRACRANIAL TUMOURS

Primary intracranial tumours show a bimodal age incidence, with a small peak in childhood at age 6–7 years, a decline until puberty, and thereafter a progressive rise in incidence to a maximum in the 5th decade. The sexes are equally affected. Apart from certain tumours such as cholesteatomas and craniopharyngiomas which arise from cell 'rests' their cause is unknown. They rarely metastasise, death resulting from the consequences of continued growth within the confined space of the skull.

About 50% of intracranial tumours are metastatic, the most frequent primary sources being lung and breast. Intracranial tumours may present with general or localised effects. Diagnosis is easy when tumours are large, but early diagnosis while the tumour is still small facilitates treatment and improves prognosis.

CT-scan and angiography are essential investigations for the diagnosis and localisation of intracranial tumours (Figs. 22.20 and 22.21).

## TUMOURS ARISING FROM THE SKULL

### Osteoma

This relatively common benign tumour is usually solitary. It usually arises in a paranasal sinus (especially the frontal sinus), or from the orbit. Osteomas usually grow outwards to produce a palpable hard mass, but may grow inwards to produce pressure on underlying brain and meninges. Osteomas growing within a sinus may

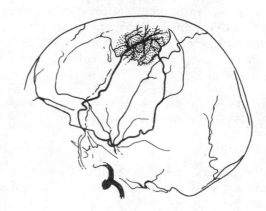

Fig. 22.21 Meningioma. Diagram of carotid angiogram.

produce obstruction and sinusitis, while those in the orbit may cause proptosis and diplopia. Symptomatic osteomas should be excised.

### Chordoma

These rare malignant neoplasms are thought to arise from embryonic remnants of the notochord. They occur in the spheno-occipital region of the skull (40%) or in the sacro-coccygeal region of the spine (60%). They are highly vascular, firm grey tumours which erode bone, and in the skull invade the optic chiasma, the sella and cavernous sinus, and displace the pons. Though malignant they are relatively slow-growing. Complete surgical removal is rarely possible, though radiotherapy may slow the growth rate and prolong life for a few years.

## Glomus jugulare tumours

These tumours arise in the middle ear and invade the posterior fossa. They often present with bleeding from the ear, and examination reveals a soft fleshy red mass protruding through the drum. Invasion of the internal jugular vein is common. Invasion of the middle ear produces tinnitus, deafness and facial paresis, while intracranial growth produces the signs and symptoms of a cerebellar pontine angle tumour.

Radical excision of the petrous and occipital bones followed by irradiation is indicated.

## Histiocytosis

In this group of disorders, comprising eosinophilic granuloma, Hand-Schuller-Christian disease and Letterer-Siwe disease, the tumours contain histiocytes, and erode bone.

Eosinophilic granuloma normally presents between the age of 8 –15 years as a solitary lesion in the skull or spine with pain, swelling, tenderness and systemic disturbance. The prognosis is good, some lesions resolving spontaneously, and others healing after curettage and/or radiotherapy.

Hand-Schuller-Christian disease becomes manifest in earlier childhood. The tumour usually involves the skull base to produce proptosis and diabetes insipidus, and occasionally causes other pituitary dysfunction. Its progress, though steady, is usually slow and relatively benign, but 25% have a poor prognosis despite radiotherapy.

Letterer-Siwe disease may be regarded as an acute form of Hand-Schuller-Christian disease. The onset is in infancy, and in addition to skull lesions, many other organs are involved. Progression is rapid, leading to death within weeks.

## Multiple myeloma

Myeloma usually presents over the age of 50, with a M:F ratio of 2:1. It is multicentric, and in addition to skull lesions, vertebrae and other bones are involved. The condition may be confused with metastases from a primary solid tumour. Systemic cytotoxic chemotherapy is indicated.

## Paget's disease (osteitis deformans)

Of unknown aetiology, this condition produces thickening, softening and deformity of bone with later dense sclerosis. The sexes are equally affected, and the condition usually begins in the 4th to 6th decades. The skull is the area most frequently affected and is enlarged and thickened. When the base of the skull is affected, encroachment on the optic or auditory foramina may produce visual or auditory disturbance. Sarcomatous change occurs in 10% of patients.

Management is usually confined to pain relief. Entrapped nerves may require surgical decompression, while radiotherapy is effective in the management of localised pain. Calcitonin is used increasingly in systemic management. Sarcomatous change is rarely resectable and has a poor prognosis.

## Metastatic tumour

The skull is a common site for metastases from cancers of the lung, breast, prostate, thyroid and kidney. The lesions are usually osteolytic, though metastases from breast and prostate may be osteoblastic. Local radiotherapy may be indicated for a rapidly enlarging metastasis.

## TUMOURS ARISING FROM THE MENINGES

### Meningiomas

These account for 20% of all brain tumours. They arise from arachnoidal cells, and are therefore most commonly found close to the intracranial sinuses; 90% occur in the supratentorial region. They are slow-growing and often highly vascular, deriving the majority of their blood supply from meningeal vessels. They are usually rounded or bosellated and imbed into the brain, but tumour cells may invade bone or spread widely over the dura (meningioma en plaque). The overlying skull may be rarefied, or thickened (hyperostosis) with production of a palpable mass.

The signs caused by meningiomas depend on their location. The parasagittal region is the commonest site for supratentorial meningiomas, and their proximity to the motor cortex results in focal seizures, particularly in the leg. They frequently invade the sagittal sinus.

Meningiomas are treated by surgical excision. If the sagittal sinus is involved, resection of the sinus with vein graft replacement is necessary to reduce the risk of recurrence.

## PITUITARY AND PARAPITUITARY TUMOURS

Pituitary tumours account for 15% of all intracranial tumours. They produce effects due partly to endocrine change and partly to local pressure (Fig. 22.22) (see Ch. 39).

### Chromophobe adenoma

This, the commonest of the pituitary tumours, is occasionally cystic due to haemorrhage. Gradual tumour growth compresses the remaining pituitary tissue producing hypopituitarism, and expands and erodes the sella turcica. Penetration of the roof of the sella causes pressure on the optic chiasma and nerves, and the characteristic visual field defect is bitemporal hemianopia.

The tumour is removed via craniotomy. Residual tumour is treated by postoperative radiotherapy.

### Eosinophilic adenoma

The adenoma is usually small — a 'microadenoma' — and exerts effects by oversecretion of growth hormone. Presentation in childhood causes gigantism, but the usual presentation is in

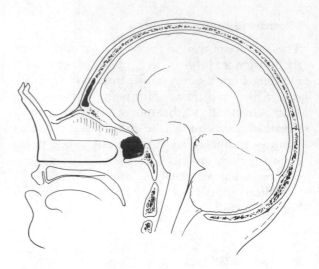

**Fig. 22.23** Trans-sphenoidal removal of pituitary tumour

middle life, causing acromegaly. The eosinophilic adenoma is not infrequently part of a chromophobe adenoma, and is then associated with the features of local expansion described above.

The tumour is usually removed by a transsphenoidal approach, leaving the rest of the pituitary intact (Fig. 22.23). Pituitary irradiation has the disadvantage that normal pituitary tissue is also destroyed. Recently, bromocryptine has been used successfully but must be continued indefinitely.

### Basophilic adenoma

These rare tumours are also small - 'microadenomas', and occur more commonly in women than men. Over-secretion of ACTH results in Cushing's disease.

The preferred treatment is trans-sphenoidal removal of the microadenoma.

### Craniopharyngoma

These tumours develop from remnants of Rathke's pouch, and present in childhood or in the elderly. Most are multicystic, and they may reach a large size. The majority lie anterior to the pituitary stalk, though some may occur within the sella.

Visual field defects occur early. Progressive growth results in hypopituitarism due to hypothalamic involvement and eventually causes signs and symptoms of raised intracranial pressure.

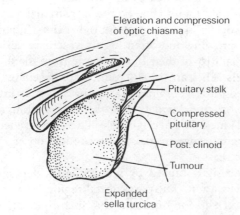

Elevation and compression of optic chiasma

Pituitary stalk

Compressed pituitary

Post. clinoid

Tumour

Expanded sella turcica

**Fig. 22.22** Pituitary tumour

Complete surgical removal is the treatment of choice for small solid tumours. If the tumour is large, and particularly if it is cystic, puncture and aspiration of the cyst contents with subsequent radiotherapy is safer and more effective.

## Cholesteatoma

The tumour is characteristically pearly-white and glistening, and is composed of layers of large finely granular cells. They may arise in the suprasellar region, but are most commonly found in the posterior fossa at the cerebellar pontine angle or within the fourth ventricle or cerebellum.

Complete removal is not often possible, but partial removal often prolongs survival.

(This condition should not be confused with cholesteoma of the middle ear.)

## Neurinomas

Neurinomas of the cranial nerves account for about 5% of primary intracranial tumours, and are almost entirely restricted to the acoustic nerve. Bilateral tumours may occur in generalised neurofibromatosis, but are rare.

The acoustic neurinoma develops within the internal auditory meatus, which it erodes and expands. The 8th and 7th nerves become stretched over the tumour as it grows into the cerebello-pontine angle (Fig. 22.24). Early symptoms are due to 8th nerve involvement, producing progressive nerve deafness, tinnitus and vertigo. Further growth produces 7th nerve compression and facial weakness, while upward extension compresses the trigeminal nerve producing diminution in facial sensation. Eventually compression of the pons and cerebellum results in ataxia and nystagmus, while gradual displacement of the brain stem angulates the aqueduct and fourth ventricle to produce internal hydrocephalus. The neurinoma may reach a large size before presenting for surgical treatment. Patients are frequently misdiagnosed as having Meniere's disease at onset.

Plain X-rays show enlargement of the internal auditory meatus, while the tumour itself is usually clearly demonstrated by CT scanning (Fig. 22.25).

Treatment consists of surgical removal via a posterior fossa approach. It is often possible to preserve the facial nerve if the operating microscope is used.

## INTRACEREBRAL TUMOURS

### Metastatic tumours

Metastatic tumours account for almost 50% of intracerebral neoplasms, the common primary sites being lung and breast. They are frequently multiple, and because of the breakdown in the blood-brain barrier are usually associated with considerable oedema.

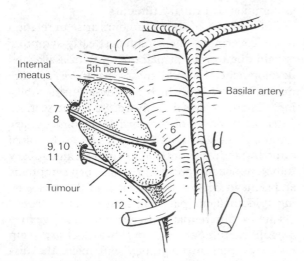

**Fig. 22.24** Right acoustic tumour in CP angle from the front

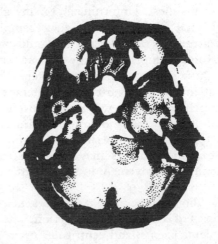

**Fig. 22.25** Right acoustic tumour. Diagram of CT scan.

Multiple metastases are inoperable, and are best treated by cytotoxic therapy or hormonal manipulation if appropriate (e.g. breast). Whole-brain radiotherapy may produce some improvement, while gross oedema can be reduced by steroids such as dexamethasone. If a metastasis is single and accessible, the patient is otherwise well and there is no evidence of wide extension of the primary tumour, surgical removal of the metastasis may be considered.

## Gliomas

Gliomas arising from the supporting cells of the brain (the glia) are much the commonest *primary* brain tumour, and account for 25% of all intra-cranial tumours. They are classified histologically into astrocytomas, oligodendrogliomas and the very rare microgliomas. *Astrocytomas* are often initially slow-growing, but may be rapidly invasive (glioblastoma multiformae). The less common *oligodendrogliomas* are slow-growing, sometimes become calcified, and have less tendency to infil-trate the brain.

Complete removal of gliomas is difficult and is often prevented by infiltration of the tumour. The cerebellar astrocytoma of childhood is an excep-tion in that removal is usually feasible and cura-tive. Gliomas confined to a single lobe may be removed by lobectomy, but more usually resec-tion is incomplete. Recurrence is common despite postoperative radiotherapy although the patient may live for several years before recurrence becomes manifest. Unfortunately, many gliomas occupy vital cerebral areas, for example the speech area, and radical removal would produce aphasia and hemiplegia — the humane surgeon rejects these patients for radical surgery. Even in such patients judicious use of radiotherapy, ster-oids and chemotherapy will prolong useful inde-pendent life for many months. Hydrocephalus may be treated by appropriate shunts, while unre-sectable cystic tumours may be aspirated with considerable improvement in the patient's condi-tion.

Some gliomas may present as emergencies with rapid onset of coma and decerebration. The use of anti-oedema agents, and ventricular drainage for hydrocephalus may improve the patient's condi-tion sufficiently to allow adequate investigation and appropriate definitive treatment.

## Ependymomas

Ependymomas arise from ependyma in the walls of the ventricles, and in the spinal cord from ependymal remnants in the central canal. They are most common in the fourth ventricle and produce hydrocephalus. They may emerge from the fourth ventricle into the cisterna and spread over the brain stem producing multiple cranial nerve palsies.

Using the operating microscope many of these tumours may be safely and completely removed.

## Medulloblastomas

These malignant tumours of childhood arise from the roof of the fourth ventricle and, like ependy-momas, tend to seed through the cerebrospinal fluid pathways, sometimes presenting with lum-bar or sacral root lesions. Treatment consists of partial removal followed by radiotherapy to the entire central nervous system.

## SPINAL TUMOURS

Primary spinal tumours are about one-sixth as common as intracranial tumours. Almost 60% are benign, and many of the remainder are suscep-tible to radiotherapy, having a better prognosis than intracranial lesions. Metastatic tumours are as common as primary tumours.

The majority of spinal tumours arise in relation to the coverings. The commonest early symptom is pain due to root displacement, with associated development of a mild spastic paraparesis, more marked in one leg, which may drag during walk-ing. There is usually disorder of micturition. Intrinsic tumours of the cord — intramedullary tumours — account for only 5% of spinal tumours and, in contrast to the extramedullary tumours, usually present with sensory symptoms and signs indicating involvement of the decussat-ing spinothalamic pain and temperature fibres.

Clinical differentiation between intra- and extra-medullary tumours is not always clear; plain radiology plus myelography will make the dis-tinction.

## Epidural tumours

90% of epidural tumours are malignant, and 75% are metastatic from a primary site elsewhere. They account for 55% of spinal tumours.

Lymphoma is the most common non-metastatic tumour, but leukaemic infiltration and myeloma also infiltrate the epidural space, producing cord compression. Metastatic carcinoma to the vertebrae may be the first manifestation of the disease, and tumour cells enter the epidural space. These lesions most commonly affect the thoracic area, and symptoms progress rapidly.

Treatment consists of decompression, laminectomy and removal of the epidural tumour, followed by local radiotherapy and systemic treatment appropriate to the primary disease.

## Intradural tumours

Accounting for 45% of spinal tumours, they are further subdivided into intradural-extramedullary (40%) and intramedullary lesions (5%). 98% of intradural tumours are primary, and 60% are benign. Progression tends to be slow in contrast to epidural lesions.

*Extramedullary tumours.* Meningiomas and Schwannomas are the common lesions. *Meningiomas* are more common in females (M:F = 1:10). They are firm hemispherical tumours, occurring most commonly in the thoracic region. They usually present after the age of 40 and compress the cord and nerve roots. Surgical removal is followed by an excellent prognosis.

*Schwannomas* affect the sensory roots more commonly than the motor roots, and tend to grow out through the intervertebral foramen and expand, producing a 'dumb-bell' tumour. They are as common as meningiomas. The much less common *neurofibroma* occurs as a part of generalised neurofibromatosis. The prognosis is excellent following removal of the tumour, although resection of the attached nerve root may be needed.

*Intramedullary tumours. Ependymomas* are the commonest intramedullary lesion, and usually affect the conus and filum terminale. They arise at the centre of the cord, and expand slowly rather than invade. Complete removal is often possible for the majority, with a good prognosis.

*Gliomas*, usually astrogliomas, are most often found in the thoracic region. They infiltrate the cord to produce a fusiform swelling. They are not usually operable, but with microscopic techniques an incomplete removal followed by radiotherapy may allow survival for 5 years or longer.

---

# MISCELLANEOUS CONDITIONS

## INVOLUNTARY MOVEMENT DISORDERS

### Parkinson's disease

Parkinson's disease affects 0.1% of the population, with an incidence of 1% in those over 50. Depigmentation of the substantia nigra occurs, and inclusion bodies are found in many neurones of the brain stem nuclei and spinal cord grey matter.

The cause is unknown in 80% of cases — *idiopathic Parkinsonism. Post-encephalic Parkinsonism* has an earlier onset than the idiopathic form. It becomes manifest 10 to 20 years after an attack of encephalitis, and is particularly associated with the world-wide epidemic of encephalitis in the 1920s. Blepharospasm and oculogyric crises are particularly common in this form of the disease.

*Arteriosclerotic Parkinsonism* occurs in an older age group and is often of sudden onset. Rigidity and akinesia are more common than tremor.

*Psychotropic drug-induced Parkinsonism* may follow administration of drugs such as the phenothiazines. The condition regresses in two-thirds of patients following withdrawal of the drug.

The onset of tremor, akinesia and bradykinesia and rigidity may be sudden or insidious. Common early complaints include a painful limb, clumsiness or weakness. Tremor is often unilateral in onset, and affects distal muscles. The fully developed clinical picture is unmistakeable, with mask-like face, flexed posture, festinating gait, and tremor. Swallowing becomes difficult, leading to drooling and respiratory aspiration, and weight loss is common. Idiopathic Parkinsonism is progressive, leading to death or severe invalidism in 15–20 years.

*Surgical treatment*. The majority of patients are treated medically, surgery being reserved for patients with severe tremor. Stereotactic radiofrequency lesions are made in the ventralis-lateralis nucleus of the thalamus, which is an important relay nucleus of the motor system. Results are good.

## Chorea

Chorea is a rapid, purposeless contraction of the face or limb muscles at rest which also interferes with voluntary movement. It may follow thrombosis of brainstem vessels. *Huntingdon's chorea* is an autosomal dominant disorder associated with progressive dementia which becomes evident in adult life. There is widespread neuronal loss in the cortex, caudate, and putamen. Though stereotactic thalamotomy will relieve chorea it is rarely undertaken.

## Choreoathetosis

Choreoathetosis with spasticity is common in young patients with cerebral palsy. Stereotactic dentatotomy converts the spastic paresis into a flaccid one, improves speech and feeding, and allows the limbs to attain greater facility.

## Torsion dystonia

The disease is characterised by sustained muscle contractions, which may be spasmodic or continuous. It usually results from birth injury or cerebral anoxia, but is occasionally inherited. Partial forms are relatively common in adults with orofacial dyskinesia and dystonia or torticollis. A good response is often obtained by stereotactic thalamotomy or dentatotomy.

## EPILEPSY

Onset of epilepsy at any age requires investigation to determine the cause. This is particularly important in *late onset epilepsy*, which is often due to a tumour or vascular lesions which may be relieved by surgery. Epilepsy may continue after removal of the cause, though it is usually easier to control, and long-term anticonvulsant therapy is mandatory.

*Idiopathic epilepsy* is usually managed satisfactorily by drug therapy, but if satisfactory control is not achieved, surgery is considered after accurate localisation of the focus of discharge. A cortical lesion may be carefully excised, using electrocorticography to ensure that the whole of the epileptic focus is removed.

*Temporal lobe epilepsy* is not infrequently associated with definite, though small, cortical or subcortical hamartomas, and if a well-localised focus can be demonstrated, temporal lobectomy gives excellent results.

For patients with *intractable grand mal seizures*, stereotactic thalamotomy is useful in a proportion of cases.

## SURGERY FOR PSYCHIATRIC DISORDERS

The surgery of mental disorder has been handicapped by indiscriminate use of gross frontal leucotomy over 30 years ago, and is only now regaining reputable status. Full cooperation with the referring psychiatrist is essential, and surgery is only recommended after frank discussion with the patient and relatives.

*Intractable anxiety states* unresponsive to medical treatment may be improved by a discrete stereotactic leucotomy which interrupts white matter pathways from various parts of the limbic lobe, such as the orbital frontal gyri.

For *aggressive disorders*, particularly those associated with temporal lobe epilepsy, stereotactic amygdalotomy is performed.

*Hyperactivity* of severe grade is difficult to manage, but stereotactic hypothalamotomy is sometimes useful.

## THE SURGICAL RELIEF OF PAIN

Intractable pain (i.e. pain not responding to routine measures) requires careful assessment before recommending procedures which themselves may be extensive or hazardous. A detailed history and examination is essential, and factors which exacerbate the pain are determined. A cause which is treatable directly may then be detected.

Full assessment of factors such as anxiety, drug dependence and attention-seeking is mandatory. Many hospitals now operate 'Pain Clinics' where patients are examined and discussed by a team of physicians, surgeons, anaesthetists and psychiatrists before management is initiated. Each case must be assessed on its own merits.

Intractable pain may be iatrogenic, and careful attention to surgical principles during operation, and adequate reassurance and information both pre- and postoperatively reduces this risk. Adequate analgesia should always be given during the painful early postoperative period, but the powerful analgesics with potent addiction risks are rarely required for more than 48 hours.

Some patients attending for pain relief merely require reassurance, others need alterations in their drug regime, while specific treatment of an underlying cause is indicated in some. If further pain-relieving procedures are needed, they should not incapacitate the patient and should aim to secure complete and long-lasting relief. Patients with incurable malignant disease and short survival prospects are not usually considered for radical surgical procedures, provided their pain can be controlled by drugs without severe side effects. Patients with longer expectation of life, or whose life expectancy is being shortened by analgesic drugs, should however be considered. The success rate is high in patients with malignant disease, possibly because they die from the disease before the pain recurs. In patients with pain from benign disease, the success rate is lower, excepting those with clear-cut conditions such as trigeminal neuralgia.

The procedures available are shown in Table 22.2.

## Peripheral neurectomy

Most nerves are mixed nerves, and although anaesthesia can be achieved by peripheral neurectomy, it is purchased at the expense of paresis and loss of normal sensation. Facial pain is an exception, as neurectomy can be performed on purely sensory nerves. Splanchnicectomy, now usually performed chemically by injection of alcohol, is sometimes helpful in the management of intractable upper abdominal pain.

**Table 22.2**

| Peripheral procedures | Central procedures |
| --- | --- |
| 1. Neurectomy | Spinal cord |
| 2. Surgical posterior rhizotomy | spinothalamic tractotomy (cordotomy) |
| 3. Intrathecal chemical rhizotomy | myelotomy |
| 4. Epidural techniques | Brain stem spinothalamic tractotomy |
| | Thalamus thalamotomy |

## Posterior rhizotomy

Posterior rhizotomy is a satisfactory procedure for pain syndromes due to direct nerve involvement but because of the extensive overlap of dermatomes (especially in the trunk), several nerve roots have to be divided to obtain a relatively small area of anaesthesia. Thus surgical rhizotomy requires extensive laminectomy and is now being replaced by *percutaneous* rhizotomy. Electrodes are introduced percutaneously into the appropriate intervertebral foramina, and the roots are subjected to radio-frequency coagulation. The procedure may be repeated, and is very suitable for patients in poor general condition.

## Intrathecal chemical rhizotomy

This is suitable for patients with pain involving a large area or multiple sites. Alcohol is effective but carries a high risk of paresis, so that its use is restricted to those already paralysed. Phenol is less risky, and pain may be controlled for many months. Hypertonic saline is the safest of all but pain relief rarely lasts for more than 3 months, and it is therefore most suitable for patients with a short life expectancy.

## Intrathecal steroids

*Local* intrathecal injection of steroids is sometimes effective in the management of chronic back pain (particularly for chronic lumbar pain from arthritis), and severe continuous pain following laminectomy. The effect is not entirely predictable, but some obtain relief of pain for 3 weeks to 6 months. The effect is presumed to be due to a local anti-inflammatory action.

## Epidural techniques

Epidural anaesthesia has become increasingly popular in recent years, and has the advantage that an epidural catheter may be left *in situ* postoperatively through which the level of analgesia may be 'topped up', avoiding the need for systemic opiates. Epidural techniques are now being utilised in the management of intractable pain but have the disadvantage of achieving only temporary relief.

*Epidural morphine.* Recent work demonstrating the presence of morphine receptors within the cord has stimulated the use of epidural morphine in the management of postoperative and chronic pain. The results are still uncertain.

*Spinothalamic tractotomy (cordotomy).* Spinothalamic tractotomy is an excellent operation for pain relief when life expectancy exceeds 6 months (Fig. 22.26). It is less satisfactory for those with pain due to benign causes. Cordotomy removes pain and temperature sensation, preserving touch. It is usually performed at the cervical level, but section at C1 is required to obtain analgesia of arm and shoulder.

The procedure is usually performed percutaneously, either using rough aiming or a stereotactic technique. Local anaesthesia is employed, and the risk of damage to motor tracts and to bladder and respiratory fibres is reduced.

*Myelotomy.* Bilateral cordotomy carries a high risk of respiratory or bladder dysfunction, and is very rarely indicated. However, by cutting the cord longitudinally in the midline one can produce bilateral analgesia by dividing the decussating fibres (Fig. 22.26). This is done as an open procedure in the lumbar region, and is useful for intractable pain following abdomino-perineal excision of the rectum. Cervical myelotomy, for pain arising at higher levels, is usually carried out by a percutaneous stereotactic technique.

*Brain stem tractotomy.* Division of the spinothalamic and trigeminal tract at the medullary level may be used to relieve widespread cervical and facial pain. The risk of operative damage to neighbouring structures is reduced if a stereotactic technique is employed.

*Thalamotomy.* Stereotactic thalamotomy is useful in patients with long-standing pain, in those in

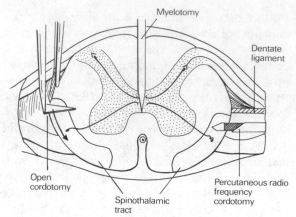

**Fig. 22.26** Spinal cord tractotomies for pain

whom the pain seems to be of central (affective) origin, and in those in whom a more peripheral procedure has failed. Alternatively, stimulating electrodes may be placed in thalamic nuclei and can be activated by the patient using a battery-operated coil placed subcutaneously.

## Additional techniques

*1. For affective pain.* Severe pain is often accompanied by emotional distress, especially in terminal malignancy, so that a technically successful pain-relieving procedure may not provide the expected relief. Addition of a simple tranquiliser may be effective, but in some patients with this so-called 'psychic' pain, stereotactic cingulotomy to interrupt circuits in the limbic system is effective.

*2. Sympathectomy.* The use of splanchnicectomy in the management of intractable abdominal pain, e.g. from chronic pancreatitis, has been mentioned. Sympathectomy is also effective in relief of *causalgia*, the burning pain and autonomic dysfunction that results from partial injury to major nerve trunks.

*3. Electroanalgesia.* Newer techniques using nerve fibre stimulation rather than destruction have been introduced, following the demonstration that stimulation of a peripheral nerve trunk reduces pain sensation over the distribution of the nerve. Activation of A fibres may interfere with the perception of a painful stimulus, possibly at spinal cord level, or there may be a release of enkephalins.

Electrodes are implanted close to the nerve trunk in question, or at higher levels in the nervous system, and activated by the patient using a small power pack when he feels the need for more analgesia. Local contact skin electrodes may be used as an alternative. Early results are encouraging, but require fuller assessment. The relationship of *acupuncture* to this technique is as yet undetermined.

*4. Hormonal ablation.* In the specific case of painful metastases from hormone-dependent tumours, particularly those arising from breast or prostate, endocrine ablation gives effective pain relief in approximately 50% of patients (p. 226).

*5. Trigeminal neuralgia.* The standard treatment of trigeminal neuralgia has been long-term use of the drug carbonazapine. However, drug reactions such as rash, drowsiness and ataxia are frequent, and pain recurrence after months or years is not uncommon. Consequently, radio-frequency trigeminal rhizotomy is now recommended for initial treatment and produces analgesia without loss of ordinary sensation in the face. The corneal reflex is preserved.

*6. Advanced oro-pharyngeal cancer.* Extensive analgesia is required. This may be achieved via a posterior fossa exposure and section of the 5th, nervus intermedius, 9th and 10th cranial nerves and the upper three cervical nerves on the appropriate side. This is a major procedure in debilitated patients and better results are obtained by stereotactic tractotomy of the trigeminal tract of the upper cervical cord under local anaesthesia.

## SURGICAL TECHNIQUES

### SURGERY OF ACCESS

While the general principles of surgical techniques apply in neurosurgery, certain requirements of access to the nervous system are peculiar to neurosurgery.

### Burrholes

Burrholes are simple skull perforations made to remove fluid, pus or blood from the cranium, or to enable instruments to be passed into the brain. The standard burrholes are made in the frontal,

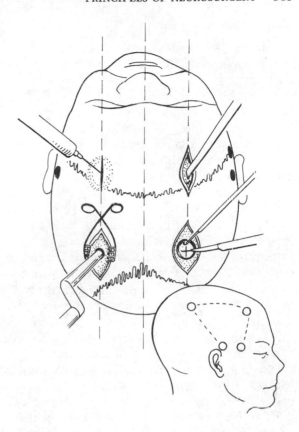

**Fig. 22.27** Standard burr holes

parietal and occipito-parietal regions along the pupillary plane (Fig. 22.27). Temporal burrholes may be made immediately above the zygoma to approach the middle meningeal artery in extradural haematoma, or directly above the root of the ear to drain a temporal lobe abscess.

After shaving the head, local anaesthetic solution with adrenaline is injected into the skin of the scalp. If the procedure is being done under general anaesthesia 1:200 000 adrenaline solution is used to assist haemostasis. An incision is now made down to bone, and the pericranium scraped away. A small self-retaining retractor is placed in the wound and the skull perforated using a brace and bit. A burr is now used to enlarge and smooth out the hole. Modern powered tools now combine these functions. The dura is now exposed, picked up with a sharp hook, and opened using a cruciate incision.

In the temporal and occipital sites, the overlying muscle additionally requires incision and retraction in order to expose the skull.

## Craniotomy

A flap of skin and skull is formed which is replaced over the defect at the end of the procedure.

The line of incision is marked out and infiltrated with a solution of local anaesthetic and adrenaline in saline. The scalp incision is made with the assistant compressing the scalp against the skull to reduce bleeding, and artery forceps or clamps are then applied to the scalp edges to prevent further bleeding. The scalp flap is elevated, and the lines of incision in the skull marked by diathermy. The pericranium is incised and scraped away from the lines of incision.

Burrholes are now made, and using a guide, a Gigli saw (Fig. 22.28) is passed under the skull between two burrholes, and the skull divided through between these points. The procedure is repeated until the bone has been completely separated from the skull. A small muscle attachment is usually left to carry the blood supply to the skull flap.

Bleeding from the exposed dura is controlled by diathermy or gelatin packs, or by dural traction achieved by suturing the periphery of the dura to the pericranium around the defect (Fig. 22.29). Raised intracranial pressure, evidenced by a tight dura, may be reduced by mannitol or by ventricular puncture.

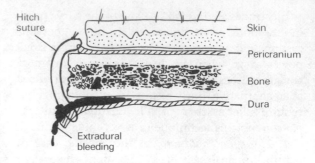

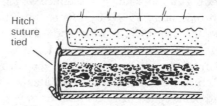

**Fig. 22.29** Control of dural bleeding with 'hitch' sutures

The dura is then opened after elevation on a small hook, and the incision extended by scissors, the brain being protected by a small swab.

## Craniectomy

In urgent situations such as the removal of an intracranial haematoma, there may not be time to 'turn a flap'. A single burrhole is made, and extended by piecemeal excision of the skull using bone forceps, making a defect referred to as a craniectomy. Such defects may be corrected at a later date by insertion of a plastic or metal mould-*cranioplasty*.

Craniectomy is always used for posterior fossa exploration, as the thick posterior neck muscles cover the defect without unsightliness.

## Laminectomy

Exposure of the spinal cord and nerves is achieved by partial or complete laminectomy.

The skin and underlying muscles are infiltrated down to the laminae with saline, adrenaline and local anaesthetic, and an incision made down to the spinous processes. A self-retaining retractor is inserted, and the paraspinal muscles separated from the processes and lamina and retracted using a larger self-retaining retractor (Fig. 22.30).

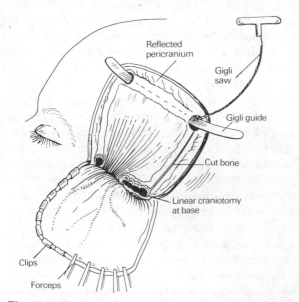

**Fig. 22.28** Turning a flap

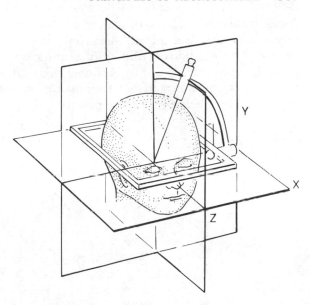

**Fig. 22.31** Principles of stereotactic apparatus

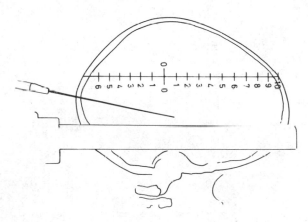

**Fig. 22.32** Stereotactic probe introduced to target

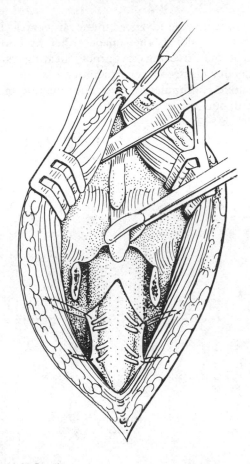

**Fig. 22.30** Laminectomy

The spinal processes over the desired length of spine are removed at their bases, and the lamina removed with bone rongeurs, while the underlying spinal dura is protected. The dura is incised longitudinally, and the cut edges sutured to the muscles.

In *partial laminectomies*, or *hemilaminectomies*, the spinal processes are preserved, while the lamina on one side is removed. In *fenestration procedures* for the removal of a prolapsed intervertebral disc, the ligamentum flavum at the appropriate site is opened, often aided by removal of a small piece of adjoining lamina, to expose the disc and nerve root.

## Stereotactic surgery

First used in the experimental animal in 1906, and introduced into clinical practice in 1947, stereotactic surgery is being increasingly used in neurosurgery, and justifies separate description.

Though the apparatus employed may seem complex, the underlying principles are simple, enabling the operator to determine the position of a point in space relative to a known reference point or points. Most stereotactic frames employ the Cartesian co-ordinate system with three mutually perpendicular planes (see Fig. 22.31). The position of a point in space can be defined in all three planes, and a probe moved precisely to that point.

The instrument is securely fastened to the skull (or spine) and using specially constructed brain or spinal stereotactic atlases, the co-ordinates of the target area are determined. Accuracy may be improved by injection of radio-opaque substances to outline the ventricles, or by obtaining electrical recordings from known areas. Under fluoroscopy, on which a measuring grid also appears, the tip of the probe may be advanced to the target area (Fig. 22.32). A lesion is then made either by cutting (leucotome), freezing (cryoprobe), heating (radio-frequency electrode), or irradiation (isotope). Alternatively, stimulating electrodes may be introduced, and left in situ if required.

# 23. The Neck

## SWELLINGS OF THE NECK

Neck swellings are classified in Table 23.1.

**Table 23.1** Classification of neck swellings (other than skin, subcutaneous tissues and lipomas)

*Midline swellings*
sublingual dermoid
thyroglossal cyst
pretracheal lymph node
subhyoid bursa
nodule in thyroid isthmus

*Lateral swellings*
1. *Anterior triangle*
   lymph nodes
   enlargement of submandibular salivary gland
   phargyngeal diverticulum
   laryngocele
   branchial cyst
   lesion lower pole parotid
2. *Posterior triangle*
   lymph nodes
   carotid body tumour
   cystic hygroma
   cervical rib

## CONGENITAL ABNORMALITIES

The mandibular region and neck develop from a series of five branchial arches during the first month of embryonic life. Each arch consists of a mesenchymal core covered by ectoderm and lined by endoderm. The arches are separated externally by four branchial clefts matched by internal evaginations, the pharyngeal pouches (Fig.23.1).

## BRANCHIAL CYST AND FISTULA

*Branchial cysts* are believed to arise from the second and third branchial arches. They are usually lined by stratified squamous epithelium but occasionally by cuboidal or ciliated columnar epithelium, suggesting that more than one developmental abnormality may result in sequestration of epithelium within the neck.

Despite its congenital origin, a branchial cyst is rarely evident before adolescence or early adult life. It presents as a deep-seated painless swelling, bulging forwards from the anterior border of the sterno-mastoid muscle at the level of the hyoid bone (Fig.23.2). The cyst may lie on either side of the neck and may on occasion be bilateral. The swelling is characteristically soft with the feel of a 'half-filled hot water bottle'. It contains opaque watery or milky fluid in which cholesterol crystals are suspended. As they contain lymphoid tissue in their walls, branchial cysts are prone to infection which tends to be recurrent. They then become tense, attached and may occasionally discharge the cyst contents to the surface.

A *branchial fistula* is less common than a branchial cyst. The external opening is usually situated at the anterior border of the lower third of the sternomastoid muscle. The fistulous track courses upwards in the line of the common carotid artery to enter the pharynx internally at the tonsillar fossa. The fistula is present at birth and intermittent mucopurulent discharge from the external opening is common.

Branchial cysts should be excised for cosmetic reasons and to prevent infective complications. A transverse incision is used. Complete removal of all epithelium is necessary to prevent recurrence and general anaesthesia is essential to allow adequate exposure.

Branchial fistulas are also excised under general anaesthesia. Complete excision of the track is

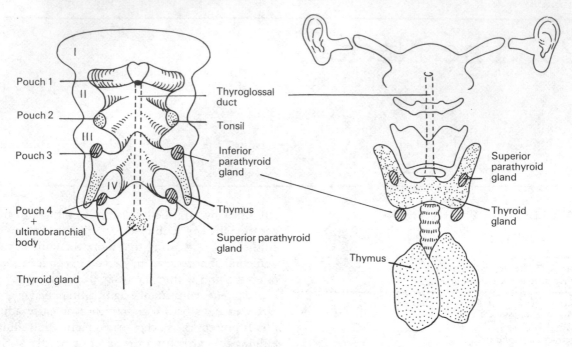

**Fig. 23.1** Embryological development of the branchial region

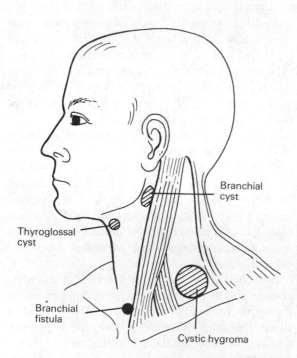

**Fig. 23.2** Surgical anatomy of the neck showing common locations for development of neck swellings due to congenital abnormalities

essential if recurrence is to be avoided and a series of horizontal 'step ladder' incisions are usually required. Some surgeons inject methylene blue into the track to aid identification.

## THYROGLOSSAL CYST

The thyroid gland develops from the embryonic thyroglossal duct (Fig.23.3). The duct commences as a median diverticulum from the floor of the developing pharynx, immediately caudal to the tuberculum impar from which the anterior two-thirds of the tongue will arise. In adult life the origin of the thyroglossal duct is marked by a small depression, the foramen caecum, on the dorsal surface of the tongue. The thyroglossal duct grows caudally as a midline blind tubular duct which finally bifurcates and gives rise to solid masses of cells which form the isthmus and both lobes of the thyroid gland. In its descent, the thyroglossal duct passes through the region in which the body of the hyoid bone is developing.

The duct normally fragments and disappears early in fetal life. Persistence of any part can give rise to aberrant masses of thyroid tissue or to thyroglossal cysts or fistulae in the midline of the neck.

excised. If there is doubt a thyroid scan is ordered before surgery is undertaken.

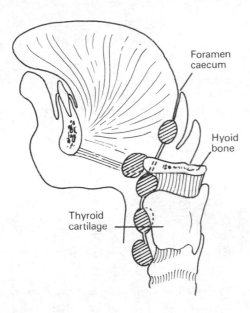

**Fig. 23.3** Diagrammatic representation of the course of the thyroglossal duct and location of thyroglossal cysts

Thyroglossal cysts are the commonest congenital abnormalities of the neck. Although present at birth they may not be noted until adolescence or even early adult life, when they present as a painless smooth and rounded swelling in the midline of the neck. The swelling is usually situated between the thyroid isthmus and the hyoid bone but may rarely be found between the hyoid and the base of the tongue. The swelling is dense and rubbery in consistency and may transilluminate. Fluctuation is seldom elicited. The cyst always moves upwards when the patient swallows or protrudes his tongue. If the contents of a thyroglossal cyst become infected and discharge to the surface, a permanent sinus track will form. A true thyroglossal fistula is rare.

Thyroglossal cysts should be excised to prevent complications and disfigurement. General anaesthesia is required and the body of the hyoid bone may have to be removed so that the thyroglossal track can be cored out as far as the base of the tongue. An ectopic thyroid gland may be mistaken for a thyroglossal cyst. As this may be the only source of thyroid hormone it must not be

## DERMOID CYSTS

Dermoid cysts result from sequestration of epidermis during fusion of blocks of embryonal tissue. They are lined by squamous epithelium with epidermal appendages and contain cheesy material produced by desquamation of epithelial cells and sometimes contain hair. They present as painless swellings of the scalp and eyebrows, and in the midline of the nose, neck and upper chest. They are generally mobile and have a doughy consistency.

'Mucous cysts' may arise from similar inclusions of mucous membrane and occur deeper in the neck or in relation to the floor of the mouth. They are often also classified as 'dermoids'.

The common dermoids are as follows:

### Submental dermoid

This is situated beneath the chin in the midline, either within or superficial to the raphe of the mylohyoid muscles. Submental dermoids resemble thyroglossal cysts but do not move on swallowing or on protrusion of the tongue.

### Sublingual dermoid

This lies beneath the tongue, protruding into the floor of the mouth. Unlike a ranula it does not transilluminate.

Dermoid cysts should be excised for cosmetic reasons and to avoid infective complications. Complete excision is essential to prevent recurrence.

## CYSTIC HYGROMA

This benign tumour of infancy is a form of lymphangioma in which soft cystic masses arise as outpouchings from the developing lymphatic system. The multilocular cysts contain clear lymphatic fluid and are lined by endothelium.

The mass is usually situated at the base of the posterior triangle of the neck behind the sternomastoid muscle (see Fig.23.2). It may extend into the axilla or mediastinum where pressure symptoms can be caused.

The majority are present at birth, and almost all will appear within two years. The lesions can grow to great size and can cause problems during delivery. Sudden increase may result from rupture during coughing or haemorrhage into the cyst.

Cystic hygroma is also found in the floor of the mouth and may be a cause of macroglossia.

On clinical examination, the cysts are characteristically soft and transilluminate readily. Small lesions may resolve spontaneously but larger lesions require surgical excision. It is not now considered wise to delay operation until the child is older as removal becomes more difficult with time. Airway obstruction, repeated inflammation or rapid enlargement are urgent indications for excision.

The aim of surgery is to remove the whole tumour mass with ligation of any divided lymphatic trunks. Complete tumour removal is not always possible as small peripheral cysts merge into surrounding normal tissues.

## STERNOMASTOID TUMOUR (CONGENITAL TORTICOLLIS)

This consists of a non-tender, hard, fusiform swelling of the lower portion of the sternomastoid muscle on one side of the neck. It may be present at birth but frequently escapes notice for some weeks.

The tumour results from ischaemic fibrosis of the sternomastoid muscle during a birth injury, and approximately one-third of children affected are breech deliveries. The tumour may resolve or progress to fibrosis with shortening of the affected muscle so that the mastoid process is pulled down towards the shoulder and the head tilted to the opposite side (Fig. 23.4). Uncorrected, the deformity becomes permanent. The child attempts to compensate by raising the shoulder on the affected side thus producing secondary cervical and thoracic scoliosis. Facial asymmetry develops later.

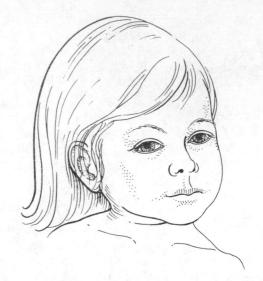

**Fig. 23.4** Deformity resulting from untreated sternomastoid tumour

Permanent deformity can be avoided by forcible rotation of the head and neck through a full range of movement several times daily. If this does not suffice the two heads of the shortened muscle should be divided above the clavicle taking care not to injure adjacent structures. The sternomastoid tumour need not be excised.

## CUT THROAT

The majority of wounds are self-inflicted. The neck is often extended during wounding so that the main blood vessels are protected from the path of the incising instrument by taut muscles. On the other hand the number of vital structures within the neck leads to a high risk of serious injury. Major vessels within the carotid sheath may be opened, the cranial nerves or brachial plexus may be torn, the trachea and even the oesophagus can be severed, and the thoracic duct may be damaged.

*Damage to the airway* poses an immediate threat to life. Aspiration of inhaled blood and secretions should be carried out urgently, and endotracheal intubation, or tracheostomy may be needed.

*Haemorrhage* requires urgent control and is the commonest cause of death following cut throat. The bleeding is frequently venous and usually follows damage to the external jugular rather than the internal jugular vein. Straining and struggling increase venous bleeding and the patient should be nursed in a slightly head-up position to reduce venous pressure. Air embolus may follow the sucking of air into the open vein should the patient be allowed to sit up or stand. Internal bleeding after a stab injury can produce subfascial haematomas, compression of neck structures and sudden haemorrhage into a pleural space.

*Infection* may complicate all forms of penetrating trauma and may be introduced by the wounding instrument or from within following penetration of the pharynx, oesophagus or upper respiratory tract. For these reasons operative treatment is essential in all wounds of the neck which penetrate the platysma. Careful wound toilet and formal surgical repair of damaged structures with adequate drainage are important steps. A broad-spectrum antibiotic should be prescribed if there is contamination or if the oesophagus or respiratory passages have been penetrated.

## ACUTE INFECTIONS IN THE NECK

Spread in cervical fascial planes is a dangerous complication of acute infections involving the neck and it is important to have a working knowledge of the fascial investments and spaces.

### The superficial cervical fascia

This is a thin lamina investing the platysma and is barely demonstrable as a separate layer. It has no surgical importance.

### The deep cervical fascia

This lies beneath the platysma, invests the neck muscles, and has considerable importance surgically (Fig. 23.5).

*The investing layer* of the deep fascia passes from the ligamentum nuchae and seventh cervical spine to invest the trapezius, crosses the posterior triangle to invest the sternomastoid, and then continues across the anterior triangle to merge with the corresponding layer from the other side.

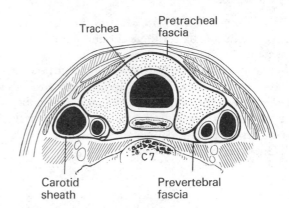

**Fig. 23.5** Diagrammatic transverse section of the neck at level of seventh cervical vertebra to show the arrangement of the deep fascia

*The carotid sheath* is a condensation of the deep cervical fascia which encloses the common and internal carotid arteries, the internal jugular vein, the vagus nerve and the ansa cervicalis. *The prevertebral lamina* of the cervical fascia covers the prevertebral muscles, then extends laterally to cover the scalene muscles as a floor for the posterior triangle. The nerves of the brachial plexus carry this fascia down behind the clavicle as the axillary sheath.

*The retropharyngeal space*. Anteriorly the vertebral fascia is separated from the pharynx by the retropharyngeal space which contains loose areolar tissue. *The pretracheal lamina* of the cervical fascia forms a thin fascial sheath which encloses the thyroid gland and attaches it superiorly to the arch of the cricoid cartilage.

The investing layer of the cervical fascia opposes the spread of infection superficially and enclosed pus tends to spread within these facial planes. Pus in the anterior triangle may spread down into the mediastinum in front of the pretracheal lamina, but the investing layer is relatively thin over this area and abscesses may point to the surface above the sternum. Pus behind the prevertebral lamina may track laterally from the spine to point in the posterior triangle, or may penetrate anteriorly to occupy the retropharyngeal space and bulge into the pharynx.

## SUPERFICIAL INFECTIONS

Superficial boils (furuncles) are common on the back of the neck and often result from minor abrasions associated with wearing a collar. Infection begins in a hair follicle and the overlying skin becomes reddened before it turns white and necrotic. Erythema, induration, pain and tenderness are common, but lymphadenitis and systemic signs of infection are rare. Most boils discharge spontaneously but incision and drainage may be required. Diabetes must be excluded if the problem is recurrent.

## Carbuncles

These also begin with hair follicle infection but this spreads to involve the dermis and subcutaneous tissues. Many of the infected extensions open to the surface as multiple discharging sinuses. There is death of the central portion of the carbuncle and a black necrotic core develops. Carbuncles are usually more extensive than their surface appearance suggests and wide excision is needed to remove all infected sinus tracts. The patient is often febrile and toxic, may prove to be diabetic, and requires antibiotics in addition to surgery.

## DEEP INFECTION

Deep cervical infections arise from a primary focus in the mouth, salivary glands, pharynx, oesophagus or larynx. Cellulitis can spread rapidly and widely beneath the investing layer of the deep cervical fascia to invove the mediastinum or compress the trachea and larynx by oedema.

*Ludwig's angina* is the term applied to infection involving the floor of the mouth and often arising from a submandibular lymph gland. There is frequently a history of faulty oral hygiene and the patient presents with swelling in the floor of the mouth or suprahyoid region of the neck, protrusion of the tongue, trismus, difficulty in speech, dysphagia and dyspnoea. Treatment consists of antibiotic therapy, bearing in mind that the organism responsible is usually a haemolytic streptococcus. Surgical incision and drainage is needed if there is any evidence of compression of respiratory or vascular structures, or oedema and fever persist for more than a few days despite energetic antibiotic therapy. Tracheostomy is required if there is airway obstruction. Future problems are avoided by attention to dental and oral hygeine and eradication of any continued focus of infection.

## CERVICAL LYMPHADENOPATHY

The neck contains many lymph nodes. Lymph from the head and neck drains into outlying groups of nodes and from there into the deep cervical chain. This chain lies in association with the carotid sheath deep to the sternomastoid muscle and receives the majority of lymphatic drainage from the head and neck. The groups of nodes and their drainage areas are shown in Fig.23.6.

Disorders affecting the cervical lymph nodes are:

*Infective*:
acute (pyogenic)lymphadenitis
chronic (granulomatous)lymphadenitis
*Neoplastic*:
primary lymphoreticular neoplasia
secondary carcinoma

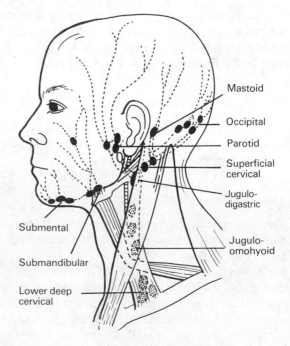

**Fig. 23.6** The lymph nodes of the head and neck

# INFECTIVE LYMPHADENOPATHY

## ACUTE LYMPHADENITIS

Infection arising at any site within the lymphatic drainage area of the cervical nodes may produce secondary cervical lymphadenitis. Staphylococcal and streptococcal infections are usually responsible. The affected nodes become enlarged and tender and the lymphadenitis often overshadows the signs and symptoms of the primary infection. Pyrexia is often marked and the systemic upset can be considerable. The lymphadenitis may settle spontaneously or progress to suppuration, spreading cellulitis and oedema. The most commonly affected nodes are the upper deep cervical (jugulodigastric) and submandibular nodes due to infection in the mouth, teeth or tonsils. Antibiotic therapy is given for severe or prolonged infections. If there is suppuration a 'collar-stud abscess' may produce a secondary subcutaneous loculus of pus and the overlying skin becomes red-hot and shiny (Fig. 23.7). Incision and drainage is indicated; the hole in the deep fascia is enlarged so that pus within the lymph node can be evacuated and drained.

## CHRONIC GRANULOMATOUS LYMPHADENITIS

Persisting infections of any type give rise to chronic cervical lymphadenitis. The term granulomatous lymphadenitis is reserved for specific infections by tuberculosis, other mycobacteria or syphilis.

### Tuberculosis

Tuberculosis of the cervical lymph nodes was common in Britain 30 years ago, usually due to infection with the human bacillus. Three types were recognised. An upper cervical (jugulodigas-tric) type associated with primary infection of the teeth or tonsil; a lower cervical (supraclavicular) type associated with a primary focus in the apex of a lung, and a generalised lymphadenopathy as part of miliary tuberculosis. Most infections were due to the human bacillus, the commonest form being that affecting the nodes of the upper neck. This condition is still seen occasionally.

The primary focus of infection is most commonly the teeth. Tubercles form in the upper deep cervical (jugulodigastric) nodes and are associated with hyperaemia and periadenitis. The lesions may resolve with fibrosis and calcification or progress to necrosis and caseation. With caseation the node breaks down and the caseous material penetrates the ensheathing layer of deep cervical fascia to produce a collar-stud abscess. The overlying skin becomes thinned and bluish-red but not hot (cold abscess).

Tuberculin testing will help establish the diagnosis. The younger the patient the greater the diagnostic significance of a positive test; repeated negative tests virtually exclude tuberculosis except in the elderly and those with severe miliary infection. Detection of calcification in the nodes on soft tissue radiology is a pointer to the diagnosis.

Treatment consists of antituberculous therapy and general measures to improve health. Local surgery is undertaken should the skin be threatened by abscess formation. Otherwise a sinus may occur and secondary infection by pyogenic organisms complicate the position. The abscess is evacuated and the opening in the deep fascia is enlarged so that all necrotic material can be curetted from the underlying lymph node. At one time excision of the infected lymph nodes was preferred but with the advent of antituberculous therapy this is now rarely practised. The wound is sutured without drainage so as to prevent secondary infection.

### Atypical mycobacterial lymphadenitis (Cat-scratch fever)

Children are commonly affected following a scratch or bite from a cat or kitten. There is acute fever and malaise accompanied by tender enlargement of regional lymph nodes. The nodes are firm but may caseate with cold abscess formation and development of a discharging sinus. Pulmonary

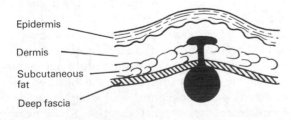

Epidermis

Dermis

Subcutaneous fat

Deep fascia

**Fig. 23.7** Collar-stud abscess

changes are rare. The tuberculin test is only weakly positive.

Treatment consists of rifampicin and if the infection is not controlled, the affected nodes are excised. Should caseation and sinus formation occur the sinus is excised and the underlying abscess is curetted.

## SYPHILIS

Cervical lymphadenitis due to syphilis is now rare. Enlarged lymph nodes in the submental or submandibular region were associated with a primary chancre of the lips or mouth, while generalised lymphadenopathy occurred in secondary syphilis.

## NEOPLASTIC LYMPHADENOPATHY

### PRIMARY LYMPHOMA

Cervical lymphadenopathy is often the first manifestation of lymphoma. For example, the patient with Hodgkins' lymphoma frequently presents with painless, discrete and rubbery nodes in the lower portion of the posterior triangle. Cervical node biopsy is required and the lymph node should be sent fresh to the histopathological department so that receptor status as well as histopathology can be determined (see p. 552).

### SECONDARY CARCINOMA

Secondary involvement of lymph nodes by metastatic tumour can occur as a result of spread from a primary tumour at any site. The affected lymph nodes are hard and often fixed to neighbouring nodes and adjacent tissues.

If the site of the primary tumour is not readily apparent it is most likely to be situated in the nasopharynx or oropharynx and thorough examination of these areas is essential. The neck and chest are X-rayed and if necessary general anaesthesia is given to allow thorough palpation and visualisation of the mouth, tongue, tonsils, nasopharynx and respiratory passages. Carcinoma arising in the stomach, lung or breast may spread to cervical nodes, particularly those of supraclavicular region. In head and neck cancer, involvement of regional lymph nodes does not imply that the disease has disseminated widely and combinations of surgery and radiotherapy may effect longstanding cure. On the other hand, involvement of cervical nodes in cancer arising in chest, breast or abdomen implies widespread dissemination and therapies become palliative rather than curative.

## CHEMODECTOMA

A chemodectoma (or carotid body tumour) is a rare cervical tumour. It is more common in places of high altitude (e.g. Peru or Mexico City), possibly because chronic hypoxia leads to carotid body hyperplasia. The tumour is a paraganglioma which arises from chemoreceptor cells within the carotid body. These are not hormonally active. Metastasis is exceptional.

There may be a familial history particularly in patients with bilateral tumours. Males and females are equally affected, the average age of presentation being in the fifth decade. The history is of a slow-growing deeply seated mass in the region of the carotid bifurcation. Characteristically the mass has some lateral but no vertical mobility. It can be felt bimanually when a finger is placed in the floor of the mouth. It may transmit pulsation but is not truly expansile. Symptoms from pressure on nearby nerves include pain in the neck or ear and hoarseness. The carotid sinus syndrome of dizziness and syncope may develop subsequently. Carotid angiograms may show lateral displacement or separation of the carotid bifurcation and a striking tumour vascularity. The angiogram also allows assessment of the adequacy of the cerebral collateral circulation.

Detection of a chemodectoma is not necessarily an indication for surgical removal, particularly in the elderly where operation can compromise the cerebral circulation. In healthy younger patients excision should be performed. The plane of dissection lies between the adventitia and media of the carotid. With care vessel continuity can be preserved. If this is not possible a temporary arterial by-pass is used while the bifurcation is resected. An autogenous vein graft is used to reconstruct the internal carotid. Radiotherapy may be of value in non-operable tumours.

# 24. Salivary Glands

## SURGICAL ANATOMY

### PAROTID GLAND

The parotid gland lies in a recess bounded by the ramus of the mandible, the base of the skull and the mastoid process (Fig. 24.1). It lies on the carotid sheath and the IXth–XIIth cranial nerves, and extends forwards over the masseter muscle. The gland is enclosed in a sheath of dense deep cervical fascia, which superficially is reinforced by platysma, making its palpation difficult. Its upper pole extends to just below the zygoma, its lower pole into the neck. The facial nerve and its branches pierce the gland and pass forwards superficial to the posterior facial vein. This 'neurovenous plane' is of surgical importance in that it divides the parotid into superficial and deep lobes.

A single duct runs from the front of the gland below and parallel to the zygomatic process. Its surface markings correspond to the middle third of a line drawn from the inferior edge of the external meatus to midway between the ala of the nose and commissure of upper lip. At the anterior border of the masseter it pierces the buccinator muscle to open into the mouth opposite the second upper molar tooth. Its anterior portion can be palpated bimanually and is readily catheterised (Fig. 24.2).

The parotid gland contains two groups of lymph nodes:

1. *the superficial pre-auricular nodes* lie immediately in front of the tragus and drain lymph from the temporal and frontal regions of the scalp, the outer eyelids and external ear; and

2. *the parotid nodes* are embedded within the

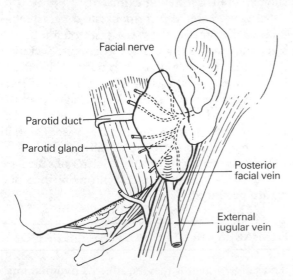

Fig. 24.1 Anatomical relationships of facial nerve

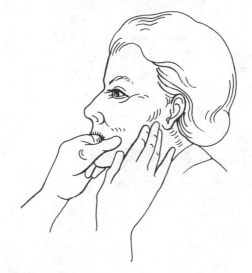

Fig. 24.2 Bimanual palpation of parotid duct

substance of the gland and drain the upper part of the nasopharynx, the soft palate and the middle ear. The gland is supplied by the auriculotemporal nerve with parasympathetic secretomotor, sympathetic vasomotor and sensory nerves.

## SUBMANDIBULAR GLAND

The submandibular (submaxillary) gland lies partly below and partly deep to the body of the mandible (Fig. 24.3). It overlaps both bellies of the digastric muscle and rests from before back on the mylohyoid, hyoglossus and pharyngeal wall. It is covered by a capsule of cervical fascia and has a deep extension between the mylohyoid and hyoglossus muscles. A duct runs forward from the deep extension to open on a visible papilla in the floor of the mouth at the side of the frenulum of the tongue (Fig. 24.4). The facial artery is closely related to the gland. It ascends in a groove at its posterior end, runs down and laterally deep to the mandible, and then crosses its lower edge at the anterior border of the masseter to enter the face. The duct intertwines with the lingual nerve, and the hypoglossal nerve runs just below the duct. Both nerves must be seen and preserved during removal of the gland. Lymph nodes draining the lateral part of the tongue and floor of mouth lie in close apposition to the gland.

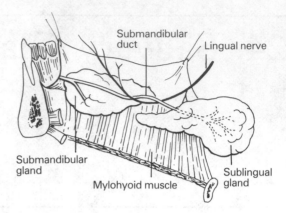

Fig. 24.4 Relationships of submandibular duct

## SURGICAL PHYSIOLOGY

Saliva has important mechanical functions; it facilitates mastication, swallowing and speech, and helps to dilute irritants in food. Although saliva contains amylase, its digestive function is negligible in man.

Saliva is secreted by the main pairs of glands, the parotid, submandibular (submaxillary) and sublingual. There are many small accessory glands beneath the buccal and palatal mucosa which secrete mucus. All of the salivary glands secrete a mixture of serous and mucous fluid but the proportions of the two differ. Parotid secretion is predominantly serous, sublingual secretion is mainly mucous, and submandibular secretion is mixed.

Saliva is secreted in response to a parasympathetic reflex initiated by the taste of food. The sight and smell of food may also initiate secretion but the importance of such conditioned reflexes has been overemphasised. The sympathetic nervous system innervates myo-epithelial cells in the salivary glands and also contributes to salivation. Local release of bradykinin causes vasodilatation which may aid in secretion of saliva.

Most texts indicate that 1–1.5 litres of saliva are produced daily, but in reality no more than 500 ml are produced.

## DISEASES OF THE SALIVARY GLANDS

The salivary glands may be affected by inflammation, obstruction and tumour. Tumours and

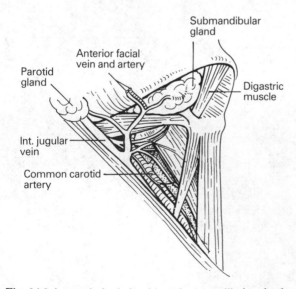

Fig. 24.3 Anatomical relationships of submandibular gland

inflammation without obstruction affect mainly the parotid, obstruction with inflammation the submandibular gland.

Because of their fascial covering, exact palpation of the salivary glands is difficult. Change in the contour of the face may be the only sign of parotid enlargement. Radiology is used to demonstrate opaque calculi and gland calcification, and the duct system can be visualised following cannulation and injection of a few ml of contrast material (Fig. 24.5). In a normal 'sialogram' the arborisations of the ducts are fine, regular and symmetrically distributed. Abnormalities include displacement, distortion, stricture, dilatation and sacculation (sialectasis).

Salivary secretions can be collected for analysis

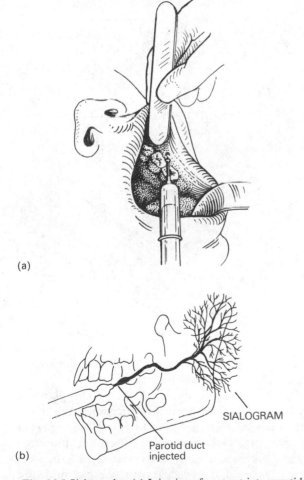

(a)

(b)

SIALOGRAM

Parotid duct
injected

**Fig. 24.5** Sialography. (a) Injection of contrast into parotid duct. (b) Parotid sialogram.

by asking the patient to spit into a container, by inserting small intraoral cups, or by cannulation of a duct. The volumetric response to a cholinergic stimulus, e.g. pilocarpine, can be measured and ionic constituents estimated.

Recently it has been found that unbound (unconjugated) steroids are secreted into the saliva in similar concentrations to those in plasma. Their measurement by radioimmunoassay may prove a useful investigation, particularly in children.

## TRAUMA TO THE SALIVARY GLANDS

The parotid gland or its duct may be damaged by facial lacerations. Damage to the gland usually causes no particular problems but duct trauma may lead to a parotid fistula or duct stricture. Awareness of the possibilty of damage to the duct followed by careful exploration of the wound and reconstitution of the duct, if damaged, are important

### Post-gustatory sweating (Frey's syndrome)

An unusual complication of parotid surgery or injury is sweating and flushing in the distribution of the auriculotemporal nerve during eating. This follows injury to the auriculotemporal nerve with subsequent aberrant regrowth of parotid parasympathetic secretomotor fibres to supply sympathetic end-organs to the skin (Fig. 24.6). The condition can be treated by division of the tympanic nerve and chorda tympani which carry the secretomotor fibres.

## INFLAMMATION OF THE SALIVARY GLANDS

### Acute parotitis

The parotid duct is normally flushed continuously by flow of secretion. Ascending infection is likely if flow becomes depressed in the elderly, debilitated and dehydrated, or following administration of anticholingeric drugs. Poor oral hygiene is an important precipitating factor. In a surgical ward the gland is most vulnerable in the postoperative period, usually in the second postoperative week. Staphylococcal infection is usually responsible and

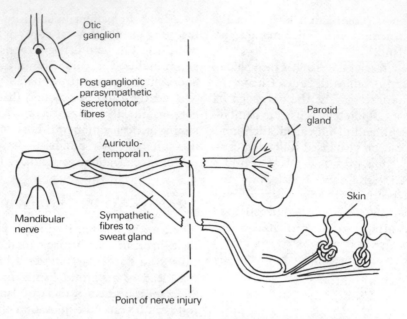

**Fig. 24.6** Cause of postgustatory sweating (Frey's syndrome). After damage to the auriculo-temporal nerve, regrowth of postganglionic fibres has been misdirected into sympathetic nerve fibres supplying skin

causes widespread patchy inflammation leading to honeycomb abscess formation.

Because the gland cannot readily expand, pain is severe. Systemic upset is marked and the patient has a swinging temperature. The parotid is tender and diffusely enlarged, forming a smooth convex swelling in front of the ear which overlies the angle of the jaw and fills the normal regional hollows. The skin becomes stretched, shiny and reddened, and trismus is marked. The duct orifice is red and patulous and there may be a purulent discharge. Gentle 'milking' pressure on the gland may evoke a gush of pus from the duct. A bacteriological swab should be taken.

*Treatment of acute parotitis.* Prophylaxis is critical. All elderly and debilitated patients who require surgery must have frequent mouthwashes and have their gums painted with a viscous antiseptic (bromoglycerol). They are encouraged to masticate, and acid drops or chewing gum are helpful stimulants to salivation. Adequate hydration must be maintained.

Should acute parotitis be suspected the patient is given full doses of a broad-spectrum antibiotic. If improvement is not marked by 48 hours and systemic signs persist, the gland should be surgi-

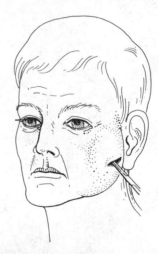

**Fig. 24.7** Drainage of a parotid abscess

cally decompressed. Signs of abscess formation are late and must not be waited for.

Decompression and drainage of the gland is achieved through a horizontal incision in the line of the body of the mandible and parallel to the facial nerve (Fig. 24.7). Forceps are used to explore the gland for pus. Drains are inserted and the skin loosely closed. Recovery is usually rapid following decompression.

## Recurrent pyogenic parotitis

Infection of the parotid with organisms of low pathogenicity (*Streptococcus viridans or pneumococcus*) can lead to recurrent attacks of subacute inflammation. A typical attack starts during a meal, the gland becoming diffusely swollen and tender. The whole gland is involved and enlarged, an important point in differentiation from parotid neoplasia. Resolution may take weeks and shrinkage of the gland follows the passage of purulent 'snowstorm' saliva. A sialogram shows clubbing and dilatation of ductules throughout the whole gland.

Treatment consists of appropriate antibiotic therapy following culture of the saliva, good oral hygiene, and instructing the patient to massage the gland forwards periodically to milk out retained secretions.

It is important to ensure that there is no duct obstruction. The duct orifice is carefully examined for obstruction by a food fragment, small calculus, ill-fitting dentures or impinging mucosal lesion. If in doubt, the duct should be explored with a fine cannula or probe, and a sialogram ordered.

## Autoimmune parotitis

The salivary glands may be chronically and symmetrically enlarged as a result of fibrosis and infiltration with lymphoid tissue, a process which also affects the lacrimal glands and the submucous glands of the mouth and upper respiratory tract. Originally described by Mickulicz, it results in cessation of secretion and a dry mouth (xerostomia) and eye (keratoconjunctivitis sicca). When associated with rheumatoid arthritis it is called Sjogren's syndrome. Tuberculosis, sarcoidosis and lymphoma must also be considered as possible causes of chronic diffuse enlargement.

## SALIVARY CALCULI

Salivary calculi are composed of calcium carbonate and phosphate, and are therefore radio-opaque. They may contain mucus, bacteria or a foreign body (e.g. toothbrush bristle) in their centre. They are most common in the submandibular gland or duct. This is believed to be due to the upward course of the submandibular duct with resulting stasis, and the higher concentration of solids in its mixed secretions. Calculus formation is more frequent in males.

The shape of a stone depends on the site of its formation. A small stone which travels along the duct and impacts at the orifice is round, but should it be trapped proximally within the duct system it becomes oval and shaped like a 'date-stone'. Some calculi remain within the gland and have a comma-shaped projection into the duct.

The stone obstructs salivary flow leading to gland enlargement which is initially intermittent and occurs during salivation. With the establishment of inflammation and fibrosis, the gland becomes permanently enlarged and solid. Occasionally a patient complains of colicky pain in the floor of the mouth. The commonest symptom is that of swelling and discomfort under the jaw during and after a meal.

The gland must be carefully palpated to detect enlargement. This is best done from behind, running the fingers backward under the ramus of the jaw. If one cannot feel the gland the patient should be asked to suck a sour sweet or drop of lemon juice and re-examined.

Bimanual palpation of the gland is performed from in front (Fig. 24.8). The fingers of one hand are placed over the gland while the index finger of the other hand is inserted into the mouth on the inner surface of the mandible and run back below and medial to its ramus.

The duct orifice is examined for redness or swelling (Fig. 24.9). Occasionally pus is seen to exude or an impacted stone may be visible. A lacrimal probe can be used to detect small stones at the orifice.

An intra-oral X-ray is ordered to demonstrate the duct and gland and show radio-opaque stones.

The treatment of a submandibular calculus depends on its site, and whether the gland is chronically enlarged. A stone in the intra-oral portion of the duct is removed through the floor of the mouth under general anaesthesia (Fig. 24.10). However, when the stone is impacted within the gland or when the gland is chronically enlarged,

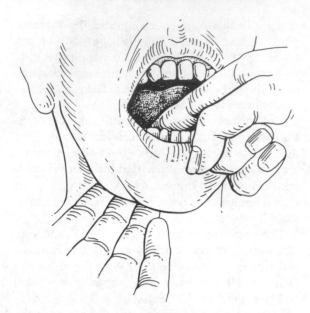

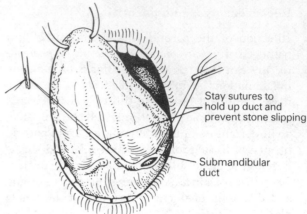

Fig. 24.10 Removal of stone from submandibular duct in the floor of the mouth

**Fig. 24.8** Bimanual palpation of submandibular gland and duct

# SALIVARY GLAND NEOPLASIA

Approximately 80% of all neoplasms of the major salivary glands are found in the parotid. The great majority of parotid tumours (roughly 85%) are benign. About half of the tumours arising in the submandibular gland are benign, and the majority of tumours of the minor salivary glands are malignant.

The great majority of benign tumours are pleomorphic adenomas. Muco-epidermoid and adenoid cystic types are now generally regarded as malignant neoplasms.

## PLEOMORPHIC SALIVARY ADENOMA (MIXED TUMOURS)

A mixed salivary tumour is an adenoma with a wide variety of histological features. It is composed primarily of epithelial glandular tissue which contains irregular spaces. In the mucoepidermoid type, epidermoid characteristics predominate and there is stratification and prickle cell formation. The epithelial elements form a mucous matrix thought originally to be cartilage and responsible for the term 'mixed salivary tumour'. There is a dense collagenous stroma, which may enclose tubules of epithelium (the so-called cylindroma) and form a dense capsule. The capsule is incomplete and portions of neoplastic

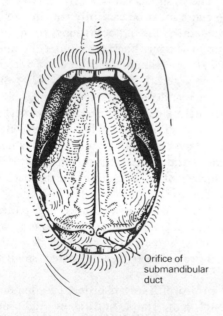

**Fig. 24.9** Site of orifice of submandibular duct

the whole gland must be removed. This is performed through an external approach, care being taken to avoid damage to the mandibular branch of the facial nerve, the lingual nerve and the hypoglossal nerve.

epithelial tissue project into the surrounding salivary tissue.

## Pleomorphic adenoma of the parotid gland

The superficial portion of the parotid gland is predominantly affected but no salivary tissue is immune. For every 100 tumours of the parotid there are 10 affecting the submandibular gland, 10 affecting the minor salivary glands (half of which are palatal), and one affecting the sublingual gland. They are found most frequently in adults of either sex aged 30–50 years. No racial differences have been described and there is no known association with antecedent disease.

The growth rate of mixed salivary tumours is extraordinarily slow and they may reach gigantic proportions. They are not frankly malignant and do not invade or metastasize. However there is a high incidence of recurrence if the lesion is incompletely excised.

Usually the patient presents with a firm swelling in the lower part of the parotid gland (Fig. 24.11). A tumour arising from the lower pole of the gland feels surprisingly superficial and 'separate' and may be mistaken for a simple dermoid or sebaceous cyst (Fig. 24.12).

## Treatment of pleomorphic parotid adenoma

Local excision or enucleation of mixed salivary tumours is associated with a high recurrence rate, although this can be reduced by postoperative radiotherapy (Fig. 24.13). Most surgeons now consider that it is better to remove that portion of the parotid which lies superficial to the facial nerve (superficial parotidectomy). The key to successful completion of this operation is definition of the facial nerve where it enters the gland and careful preservation of its branches. In expert hands the operation gives excellent results.

## Pleomorphic adenomas in other salivary glands

A mixed tumour affecting the submandibular gland forms a hard nodular swelling of the gland.

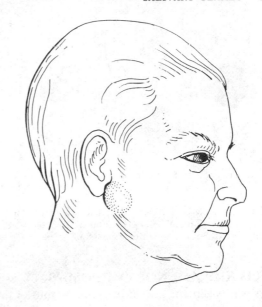

**Fig. 24.11** Typical mixed tumour of the parotid

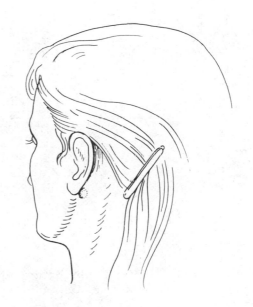

**Fig. 24.12** A diagnostic trap – a 'sebaceous' cyst at the lower angle of the jaw which is in fact a mixed parotid tumour

The entire gland should be removed. Tumours of ectopic salivary tissue occur within the mouth, particularly on the palate and form a lobular firm submucous swelling. They are commonly of cylindromatous type and particularly prone to recur. They should be excised widely and adjuvant radiotherapy considered.

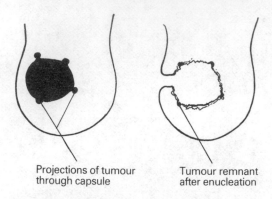

Projections of tumour
through capsule

Tumour remnant
after enucleation

**Fig. 24.13** Enucleation of parotid tumour: the reason for recurrence. (a) Tumour before enucleation. (b) Projections of tumour tissue remaining after enucleation

## SALIVARY ADENOLYMPHOMAS

This is a rare benign solid or cystic tumour of the parotid which may affect males late in life. It is slow-growing and characteristically soft when cystic. Such tumours contain creamy material and epithelial elements which may form papillary projections and which are associated with a mixed lymphoid stroma. The tumour feels superficial and is freely mobile. Some believe that it arises from heterotopic salivary tissue in lymph nodes.

## ANAPLASTIC CARCINOMA

Frankly malignant tumours of the parotid occur at a later age than mixed tumours, grow faster and invade surrounding tissues. They form a stony-hard fixed mass which is associated with pain in temple and scalp corresponding to the distribution of the auriculotemporal nerve. Facial palsy due to invasion of the facial nerve is typical. Complete surgical removal, combined with radiotherapy, offers the only hope of cure but is rarely possible.

# 25. Face, Mouth and Tongue

## CONGENITAL ABNORMALITIES

### CLEFT LIP AND CLEFT PALATE

The upper lip and palate form by fusion of the median *premaxillary process* with the lateral *maxillary processes* (Fig. 25.1). The developing palate becomes confluent with the lower border of the midline primitive nasal septum. Failure of fusion of their component parts gives rise to cleft lip, cleft palate, or some combination of the two in approximately 1 in 1000 live births. The reasons for failure of fusion are unknown, but for some reason cleft lip alone is commoner in males while cleft palate alone is commoner in females. Clefts of the palate are found in 40% of children born with the Pierre Robin syndrome, a congenital abnormality characterised by a small mandible, backward displacement of the chin, and a tendency of the tongue to prolapse into and occlude the pharynx.

Rarer congenital abnormalities of the face and lips include aplasia or hypoplasia of the premaxillary process (the true hare-lip as seen in rodents), median clefts of the lower lip due to failure of fusion of the two parts of the mandibular (first branchial) arch, and lateral clefts of the face extending from the angle of the mouth (macrostoma).

By definition, the *primary palate* consists of the upper lip and alveolar ridge, while the *secondary palate* comprises the definitive hard and soft palate. Clefts can thus be classified into *partial* or *complete* clefts of the primary or secondary palate or both (Fig. 25.2). Partial midline clefts of the secondary palate may involve both hard and soft

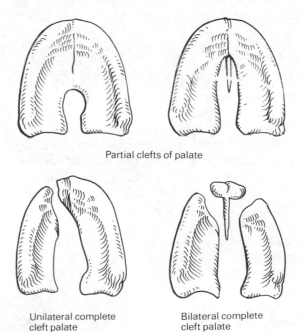

Partial clefts of palate

Unilateral complete cleft palate

Bilateral complete cleft palate

**Fig. 25.2** Types of cleft palate

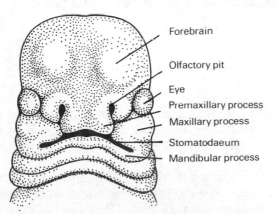

Forebrain

Olfactory pit

Eye
Premaxillary process
Maxillary process

Stomatodaeum
Mandibular process

**Fig. 25.1** The development of the lips and mouth

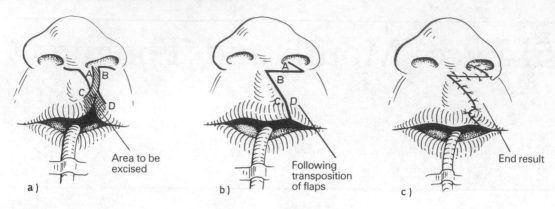

Fig. 25.3 Repair of cleft lip

palate, or merely consist of clefts of the the uvula. Cleft palate in association with cleft lip is three times more common than cleft palate alone, and usually takes the form of a unilateral complete cleft of both primary and secondary palate.

## Clinical features

The defect is obvious on inspection and difficulty in suckling is usual. Uncorrected, the abnormalities lead to permanent disfigurement, speech impediment, persistent dental abnormalities, and troublesome rhinitis and sinusitis.

## Treatment

Special teats, syringes or spoons are used to feed the infant in preparation for surgery.

*Cleft lip*. Operation is best deferred until the child is 3–6 months old. Cosmetic closure of the defect involves freeing the lip from the underlying maxilla, freshening the edges of the cleft, and apposing them by meticulous suture (Fig. 25.3). Some form of Z-plasty is often needed to increase the vertical length of the lip and restore facial symmetry.

*Cleft palate*. Surgery should be undertaken before the child begins to speak, but is best deferred until the age of 12-18 months. This means that endotracheal anaesthesia can be employed and that the affected structures have grown sufficiently to facilitate surgery. Operation aims at closing the palatal defect to separate the oral and nasal cavities, and lengthening the palate

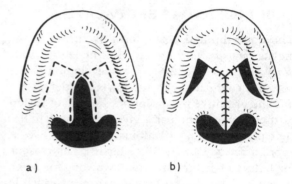

Fig. 25.4 Repair of cleft palate

so that the nasopharynx can be occluded during phonation (Fig. 25.4).

The surgery of cleft lip and cleft palate is specialised. Excellent cosmetic and functional results are obtainable only if operation is undertaken by a surgeon skilled and experienced in the techniques available.

## DERMOID CYSTS

These congenital abnormalities result when a portion of skin becomes detached and buried beneath the line of fusion of two skin processes during development. The cyst wall consists of all layers of skin, including epidermal appendages. The cyst contains sebaceous material but for some reason never contains hair.

Dermoid cysts may occur in the floor of the mouth, and although congenital, seldom present before the age of 10 years. They can lie above or below the mylohyoid muscle, and so may bulge into the floor of the mouth or to the exterior. The cyst is commonly midline but may be deviated to one side. Cysts bulging into the floor of the mouth are opaque, in contrast to ranulae which are translucent.

The patient usually presents with a persistent painless swelling. Operation is advised to establish the diagnosis, remove anxiety, and restore cosmetic appearances. The cyst is usually removed through an incision beneath the mandible.

*External angular dermoid.* See page 185.

## CONGENITAL SINUSES OF THE LOWER LIP

This condition tends to run in families but cannot be explained embryologically. Two blind pits are found, one on either side of the midline, on the vermilion-skin border of the lower lip. The pits are lined by squamous epithelium and have numerous mucous glands near their blind ending. The pits traverse the orbicularis oris muscle to terminate beneath the mucous membrane of the mouth. Complete excision is indicated.

## CONGENITAL ABNORMALITIES OF THE TONGUE

*Macroglossia* or enlargement of the tongue may be congenital or acquired (cretinism). *Bifid tongue* is an extremely rare but readily correctable anomaly.

*Ankyloglossia* or tongue-tie results when the lingual frenulum is too short. Although often a source of maternal anxiety during infancy, the abnormality rarely gives rise to speech impediment and division of the frenulum is seldom necessary.

The thyroglossal duct commences at the foramen caecum at the junction of the anterior two-thirds and posterior one-third of the tongue. *Thyroglossal cysts* (see p.320) occasionally cause a persistent swelling in this region, and may have to be excised. Failure of descent of the thyroid *(lingual thyroid)* is an extremely rare condition in which the thyroid tissue remains attached to the base of the tongue. The anomaly must be borne in mind when considering removal of any swelling in this region.

## ACQUIRED CYSTS OF THE MOUTH

### RETENTION CYSTS

Small fluid-filled transparent retention cysts commonly occur on the lower lip. They are usually bluish in colour and result from plugging of mucous glands. They are not tender unless infected and the patient usually presents because of the deformity. The cysts can be excised or marsupialised (see below).

### RANULA

A ranula is a thin-walled retention cyst arising from the floor of the mouth. It is caused by obstruction and degeneration of a mucous gland or sublingual salivary gland. The swelling is usually located beneath the tongue, grows slowly, and may burst and recur. The ranula contains thick crystal-clear fluid. Because of its thin wall, the swelling is translucent. It is mainly if not entirely unilateral, and the submandibular duct and lingual vein are often visible, stretched over the swelling. *Plunging ranula* is a rare variant in which a deep prolongation of the cyst may be apparent in the neck. A ranula is painless unless infected, and the patient usually presents because of the swelling.

Excision is usually impossible because of the thin wall, and *marsupialisation* is the treatment of choice. In this technique, the protruding cyst wall is excised and the cut edge of the cyst wall is sutured to the surrounding cut edge of mucous membrane (Fig. 25.5). The submandibular duct is carefully preserved during surgery.

## TRAUMA TO THE MOUTH

### LACERATIONS OF THE LIP

Lacerations frequently extend through the full thickness of the lip, dividing fibres of the orbicularis oris muscle and the internal mucous membrane. The laceration tends to gape because of the muscle pull, giving rise to an erroneous impression of tissue loss. Profuse bleeding can be arrested by compression of tissues on either side

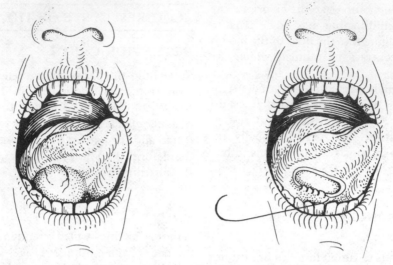

**Fig. 25.5** Ranula and its treatment by marsupialisation

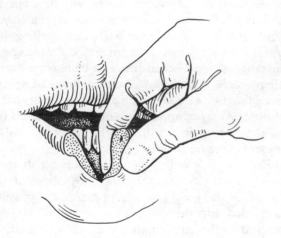

**Fig. 25.6** Compression of lip to arrest haemorrhage

of the tear between thumb and forefinger (Fig. 25.6). Copious irrigation is followed by debridement, meticulous haemostasis and suture. The muscle layer and mucosa are opposed with an absorbable material such as polyglycolic acid (Dexon), while the skin is approximated with 5–0 silk or Prolene sutures. It is essential to re-align the vermilion-cutaneous junction accurately.

All wounds involving the inner surface of the oral cavity may become contaminated with Vincent's spirochaetes, fusiform bacteria and a variety of pathogenic anaerobes. It is advisable to cover all such wounds with a 5-day course of penicillin. Similarly, all wounds resulting from human bites should receive penicillin cover.

## LACERATIONS OF THE TONGUE

Tongue lacerations bleed copiously and are sometimes inaccessible. All but the most major wounds can usually be repaired under local anaesthetic using a solution of 1% lignocaine with 1 in 100 000 adrenaline. A temporary transfixion stitch through the anaesthetised tongue tip serves as a useful retractor to improve access. Individual bleeding points are ligated with polyglycolic acid ligatures, and the tongue muscle and mucosa are brought together by polyglycolic acid sutures with buried knots. As with lip lacerations, a 5-day course of penicillin is advisable.

## PERFORATION OF THE PALATE

Although all age groups may sustain this injury, it is seen most often in small children who fall while carrying a rigid object such as a pencil in the mouth. If the object is impacted, the depth of penetration should be established radiologically before its removal. A neurosurgical opinion is sought if the object has penetrated the base of the skull, but this is rarely the case. The palatal perforation is not closed surgically as most will close spontaneously under antibiotic cover.

## BURN INJURY

### Thermal burns

Thermal burns of the lip usually involve both skin and mucosal surfaces, but are managed in the same way as all skin burns (Ch. 13). Thermal burns within the mouth result from inhalation of smoke and fumes, or accidental ingestion of hot liquids and solids. They are seldom deep and are usually managed by regular mouthwashes and analgesia.

### Chemical burns

Chemical burns of the lips and mouth are caused by accidental or deliberate (suicidal) ingestion of caustic chemicals, and are typically deep, penetrating and extensive. Emergency treatment consists of copious irrigation of the mouth with cold tap water for up to 12 hours. Water dilutes and washes away the chemical, and decreases tissue damage due to exothermic reaction between caustic alkali and tissue fat.

Antibiotics are essential to reduce secondary infection, and steroids may be of value in reducing tissue oedema and inflammatory reaction. The patient is nursed with the head elevated to reduce oedema, and tracheostomy may be needed if there is extensive injury to the mouth and pharynx.

### Electrical burns

Electrical burns of the mouth are seen occasionally in small children who have bitten through a flex or sucked a live wire. Saliva short-circuits the terminals within the mouth and deep coagulation necrosis results. Treatment is initially conservative with antibiotic cover. Debridement is limited to obviously dead and necrotic tissue.

## DISLOCATION OF THE JAW

### Anterior dislocation

This is relatively common and usually bilateral. It follows opening of the mouth too widely as in yawning or dental extraction, and may result from a blow on the jaw while the mouth is open. In bilateral dislocation, the mandible is displaced forwards, while in unilateral dislocation it is pushed over to the affected side. The mouth is held open and the patient complains of pain, inability to talk, and inability to swallow. Treatment consists of downward traction on the mandible with backward displacement, and may be possible without general anaesthesia in some patients.

### Superior dislocation

This may follow major trauma. The condyle of the mandible is driven upwards and forwards through the base of the skull causing variable degrees of brain damage.

### Posterior dislocation

This is relatively uncommon and follows trauma to the mandible while the jaws are closed. Fracture of the tympanic plate is inevitable and the condyle enters the external auditory meatus where it can be seen with an auroscope.

## FRACTURES OF THE JAWS

### Mandibular fractures

Fractures of the *mandible* are common. Of the bones of the facial skeleton, only those of the nose are fractured more frequently. Mandibular fractures may involve the body, angle, ramus, condylar neck or condylar process (Fig. 25.7). They result from direct or indirect injury, and are a common consequence of fighting or road traffic

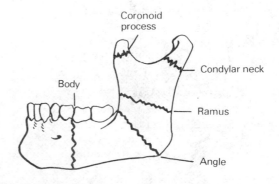

Fig. 25.7 Sites for fractures of the jaw

accidents. The fractures are frequently multiple and comminuted, and are often associated with injury to other areas of the facial skeleton. Fractures lying in front of the third molar tooth are invariably compound into the mouth.

The patient gives a history of injury and complains of pain, tenderness and swelling. He is often unable to close the mouth and may have anaesthesia over the lower lip if the mental branch of the inferior dental nerve has been damaged. Oedema is marked and develops rapidly, often masking displacement. The fragments are often displaced by the initial injury or pulled apart by the upward pull of masseter and temporalis, and the downward pull of genio-glossus and genio-hyoid (Fig. 25.8).

The diagnosis is usually obvious clinically but can be missed if displacement is minimal and swelling is marked. Point tenderness at the fracture site and crepitus or movement on bimanual examination are valuable clinical signs. X-rays confirm the diagnosis. Additional oblique views and tomograms may be needed to define fractures involving the condyle.

The muscles attached to the mandible are strong and have considerable leverage, so that strong fixation is usually needed to maintain reduction. This is usually achieved by some form of interdental wiring under nerve block anaesthesia. Fractures in edentulous patients can be man-

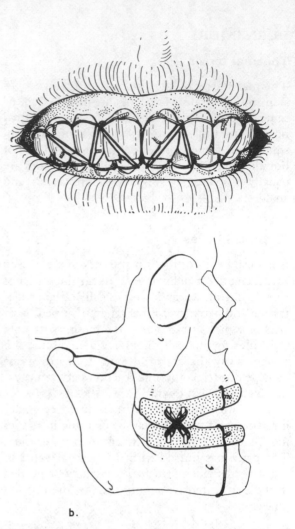

**Fig. 25.9** Fixation in jaw fractures. (a) Interdental wiring. (b) Fixation in edentulous jaw.

aged by using dentures or dental splints wired to the mandible and then fixed to the overlying maxilla. Such intermaxillary elastic traction is useful in all patients as a means of reinforcing immobilisation and ensuring that normal dental occlusion is restored (Fig. 25.9). Fixation is usually maintained for 6 weeks.

Open reduction is indicated when marked displacement cannot be reduced or maintained by simple intermaxillary fixation. The fragments are wired or plated together, and then fixed to the maxilla.

At one time, all teeth lying in the fracture line were removed on the premise that devitalised teeth were a potential source of infection, leading

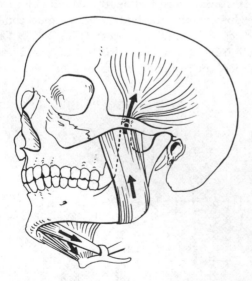

**Fig. 25.8** Muscles causing displacement of jaw fractures

to osteomyelitis and delayed or non-union. It is now recognised that many such teeth can be saved by conservative management, although antibiotic cover is advisable. When there are missing teeth a chest X-ray is essential to exclude aspiration. Condylar fractures are also treated by intermaxillary fixation. This should not be prolonged for over 3 weeks for fear of ankylosis at the temporomandibular joint. Open reduction of condylar fractures is only indicated when there is marked displacement of the condyle in young children. This is rare.

## Maxillary fractures

Fractures of the *maxilla* are much less common than those of the mandible. The membranous bone of the maxilla has great capacity to absorb the force of deceleration injuries, and so protect the brain from lethal injury. The muscles attached to the upper jaw have less strength and leverage than those of the mandible, so that less strong fixation is needed when maintaining reduction of maxillary fractures.

The fractures range in severity from simple undisplaced fractures through the alveolar ridges to extensive displacement of the middle third of the face with fractures involving the orbit, zygomatic process or frontonasal bones (Fig. 25.10). Airway obstruction may necessitate emergency tracheostomy, and major bleeding may have to be arrested urgently.

As with mandibular fractures, oedema may mask the true extent of bony displacement and careful palpation is needed to elicit crepitus and mobility of the maxilla. X-rays are an essential part of assessment and must include postero-anterior views taken with the head in the Waters position to display the maxilla, orbits and zygomatic arches (Fig. 25.11).

Unilateral undisplaced fractures may be treated by intermaxillary wiring, but open reduction and direct wiring of the fragments is needed in most cases. Reduction and fixation can be delayed for up to 14 days if other injuries take precedence but occlusion should be restored as quickly as possible. Complicated fractures may require additional splinting from a head cap and supporting wiring from intact facial or cranial bones.

## INFECTIONS OF THE ORAL CAVITY

### NON-SPECIFIC GINGIVITIS AND STOMATITIS

These conditions are encountered in surgical patients who are dehydrated, febrile and ill-nourished. Poor oral hygiene is a major predisposing factor. Carious jagged teeth, ill-fitting dentures

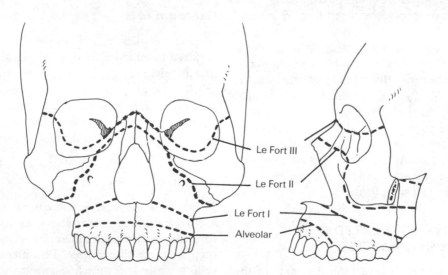

**Fig. 25.10** Maxillary fractures (Le Fort's classification)

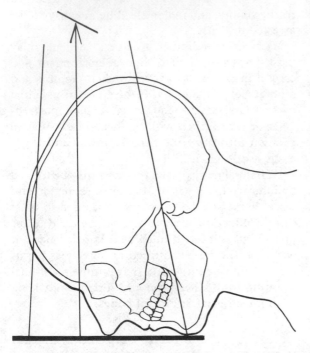

**Fig. 25.11** Waters position — patient on X-ray table with head in correct position

and heavy smoking favour development of infection.

The organisms responsible are normal mouth commensals. The oral mucosa becomes reddened and dry, the tongue is swollen and furred, and halitosis is prominent. The patient complains of discomfort and pain on eating, particularly when the condition progresses to ulceration. Fever and malaise are common.

This type of stomatitis is largely preventable if dehydration is avoided and oral hygiene is maintained by regular mouthwashes in patients unable to eat and drink. Established stomatitis is treated by removing any obvious precipitating cause, hydrating the patient, providing regular mouthwashes, and promoting flow of saliva by chewing-gum once the patient is hydrated. The condition should respond promptly to this management and antibiotics are rarely indicated.

## ULCERATIVE STOMATITIS (SYN. VINCENT'S STOMATITIS)

Vincent's stomatitis is now rare. Any area of the mouth may be affected but the gums are usually most severely involved. The affected regions become reddened, swollen and ulcerated, the ulcers being covered by a grey-yellow slough.

The condition is painful, interferes with eating, and gives rise to fever, malaise and headache. Halitosis is pronounced.

Smears from the ulcers reveal large numbers of fusiform bacilli and spirochaetes, but it is unlikely that specific infection by these organisms is responsible. The condition does not affect edentulous patients and it is thought that faulty oral and dental hygiene diminishes local resistance to infection by mouth commensals. Other promoting factors include debilitation, vitamin deficiencies and dehydration.

The condition is treated by systemic penicillin for 5 days or by a 5-day course of metronidazole in a dose of 200 mg three times a day. Broad-spectrum antibiotics are avoided so as not to precipitate monilial overgrowth (see candidiasis, below). Faulty oral and dental hygiene is corrected, dehydration rectified and adequate nutrition ensured.

### Vincent's angina

This is a similar condition which affects the fauces and gives rise to great pain and difficulty in swallowing. Respiratory obstruction may occur.

### Cancrum oris

A rare complication of stomatitis in debilitated children in which ulcerative stomatitis progresses to full-thickness gangrene and destruction of the cheek. The gangrenous area is excised, penicillin is administered, and the state of nutrition and oral hygiene is improved. Cancrum oris is usually a pre-terminal event and carries a grave prognosis.

### Aphthous ulceration

Aphthous ulceration is a common complaint in normal individuals. It is also seen occasionally in surgical patients with inflammatory bowel disease such as ulcerative colitis. The ulcers are small, yellow-white and punched-out with a surrounding halo of erythema. Their aetiology is unknown but an association with mental stress or food allergy has been suggested.

Treatment may be unnecessary but some patients find that sucking pellets containing 2.5 mg of hydrocortisone or local anaesthesia gives relief from discomfort.

## CANDIDIASIS (SYN. THRUSH)

Infection with the fungus *Candida albicans* is seen in surgical patients as a complication of prolonged administration of broad-spectrum antibiotics. It is also associated with debilitating disease, corticosteroid therapy and immuno-suppressive therapy.

Small white flecks resembling milk curds are seen throughout the oral cavity and may involve the pharynx, oesophagus and trachea. The flecks adhere to the underlying mucosa but can be scraped away to reveal underlying erythematous mucosa. The plaques coalesce to form sheets, and the associated discomfort may interfere markedly with eating.

The diagnosis is confirmed by microscopic examination of mouth scrapings. Antibiotics and steroids are discontinued if this is feasible, and nystatin is given in the form of suspension or lozenges (500 000 units four times a day for 4 days). Oral hygiene is further promoted by mouthwashes.

Painting the mouth with gentian violet is probably of no value, but amphotericin B can be considered as an alternative to nystatin in patients with generalised candidiasis.

## ACTINOMYCOSIS

*Actinomyces israeli* is an anaerobic organism normally present as a mouth commensal. Carious tooth sockets and local trauma such as dental extraction allow the organism access to the tissues. All forms of actinomycosis are rare, and cervicofacial actinomycosis is found mainly in patients who have neglected oral and dental hygiene.

The gum becomes indurated and a nodule or nodules develop in the external aspect of the lower jaw. The overlying skin becomes bluish in colour and diffusely indurated. Pus is usually discharged intermittently from multiple sinuses. The cervical lymph nodes may remain normal: enlargement usually denotes secondary bacterial infection.

The diagnosis should be suspected whenever infection in and around the mouth does not heal promptly and runs a relapsing course. Microscopic examination of the pus reveals typical 'sun-ray' granules consisting of a mass of radiating Gram-positive mycelial filaments (Fig. 25.12). Fresh mycelial threads may exhibit Gram-negative expanded ends or 'clubs'. The mycelia are surrounded by the pus of secondary bacterial infection.

Treatment consists of attention to oral and dental hygiene, coupled with a 6-week course of penicillin in large doses.

## OTHER FORMS OF SPECIFIC ORAL INFECTION

Syphilitic and tuberculous ulcers are now rare.

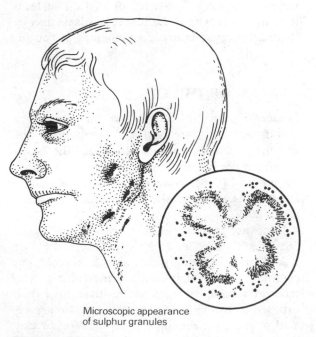

Microscopic appearance of sulphur granules

**Fig. 25.12** Actinomycosis

## PREMALIGNANT AND MALIGNANT CONDITIONS

### LEUKOPLAKIA

Leukoplakia is a precancerous condition caused by longstanding irritation of the tongue, lips and buccal mucosa. Its development is prompted by tobacco smoking, trauma from carious teeth and ill-fitting dentures, ingestion of hot liquids and spices, and the chewing of tobacco and betel nuts. 50% of all oral cancers arise in patients with pre-existing leukoplakia.

Leukoplakia commences as a redness of the mucosa followed by induration and hyperkeratosis. The hyperkeratotic areas are seen as white patches from which the name leukoplakia derives. Desquamation exposes sensitive red areas resembling raw beef. Candida infection is commonly associated with leukoplakia and is a cause of chronic ulceration. Hyperkeratosis may proceed to papillomatous proliferation and fissuring, cancer tending to arise in such fissured areas.

Leukoplakia must be observed regularly. Known aetiological factors are removed. Suspicious thickened areas should be biopsied.

Small nodular areas should be excised but widespread surgical excision of affected surfaces is no longer practised. Diffuse leukoplakia may be treated by cryotherapy. Radiotherapy is contra-indicated.

### CANCER OF THE LIP

Some 95% of lip cancers are squamous cell lesions while 5% are basal cell carcinomas. The tumours virtually always arise on the skin-vermilion border, and the great majority occur on the lower lip. Men are much more commonly affected than women, the male:female ratio being about 20:1.

Exposure to sunlight is the major aetiological factor and outdoor workers are particularly at risk. The neoplasm is rare among negroes but common among fair-skinned individuals who tend to freckle or burn rather than tan when exposed to sunlight. Pipe smoking is also associated with lip cancer: pipe stems of wood or clay were particularly dangerous in that they soaked up the tobacco tars and were in effect applications of a hot moist tar 'poultice' to the lip. The association between cigarette smoking and lip cancer is less strong than the association with cancer of the mouth, larynx or lungs.

Leukoplakia precedes development of lip cancer in one-third of patients. The lip mucosa thins, becomes pale, and then becomes hyperkeratotic with the formation of a white, cracked and fissured film.

Metastases are to the lymph nodes. The incidence increases with tumour size, although some cancers attain large size without having metastasised. Spread from lower lip tumours is to the submental nodes on the side of the lesion. Spread to the contralateral submental nodes is unusual unless the primary cancer crosses the midline. Lesions of the upper lip spread first to involve the submandibular nodes.

Cancers on either lip spread ultimately to involve the jugular chain and the mandible may be involved by spread through the mental foramen. As with all cancers in and around the mouth, widespread lymphatic or bloodstream dissemination is exceptional.

*Clinical features.* The diagnosis is usually obvious. Bidigital examination of the floor of the mouth and thorough examination of the neck is performed to determine extent. A biopsy is essential.

*Treatment.* Small lesions are excised using a V-shaped incision with immediate repair (Fig. 25.13). As surgical removal of larger lesions entails the use of flaps to reconstitute the lip, they are usually treated by radiotherapy. Extensive

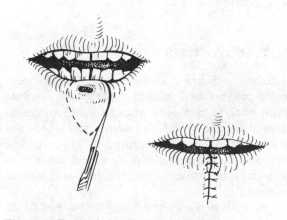

**Fig. 25.13** Excision of malignant ulcer of lip

lesions with neck metastases are treated by irradiation followed by block dissection of the neck.

There is debate as to the best course of management in patients with large primary lesions but no obvious nodal metastases. Prophylactic block dissection of the neck will reveal unsuspected micrometastases in a proportion of cases, but neck dissection is best deferred until affected nodes are detected clinically. Nodal metastases are likely to declare themselves clinically within 2 years.

Lesions smaller than 1 cm carry an excellent prognosis with a 5-year survival of 90% after treatment. Neglected larger lesions fare less well but radical treatment is still worthwhile. In such cases a 5 year survival rate of about 50% can still be achieved.

## CANCER OF THE TONGUE AND ORAL CAVITY

Oral and lingual cancer have become less common over the past 50 years but still account for about 5% of all malignancies. Detection is relatively simple in that all of the lesions except those of the posterior one-third of the tongue are readily accessible to the examining eye or finger. Nevertheless these lesions are often neglected or overlooked at an early stage of development when eradication would be simple.

The following generalisations apply to oral and lingual cancers:

1. The great majority (over 90%) are squamous cell lesions with pleomorphic salivary adenomas accounting for most of the remainder.

2. The male:female ratio (at one time 10:1) has fallen to between 2–4:1.

3. Oral cancer is uncommon before the age of 45 years but its incidence rises steadily with age thereafter. 50% occur in those over 70 years of age.

4. Oral cancer spreads by local infiltration and lymphatic spread to nodes in the head and neck. Widespread metastases via lymphatics and bloodstream are exceptional.

5. Surgery and radiotherapy are equally effective in treatment: the choice of therapy is determined by technical and local considerations.

6. Death results not from the effects of carcinomatosis but from the complications of the primary tumour and its nodal metastases.

### Aetiological factors

*Tobacco smoking* is a recognised aetiological factor and pipe and cigar smoking raise the risk of developing oral and lingual cancer by a factor of three. The risk is particularly high in those areas of the world, e.g. the Andra Pradesh region of India, where cigars are smoked with the lighted end inside the mouth. Chewing tobacco is also carcinogenic. *Betel nut* chewing is said to be associated with an increased risk but it now seems that it is the combination of betel nut with tobacco chewing which is responsible. In those parts of India where this is popular, oral and lingual cancer represents one third of all malignancies amongst individuals indulging in this habit. *Heavy alcohol consumption* is also thought to be an aetiological factor. In heavy smokers and drinkers the incidence is increased 15-fold. *Poor oral hygiene* has been incriminated, but this is often associated with other known aetiological factors. *Syphilitic glossitis* is now relatively rare but is a definitive risk factor. The tongue becomes scarred and fibrotic, with formation of longitudinal fissures and thickened plaques on which cancer develops. At one time, 20% of all males with lingual cancer had pre-existing syphilitic glossitis.

### Cancer of the tongue

*Anterior two-thirds of the tongue.* Cancer commonly arises at the tip or on one of the free borders, and often develops in an area of hyperkeratosis, typically appearing as a raised ulcer with overhanging edges. Infiltration of the underlying muscle is often extensive and the tongue becomes indurated and fixed. Lingual cancer arising on a background of syphilitic glossitis commences on the dorsal surface of the tongue.

Almost half of the patients with lingual cancer will have neck node metastases by the time of presentation. Lesions on the tip metastasise to the submental nodes and may give rise to bilateral nodal involvement. Lesions on the edge of the tongue spread to ipsilateral submandibular nodes. Nodes at the angle of the mandible are invariably associated with periosteal seedlings.

The primary tumour may be treated by surgery (Fig. 25.14) or radiotherapy. Resection of part of the body of the mandible is essential if it is in

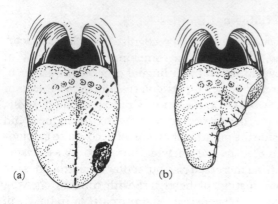

(a)          (b)

**Fig. 25.14** Operation for cancer of tongue. (a) anterior third, (b) posterior two-thirds

contact with the primary tumour. Some surgeons advocate routine block dissection of lymph nodes in the neck; most prefer to perform this procedure only when nodes are palpable. The effect of prophylactic radiotherapy to the neck nodes is under study.

Approximately one-third of all patients with tongue cancer (50% of those with no nodal involvement) will survive for 5 years after treatment.

*Posterior one-third of tongue.* Lesions of the posterior one-third of the tongue tend to be more malignant than those situated anteriorly. They spread more rapidly to the cervical nodes, and may metastasise to more distant sites. As the cancer is relatively inaccessible it is often overlooked until there is pain or difficulty on swallowing, enlargement of cervical lymph nodes, or weight loss. Ulceration of the tumour causes pronounced halitosis.

Because of its late presentation, treatment is a problem. Surgical eradication usually entails complete loss of the tongue and radiotherapy is more commonly advised. Palpable neck nodes should be resected *en bloc*.

Five-year survival rates are very low.

## CANCER OF THE ORAL CAVITY

Cancer of the *floor of the mouth* tends to spread around the inner aspect of the mandible and can involve the entire floor of the mouth by the time of presentation. Cancer of the *gingivae* usually presents as a tender mass with loosening of adjacent teeth, and can be mistaken for an abscess or cyst. Cancer of the *buccal mucosa* may penetrate the cheek and create an orocutaneous fistula.

All of these forms of cancer spread to involve cervical lymph nodes. Radical neck dissection may be indicated in addition to wide excision primary tumour. Pre-operative radiotherapy may be used to try to minimise the extent of surgical resection. Associated resection of part of the mandible or maxilla may be needed if the tumour lies adjacent to bone.

The results of surgery depend on the extent of tumour spread but in general these forms of oral cancer have a 5-year survival rate of only 40%.

## MIXED SALIVARY TUMOURS

As described in Chapter 23, pleomorphic salivary adenomas can arise from accessory salivary glands distributed throughout the oral cavity. Such tumours more often have malignant characteristics than pleomorphic adenomas within the parotid. They should be excised widely to prevent recurrence.

# 26. The Oesophagus

## SURGICAL ANATOMY

The oesophagus is a hollow muscular tube which extends from the termination of the pharynx (C6) to the oesophago-gastric junction (Fig. 26.1). It has cervical, thoracic and abdominal portions and is 25 cm long, the final 2–4 cm lying within the abdomen. The muscle coat comprises an inner circular and outer longitudinal layer; the muscle fibres are striated in the upper third with a gradual transition to smooth muscle below that level. The oesophageal lumen is lined by squamous epithelium which, on occasions, contains islands of ectopic gastric mucosa. The distal 1–2 cm of oesophagus is lined by columnar epithelium. The submucosa contains numerous mucous glands, a rich lymphatic network and the neural plexus of Meissner. Auerbach's neural plexus is found between the two muscle layers.

There are two oesophageal sphincters. The *upper oesophageal sphincter* is 3–4 cm long and is formed by the cricopharyngeus muscle and first few centimetres of oesophagus. It is closed at rest to prevent air from entering the oesophagus, but opens on swallowing. The *lower oesophageal sphincter* cannot be defined anatomically but is detected as a high pressure zone on manometry. The sphincter is tonically closed at rest, is 3–5 cm long, and is located in the region of the oesophageal hiatus in the diaphragm.

Three areas of oesophageal narrowing can be demonstrated on barium swallow and are often seen during endoscopy. They are situated: 1. at the beginning of the oesophagus, 2. as it passes to the right of the aortic arch and behind the left bronchus, and 3. as it traverses the oesophageal hiatus of the diaphragm.

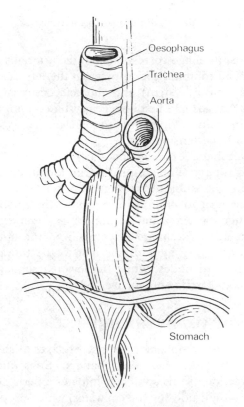

**Fig. 26.1** The relationships of the oesophagus

The oesophageal hiatus consists of an encircling noose of muscle drawn mainly from the right diaphragmatic crus with a variable contribution from the left crus (Fig. 26.2). The lower oesophagus and oesophago-gastric junction are held loosely in the hiatus by a condensation of fascia known as the phreno-oesophageal ligament.

The oesophagus receives arterial blood from the gastric and phrenic vessels below, from the aortic and bronchial vessels in the thorax, and from the inferior thyroid arteries in the neck.

347

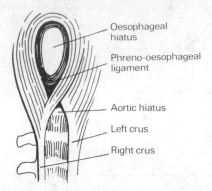

Fig. 26.2 The anatomy of the oesophageal hiatus

Venous drainage corresponds to the arterial supply. The communication between the left gastric veins (portal system) and thoracic oesophageal veins (azygos and hemi-azygos system) is important in the development of oesophageal varices in portal hypertension.

Lymphatic drainage does not correspond to blood supply. The lymphatics run longitudinally within the submucosa before penetrating the muscle coat to drain into regional lymph nodes. Submucosal extension of tumour is common in oesophageal carcinoma. Lymph from the upper and mid-oesophagus drains first to the thoracic and cervical nodes, while the lower oesophagus drains to gastric and coeliac nodes.

## SURGICAL PHYSIOLOGY

The upper oesophageal sphincter relaxes to allow entry of food from the pharynx. Subsequent contraction of this sphincter initiates a peristaltic wave (amplitude 50–100 cm water) which propels food distally. The lower oesophageal sphincter relaxes as the wave approaches and food passes into the stomach. Passage of the peristaltic wave can be monitored by recording luminal pressure at varying levels in the oesophagus (see Fig. 26.3).

Resting pressure within the thoracic oesophagus reflects intra-thoracic pressure and mean values are sub-atmospheric. Intra-abdominal pressure exceeds atmospheric pressure but reflux of gastric content is normally prevented by the lower oesophageal sphincter. A number of mechanical factors may contribute to gastro-oesophageal competence; they include the diaphragm, the prominent folds of gastric mucosa (mucosal rosette) at the oesophago-gastric junction, and the oblique entry of the oesophagus into the stomach with creation of a flap-valve effect.

The vagus may affect peristalsis in the body of the oesophagus and influences the lower oesophageal sphincter. However, sphincter tone is not abolished by vagal or sympathetic denervation and the sphincter continues to relax on swallowing. Sphincter tone is increased by gastrin and reduced by secretin and cholecystokinin, although it is now considered that these are pharmacological rather than physiological effects.

## SYMPTOMS OF OESOPHAGEAL DISEASE

There are three principal symptoms of oesophageal disease:

### Dysphagia

Difficulty in swallowing is usually an indication of organic disease and requires urgent and careful investigation. Some patients localise the site of their obstruction accurately but in many cases localisation is poor. For example, the patient may indicate that food sticks at the level of the suprasternal notch when the lesion is located at the lower end of the oesophagus. It is important to establish the length of history, whether dysphagia is intermittent, constant or progressive, and whether liquids and solids are equally affected. Patients with oesophageal obstruction may complain of *hiccough* during eating. The mechanism responsible is uncertain but the symptom may predate the onset of dysphagia by several weeks.

Some of the main causes of dysphagia are shown in Table 26.1; peptic oesophagitis and carcinoma are common causes of this symptom.

*Globus hystericus* is often confused with dysphagia. The patient feels as if there is a lump in the throat or upper oesophagus, but on close questioning the symptom is often found to be more troublesome between meals than during eating. The symptom is associated with nervous tension and has no organic cause. However, it may prove difficult to distinguish clinically between globus hystericus and dysphagia, and the

**Table 26.1** Causes of dysphagia

|  | Intraluminal | Intramural | | Extrinsic |
|---|---|---|---|---|
| Pharynx and upper oesophagus | Foreign body | Mucosal | Pharyngitis<br>Tonsillitis<br>Moniliasis<br>Sideropenic web<br>Corrosive poisons<br>Carcinoma | Thyroid enlargement |
|  |  | Muscular |  | Pharyngeal pouch |
|  |  |  | Myasthenia gravis |  |
|  |  | Neurological | Bulbar palsy |  |
| Body of oesophagus | Foreign body |  | Corrosive poisons<br>Peptic oesophagitis<br>Carcinoma | Mediastinal lymphadenopathy<br>Aortic aneurysm<br>Dysphagia lusoria |
| Lower oesophagus | Foreign body | Mucosal | Corrosive poisons<br>Peptic oesophagitis<br>Carcinoma | Unfolded aorta<br>Para-oesophageal hernia |
|  |  | Muscular | Oesophageal spasm<br>Scleroderma |  |
|  |  | Neurological | Achalasia<br>Post-vagotomy |  |
| Gastric |  |  | Carcinoma |  |

former diagnosis can only be accepted after organic disease has been excluded by rigorous investigation.

## Pain

*Heartburn* is a retrosternal burning discomfort or pain associated with gastro-oesophageal reflux. The pain may radiate up to the neck and jaws, through to the back, or down the arms. It is often brought on by recumbency (as in bed at night) or stooping, occurs soon after meals, and may be precipitated by hot liquids or fruit juice. The pain can usually be reproduced by instillation of 0.1 M HCl (or the drinking of pineapple juice) and is usually relieved by alkali. However, acid is not essential for the production of heartburn and the symptom may occur after total gastrectomy and in patients who are achlorhydric. Alkaline bile reflux may be responsible for heartburn in such individuals. Although conditions which cause reflux oesophagitis usually produce heartburn, the symptom has an inconstant relationship with endoscopic and histological evidence of inflammation. Oesophageal motor abnormalities are also associated with production of heartburn but the exact relationship between the two is uncertain.

*Oesophageal spasm* is thought to produce a diffuse gripping retrosternal sensation or pain which may resemble angina pectoris or heartburn. However, the pain of spasm is not related to exercise and, in contrast to heartburn, it is unaffected by posture or ingestion of alkali.

## Regurgitation

Some patients with oesophageal obstruction complain of food regurgitation rather than dysphagia. The patient often states that he vomits, but careful questioning reveals that there is no associated nausea and that the 'vomiting' is effortless. The patient spits out food rather than vomits, and the 'vomitus' usually consists of undigested food uncontaminated by gastric juice or bile. Nocturnal reflux and aspiration of food may wake the patient with coughing fits, and can cause aspiration pneumonia which so dominates the clinical picture that the primary problem is easily overlooked.

## INVESTIGATION OF OESOPHAGEAL DISEASE

A careful history and thorough physical examination are essential when oesophageal disease is suspected. Most of the oesophagus is inaccessible to clinical examination but particular attention is paid to palpation of the neck, chest and upper abdomen.

A *chest X-ray* may raise suspicion of oesophageal disease by revealing enlarged mediastinal lymph nodes, evidence of aspiration pneumonia, or even pulmonary metastases. The gastric air bubble is seen within the chest in some patients with hiatus hernia, and is occasionally indented by tumour arising in the region of the cardia. Following oesophageal trauma, air may be seen in the mediastinum and root of the neck.

*Barium swallow and meal* are essential investigations and *cine radiography* often assists in the assessment of motility disorders.

*Endoscopy* is mandatory, even when the diagnosis appears certain on radiological grounds; unsuspected additional pathology may be revealed, as for example the presence of early carcinoma in a patient with long-standing hiatus hernia. The oesophagus, stomach and proximal duodenum are inspected and all suspicious lesions are biopsied. The flexible fibre-optic endoscope has largely replaced the rigid oesophagoscope in that it is less uncomfortable for the patient, carries less risk of oesophageal perforation and allows inspection of the entire stomach and proximal duodenum. Fibre-optic endoscopy suffers from the limitation that only small mucosal biopsies can be obtained and submucosal extension of cancer may escape detection.

*Oesophageal pressure recordings* may aid the detection and assessment of abnormal motility. Pressure readings are obtained from a series of fine tubes perfused with saline and bound together so that their openings are 5 cm apart (Fig. 26.3). The assembly can be used to detect the lower oesophageal sphincter and measure sphincter pressure, or to monitor propulsion of the peristaltic wave during swallowing. Abnormal motility patterns are a feature of achalasia, diffuse oesophageal spasm and scleroderma (see below).

*Bernstein's test* entails passing a narrow-bore nasogastric tube into the lower oesophagus and infusing 0.1 M HCl. This reproduces the patient's symptoms if they are due to reflux oesophagitis, but false positive and false negative results are not uncommon (Fig. 26.4).

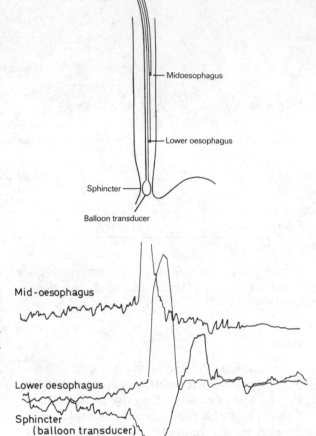

**Fig. 26.3** Recording of intraoesophageal pressure. (a) Balloon-covered differential transformer and open-tipped tubes (arrows) used in the measurement of oesophageal and sphincter pressures. (b) Deglutitive response of inferior oesophageal sphincter in healthy subject. Note that relaxation precedes arrival of peristaltic wave in sphincter.

*pH measurements* can be made using an intraluminal electrode and are used to detect gastro-oesophageal reflux. In an extension of the Bernstein test, the electrode can also be used to determine the number of swallows needed to clear acid from the lower oesophagus.

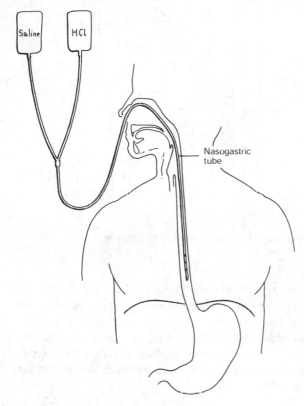

Saline    HCl

Nasogastric
tube

**Fig. 26.4** Bernstein's test (the two bottles, one containing HCl and the other not, are to allow interchange of infusion without the knowledge of the patient)

## DISORDERS OF OESOPHAGEAL MOTILITY

### Abnormalities of the upper oesophageal sphincter

Lack of co-ordination between pharyngeal contraction and relaxation of the upper oesophageal sphincter is implicated in dysphagia due to myasthenia gravis and bulbar palsy, and may follow extensive surgery in the oropharyngeal region. Oesophageal manometry can define those patients in whom cricopharyngeal myotomy will be of value. Abnormal motility has also been incriminated in the development of pharyngo-oesophageal diverticulum (see p. 353).

### Achalasia of the cardia

Achalasia is the commonest oesophageal motility disorder although its annual incidence is less than 1 per 100 000 individuals. Males and females are affected with equal frequency and while the disease occurs in all age groups, it is most common in patients between 30 and 60 years of age. The cause of achalasia is unknown but it has a neurogenic basis in disintegration or absence of Auerbach's plexus. Degenerative changes have also been demonstrated in the vagal branches to the lower oesophagus, and degeneration of the myenteric plexus may be secondary to lesions in the vagus or brain stem.

Infection with *Trypanosoma cruzi* (Chagas disease), prevalent in South America, causes degeneration of Auerbach's plexus and leads to motor changes indistinguishable from those of achalasia.

Manometric studies in achalasia reveal that motility is disordered throughout the oesophagus; resting pressure in the body of oesophagus is high, propulsive peristalsis is absent, and the lower oesophageal sphincter fails to relax on swallowing.

*Clinical features.* Dysphagia is the cardinal symptom and is at first intermittent but usually becomes progressive. It may be aggravated by anxiety or fatigue, is often worse with liquids as opposed to solids, and may be more troublesome with cold food. Gravity rather than peristalsis is responsible for food leaving the oesophagus, and the patient may develop tricks to aid oesophageal emptying. For example, he may stand while eating or drinking, and may force food through the oesophagus by expiring forcibly against a closed glottis. Marked weight loss occurs if dysphagia is severe.

Food regurgitation is common and occurs during sleep. Repeated bouts of aspiration pneumonia may lead to pulmonary fibrosis. Retrosternal pain occurs in about 25% of patients and is described as bursting or burning, with radiation to the neck, throat, back or arms. Hiccough may predate dysphagia.

Minor mucosal erosions of the oesophagus are common but peptic ulceration is exceptional. Carcinoma can develop in long-standing achalasia, even after successful surgical treatment. Its development is insidious and the resulting oesophageal obstruction may be attributed to the dysphagia of achalasia, leading to late diagnosis of cancer at an inoperable stage.

*Diagnosis.* Barium swallow reveals gross distension and/or tortuosity of the oesophagus, with a conical narrowing at the cardia leading to a

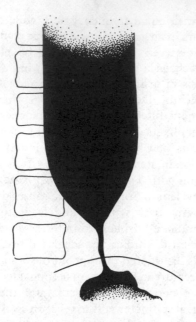

**Fig. 26.5** The radiological appearance of achalasia of the cardia ('rat-tail')

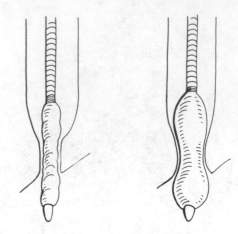

**Fig. 26.6** Hydrostatic dilation of achalasia

string-like passage to the stomach (Fig. 26.5). Cine-radiology shows irregular disorganised contractions of the body of oesophagus and failure of relaxation of the lower oesophageal sphincter. Despite classical radiological appearances, endoscopy is essential to exclude carcinoma or benign oesophageal stricture.

Manometry confirms the lack of propulsive peristalsis and failure of relaxation of the lower oesophageal sphincter. The denervated oesophagus is hypersensitive to subcutaneous injection of small doses of the parasympathomimetic drug methacholine, but in practice this test is rarely necessary.

*Treatment.* Diet and drugs are ineffective in the treatment of achalasia. Forcible dilatation by hydrostatic (Fig. 26.6), pneumatic or mechanical means will relieve symptoms in about 80% of cases, but complications (notably oesophageal perforation) occur in 5%. Repeated dilatations may be necessary. Cardiomyotomy is employed if dilatation fails, and many surgeons now regard this operation as the primary treatment of choice. The oesophagus is usually approached through the thorax; a 10-12 cm longitudinal incision is made through the oesophageal musculature without breaching the mucosa (Fig. 26.7) and taking

care to preserve the vagus nerves. The incision is extended on to the stomach, but this should not exceed 1 cm. Good to excellent results are obtained in 90% of patients, but the results can be marred by gastro-oesophageal reflux with stricture formation if the incision is extended too far distally.

## Diffuse oesophageal spasm

This disease differs from achalasia in that the lower oesophageal sphincter is hypertensive in addition to failing to relax. Hypermotility of the body of the oesophagus leads to repeated spasmodic contractions. The cause of diffuse oesophageal spasm is unknown.

Pain is the cardinal clinical feature and varies in severity from retrosternal discomfort to severe colicky retrosternal pain which may radiate widely and mimic angina pectoris. The pain is frequently provoked by eating but sometimes occurs spontaneously and may wake the patient at night.

Barium swallow reveals a 'corkscrew oesophagus' in 50% of cases, the appearances being due to indentation of the lumen by contracted muscle bundles (Fig. 26.8). Manometry demonstrates that oesophageal peristalsis is replaced by simultaneous repetitive contractions, and may show that the lower oesophageal sphincter is hypertensive with failure to relax on swallowing.

Patients with such abnormal motility are treated by a long myotomy which may extend

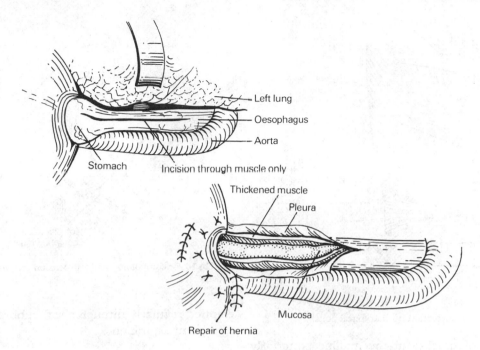

**Fig. 26.7** Cardiomyotomy (Heller's operation)

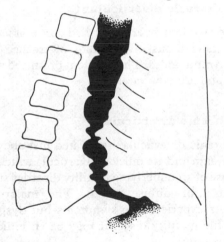

**Fig. 26.8** 'Corkscrew' oesophagus as seen on barium swallow

from above the aortic arch to the cardia. The length of incision is determined by the extent of manometric abnormality.

### Miscellaneous motility disorders

Abnormal oesophageal motility leads to dysphagia in a number of collagen diseases and neuromuscular disorders. Scleroderma is probably the commonest, its oesophageal manifesta-

tions being characterised by fragmentation of submucosal connective tissue and smooth muscle atrophy. The lower oesophageal sphincter is incompetent leading to reflux oesophagitis, stricture and dysphagia. Associated fibrosis leads to shortening of the oesophagus and a hiatus hernia. Motor failure can be confirmed manometrically and radiologically.

Treatment consists of medical measures to combat reflux oesophagitis, forcible dilatation if a stricture forms, and an anti-reflux procedure if these measures fail (p. 356).

## OESOPHAGEAL DIVERTICULA

Diverticula of the oesophagus can be classified according to their location (pharyngo-oesophageal, mid-thoracic or epiphrenic), their mode of formation (pulsion or traction), and as true or false depending on whether they contain all or only some layers of the oesophageal wall.

### Pharyngo-oesophageal diverticulum (syn. pharyngeal pouch)

This is the commonest type of diverticulum affecting the oesophagus. It arises as an out-

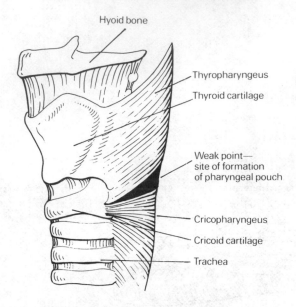

Fig. 26.9 Site of formation of pharyngeal pouch

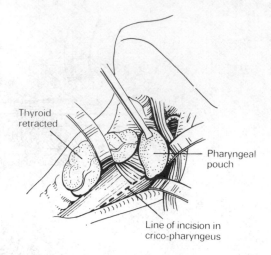

Fig. 26.10 Cricomyotomy and 'suspension' of pharyngeal pouch

pouching of mucosa in the midline posteriorly between the oblique fibres of the crico-pharyngeus and the lower border of the inferior constrictor of the pharynx (Fig. 26.9). Development of the diverticulum is associated with inco-ordination between contraction of the pharynx and relaxation of the upper oesophageal sphincter. As the pouch enlarges it grows downwards to form a blind sac, the opening of which is in line with the lumen of the upper oesophagus.

*Clinical features.* The patient is usually elderly and complains of dysphagia due to the pouch filling with swallowed food and obstructing flow down the oesophagus. Noisy gurgling during deglutition is common, and nocturnal regurgitation is associated with pulmonary aspiration and fibrosis.

The pouch may be palpable as a soft swelling in the neck and its presence is confirmed by barium swallow. Oesophagoscopy is advised to exclude a carcinoma in the pouch.

*Treatment.* Treatment consists of excision of the pouch alone or combined with cricopharyngeal myotomy. Alternatively, crico-pharyngeal myotomy may be combined with 'suspension' of the pouch to ensure adequate drainage (Fig. 26.10). Recurrence is exceptional after adequate treatment.

In those unfit for operation, the pouch is emptied regularly through a soft rubber catheter to prevent aspiration.

## Mid-thoracic diverticulum

These traction diverticula used to be associated with tuberculous involvement of tracheo-bronchial lymph nodes. They seldom produced symptoms and are now rare.

## Epiphrenic diverticulum

Epiphrenic diverticula are located just above the diaphragm and are pulsion diverticula which arise because of an underlying motility disorder such as achalasia or diffuse spasm. The majority of patients experience no symptoms but dysphagia from the motility disorder may be an indication for myotomy.

## HIATUS HERNIA AND OESOPHAGITIS

Herniation of a portion of the stomach through the oesophageal hiatus in the diaphragm is common, particularly in later life. It must be emphasised that hiatus hernia is not necessarily associated with symptoms; conversely, reflux oesophagitis often occurs in the absence of demonstrable gastric herniation.

There are two main types of hiatus hernia. Sliding hiatus hernia is common (95% of cases)

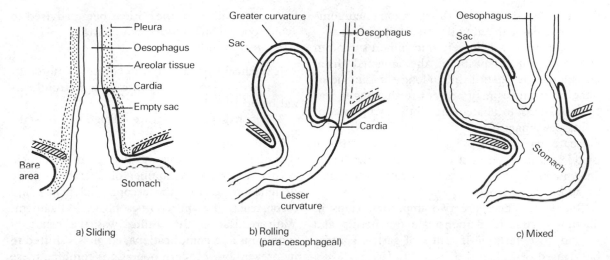

**Fig. 26.11** Types of hiatus hernia

whereas para-oesophageal (or rolling) hiatus hernia is rare (less than 5% of cases). Mixed hiatus hernia in which there is both a sliding and rolling component is exceptional (Fig. 26.11).

## Sliding hiatus hernia

*Pathological anatomy.* As intra-abdominal pressure normally exceeds intra-thoracic pressure, herniation of the stomach upwards is facilitated. Any additional increase in intra-abdominal pressure (as occurs during stooping, straining, coughing and in pregnancy) favours herniation. The phreno-oesophageal ligament becomes attenuated and allows the upper stomach to pass through the hiatus in a concentric fashion. Once herniation has occurred the oesophago-gastric junction slides upwards and downwards through the hiatus (hence the term 'sliding hiatus hernia').

Provided the lower oesophageal sphincter remains competent, herniation does not lead to reflux of gastric contents and oesophagitis. Should reflux occur, the resulting inflammation and fibrosis may prevent further movement of the oesophago-gastric junction, leading to a fixed concentric hiatus hernia with shortening of the oesophagus (Fig. 26.12).

*Clinical features.* The majority of patients have no symptoms referrable to their hiatus hernia and the condition is frequently discovered coincidentally during upper gastrointestinal radiology or

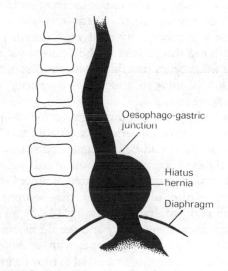

**Fig. 26.12** Radiological appearance of a 'short oesophagus'

endoscopy. It is the development of reflux oesophagitis which produces the cardinal symptom of heartburn. Heartburn occurs soon after meals, particularly large ones, is often promoted by stooping or recumbency, and is relieved by antacids. Patients may have learned to avoid tight clothing and to sleep with the head of the bed elevated to minimise symptoms.

The patient may complain of waterbrash and reflux of bitter irritating fluid into the pharynx and mouth. In waterbrash the mouth suddenly fills with clear tasteless fluid, probably from paroxysmal excessive salivation. Regurgitation of fluid and food may be associated with aspiration pneumonitis, particularly if reflux occurs during sleep.

Dysphagia is a relatively uncommon symptom and may reflect spasm of the inflamed distal oesophagus or stenosis due to long-standing oesophagitis. Stenosis may prevent further regurgitation and lead to abatement of the symptoms of reflux oesophagitis.

Acute haemorrhage is unusual, but chronic blood loss is a common cause of iron deficiency anaemia in elderly patients with reflux oesophagitis and hiatus hernia.

*Diagnosis.* There are two important steps in diagnosis; first to demonstrate the hernia and second, to determine if reflux of gastric content has caused oesophagitis.

The hernia may be evident on an ordinary barium swallow and meal but in many patients it only becomes apparent when intra-abdominal pressure is increased by applying external pressure, placing the patient in the head-down position, or asking him to strain. Oesophagitis may be suspected if there is mucosal irregularity with oesophageal spasm.

Endoscopy is the key investigation for oesophagitis, the mucosa appearing red, friable and haemorrhagic. It should be biopsied. Endoscopy also allows the exclusion of carcinoma in patients with stenotic lesions, and the definition of other lesions such as peptic ulceration of the oesophagus, stomach and proximal duodenum.

Oesophageal manometry and the Bernstein test may aid evaluation of patients with an atypical presentation but are not essential as routine investigations. A cholecystogram (or ultrasonic scan) should be performed to exclude gallstones.

*Management.* Asymptomatic hiatus hernia does not require treatment. Reflux oesophagitis is managed in the first instance by conservative measures which are successful in 85% of cases. These include weight reduction, avoidance of tight clothing and stooping, elevating the head of the bed at night (either by blocks or by increasing the number of pillows), stopping cigarette smoking, and pharmaceutical agents to neutralise gastric contents (antacids) or reduce the secretion of acid (cimetidine). Anticholinergic drugs are contraindicated as they promote gastric stasis and may increase reflux. Large meals are replaced by more frequent small ones, the patient being advised to avoid foods which induce symptoms.

Surgery is indicated if:

1. medical measures fail to control symptoms
2. there is evidence of continuing gastrointestinal blood loss
3. dysphagia and stricture formation are established

In the past, emphasis was placed on anatomical hernia repair and a number of operations were designed to narrow the oesophageal hiatus and reconstruct the phreno-oesophageal ligament. With realisation that reflux was the cause of symptoms and complications, emphasis shifted to its prevention. Modern operations combine these two principles.

Most surgeons now favour the operation of fundoplication as described by Nissen. The operation can be performed through the chest or through the abdomen. The mobilised fundus of the stomach is 'wrapped around' the lower oesophagus so that the oesophago-gastric junction and lower oesophagus are enclosed in a tunnel of stomach (Fig. 26.13). As pressure rises within the stomach, the enclosed segment of lower oesophagus is compressed and reflux is prevented.

The margins of the oesophageal hiatus are approximated behind the oesophagus so that the fundoplication is retained below the diaphragm. However, this is not essential in that reflux is still prevented if the fundoplication is left within the chest.

Approximately 90% of patients are rendered symptom-free and recurrence of reflux symptoms is uncommon. The 'gas-bloat' syndrome with inability to belch or vomit is experienced by about 10% of patients following fundoplication. This syndrome may improve with time and is minimised by avoiding large meals. Measures designed to reduce gastric acid-pepsin secretion (e.g. truncal vagotomy and drainage, highly selective vagotomy) are unnecessary unless the patient has associated peptic ulceration.

## Para-oesophageal hernia

*Pathological anatomy.* There is usually a wide defect in the oesophageal hiatus lying to the left of

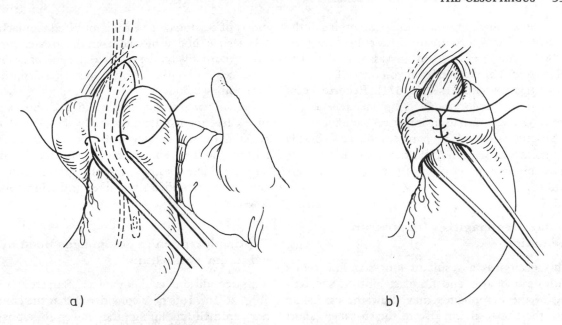

**Fig. 26.13** Fundoplication. (a) Fundus wrapped around lower oesophagus. (b) Sutures in position.

the oesophagus. The fundus of the stomach passes upwards into a well-defined hernial sac lined by peritoneum, and the greater curve rolls upwards into the chest as the hernia enlarges. In time the entire stomach may roll into the chest so that the cardia and pylorus are approximated, the stomach appearing upside down when examined radiologically (Fig. 26.14).

*Clinical features.* The patient is frequently middle-aged or elderly, and herniation occurs without a recognisable precipitating cause. Symp-

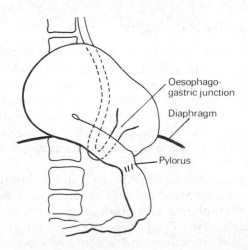

**Fig. 26.14** An 'upside-down' stomach

Oesophago-
gastric junction

Diaphragm

Pylorus

toms of reflux are exceptional, the patient usually experiencing discomfort or pain from distension of the thoracic portion of the stomach by food. The pain is deep seated within the chest, often described as crushing, and closely related to meals. Flatulence with belching is common and probably reflects attempts by the patient to gain relief. Weight loss and malnutrition may supervene as the patient cuts down on food intake to avoid symptoms.

Incarceration, pressure necrosis, gangrene and rupture can complicate para-oesophageal herniation, and lead to an acute illness with potentially fatal rupture of gastric contents into the mediastinum. Peptic ulceration, due possibly to inadequate drainage, may occur in the incarcerated stomach and in turn can be complicated by perforation or bleeding.

*Diagnosis.* The diagnosis is often apparent on chest X-ray which reveals a gas bubble and fluid level in the entrapped thoracic portion of stomach. The diagnosis is confirmed by barium meal examination. Endoscopy is not essential but may be used to exclude reflux oesophagitis.

*Management.* There is no medical management for para-oesophageal hiatus hernia and surgery is advised in all cases to relieve symptoms and avoid complications. The hernia can usually be reduced by an abdominal approach and the margins of the hernial defect approximated. An anti-reflux procedure is unnecessary but any associated gastric ulcer should be treated by vagotomy and drainage or gastric resection (see p. 371). Recurrence of herniation is uncommon. Symptoms are relieved promptly, and nutrition improves rapidly.

Strangulation of a para-oesophageal hernia necessitates emergency thoracotomy and gastric resection may be required if gangrene has supervened.

## Reflux oesophagitis with stricture formation

This occurs as a result of long-standing reflux with oesophagitis and fibrosis. Fibrotic shortening of the oesophagus may draw the cardia up into the chest, giving rise to the so-called 'short oesophagus'. This was once believed to be congenital. Heartburn is the dominant clinical feature of reflux oesophagitis but is replaced by dysphagia with stricture formation.

Dilatation alone does not prevent continuing gastro-oesophageal reflux and stricture recurrence is common. A trial of dilatation and intensive medical therapy is used in some centres as a first-line treatment of oesophageal stricture, but is reserved in others for frail or elderly patients. Dilatation followed by a surgical anti-reflux procedure is used when more conservative measures fail to produce relief.

Dilatation may be undertaken by passing a rigid oesophagoscope to the site of narrowing, and passing bougies of increasing diameter through the stricture. This can be facilitated by asking the patient to swallow a piece of string on the previous evening which will mark the path to be followed. Preferably, a fibre-optic endoscope can be used to pass a fine guide wire through the stricture under vision. The endoscope is then withdrawn and a series of flexible sounds are passed over the guide wire to dilate the narrowed area.

Rigid tough strictures may fail to respond to dilatation and an operation, which should include an anti-reflux procedure, may be needed. This may be:

*Resection.* The strictured portion of oesophagus is resected and continuity is restored by anastomosis of oesophagus to the mobilised stomach or to a gastric tube fashioned from the greater curvature. Alternatively, the resected portion of oesophagus can be replaced by a pedicled length of jejunum or colon.

*Fundal patch technique* (Fig. 26.15). Short strictures are opened longitudinally and the defect covered by the serosal surface of the mobilised gastric fundus. The fundus is sutured in place and its incorporated serosal surface becomes covered by stratified squamous epithelium within 3 weeks.

## Peptic ulceration in oesophagus lined by columnar epithelium

This condition is known as Barrett's ulcer (Fig. 26.16). It is now considered that the columnar epithelium lining the lower oesophagus represents a metaplastic response to persistent gastro-oesophageal reflux, and is not a congenital anomaly. Ulceration occurs at the squamocolumnar junction and may be complicated by bleeding, perforation or stricture formation. An associated hiatus hernia is common. The abnormal epithelium should be regarded as premalignant since adenocarcinoma develops in 10% of patients.

Elective surgery is advisable and consists of dilatation of any associated stricture with an anti-reflux procedure. Perforation or bleeding may require emergency oesophageal resection.

## Corrosive oesophagitis

This occurs most commonly in young children who accidentally swallow household caustics, corrosives and bleaches, and is no longer a common method of suicide. Necrosis and perforation of the oesophagus or stomach may occur, and strictures form in approximately 20% of surviving patients. Strictures are frequently multiple and extensive.

*Immediate management.* 1. Water is given to dilute the corrosive agent. If its nature is known, a dilute solution of acid or alkali may be used for neutralisation. The passage of a tube for gastric lavage is contraindicated because of the risk of perforation.

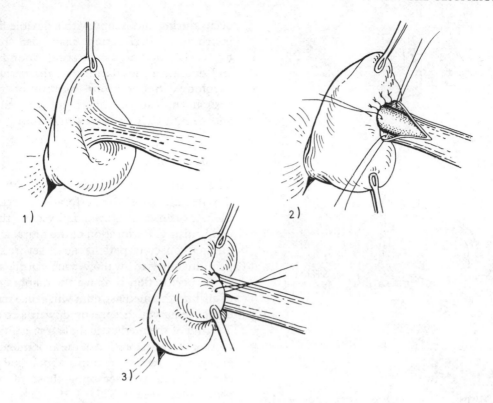

**Fig. 26.15** A fundal patch

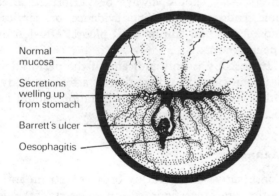

**Fig. 26.16** Endoscopic appearance of a Barrett's ulcer

Labels on figure: Normal mucosa; Secretions welling up from stomach; Barrett's ulcer; Oesophagitis

2. Steroids and a broad spectrum antibiotic are commenced immediately and continued for 3 weeks. The patient is carefully observed for signs of oesophageal or gastric necrosis and perforation.

3. Early gentle endoscopy under general anaesthesia is advised to assess the severity of the damage, but is unnecessary if associated respiratory symptoms suggest severe oesophageal injury.

4. Early feeding is encouraged in patients without perforation, as food is a natural form of bouginage.

5. Barium studies are repeated at intervals for 12 months to detect stricture formation. The return of dysphagia indicates a stricture and is an indication for repeat radiology.

*Management of strictures.* Mild early stricture formation will sometimes respond satisfactorily to a single dilatation. Established strictures require multiple dilatations and patients may require a feeding gastrostomy. In these patients retrograde bouginage through the gastrostomy is possibly safer than bouginage by the usual route.

Patients with extensive or multiple strictures require surgical treatment. Extensive peri-oesophageal scarring makes resection difficult and the oesophagus is better bypassed. The right or left colon can be used, the upper anastomosis being made in the neck (Fig. 26.17). The segments are long and the blood supply may be impaired, resulting in potentially lethal ischaemic necrosis in the upper portion of the segment.

Alternative forms of bypass utilise a microvas-

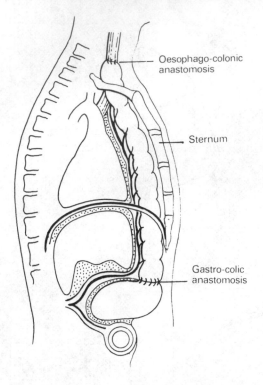

Fig. 26.17 Bypass of the oesophagus using a loop of colon

cular anastomosis between a neck vessel (eg inferior thyroid artery) and the pedicle of a segment of gut. Alternatively, one may construct a buried skin tube to connect the pharynx and abdominal oesophagus.

Patients with corrosive strictures of the oesophagus have a high risk of developing oesophageal carcinoma and should be kept under long-term review. For this reason, many surgeons favour resection in patients requiring operation for corrosive stricture. Carcinoma developing in oesophageal strictures appears less aggressive than the usual oesophageal carcinoma.

## OESOPHAGEAL PERFORATION

Perforation of the oesophagus may be caused accidentally at endoscopy, bouginage or the forcible passage of a wide-bore gastric lavage tube. Perforation is particularly liable to occur at the pharyngo-oesophageal junction (due to spasm of the cricopharyngeus muscle) or at the lower end of the oesophagus. Perforation is more common during passage of rigid oesophagoscopes but can

occur during endoscopy with a flexible fibre-optic instrument. Perforation may also be caused by foreign bodies, penetrating wounds, trauma and operative mobilisation of the oesophagus at vagotomy. Spontaneous rupture of the lower oesophagus can be caused by forceful retching and vomiting (Boerhaave syndrome).

### Clinical features

The severity of the clinical signs is influenced by the site and size of the perforation. Perforation in the neck causes surgical emphysema, throat pain and bruising. Perforation of the thoracic oesophagus in a conscious patient causes severe substernal pain, inability to swallow, tachycardia and fever. If the perforation is above the diaphragm escape of air into the mediastinum will cause mediastinal emphysema which spreads upwards to the neck. Tearing of the mediastinal pleura results in pneumothorax. A perforation of the abdominal oesophagus will produce acute upper abdominal pain with clinical features resembling those of perforated peptic ulcer (see p. 377).

Awareness of the diagnosis is essential and a chest X-ray should always be performed after rigid endoscopy, seeking evidence of cervical and mediastinal emphysema, pleural effusion or pneumothorax.

Endoscopy is only indicated if the perforation has been caused by ingestion of a foreign body. Otherwise, the site of the perforation should be localised by a gastrografin swallow.

### Management

Conservative treatment by broad spectrum antibiotics and insertion of a nasogastric tube is indicated for perforations of the cervical oesophagus. Drainage of the retro-oesophageal space through an incision in the neck may also be required. Perforation of the thoracic oesophagus demands immediate thoracotomy with repair of the perforation, or if necessary, resection of the affected segment. A patch of gastric fundus may be used to close the defect. The mediastinum and pleura should be drained. Provided operation is undertaken promptly and there is no sinister underlying cause, the prognosis is good.

## OESOPHAGEAL WEB

A fibrous web at the entrance of the oesophagus is the cause of the dysphagia which occurs in the Paterson-Kelly syndrome. Typically this occurs in middle-aged edentulous women and is associated with atrophic mucosa, anaemia and spoon-shaped fingers with brittle nails. However, all features of the syndrome are not necessarily present.

The presence of a web is confirmed by barium swallow and oesophagoscopy. Treatment consists of its disruption and correction of anaemia if present. As the atrophic mucosa is prone to malignancy, patients must be kept under regular supervision.

## TUMOURS OF THE OESOPHAGUS

### Benign tumours

Benign tumours of the oesophagus are rare accounting for less than 1% of all oesophageal neoplasms. The majority are asymptomatic but dysphagia and bleeding may occur. Leiomyoma is the commonest benign tumour and is detected radiologically as a filling defect covered by intact mucosa. Local resection is indicated. Other benign neoplasms include fibrovascular polyps and lipomas for which endoscopic removal may be feasible. Lipomas may also be intramuscular and require surgical removal.

### Carcinoma of the oesophagus

The incidence of oesophageal carcinoma varies widely throughout the world. It is particularly common in the Far East, Iran, Africa and the West Indies. In Europe it is a relatively rare form of cancer and in Scotland accounts for just over 1% of all cases of malignancy.

Oesophageal cancer is rare before the age of 40 years. Thereafter its incidence increases progressively and is greatest in those over 70 years. Men are more commonly affected than women except for hypopharyngeal cancer which is more common in women.

*Aetiology*. The aetiology of oesophageal cancer remains unknown but chronic irritation, alcohol, tobacco chewing and smoking are risk factors. Hot spicy foods are also believed to favour development of the disease. Other dietary factors include nitrosamines and the aflatoxin of the mould *Aspergillus flavus* which can affect nuts and seeds stored in damp conditions. Nutritional and dietetic deficiency has also been implicated.

Local conditions associated with an increased risk of oesophageal cancer include the Paterson-Kelly syndrome, achalasia, hiatus hernia and corrosive strictures.

*Pathology*. The majority of oesophageal cancers are of squamous type. Eighty per cent of such epidermoid tumours occur in the middle third of the oesophagus, the remainder being distributed between the upper and lower thirds. Adenocarcinomas may arise in columnar epithelium in the lower oesophagus. These adenocarcinomas usually arise from the upper stomach and extend upwards to involve the oesophagus.

Oesophageal cancer may become manifest as a polypoidal, ulcerating or hard infiltrating growth which spreads along the oesophageal mucosa and submucosa and invades adjacent structures.

*Clinical features*. Progressive dysphagia (first for solids and then for liquids) and weight loss are typical features. Excessive salivation, aspiration pneumonia, anaemia and lassitude are late effects. The tumour may also erode into a bronchus to establish an oesophago-bronchial fistula, perforate into the mediastinum, or infiltrate the recurrent laryngeal nerves to cause hoarseness. Distant metastases are rare.

As the oesophagus lies deeply within the thorax, clinical examination is rarely helpful. However, the lower neck and upper abdomen should be carefully palpated for lymph-node enlargement, a tumour mass, and hepatomegaly. Barium swallow usually reveals an irregular filling defect or localised stricture of the oesophagus (Fig. 26.18). The oesophagus above the tumour does not dilate to the extent seen in achalasia. Endoscopy demonstrates an oedematous and friable oesphagus above the tumour. The cancer usually forms a hard occluding mass which prevents further advancement of the instrument. Its upper level is noted and a biopsy is taken.

*Management*. Oesophageal cancer can be managed by resection, by irradiation, or by a combination of both according to the extent of the site

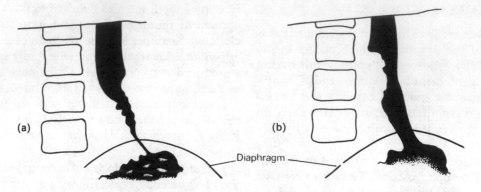

**Fig. 26.18** Radiological features of oesophageal carcinoma. (a) Long, irregular stricture. (b) Irregular filling defect.

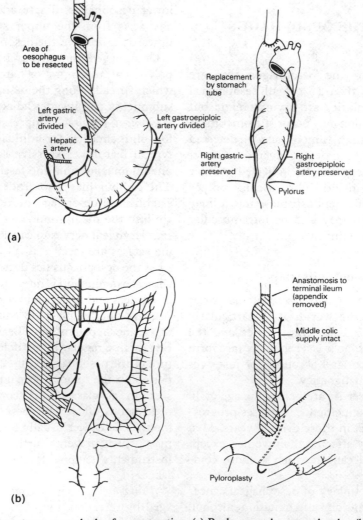

**Fig. 26.19** Total oesophagectomy — methods of reconstruction. (a) Replacement by stomach tube. (b) Replacement by colon.

of the lesion. Tumours of the upper third of the oesophagus are generally treated by radical radiotherapy, those of the lower third by surgery, and those in mid-oesophagus by either modality. Some surgeons prefer to perform a total oesophagectomy in all cases, bringing a tube of stomach or colon up to the neck to anastomose to the pharynx (Fig. 26.19).

In patients with non-resectable cancer, dysphagia can be relieved by insertion of a Celestin or similar tube (Fig. 26.20) to ensure that the patient can swallow and maintain nutritional intake. Alternatively, the obstructing cancer can be by-passed by bringing up a loop of jejunum to the oesophagus above the lesion.

Resectability and prognosis are influenced by tumour size; 50% of tumours under 5 cm in length have lymph node involvement whereas 90% of those longer than 5 cm have nodal deposits. Oesophago-tracheal fistula and hoarseness are signs of inoperable disease, and resection is seldom worthwhile in patients with metastatic spread. Of 100 patients presenting with oesophageal cancer, 60 will undergo surgical exploration, of whom only 40 will undergo resection.

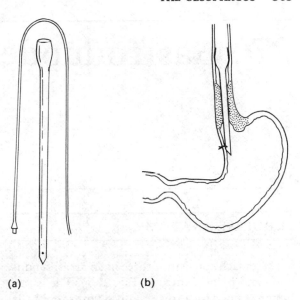

(a)                              (b)

**Fig. 26.20** (a) Celestin tube and guide, (b) Celestin tube in position.

Resection carries an operative mortality of 10–20%. The overall one-year survival following diagnosis of oesophageal cancer is 20%; the 5-year survival is less than 5%.

# 27. Gastroduodenal Disorders

## SURGICAL ANATOMY

The stomach consists of three main areas: fundus, body and pyloric antrum (Fig. 27.1). The gastric lumen is lined by a row of tall columnar epithelial cells which commence abruptly at the cardia at the point of termination of the stratified squamous epithelium of the oesophagus. The gastric epithelium is pitted throughout by the opening of gastric glands. These glands are of three types:

The *cardiac glands* which secrete mucus and electrolytes, and occupy a small ring around the oesophago-gastric junction.

The *gastric glands* which occupy the entire fundus and body of the stomach, taking up some 75% of gastric mucosal surface area. There are at least five types of cell lining these glands. *Mucous neck cells* lie in the narrow neck beneath the gastric pits. *Undifferentiated neck cells* divide throughout life to replenish the surface epithelium and oxyntic glandular cells. *Parietal cells* produce $H^+$ and intrinsic factor and are most numerous in the upper half of the glands. *Peptic*

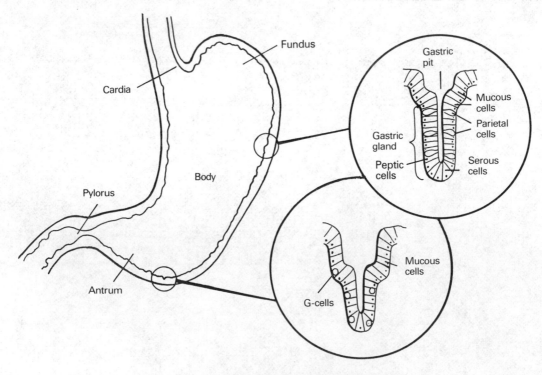

**Fig. 27.1** Anatomy of the human stomach

*cells* secrete pepsinogen and are most numerous in the lower half of the glands. A number of *endocrine cells* are found between the peptic cells but their physiological function is uncertain (Fig. 27.1).

The *pyloric glands* occupy the antrum and are separated from the oxyntic gland area by a transitional zone. The glands are lined by cells resembling mucous neck cells which secrete mucus and electrolytes, and by G-cells which produce the hormone gastrin.

## Nerve supply

The stomach receives its autonomic nerve supply from the vagus nerves and from the sympathetic nervous system. The left and right vagus nerves form an anterior and posterior oesophageal plexus on the mid-oesophagus, each plexus containing fibres from both nerves (Fig. 27.2). Each plexus forms a vagal trunk just above the diaphragm and the anterior and posterior trunks enter the abdomen by passing through the diaphragm with

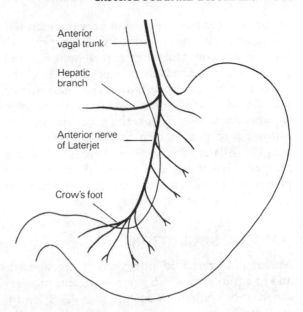

**Fig. 27.3** Anatomy of anterior vagus nerve

the oesophagus. The anterior trunk gives off a hepatic branch and then descends along the lesser curvature to supply the front wall of the stomach (Fig. 27.3). The posterior trunk gives off a coeliac branch on entering the abdomen and then descends along the posterior aspect of the lesser curve supplying the back wall of the stomach (Fig. 27.2). Approximately 80% of vagal fibres are afferent, and almost two-thirds of the fibres entering the abdomen innervate the stomach. The remaining one-third pass in the hepatic and coeliac branches to innervate the liver, gallbladder, pancreas, small intestine and large intestine as far as the distal transverse colon.

Sympathetic post-ganglionic fibres pass from the coeliac ganglion and reach the stomach by accompanying the gastric arteries.

## SURGICAL PHYSIOLOGY

### GASTRIC MOTILITY

After ingestion, food is stored in the stomach where it is ground, mixed and prepared for controlled release into the duodenum. Receptive relaxation is the process by which the body and fundus of stomach relax to accommodate increasing

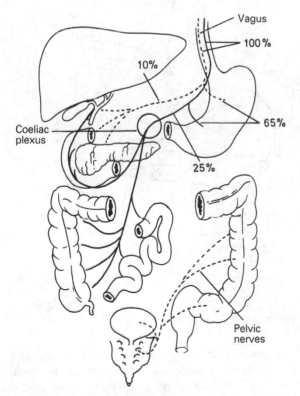

**Fig. 27.2** Distribution of abdominal parasympathetic nerves

volumes of food without major pressure increase. The antrum is not concerned with receptive relaxation but powerful antral contractions mix and grind the food, and then expel food into the duodenum as the pylorus relaxes. The intrinsic neural plexuses (myenteric and submucosal) play an important role in governing gastric motility but are regulated in turn by the extrinsic nerve supply. Bilateral truncal vagotomy abolishes receptive relaxation and greatly diminishes the power of antral contraction. The sympathetic nerves inhibit gastric motility.

## GASTRIC SECRETION

Mucus is secreted by all regions of the stomach and in addition to serving as a lubricant, protects the surface epithelium against auto-digestion by acid and pepsin.

Gastric acid and pepsin secretion is not essential for protein digestion as great quantities of proteolytic enzymes are secreted by the pancreas. Four substances normally present in the body are capable of stimulating gastric secretion. *Calcium* acts as a stimulant to acid, pepsin and gastrin secretion when there is hypercalcaemia but is not a normal physiological stimulant. *Acetylcholine* and *gastrin* have established physiological roles as secretory stimulants, while *histamine* has strong claims for a physiological role. Acetylcholine acts as a neurocrine regulator and mediates vagal stimulation. Gastrin serves as a conventional endocrine regulator and is carried by the blood stream from antrum to body of stomach, while histamine is probably released from cells in the immediate vicinity of parietal and peptic cells, and acts as a *paracrine* regulator. The parietal and peptic cells possess separate receptor sites for acetylcholine, gastrin and histamine, but the action of each chemical is potentiated by a tonic effect of the other two. This means that surgical vagotomy not only removes stimulation by acetylcholine, it also reduces the efficacy of gastrin and histamine as stimulants (Fig. 27.4).

### Control of gastric secretion

The stimulation of gastric secretion is usually divided into three phases (Fig. 27.5).

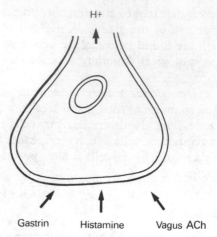

Hydrochloric acid secreted in response to various stimuli

**Fig. 27.4** Interactions of gastric hormones and parietal cell

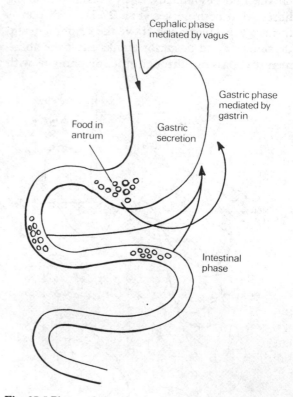

**Fig. 27.5** Phases of gastric secretion

*Cephalic (neural) phase.* The sight, smell, taste and even the thought of food activates the vagal centre. Impulses then pass down both vagal nerves to stimulate the parietal and peptic cells directly by releasing acetylcholine, and indirectly by releasing gastrin from the antrum. The indirect mechanism is less important than the direct one.

*Gastric phase.* Food in the stomach initiates acid and pepsin secretion by releasing gastrin from G-cells in the antrum. Antrectomy without vagotomy reduces the maximal acid response to histamine by 50–80%. Protein constituents are particularly effective releasers of gastrin. Luminal pH regulates the gastric phase in that gastrin secretion is reduced by antral acidification; the gastrin response to a protein meal when luminal pH is 2.5 is 80% less than that at pH 5.5. This inhibitory feedback mechanism is important in preventing inappropriate acid and pepsin secretion.

Gastric distension also stimulates gastric acid and pepsin secretion. Local intramural reflexes involving acetylcholine release are probably responsible.

*Intestinal phase.* This phase commences as food enters the duodenum and persists for some hours after a meal. The mechanism responsible is uncertain but may involve release of gastrin from cells in the duodenum, release of other hormones from the small intestine, or neural reflexes. Increased acid secretion follows extensive resection of the small intestine, suggesting that important inhibitory mechanisms are also triggered by food in the intestine.

## PEPTIC ULCERATION

Peptic ulceration results from an imbalance between gastric secretion and the ability of the mucosa of the upper gastro-intestinal tract to withstand peptic digestion. The proteolytic enzyme pepsin is responsible for mucosal digestion and ulceration; acid secretion is important only in that it provides an environment conducive to peptic activity. Pepsin enjoys optimal activity at around pH 2, is inactive when pH exceeds 4.8, and is irreversibly inactivated above pH 7.

Excessive or inappropriate acid and pepsin secretion is implicated in duodenal ulceration in that the mean maximal secretory capacity of duodenal ulcer patients exceeds that of normal subjects (Fig. 27.6). However, there is considerable overlap between the groups and many individuals with duodenal ulceration have secretory capacities within the normal range. Hypersecretion is not of primary importance in the development of gastric ulceration. Many patients have normal or reduced secretory capacity (Fig. 27.6). Defective mucosal defence is believed to be a major factor leading to ulceration in such individuals. However, ulceration does *not* occur in the absence of acid and pepsin secretion. At least some secretion is essential to exploit defective or damaged mucosal defences and cause ulcer formation.

Peptic ulceration produces a wide spectrum of clinical disorders. For example, the ulcer may be acute or chronic, may heal spontaneously or exhibit alternating periods of remission and exacerbation. It may also give rise to complications such as bleeding, perforation or stenosis. Stress ulceration is an acute form of gastric or duodenal ulceration encountered during severe illness or injury, and will be considered separately.

## SITES OF PEPTIC ULCER

Peptic ulceration occurs in the duodenum, stomach, oesophagus and jejunum, and rarely in association with a Meckel's diverticulum containing ectopic acid-secreting mucosa (Fig. 27.7). (See p. 396)

### Duodenum

Ulceration of the first part of the duodenum is the commonest form of peptic ulcer. Ulceration of other parts of the duodenum is exceptional, but may occur in the rare Zollinger-Ellison syndrome (p. 385).

### Stomach

Gastric ulceration is the second commonest form of peptic ulcer. Three types of gastric ulcer are described (Fig. 27.8).

*Type I* or primary gastric ulcers account for the majority and arise because of damaged mucosal defences. The ulcer is often on the lesser curve, is usually associated with gastritis, and develops at

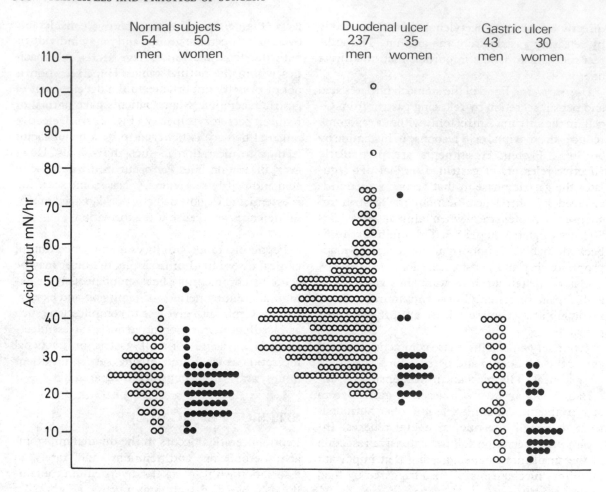

**Fig. 27.6** Maximal acid secretion in normal males and in patients with duodenal and gastric ulcer

the junction between acid secreting and non-acid secreting mucosa.

*Type II* or secondary gastric ulcers are found in association with duodenal ulcers and arise because of gastric stasis due to duodenal deformity.

*Type III* ulcers are found in the pyloric channel or immediate pre-pyloric area and are believed to have more in keeping with duodenal than gastric ulceration. Thus they are associated with normal or increased levels of gastric secretion.

### Oesophagus

Oesophageal ulceration is relatively rare and is due to reflux of acid and pepsin from the stomach (p. 354). These ulcers are small and superficial unless they occur on columnar mucosa when they may be large and penetrating.

### Jejunum

Jejunal ulceration is uncommon. It occurs as a form of recurrent ulceration when gastric contents have been diverted into the jejunum by gastro-jejunal anastomosis, and may be a manifestation of the Zollinger-Ellison syndrome.

### SYMPTOMS OF PEPTIC ULCERATION

The clinical features of peptic ulceration are dominated by epigastric pain. As the stomach and duodenum, in terms of their visceral embryonic innervation are midline structures, the pain is felt in

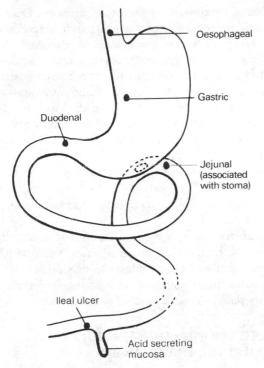

**Fig. 27.7** Sites of peptic ulceration

the mid-line of the epigastrium and is of vague, boring and deep-seated type.

The main characteristics of peptic ulcer pain are:

1. *Periodicity.* 'Good spells and bad spells' are typical. Usually symptoms occur every 3–6 months and last for 7–10 days but the time, both of the attacks and periods of remission, is variable. No clear explanation has yet been given for this typical pattern.

2. *Relationship to food.* During an attack, the pain of peptic ulceration is related to food. Typically, the pain occurs when the stomach is empty and is relieved within minutes of taking food. It is truly a 'hunger pain'. If symptoms are severe, the pain wakens the patient during the night usually around 2.00–3.00 am when, as at other times, a drink of milk will rapidly abate the symptoms. Alkali has a similar effect.

3. *Accompanying symptoms.* Pain apart, peptic ulcer causes symptoms of hyperacidity with heartburn (burning pain in the midline of the lower chest), water-brash (sudden flow of saliva) and a general feeling of upper abdominal unease. Vomiting of small quantities of fluffy secretions tinged with food-stuffs often relieving the pain is typical. A feeling of fullness accompanied by inability to eat large quantities of food is a common symptom which can cause embarrassment.

4. *Vomiting* is of two types: 'retention vomiting' due to pyloric obstruction occurs after a long period of peptic ulcer symptoms, and that during an acute attack (as described above). The latter is more common.

## Treatment

The initial treatment of the patient with peptic ulcer is medical and has been revolutionised by the

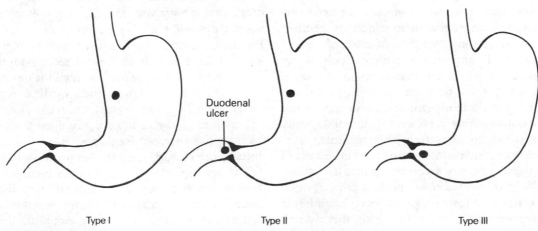

**Fig. 27.8** Types of gastric ulceration

introduction of drugs effectively inhibiting gastric acid secretion.

Peptic ulcer patients come under the care of the surgeon in the following circumstances:

1. For the management of ulcer disease suspected or diagnosed by general practitioners and other hospital physicians.

2. For consideration of surgical treatment in patients failed on medical management.

3. For the management of emergency complications of peptic ulcer, namely bleeding, perforation or stenosis.

4. For the management of the long-term complications of previous ulcer surgery.

5. When stress ulceration develops in patients as a consequence of injury, operation or severe illness.

6. To undertake endoscopy to establish the diagnosis.

## ELECTIVE SURGICAL MANAGEMENT OF PEPTIC ULCERATION

Patients may be referred directly to the surgeon by their general practitioner or referred for surgery by a physician. Patients coming to hospital for the first time may have had little or no investigation of their symptoms, whereas patients referred by a physician have usually undergone thorough investigation and a trial of medical management. Regardless of the mode of referral, the surgeon must address the following issues:

1. *Is the diagnosis of peptic ulcer correct and have all necessary investigations been completed?*

*Barium meal examination* must have been carried out in all cases, bearing in mind that the ulcer may not be seen in some 25% of cases.

*Endoscopy* is indicated in patients with 'X-ray negative dyspepsia' and is mandatory in all cases of gastric ulcer so that the ulcer can be inspected and biopsied to exclude malignancy. Endoscopy is not carried out routinely in patients with radiologically proven duodenal ulceration, although many surgeons recommend endoscopy to detect unsuspected oesophageal lesions or secondary gastric ulceration.

*Acid secretory studies* are no longer performed as a routine. Most surgeons have abandoned selective surgery policies in which the type of operation performed was determined by the patient's maximal acid secretory capacity. Determination of basal acid output and maximal response to pentagastrin was once used to diagnose the Zollinger-Ellison syndrome and to exclude achlorhydria in patients thought to have benign gastric ulceration. However, gastrin radioimmunoassay has replaced secretory studies in diagnosis of the Zollinger-Ellison syndrome, while endoscopy is now used to inspect and biopsy all gastric ulcers to exclude malignancy.

*Serum gastrin levels* are measured under fasting conditions and in response to secretin injection whenever the Zollinger-Ellison syndrome is suspected (p. 385).

*Oral cholecystography* or ultrasonic scan may be advisable because of the frequency with which peptic ulcer and cholelithiasis co-exist.

2. *Are there sufficient indications for surgical rather than continued medical management?*

## INDICATIONS FOR SURGERY IN DUODENAL ULCERATION

### Failure of medical management

Reduction of gastric secretion and ulcer healing can now be achieved in the majority of patients by the histamine $H_2$-receptor antagonists cimetidine or ranitidine. However, while these drugs speed ulcer healing and can sustain remission, they do not remove the underlying ulcer diathesis. Although cimetidine appears to be a relatively safe drug, the consequences of long-term therapy are as yet unknown, and most physicians are reluctant to prescribe more than two 6-week courses of the drug, or to persist with maintenance therapy (400 mg nocte or 400 mg bd) for more than 12 months. For these reasons surgery is usually recommended when cimetidine fails to control ulcer symptoms (uncommon), when a patient is unwilling or unable to comply with the prescribed medical regime (uncommon), or when symptoms recur after two full courses of the drug or a sustained period of maintenance therapy. Ranitidine has been introduced more recently, and similar principles apply.

The severity of symptoms varies considerably from patient to patient and the duration of history alone should not necessarily influence the decision to advise surgery. Patients should no longer have to 'earn their operation' by years of discomfort and misery. Factors which favour early recourse to operation include:

1. Onset in adolescence.
2. Strong family history of duodenal ulceration.
3. High levels of acid secretion.
4. A previous complication (see below).
5. Occupational factors. Loss of time from work is usually regarded by patient and surgeon as a factor favouring operation. In the Armed Forces, peptic ulceration leads to automatic downgrading with adverse effects on promotion prospects. Patients likely to spend long periods without easy access to medical care should be advised to have surgery.
6. Intercurrent disease (patients who require long-term anticoagulant or steroid therapy and who have an ulcer should have this treated surgically prior to starting therapy if this is feasible).

### Development of complications

Previous perforation or ulcer bleeding are strong indications for elective operation in patients with recurrent symptoms. Pyloric stenosis is an absolute indication for surgery. Patients with combined duodenal and gastric ulcers are advised to have operation because the response to medical management is usually poor.

### Psychological factors

Patients with marked psychological disturbance or personality disorder pose a difficult problem in management, and some surgeons are reluctant to recommend operation. However, the prospects for ulcer healing after operation are just as good as in other patients, and this group should not be denied surgery. It is essential to make certain that the patient's symptoms are due to duodenal ulcer, and this requires endoscopic visualisation of an active ulcer crater during a symptomatic period. All concerned must be made aware of the fact that surgery is unlikely to influence the underlying psychological problem, and continued collaboration with a psychiatrist may be necessary.

## INDICATIONS FOR SURGERY IN GASTRIC ULCERATION

Patients with gastric ulceration are more likely to require operation than those with duodenal ulcer. Indications for surgery include:

### Suspicion of malignancy

Ten per cent of ulcers diagnosed as benign on barium meal examination prove to be malignant. Malignant transformation of a benign peptic ulcer is now considered unlikely, and many cases of 'malignant transformation' merely reflect failure to detect the underlying malignant nature of the ulcer. Endoscopic inspection and multiple biopsies to exclude malignancy are essential prerequisites of the medical treatment of gastric ulceration, and any course of treatment must be followed by full reassessment to reduce diagnostic error. Ulcers at sites other than the lesser curvature are regarded with particular suspicion, but vigilance cannot be relaxed when the ulcer is located on the lesser curve.

### Failure of medical management

Failure of ulcer healing after a 6-week course of therapy suggests that there may be underlying malignancy and is a strong indication for surgery.

### Recurrence of ulceration

This is a strong indication for operation.

### Development of complications

Previous perforation or bleeding, or the development of fibrous contraction — 'hour-glass stomach', are indications for operation.

## INDICATIONS FOR SURGERY IN ENDOCRINE ADENOPATHIES

Peptic ulceration occurs in some 15% of patients with hyperparathyroidism and may be due to hypergastrinaemia and gastic hypersecretion consequent on hypercalcaemia. In the majority of cases, the peptic ulcer heals following surgical treatment of hyperparathyroidism, and direct ulcer surgery is only indicated if ulceration persists. The surgical management of the Zollinger-Ellison syndrome is discussed below (p. 385).

## PREPARATION FOR ELECTIVE OPERATION

The patient is prepared as for all elective major abdominal operations. A nasogastric tube is passed on the morning of operation to ensure that the stomach remains empty, to aid the surgeon in mobilisation of the oesophagus for vagotomy, and to prevent post-operative gastric distension.

The patient is warned to expect a hospital stay of some 7–10 days and should remain off work for about 6 weeks.

## PRINCIPLES OF SURGERY

The aim of surgery is to reduce acid and pepsin secretion to levels no longer associated with peptic ulceration. The ideal operation should achieve this consistently and safely, and give rise to an acceptably low incidence of post-operative side effects. A number of operations are available for the surgical cure of gastric and duodenal ulcer but no one operation is ideal and different surgeons may vary in their choice of procedure.

## OPERATIONS AVAILABLE FOR ELECTIVE MANAGEMENT OF DUODENAL ULCER

### Truncal vagotomy and drainage

Division of the anterior and posterior vagal trunks just beneath the oesophageal hiatus reduces acid and pepsin secretion at the expense of impaired receptive relaxation and diminished antral motility. These undesired effects led to significant stasis in approximately half of the patients subjected to truncal vagotomy alone, and for this reason truncal vagotomy was combined routinely with a procedure to facilitate gastric drainage and prevent stasis. The drainage procedure may consist of pyloroplasty or gastroenterostomy (Fig. 27.9). Gastroenterostomy is preferred if there is marked duodenal inflammation or scarring, but otherwise there is little to choose between the two procedures, and pyloroplasty is generally preferred.

Truncal vagotomy and drainage is safe in that the operative mortality is below 1%, but approximately 5–10% of patients develop recurrent ulceration (see below). Failure to define and divide all vagal trunks is usually responsible. The integrity of the vagus can be tested by the induction of insulin hypoglycaemia, which with intact vagi stimulates a brisk secretory response (Fig. 27.10).

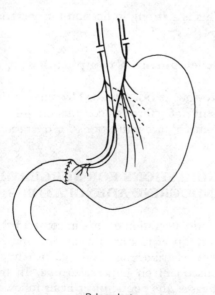
Pyloroplasty

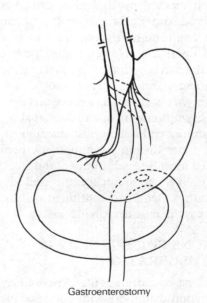
Gastroenterostomy

**Fig. 27.9** Truncal vagotomy and drainage

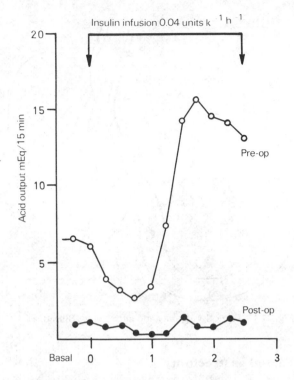

Fig. 27.10 Insulin test of gastric secretion (time in hours)

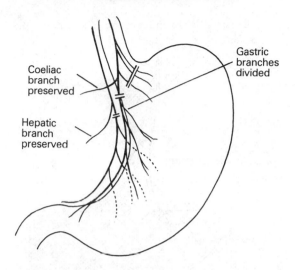

**Fig. 27.11** Selective vagotomy

Post-operative insulin tests show that vagotomy has been incomplete in some 30–40% of patients. The best method of administering insulin is by the intravenous infusion of a constant dose (0.04 unit/kg body wt/hr). However the insulin test is often unpleasant for the patient, is potentially dangerous, and is no longer performed routinely.

In addition to gastric denervation, truncal vagotomy denervates the other abdominal organs supplied by the vagus. Diarrhoea may follow vagotomy and drainage, although it poses a serious problem in only some 3% of patients. At one time, diarrhoea was considered to be a consequence of the vagotomy but it is now thought more likely to be due to the drainage procedure and uncontrolled gastric emptying. The dumping syndrome may also occur from this cause (see p. 382). Bilious vomiting is a common side effect of truncal vagotomy and drainage and results from regurgitation of bile through the pyloroplasty or gastroenterostomy.

Despite these shortcomings, its relative safety and ease of performance have made truncal vagotomy and drainage the standard duodenal ulcer operation in this country.

## Selective vagotomy and drainage

This operation was introduced to avoid vagal denervation of abdominal organs other than the stomach in the hope that the incidence of side effects would be lower than that following truncal vagotomy. Only the gastric branches of the vagus were divided (Fig. 27.11) and it was hoped that the more detailed dissection needed would ensure complete gastric vagotomy and a reduced incidence of recurrent ulceration. These hopes have not been realised, and this operation is now seldom performed.

## Highly selective vagotomy (proximal gastric vagotomy)

In Edinburgh and some other centres, this operation is now the most frequently performed elective operation for duodenal ulcer. Only those vagal fibres innervating the body of stomach are divided while those supplying the antrum and other abdominal organs are spared (Fig. 27.12). Acid and pepsin secretion are reduced to about the same extent as after truncal vagotomy, but the antrum and pylorus remain innervated so that there is no need to carry out a drainage procedure. The operation is safe, the incidence of side effects such as diarrhoea, bilious vomiting and dumping is minimal, and in experienced hands the rate of recur-

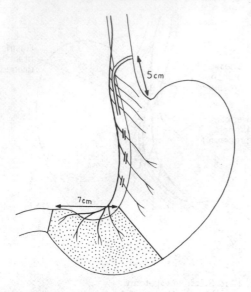

**Fig. 27.12** Highly selective vagotomy

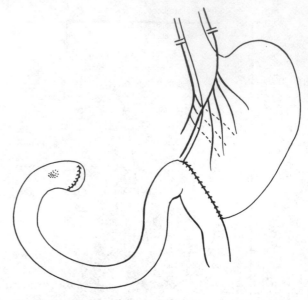

**Fig. 27.13** Truncal vagotomy and antrectomy (Billroth II)

rent ulceration is reported to be no greater than that of truncal vagotomy and drainage (Table 27.1).

## Truncal vagotomy and antrectomy

As vagal denervation is combined with removal of the major gastrin-producing area, this operation has a recurrent ulcer rate of only 1%. It is associated with a greater operative mortality than truncal vagotomy and drainage or highly selective vagotomy. The incidence of other side effects is similar to that of truncal vagotomy and drainage (Table 27.1).

Intestinal continuity after antrectomy is restored by gastro-duodenal (Billroth I) or gastro-jejunal anastomosis (Billroth II) (Fig. 27.13).

## Partial gastrectomy

Partial gastrectomy was once the standard operation for duodenal ulcer but has been largely superseded by the various operations involving vagotomy. The operation consists of removing the antrum plus a proportion of the body of the stomach, leaving only 1/4 to 1/3 of the stomach in place. Intestinal continuity is restored by gastro-jejunal anastomosis (Fig. 27.14). The more extensive the resection, the lower the risk of recurrent ulceration. The surgeon has to balance the desire to avoid recurrence against the undesirable consequences of a small gastric remnant (see p. 382). Partial gastrectomy carries an overall operative mortality of at least 2% (Table 27.1). Leakage

**Table 27.1** Results of surgery for duodenal ulcer

| Criterion | | Operation | | |
|---|---|---|---|---|
| | HSV | TV+D | TV+A | PG |
| Operative mortality | 0.3% | 0.6–0.8% | 1–1.5% | 2% |
| Satisfactory long-term results (Visick grade I & II) | 86% | 75% | 85% | 75% |
| Recurrent ulceration | 10% | 10% | 1% | 3% |

Key    HSV = highly selective vagotomy
       TV+D = truncal vagotomy and drainage procedure
       TV+A = truncal vagotomy and antrectomy
          PG = partial gastrectomy

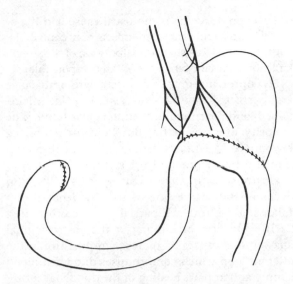

**Fig. 27.14** Partial gastrectomy for duodenal ulcer (Polya or Billroth II)

from the duodenal stump after Billroth II procedures is the commonest cause of death.

# OPERATIONS AVAILABLE FOR THE ELECTIVE MANAGEMENT OF GASTRIC ULCER

## Type I gastric ulcer

The choice rests between Billroth I partial gastrectomy (Fig. 27.15) and truncal vagotomy with drainage. Partial gastrectomy reduces acid and pepsin secretion by removing about 60% of the stomach including the ulcer. The results of the operation are usually excellent. Operative mortality is acceptable and recurrent ulceration is rare (Table 27.2). As the ulcer is removed for complete histological examination, there is no risk of leaving a malignant ulcer *in situ*.

Truncal vagotomy and drainage is a less certain method to reduce acid and pepsin secretion and recurrent ulceration follows this operation in 10% of patients (Table 27.2). The operation carries a lower operative mortality than partial gastrectomy but there is a real risk that a malignant ulcer may be missed and left *in situ*. If truncal vagotomy and drainage is employed, the stomach must be opened and the ulcer subjected to multiple biopsy or excision.

Most surgeons now favour partial gastrectomy

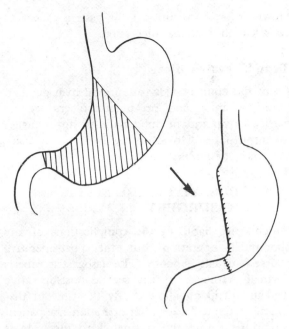

**Fig. 27.15** Partial gastrectomy for gastric ulcer (Billroth I)

**Table 27.2** Results of surgery for gastric ulcer

| Criterion | Operation | |
| --- | --- | --- |
| | TV+D | PG |
| Mortality | 1.5% | 2% |
| Satisfactory long-term results (Visick grade I & II) | 70% | 75% |
| Recurrent ulceration | 10% | 3% |
| Risk of retained cancer | ? | 0 |

*Key* TV+D = truncal vagotomy and drainage procedure
PG = partial gastrectomy

for gastric ulceration because of the risks of malignancy. Truncal vagotomy and drainage is usually reserved for poor risk patients, or those in whom the ulcer is situated so high on the lesser curvature that gastric resection would be extensive or difficult and incur serious risk of complications.

Highly selective vagotomy is not generally recommended for gastric ulceration.

## Type II gastric ulcer

The gastric ulcer is secondary to duodenal ulceration and the surgeon carries out the operation he favours for duodenal ulcer. If the gastric ulcer is to be left *in situ*, adequate biopsy is advised.

However it is exceptional for gastric cancer to coexist with duodenal ulceration.

### Type III gastric ulcer

From the point of view of surgical management, pyloric channel and pre-pyloric ulcers are regarded as variants of duodenal ulcer for management purposes. However highly selective vagotomy is not suitable.

## POSTOPERATIVE CARE AFTER GASTRIC SURGERY

Patients are liable to the complications of any abdominal operation but the post-operative course is usually smooth. The nasogastric tube is normally removed by the second post-operative day and drinking allowed. By the time of discharge at about 1 week after operation, the patient should be eating the normal ward diet. He is advised initially to eat small meals at frequent intervals, rather than attempt two or three large meals in the course of a day. 'Ulcer diets' are not necessary after operation. No restrictions are placed on food content. However, the patient with an anastomosis should be warned to avoid fruits such as orange with a strong pith. The pith may pass undigested through a wide or incontinent gastric outlet and occlude the small intestine, a 'bolus' obstruction.

## SPECIFIC COMPLICATIONS OF SURGERY FOR PEPTIC ULCERATION

The following complications may arise in the immediate post-operative period:

*Chest infection.* This is common because the upper abdominal incision restricts lung expansion and coughing, and many ulcer patients are cigarette smokers.

*Suture line haemorrhage.* This occurs during the first 24 hours after operation and is recognised by bright blood in the nasogastric aspirate. It usually ceases spontaneously, but transfusion may be needed. Re-operation is rarely required.

*Stomal hold-up* with obstruction of the gastric outlet is suspected if the patient continues to have large volumes of nasogastric aspirate. An X-ray examination with gastrografin will confirm stomal obstruction. Oedema is the usual cause and hypoproteinaemia and electrolyte upsets may contribute. Mechanical factors such as malposition of the stoma, kinks or adhesions are occasionally responsible.

Hypoproteinaemia and electrolyte imbalance are corrected, nasogastric aspiration is maintained, and parenteral nutrition is instituted. The majority of cases settle, but hold-up persisting beyond 10 to 14 days usually requires re-operation and refashioning of the stoma.

*Anastomotic leakage.* This is most likely to occur at the suture line of the duodenal stump following Billroth II partial gastrectomy (Fig. 27.16). Oedema or kinking at the gastro-jejunal anastomosis causes an increase in pressure in the afferent loop which compromises duodenal blood supply and impairs healing of the duodenal suture line. Duodenal stump 'blow-out' is evident on the 4th or 5th day after operation. The patient looks and feels unwell, experiences pain in the right hypochondrium with pyrexia, and discharges bile-stained fluid through the wound or drain track. Local adhesions usually prevent generalised peritonitis, but subphrenic or subhepatic abscess formation is common and a fistula forms.

The principles of management of a duodenal fistula are:

1. Ensure that *external drainage is adequate* and that duodenal content is not accumulating within the abdomen. Re-operation may be needed to place a large drain down to or in to the leaking duodenum. Repair of the fistula is usually not feasible at this stage.

2. *Maintain fluid and electrolyte balance* by recording daily fluid and electrolyte intake and

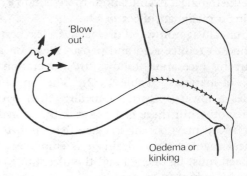

**Fig. 27.16** Duodenal fistula following Billroth II gastrectomy

loss, and by establishing an intravenous infusion. The volume of fistula loss varies greatly but may exceed 3 litres a day.

3. *Prevent erosion of the skin* around the fistula site by the proteolytic enzymes in pancreatic juice. The skin is protected by applying a stom-adhesive pad and attaching a colostomy bag to collect the fistula fluid. Alternatively, a sump suction drain may be placed in the fistula track.

4. *Maintain nutritional intake.* Oral intake may be continued when the output from the fistula is small and this may be supplemented by an elemental diet. If the volume of output increases, food residue appears in the discharging fluid or the patient is progressively losing weight and well-being oral intake is stopped and parenteral nutrition given.

5. Ensure that there is *no distal hold-up* preventing healing of the duodenum.

In the majority of patients, the fistula will heal on conservative management within 2 weeks. Failure to heal suggests persisting afferent loop obstruction and contrast radiology followed by re-operation may be required.

## COMPLICATIONS OF PEPTIC ULCERATION

### HAEMORRHAGE

Bleeding occurs in about 20% of ulcer patients, and peptic ulcer is the commonest cause of acute upper gastro-intestinal blood loss. This topic is considered on p. 390.

### PERFORATION

#### Clinical features

Perforation of a duodenal ulcer is ten times more common than perforation of a gastric ulcer. No age group is immune but the peak incidence lies in the 4th and 5th decades of life. Perforation can occur without significant preceding dyspepsia and may be stress related. Alternatively, the patient may have had a long dyspeptic history with previous episodes of bleeding or perforation.

Treatment is influenced by whether the ulcer is 'acute' or 'chronic'. As an arbitrary working rule a

duodenal ulcer is regarded as chronic when the dyspeptic history exceeds 3 months. A gastric ulcer which perforates is regarded as chronic.

Clinically, perforation of a peptic ulcer usually presents as an acute abdominal catastrophe with sudden severe epigastric pain which rapidly becomes generalised throughout the abdomen. The precise time of onset is clearly recalled. Retching may have occurred at the onset of pain but vomiting is rare.

The patient lies still, being afraid to move for fear of exacerbating the pain. Abdominal tenderness, guarding, and board-like abdominal rigidity are characteristic and denote peritonitis. In some patients the full clinical picture does not develop. Because the perforation is sealed rapidly by omentum, the signs remain localised. In others, fluid leaking from the perforation down the right paracolic gutter produces clinical findings resembling those of acute appendicitis (Fig. 27.17).

Leaking gastric and duodenal fluid is irritant and causes a chemical peritonitis with marked exudation of fluid. This dilutes the leaking content so that abdominal pain and other signs often lessen after some hours. The peritoneal fluid is

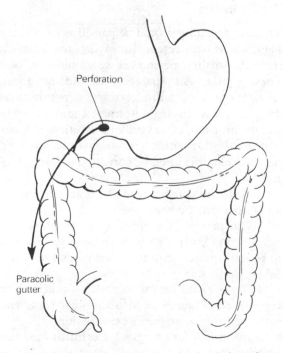

**Fig. 27.17** Perforated duodenal ulcer showing leakage down the paracolic gutter

initially sterile but secondary bacterial invasion occurs within 6 hours. Bacterial peritonitis follows.

The overall mortality of perforated peptic ulcer is about 10%. This increases with delay in diagnosis and management. Mortality is greatest in the elderly and those ill from intercurrent disease.

The clinical diagnosis is confirmed in approximately two-thirds of patients by the presence of air beneath the diaphragm on a chest X-ray or erect abdominal films. Lateral decubitus films may also reveal free peritoneal gas and are of particular value in shocked or debilitated patients. Absence of peritoneal gas does not rule out a perforation. If the diagnosis is in doubt, e.g., when the perforation is into the lesser sac or rapidly seals when air is not seen on a plain X-ray, an emergency gastrografin series should be ordered.

Acute pancreatitis should always be considered in the differential diagnosis of a perforated ulcer. The serum amylase concentration should be determined, remembering that moderate elevation may occur in a perforation.

## Management

A nasogastric tube should be passed as soon as the diagnosis is suspected. Emptying the stomach prevents further peritoneal contamination and relieves pain. An analgesic should be given, haematology, urea and electrolyte concentrations checked, blood group determined and an intravenous infusion of crystalloid solution is commenced. If the patient is seriously shocked on presentation, this must be corrected before operation.

*Conservative management.* Perforated peptic ulcer is managed by *operation* unless:

1. The patient is extremely ill on admission, there having been a long delay between perforation and diagnosis with the development of bacterial peritonitis.

2. The perforation has sealed, as indicated by an absence of generalised abdominal signs and confirmed by gastrografin examination.

3. Facilities for surgical treatment are not available.

Then the patient should be managed conserva-

tively by regular nasogastric aspiration, intravenous fluid therapy, cimetidine infusion, and broad spectrum antibiotic cover if there are signs of peritonitis. Conservative management was once a popular alternative to operation and gave comparable results in terms of mortality. However, there was a higher incidence of subphrenic or local abscess after conservative management, and on occasions a more serious cause of peritonitis, e.g. strangulated bowel, was wrongly treated. Operation is now preferred.

## Operative management of perforated duodenal ulcer

*Simple closure.* The abdomen is opened through a short right paramedian or midline incision. All foreign material is aspirated from the peritoneal cavity, the peritoneum is lavaged with saline, and the perforation is closed by three catgut sutures incorporating a tag of omentum (Fig. 27.18). The abdomen is then closed without drainage.

Following simple closure of an *acute ulcer*, one-third of patients have no further dyspepsia, one-third experience mild symptoms easily controlled medically, and one-third eventually require definitive ulcer operation.

*Vagotomy and pyloroplasty.* Simple closure of a chronic ulcer is likely to be followed by recurrent dyspepsia requiring later definitive surgery. It is better to carry out definitive surgery at the emergency laparotomy. Truncal vagotomy and

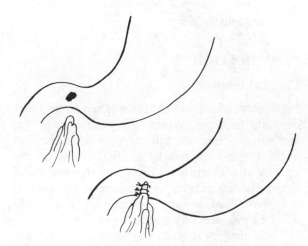

**Fig. 27.18** Closure of perforation

pyloroplasty is then the procedure of choice. The perforation is excised or incorporated into the pyloroplasty. If gross scarring or duodenal friability makes pyloroplasty difficult, a gastro-jejunostomy is performed after closure of the perforation.

Emergency definitive surgery is not advised: 1. in poor risk patients with severe intercurrent disease; 2. when the perforation is more than 12 hours old and bacterial contamination is likely to be heavy; 3. when an experienced surgeon or anaesthetist is not available. Age by itself is not a contra-indication. Given correct patient selection and appropriate surgical expertise, the mortality of an emergency vagotomy and pyloroplasty should be no greater than that of simple closure.

## Operative treatment of perforated gastric ulcer

Perforated peptic gastric ulcers are usually chronic and definitive surgery is preferred to simple closure. Approximately 15% of perforated gastric ulcers are malignant and provided an experienced team is available, Billroth I gastrectomy is the procedure of choice. Excision of the ulcer with truncal vagotomy and pyloroplasty is a satisfactory alternative in those cases where the position of the ulcer makes gastrectomy difficult.

Simple closure after adequate biopsy of the ulcer is justifiable in poor risk patients, but endoscopic follow-up for ulcer recurrence is mandatory.

## PYLORIC STENOSIS

The stenosis is usually located in the first part of the duodenum rather than at the pylorus, but the term pyloric stenosis is time honoured (Fig. 27.19). Obstruction may result from oedema during an acute exacerbation of ulceration, from fibrous scarring during repair or from a combination of the two. Muscle spasm may play a role in some patients, notably those in whom the ulcer is located within the pyloric channel. Pyloric stenosis is less common than ulcer bleeding or perforation.

A rare form of pyloric stenosis due to hypertrophy of the pyloric musculature which is unassociated with peptic ulceration also occurs in adults. This may be a mild and chronic form of congenital

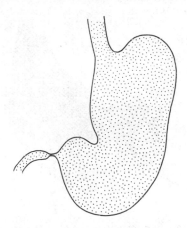

**Fig. 27.19** Pyloric stenosis — appearance at operation

pyloric stenosis in infants. Hypertrophy of the pyloric musculature is also a consequence of true pyloric ulcer.

## Clinical features

The symptoms of pyloric stenosis are insidious and consist of upper abdominal distension following meals, eructations and bad breath. Intermittent bouts of diarrhoea may occur. The character of the peptic ulcer pain may change, initially becoming continuous and intractable and later less intense or even disappearing. Vomiting occurs late, and classically is of retention type. Every day or two, and usually in the evening, the patient vomits copious quantities of gastric juice containing partially digested food which he recognises to have eaten some hours or days before. The site of the obstruction is reflected by the fact that the vomitus never contains bile.

On examination the classical clinical feature is that of gastric distension. The stomach may be visibly enlarged and gentle side-to-side shaking of the patient elicits a succussion splash. In long standing stenosis from duodenal ulceration visible peristalsis is not a feature. A plain abdominal X-ray may show a large fluid-filled stomach. This is confirmed by a barium meal which will show a grossly distended stomach, hypertrophied mucosa and mixing of barium and retained foodstuffs to give a frothy or thumb-print appearance (Fig. 27.20). Late films show a gastric sump in the pelvis.

Pyloric obstruction may also be caused by

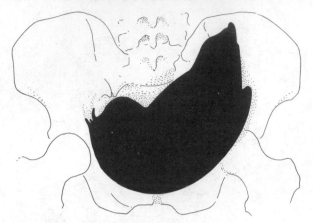

**Fig. 27.20** Barium meal appearance of pyloric stenosis

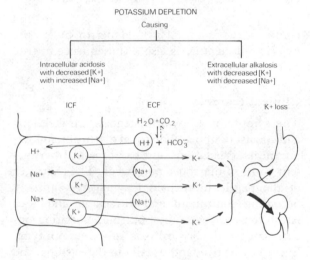

**Fig. 27.21** Effect of potassium depletion

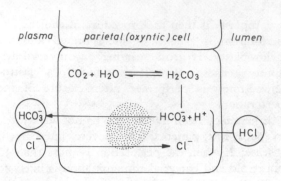

**Fig. 27.22** Initial biochemical changes in pyloric stenosis showing transfer of electrolytes across cells

conditions other than chronic duodenal ulcer, e.g. a distal carcinoma. The cause of the obstruction is not always obvious on barium studies or on endoscopy and definition of the cause may have to await laparotomy.

## Biochemical changes

The initial biochemical changes in long-standing pyloric stenosis are due to starvation. Sodium is retained by the kidney, and water and salt balance is preserved. However, the obligatory excretion of potassium leads to hypokalaemia. Intracellular potassium is lost, and replaced by sodium and hydrogen ions so that there is an intracellular acidosis and extracellular alkalosis (Fig. 27.21).

With vomiting there is loss of acid gastric juice, this leading to intensification of the alkalosis and hypokalaemia and loss of salt and water (Fig. 27.22). The patient becomes severely dehydrated. Chloride ion also is lost and replaced by bicarbonate. The urine is alkaline.

As stores of potassium become progressively exhausted the kidney excretes hydrogen ion rather than potassium and paradoxical aciduria may occur. This is a sign of severe biochemical upset.

If the obstruction is due to a carcinoma, there is likely to be hypochlorhydria of the gastric juice so that the disturbance of acid-base balance is less.

Loss of protein leads to hypoproteinaemia. As this is a hazard to healing after surgery the plasma proteins must always be estimated pre-operatively.

## Treatment

The treatment of pyloric stenosis is surgical relief of the obstruction. This is not an emergency procedure and some days of preparation for operation are usual. Dehydration, electrolyte and acid-base balance are corrected by the intravenous infusion of saline and potassium chloride monitored by urine volume, serum levels of electrolytes and blood gas estimations. Anaemia is present in about one in four patients with pyloric stenosis and should be rectified.

A large bore (32 FG) nasogastric tube is passed to empty the stomach of food residue and allow lavage. Once the aspirate is clear the tube can be replaced by one of smaller diameter which is kept in place until operation. Regular aspiration avoids gastric distention and allows the gastric muscle to regain tone.

Operation is usually undertaken after some 4–5 days of intravenous therapy and aspiration. Truncal vagotomy and gastrojejunostomy is the procedure of choice. If pyloric carcinoma is found this should be resected.

Nasogastric intubation is continued for some days after operation, to avoid gastric retention and encourage the gastric muscle to regain tone.

## LONG-TERM COMPLICATIONS OF PEPTIC ULCER SURGERY (Table 27.1)

### Recurrent ulceration

*Duodenal ulcer.* The incidence and site of recurrent ulceration after surgery for duodenal ulcer is influenced by the type of operation employed. If this were a pyloroplasty or gastro-duodenal anastomosis, recurrent duodenal ulceration may occur whereas following a gastro-jejunal anastomosis the ulcer is on the jejunal side of the anastomosis. The ulcer recurs because the initial operation failed to sufficiently reduce acid and pepsin secretion. Recurrent ulcer is associated with renewal of ulcer symptoms but the periodicity of the pain may be atypical. Barium studies may be difficult to interpret because of the previous surgery and endoscopic examination is essential.

Re-operation is advisable, the aim being to ensure that acid and pepsin secretion are reduced further. Patients with recurrence after vagotomy and drainage or highly selective vagotomy are treated by attempting to complete the vagotomy in association with antrectomy. Recurrence after partial gastrectomy is best dealt with by the addition of a truncal vagotomy. Recurrence after truncal vagotomy and antrectomy is rare and is treated by searching for intact vagal fibres and more extensive gastric resection. Although rare, the Zollinger-Ellison syndrome may present as recurrent ulceration. A fasting gastrin level should be measured routinely to exclude this possibility.

Long-term therapy with histamine $H_2$ antagonists may be employed in those patients unfit for, or who refuse, further surgery.

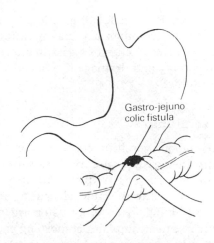

**Fig. 27.23** Gastro-jejuno-colic fistula

Ulcers at the anastomotic site may be associated with the use of non-absorbable sutures at the initial operation. The levels of acid and pepsin secretion are not high. On endoscopy a suture is seen in the base of the ulcer, removal of which results in healing. Some now recommend that only absorbable sutures are used in gastric anastomoses.

In addition to causing renewed pain and dyspepsia, recurrent ulcers may be complicated by bleeding, perforation or the development of gastro-jejuno-colic fistula. Bleeding and perforation occur more frequently than with primary ulcers, but fistula formation is relatively rare. This usually arises after gastro-jejunal anastomosis, particularly when the anastomosis has been retro-colic. The communication between stomach and large bowel allows colonisation of the stomach and small bowel by faecal organisms which produces severe diarrhoea and malabsorption, and leads to rapid weight loss. Only small amounts of food pass directly from stomach to colon so that the diagnosis is confirmed most readily by barium enema.

Should a fistula form, early operation after bowel preparation is indicated. The fistula is disconnected, the colon repaired, and an appropriate recurrent ulcer operation is carried out. These aims are usually achieved at one operation, but preliminary transverse colostomy may be required to divert the faecal stream, relieve symptoms and allow nutritional status to improve in poor risk patients (Fig. 27.23).

*Gastric ulcer*. Recurrence of gastric ulcer after gastrectomy is uncommon and may indicate further resection. Recurrence of a gastric ulcer after truncal vagotomy and drainage is treated by partial gastrectomy.

## Bilious vomiting

Occasional bilious vomiting occurs in about 30% of patients after gastric surgery. In a small proportion the vomiting is frequent and persistent due to bile reflux into the stomach causing severe gastritis. Bile lying in an empty stomach overnight gives rise to a complaint of morning nausea. Vomiting is often precipitated by eating a cooked breakfast. Many patients with bilious vomiting are heavy smokers and/or drinkers.

Abstinence or moderation is the single most effective measure in its management.

In a few patients, bilious vomiting is the result of afferent loop obstruction after a gastro-jejunal anastomosis, pressure building up in the loop causing colicky upper abdominal pain. When the obstruction is overcome bile and pancreatic juice are discharged rapidly into the stomach and vomited.

Persistent, troublesome, bilious vomiting may respond to antacid or cimetidine therapy, thus reducing the amount of acid available to exploit the damaged gastric mucosal defences. Metoclopramide improves gastric emptying. If such medical management fails to relieve symptoms an operation to divert bile from the stomach, e.g. by a Roux-en-Y anastomosis, may be necessary (Fig. 27.24).

Following operations for ulcer, there is an increased incidence of gastric carcinoma in which chronic biliary gastritis ulcer has been implicated. Highly selective vagotomy is not associated with increased biliary reflux but it is not yet known if the risk of carcinoma is lower in this group.

## Food vomiting

Vomiting of food may be due to fibrosis and narrowing of the stoma or to faulty siting of a gastroenterostomy. A diagnosis of stomal malfunction can be confirmed radiologically or endoscopically. Revisional surgery is required.

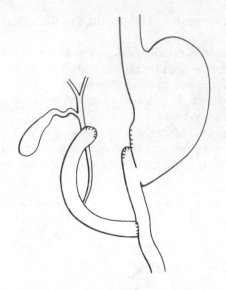

**Fig. 27.24** Roux-en-Y operation for bilious vomiting

Occasional patients develop gastric hypotonia despite an adequate anastomosis. Food vomiting may be relieved by metoclopramide, an antiemetic which co-ordinates and improves gastric emptying.

## Dumping

The dumping syndrome consists of uncomfortable epigastric fullness after food associated with flushing and sweating, marked lassitude, increased peristalsis with borborygmi, and sometimes diarrhoea. These symptoms commence within 10 to 15 minutes of eating and usually settle within 30 to 60 minutes. The patient frequently has to lie down until symptoms pass.

Epigastric fullness after eating an average-sized meal occurs in about 40% of patients after gastric surgery. Impaired receptive relaxation is believed to be responsible. This symptom alone does not constitute dumping. It usually improves spontaneously in a few months and can be avoided by taking small meals without fluids.

The dumping syndrome proper is due to rapid emptying of hyperosmolar solutions, particularly of carbohydrates, into the small bowel (Fig. 27.25). It can be induced by jejunal instillation of hypertonic glucose and is believed to be due to the osmotic attraction of large amounts of fluid into the

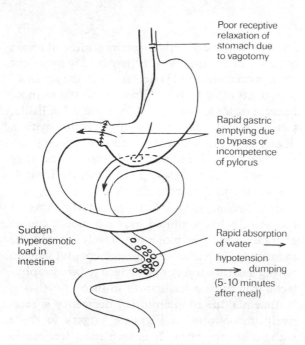

Poor receptive relaxation of stomach due to vagotomy

Rapid gastric emptying due to bypass or incompetence of pylorus

Sudden hyperosmotic load in intestine

Rapid absorption of water →

hypotension

→ dumping (5-10 minutes after meal)

Fig. 27.25 Dumping syndrome

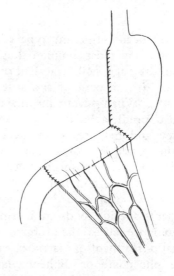

Fig. 27.26 Jejunal interposition

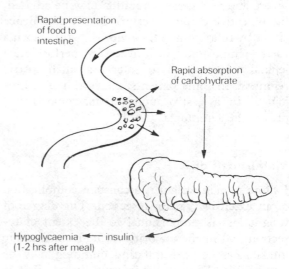

Rapid presentation of food to intestine

Rapid absorption of carbohydrate

Hypoglycaemia ← insulin (1-2 hrs after meal)

Fig. 27.27 Hypoglycaemic syndrome after gastrectomy

lumen of the small bowel. There is transcellular flux of potassium and other ions and extracellular fluid volume is reduced. Distension of the jejunum creates a sensation of fullness and stimulates peristalsis. Release of 5-hydroxytryptamine and bradykinin also may be implicated.

The symptoms of dumping may be ameliorated by reducing the size of meals which are taken more frequently, reducing carbohydrate consumption, and avoiding liquids during meals. Otherwise the medical treatment of dumping has proved unsatisfactory. If troublesome symptoms persist after dietary modification, operation may be required. This consists either of converting the gastro-jejunal to a gastro-duodenal anastomosis or, if the gastric remnant is small, interposing a segment of jejunum between stomach and duodenum (Fig. 27.26). It is advisable to wait for at least a year after the primary operation as (i) symptoms often improve spontaneously; (ii) the long-term results of surgery for dumping are disappointing.

## Reactive hypoglycaemia

Reactive hypoglycaemia was once erroneously known as 'late dumping', but this term is no longer used. Rapid absorption of glucose from the upper small bowel produces hyperglycaemia and causes excessive insulin secretion, and reactive hypoglycaemia (Fig 27.27). Tremor, tachycardia, palpitation and sweating develop about 90 to 120 minutes after a meal, and are potentiated by exercise. Approximately 5 to 10% of patients experience this symptom at some time after surgery, but in the great majority such hypoglycaemia is mild, transient and easily avoided.

Patients are advised to reduce carbohydrate consumption and to carry glucose sweets to take if symptoms arise. Revisional surgery is rarely required.

## Diarrhoea

Diarrhoea may occur after any type of gastric operation, but is now most common after truncal vagotomy and drainage. Mild transient diarrhoea occurs in over 20% of patients and severe diarrhoea in 3–4%. When severe the diarrhoea is episodic and unpredictable. It is associated with great urgency and may result in incontinence disrupting the patient's professional and social life. Steatorrhoea and malabsorption are rare.

The cause is not certain but loss of gastric continence is now considered to be a major factor. In some patients specific foods are incriminated, and their avoidance 'cures' the problem.

Symptomatic treatment of diarrhoea with kaolin, codeine phosphate or diphenoxylate with atropine (Lomotil) is of value. If diarrhoea is severe and refractory, operation may be advised, the objective being to restore gastric continence either by refashioning the pylorus, taking down a gastro-jejunostomy, or if necessary, performing a jejunal transposition to enlarge a small gastric remnant. In some patients, converting a gastro-jejunal to a gastro-duodenal anastomosis improves the symptoms.

## Malabsorption

Failure to gain weight is a constant complication of an extensive gastric resection. The degree of weight loss is proportional to the extent of resection and in the majority is due to inadequate intake. Fear of precipitating dumping may be responsible. Dietary advice may be all that is required.

True malabsorption with steatorrhoea and weight loss is relatively rare. It may be caused by lactose intolerance, the blind loop syndrome or a gastro-jejuno-colic fistula.

The blind loop syndrome is encountered occasionally after Billroth II gastrectomy or gastrojejunostomy with vagotomy. The diagnosis is confirmed by the demonstration of high jejunal bacterial counts and a good response to antibiotics. Conversion of the gastro-jejunal to a gastro-duodenal anastomosis, or replacement of a gastrojejunostomy with a pyloroplasty can give permanent relief.

## Anaemia

Iron deficiency anaemia is common after all forms of peptic ulcer surgery. It is particularly prevalent after gastrectomy and is detectable in the majority of patients after 10 years. Premenopausal women, because of menstrual blood loss, are more liable. Causes are: 1. patients leaving hospital with a degree of anaemia due to operative or pre-operative blood loss; 2. reduced acid secretory capacity with less efficient absorption of dietary iron; 3. chronic blood loss from gastritis.

Any patient who is anaemic at the time of hospital discharge should have a 3-month course of oral iron. Haemoglobin levels should be monitored thereafter. All premenopausal women having gastric surgery are advised to take prophylactic iron during one month in three.

Anaemia due to vitamin $B_{12}$ deficiency is relatively uncommon after gastric surgery in those without steatorrhoea. It is seen most frequently after gastric resection but can occasionally follow truncal vagotomy and drainage, and may complicate gastritis. Parenteral vitamin $B_{12}$ administration is required for life.

## Calcium malabsorption

This may develop in association with steatorrhoea, but also may occur 10–15 years after operation in some patients without steatorrhoea. Partial gastrectomy enhances calcium malabsorption and postmenopausal women who frequently lack calcium are particularly prone to develop osteomalacia. For this reason, partial gastrectomy should be avoided in female patients if possible.

## Tuberculosis

Patients with a history of tuberculosis are prone to relapse following gastric resection and must be carefully followed up.

## STRESS ULCERATION

Acute superficial ulcers may develop in the stomach or duodenum after operation, injury or severe illness. The ulcers are frequently multiple, are usually small, and are sometimes described as erosions. The cause of stress ulceration is not clear but reduced mucosal resistance is probably important. Resistance is impaired during periods of ischaemia because of reduced gastric mucosal blood flow, by bile reflux, by exposure to drugs such as aspirin or indomethacin, and by increased output or administration of glucocorticoids.

Ulceration of the duodenum in burned patients (Curling's ulcer) or of the stomach and duodenum after neurosurgical illness or operation (Cushing's ulcer) are specific forms of stress ulceration. Cushing's ulcers are unusual in that gastric secretion is increased, possibly because of increased vagal activity associated with increased intracranial pressure.

All forms of stress ulceration can cause bleeding which may be life-threatening. Except in Cushing's and Curling's ulcers perforation is uncommon because of the superficial nature of the lesions. Suppression of gastric secretion by cimetidine or continuous administration of alkali in high dosage is of value in prevention and treatment of stress lesions, and surgery should be avoided if at all possible.

If bleeding fails to respond to medical management, operation usually consists of vagotomy and drainage. Vagotomy reduces gastric secretion and favours the opening of arterio-venous shunts which divert blood from the engorged mucosa. The management of bleeding is discussed in detail on p. 390.

# ZOLLINGER-ELLISON SYNDROME (GASTRINOMA)

The Zollinger-Ellison syndrome is a rare entity in which autonomous secretion of gastrin leads to gastric hypersecretion and a fulminant form of peptic ulceration (Fig. 27.28). The tumour (gastrinoma) usually arises from gastrin-secreting cells (G cells) in the islets of the pancreas but also may arise in the stomach or duodenum. About two-thirds of gastrinomas are malignant, and more than three-quarters of patients have multiple tumours.

Men are more commonly affected than women

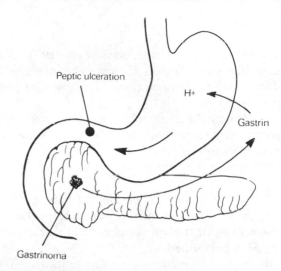

Fig. 27.28 Zollinger-Ellison syndrome

(M:F, 3:2) with a peak incidence between 20 and 50 years of age.

G-cell hyperplasia is a very rare condition in which hypergastrinaemia is due to hyperplasia of G-cells in the antrum, and not to tumour formation.

## Clinical features

The classical presentation is one of severe fulminating ulcer dyspepsia refractory to routine forms of therapy. Many patients first have only mild dyspepsia which is slowly progressive. Bleeding (33%), perforation (25%) and pyloric obstruction (10%) are common. Ulceration often occurs at more than one site in the stomach, duodenum or proximal jejunum.

One third of patients have diarrhoea. This is usually due to underlying steatorrhoea caused by destruction of lipase by the high luminal acid content of the small bowel, and should be distinguished from the watery diarrhoea of the WDHA syndrome (p. 516). Diarrhoea may be the first symptom of a gastrinoma.

One quarter of gastrinoma patients have other endocrine abnormalities. Parathyroid adenomas commonly co-exist and in some patients there is multiple endocrine adenomatosis (see p. 583).

## Diagnosis

A high index of suspicion is essential if the diagnosis is to be established or even entertained before primary operation. This should be prompted by:

1. Chronic duodenal ulceration associated with gastric hypersecretion and a ratio of basal to maximal acid output which exceeds 0.6:1.

2. Duodenal ulceration occurring in childhood or youth.

3. Stomal ulceration developing rapidly after surgery for duodenal ulcer, particularly when a gastrectomy or truncal vagotomy and antrectomy has been performed.

4. Peptic ulceration involving unusual sites such as the distal duodenum or jejunum.

5. Peptic ulceration associated with unexplained diarrhoea.

6. Associated endocrine abnormalities such as hyperparathyroidism.

Gastric secretory studies are no longer the mainstay of diagnosis. Emphasis now is placed on radioimmunoassay of gastrin in the circulating blood. The normal value for fasting serum gastrin levels in most laboratories is below 150 ng/l. All gastrin values above this level are viewed with suspicion. The higher the fasting gastrin, the more likely the diagnosis of gastrinoma, and levels in excess of 500 ng/l are strongly suggestive. Provocation tests may be employed for confirmation. A rapid bolus intravenous injection of secretin causes a marked rise of serum gastrin in gastrinoma patients.

Selective angiography may help to localise the tumour and detect hepatic metastases. Selective venous sampling using a catheter passed through the liver into the splenic vein is also useful in detecting high local venous gastrin levels and so localising tumour deposits.

Before accepting the diagnosis of a gastrinoma, other causes of hypergastrinaemia should be excluded. These are:

Pernicious anaemia
Achlorhydria or hypochlorhydria due to gastritis
Gastric outlet obstruction
Short bowel syndrome
Renal insufficiency

## Management

The availability of the histamine $H_2$-receptor antagonist cimetidine has offered a feasible alternative to surgery in many patients. Although doses of the order of 2400 mg/day may be required, gastric hypersecretion can usually be controlled.

Ideally an attempt should then be made to resect the tumour and so remove the cause of the hypergastrinaemia. However this is frequently thwarted by the fact that the majority of tumours are multiple and/or malignant.

If the acid hypersecretion cannot be controlled with cimetidine, total gastrectomy is likely to prove necessary. Following this operation 60% of patients survive 5 years and 40% 10 years, the pancreatic tumour often remaining stable or even, on rare occasions, regressing. Cytotoxic therapy with streptozotocin may be of some value for the treatment of malignant disease.

# GASTRIC NEOPLASIA

## BENIGN GASTRIC NEOPLASMS

Benign tumours of the stomach may arise from epithelial or mesenchymal tissue. Adenomatous polyps are the most common neoplasm to arise from epithelium and may be single or multiple. The risk of malignant transformation increases with polyp size and when there are multiple polyps.

Leiomyoma is the commonest benign mesenchymal tumour. Neurogenic tumours, fibromas and lipomas are rare.

Benign tumours are frequently discovered as an incidental finding on barium meal examination, but may give rise to bleeding or intermittent pyloric obstruction with vomiting. Intussusception through the pylorus is exceptionally rare. The benign nature of the polyp is confirmed by endoscopy with biopsy. Some pedunculated polyps can be removed through the endoscope using a diathermy snare, but operative removal is indicated for the remainder in view of the risk of malignant transformation. Multiple polyps are treated by gastric resection, and total gastrectomy is required on rare occasions for diffuse gastric involvement.

# MALIGNANT GASTRIC NEOPLASMS

## Cancer of the stomach

The stomach is the second commonest site for cancer of the gastro-intestinal tract. In Great Britain, 50–60 persons per 100 000 per annum are affected by the disease which accounts for 10% of cancer deaths. Present day methods of treatment have done little to alter its appalling mortality, less than 10% of all patients surviving for 5 years.

Cancer of the stomach is curable by surgery only if it is confined to the stomach wall. Such favourable cases are relatively uncommon and generally detected only through the screening of normal persons. By the time most patients experience symptoms related to the disease it already has spread through and beyond their stomach and cure by local treatment is no longer possible, though considerable palliation of symptoms may be achieved.

In an attempt to improve the serious mortality of gastric cancer, air contrast barium studies and endoscopy are being used to screen asymptomatic persons. Lesions can be detected which are confined to the mucosa and which, following gastrectomy, have a high likelihood of cure. Recent survival figures from Japan where screening is widely practised suggest that 95% of such patients live for 5 years or more.

In Britain, routine screening for gastric cancer is limited to those at high risk, eg with atrophic gastritis or pernicious anaemia, in whom annual contrast barium endoscopy should be arranged.

*Aetiological factors.* There are marked geographical differences in the incidence of gastric cancer. In Japan, Iceland, South America and East Europe it is much more common than in the UK or North America. There may also be differences in incidence within a country. In England and Wales the line between the Severn and the Wash divides the country into northern high incidence and southern low incidence areas.

It is believed that these differences are due to environmental factors, a view supported by the striking reduction in incidence in the United States during the past 40 years. A similar trend has occurred in Britain in which the peak incidence for the disease occurred in the decade 1930–1940.

Cancer of the stomach is twice as common in males as in females and most common in unskilled social groups. Its incidence increases with age although 1 in 15 cases still occur in patients under 40 years of age.

Certain occupations increase the risk of gastric cancer. Miners, rubber and asbestos workers are prone to develop the disease.

Family history is relevant. Blood relatives of patients with the disease are at increased risk. Those of blood group A are more prone to develop gastric cancer than other blood-group types.

The incidence of gastric cancer is increased by three or four times in patients with pernicious anaemia, or other atrophic states affecting the gastric mucosa. Hypochlorhydria by altering the distribution of bacteria in the gastro-intestinal tract is believed to be one factor. Intestinal metaplasia of the gastric mucosa is another. Adenomatous gastric polyps, particularly when multiple, are prone to become malignant. A recent figure suggests that the incidence may be as high as 20%.

A benign gastric ulcer occasionally undergoes malignant change but, in general, the relationship between benign and malignant ulceration is not strong. Surgery for peptic ulcer does increase the risk of gastric cancer, believed again to be associated with reduction in acid secretion. The incidence of gastric cancer in patients treated by long-term antisecretory drugs is under review.

The main factors which lead to the development of gastric cancer are believed to be dietary in origin. For example, an association between human cancer of the stomach and a high intake of nitrate salts has been described. On reduction to nitrites by bacterial action, N-nitrosation of amino compounds occurs in the stomach to form N-nitroso compounds (nitrosamines) which are known to be carcinogenic. Bacteria also catalyse the N-nitrosation of secondary amine groups, a factor of particular importance in the achlorhydric stomach.

## Pathology

Cancers of the stomach are adenocarcinomas derived from mucus-secreting cells of gastric glands. They can occur in any part of the stomach but are most common in the pyloric antrum. They are classified as 1. ulcerating; 2. proliferating (encephaloid or polypoidal); and 3. infiltrating depending upon the degree of penetration of the gastric wall and growth into the lumen. Combinations of these types occur. Diffuse infiltration of the whole of the stomach accompanied by a fibrous reaction causes so-called 'leather-bottle stomach' (linitus plastica).

Spread of a gastric cancer occurs by:

1. Direct extension to neighbouring organs (e.g. liver, pancreas, colon).

2. Transcoelomic spread within the peritoneal cavity to form seedling deposits on peritoneal and omental surfaces, on the ovaries (Krukenberg tumour) and in the recto-vesical pouch (forming a so-called rectal 'shelf').

3. Lymphatic spread to regional lymph nodes in the perigastric tissues along the splenic and hepatic vessels, and in the porta hepatis. Occasionally the disease spreads along the course of the thoracic duct to involve the left supraclavicular nodes and form a hard mass in the neck.

4. Blood-borne spread via the portal vein to the liver and occasionally to the lungs and other sites.

As with cancers elsewhere lymph node involvement is a bad prognostic sign. When a tumour is confined to the gastric wall, 5-year survival after resection approximates 45%. Involvement of local lymph nodes reduces this figure to under 20%.

An international system of clinical and pathological staging using TNM categories is described but is not commonly used in this country.

## Clinical features

The classical symptoms of gastric cancer — anorexia, vomiting, anaemia, eructation, ill-health and loss of weight — are those of late disease.

Early symptoms are referable to the gastrointestinal tract and similar to those caused by a variety of minor digestive ailments. Epigastric pain, vague indigestion or fullness are typical. A history of recurrent dyspepsia or relief by alkali does not rule out the diagnosis of cancer.

Frank haemorrhage from a gastric cancer is rare. Slow oozing of blood from its surface is common and causes anaemia with lassitude, pallor and breathlessness. Anaemia should never be treated without investigation for chronic blood loss.

Rarely, the initial symptoms of a gastric cancer can be acute with pyloric hold-up, perforation or severe haemorrhage. In some cases, the first symptom may be caused by metastatic deposits, e.g. in the liver, supraclavicular nodes or peritoneal cavity.

*Clinical signs.* Those with symptoms of early disease do not usually have clinical signs. In such patients the faeces must be tested for occult blood.

By the time most patients are referred to hospital, loss of weight is obvious. An epigastric mass may be found on abdominal examination. The liver, supraclavicular nodes and pelvic floor must be carefully examined for metastatic disease.

A full blood examination is requested and a barium meal arranged. Air-contrast studies are now routine in patients in whom gastric cancer is suspected.

In an established tumour, ulceration, a filling defect and rigidity of the stomach wall are typical features of the disease. In linitus plastica, the stomach is contracted to a narrow rigid tube which empties rapidly into the duodenum.

Early lesions form a mucosal 'plaque', a small superficial ulcer or disrupted mucosal folds. These appearances are detected only by air-contrast techniques.

Differentiation of a malignant from a benign gastric ulcer on radiological grounds can prove difficult. Irregularity of the base, interruption and rigidity of the mucosal folds, and a crater which does not penetrate beyond the confines of the stomach are signs suggesting cancer. Ulcers on sites not usually affected by peptic ulceration, e.g. greater curve, are also suspicious.

All patients with X-ray suspicion of cancer of the stomach should be gastroscoped and the lesion biopsied. It is also advisable to gastroscope all patients over middle age with recent dyspepsia and a negative barium examination. Smears of surface cells for cytological examination may be made by brushing the gastric mucosa through the endoscope. Gastric secretion studies and blind cytology (e.g. by gastric lavage) are no longer used for diagnosis.

*Differential diagnosis.* A carcinoma of the stomach must be differentiated from other infiltrating lesions. Of particular importance is non-Hodgkins lymphoma which may cause a large apparently inoperable tumour which, nevertheless, is amenable to therapy. Giant hypertrophy of the gastric mucosa may be associated with clinical and radiological features similar to cancer. In cases of doubt, gastroscopy should be performed.

## Treatment

The primary treatment of gastric cancer is surgical. Unless there is gross clinical evidence of metastatic disease, or general illness contraindicates surgery, the abdomen should be explored.

The first duty of the surgeon is to confirm the diagnosis. This is usually obvious but a small lesion may be difficult to palpate through the gastric wall. Opening the stomach (gastrotomy) and palpation within the lumen is advocated but is no substitute for precise pre-operative definition of the lesion by endoscopic biopsy.

Next, the surgeon should determine the extent of the disease. Peritoneal seedlings of tumour, ascites and gross liver metastases indicate that this is advanced and that operation will not be curative. Small liver metastases and extensive lymph node invasion are also signs of incurable disease but if the patient has obstructive symptoms, surgical removal of the tumour may be worthwhile. In this situation, some surgeons perform a simple bypass procedure (gastroenterostomy), but the palliation achieved is poor. Histology (if not previously available ) is mandatory even in apparently inoperable cases as if the diagnosis proves to be that of lymphoma, radiotherapy and/or chemotherapy can give excellent remission of disease.

In the absence of obvious spread to other sites, gastric resection should be performed, unless the cancer is so fixed to surrounding structures that it is irremovable.

## The operation

The standard operation for cancer of the distal stomach is a partial gastrectomy removing the distal three-quarters of the stomach and the first 2–3 cm of the duodenum. As regional lymph nodes should be included with the specimen, blood vessels are ligated and divided at their origins and the omentum removed with the stomach. A gastro-jejunal (Polya) reconstruction is usual.

For cancers of the body of stomach, or the cardia, a total gastrectomy will be required including removal of the lower 2–3 cm of the oesophagus. In some cases this is combined with resection of the spleen and the distal pancreas. Reconstruction consists of anastomosis of a loop of proximal jejunum to the oesophagus usually by the Roux-en-Y technique. The length of ascending limb should exceed 45 cm to prevent alkaline oesophagitis. Total gastrectomy is best performed through a thoraco-abdominal approach, extending the abdominal incision over the costal margin, opening the chest and dividing the diaphragm down to the oesophageal hiatus.

## Adjuvant therapy

Radiotherapy has little place in the management of adenocarcinoma of the stomach. Combination chemotherapy may achieve remissions in some patients with advanced disease and adjuvant chemotherapy at the time of primary surgery is under study.

## Gastric lymphoma

Lymphomas account for 2% of all malignant gastric tumours. The presenting symptoms and signs resemble those of gastric carcinoma but are often mild relative to the size of the neoplasm. The tumour may be misdiagnosed radiologically as gastric cancer and endoscopy with biopsy is essential.

Radical subtotal gastrectomy followed by radiotherapy results in a 5-year survival rate approaching 50% if lymphoma is localised, and tumour size should not be taken as a contra-indication to surgery. If local extension prohibits resection, radiotherapy often gives worthwhile palliation, while diffuse disease may respond to chemotherapy.

## Gastric leiomyosarcoma

These tumours account for less than 1% of malignant gastric neoplasms. The lesion may protrude into the gastric lumen, remain within the gastric wall, or even bulge into the peritoneal cavity. The luminal surface frequently ulcerates due to central necrosis and bleeding is common.

The tumour grows slowly and metastasises late. The 5-year survival rate is around 50% after partial gastrectomy. The tumours are not radio-sensitive so that prognosis is poor if the lesion cannot be resected.

# UPPER GASTRO-INTESTINAL HAEMORRHAGE

Bleeding from the upper gastro-intestinal tract is common. If mild and chronic, it may go un-noticed for many months until the development of anaemia raises the suspicion of chronic blood loss. If severe, it can cause acute hypovolaemia and shock requiring urgent treatment in hospital. The blood may be vomited (haematemesis) when it is bright red and fluid, coffee-ground, or contains clots. Alternatively, should it pass down the gastro-intestinal tract and be excreted in altered form in the faeces, it is black and treacly (melaena).

## CAUSES

Peptic ulceration of the stomach or duodenum or gastritis with erosions are responsible for the majority of massive upper gastro-intestinal bleeds. Oesophageal varices complicating portal hypertension and Mallory-Weiss tears at the gastro-oesophageal junction account for most of the remainder. A rare cause of acute bleeding is a chronic gastric ulcer complicating a para-oesophageal hernia. Sliding hiatus hernia with erosive oesophagitis may cause chronic bleeding but not acute haemorrhage.

## PRINCIPLES OF MANAGEMENT

There are three vital steps in the care of a patient with massive gastrointestinal haemorrhage:

1. Early replacement of blood volume so that exsanguination is prevented and hypovolaemia promptly corrected.
2. Detection of the nature and site of the bleeding lesion.
3. Control of the bleeding point.

It is important to appreciate that all patients with an acute upper gastro-intestinal bleed, even if apparently minor, should be referred urgently to hospital for investigation and treatment. Any minor bleed may become major within a few hours, causing severe hypovolaemia and shock. Ideally, all patients should be admitted under the care of a haematemesis team which includes a surgeon. Otherwise, delay in reaching a diagnosis or failure to appreciate a serious risk of exsanguinating haemorrhage and the need for surgery, may compromise survival. Severe bleeding into the gastro-intestinal tract is not directly visible but this must not detract from a sense of urgency in management.

Steps in the management of the patient are as follows:

## HISTORY

A history of peptic ulceration, of liver disease or of previous operations may prove helpful in suggesting a likely source of bleeding. A recent story of severe vomiting may indicate the likelihood of mucosal tears in the region of the cardia (Mallory-Weiss syndrome). Previous upper gastro-intestinal barium studies may have shown a chronic peptic ulcer or duodenal scarring.

The ingestion of non-steroidal anti-inflammatory compounds (e.g. aspirin or indomethacin), steroids or anticoagulants predisposes to gastro-intestinal haemorrhage, and specific enquiry must be made. Recent or chronic alcohol abuse is also important. However, the history is not always helpful and may even be misleading. No less than 40% of patients with known upper gastro-intestinal disease will prove to have bled from another cause or from a different site.

## Clinical examination

A thorough clinical examination is mandatory. Particular attention is paid to determine whether signs of chronic liver disease (liver palms, spider naevi, jaundice) and/or portal hypertension (palpable spleen, ascites, distended collaterals) are present. It is also important to seek evidence of such rare conditions as hereditary telangiectasia.

## The degree of blood loss

An important part of initial clinical assessment is to determine the likely loss of blood. This is frequently under-estimated so that blood replacement is often too little, too late and too slow.

Pallor, tachycardia, hypotension or anaemia indicate a loss of at least 1 litre and the need for transfusion.

## Initial manoeuvres

The objective of immediate treatment is to restore the circulation and provide a reserve against continued or recurrent bleeding. An intravenous line is immediately established and 1 litre of crystalloid solution (saline or Ringer lactate) infused while the patient is grouped and cross-matched. Urea, electrolyte and haemoglobin concentrations and packed cell volume are measured. A platelet count and prothrombin ratio should be requested on the first blood sample. $Pa_{O_2}$, $Pa_{CO_2}$ and $H^+$ concentrations are determined if the patient is severely shocked.

Pulse and blood pressure are monitored and if the patient is consistently hypotensive, a central venous line and urinary catheter are inserted. A large size nasogastric tube is introduced and intermittent suction is instituted. This helps to prevent aspiration of gastric contents and may detect fresh bleeding. As the stomach may contain blood clot, it is important to maintain patency of the tube by repeated irrigation with saline.

## Replacement of blood volume

As soon as it is available whole blood is infused through a free-flowing line. Pulse rate, CVP and arterial blood pressure must be adequate as judged by monitoring of volume and rate. If the patient is elderly, has cardiac failure or chronic respiratory disease, monitoring of pulmonary wedge pressure by a Swan-Ganz catheter may prevent pulmonary overload. If massive blood replacement is required, the blood must be warmed adequately and citrate acidaemia avoided by monitoring blood gases and pH, and administering bicarbonate if necessary.

Impaired haemostasis is anticipated in patients needing massive transfusion and in those with deranged liver function. The administration of stored blood quickly results in deficiencies of labile factors V and VIII but these defects can be restored by fresh frozen plasma (FFP); 1 pack for every 3 litres of blood transfused. Clotting screens to determine thrombin time, prothrombin time, kaolin-cephalin coagulation time and platelet count are of value in patients with massive bleeding. Vitamin $K_1$ is given routinely to all patients who are jaundiced or when the prothrombin time is prolonged (5–50 mg IV). FFP is needed in patients with liver disease unresponsive to vitamin K.

Urine output is monitored and an output of more than 40 ml/hour maintained by restoration of circulating blood volume.

It should again be stressed that all patients admitted to hospital with major upper gastrointestinal bleeding should be seen by a surgeon shortly after admission. This enables a balanced decision to be taken regarding further management and allows optimal timing of surgery if operation is required to control haemorrhage.

## Detection of nature and site of the bleeding lesion

As soon as the blood volume has been restored, an attempt should be made to detect the site of bleeding, even if the patient appears to have settled completely. Patients rarely die from their initial bleed but the death rate from recurrent haemorrhage is significant and the opportunity to determine the source of bleeding must not be lost. As indicated above, a history of chronic peptic ulceration or radiological demonstration of a longstanding lesion, e.g. duodenal scarring, is not always helpful in defining the cause of bleeding. At one time a barium meal was used as the standard investigation for acute haemorrhage but most clinicians now believe that the place of barium studies lies in detecting chronic gastro-intestinal disease and not a site of bleeding. As barium in the gastro-intestinal tract compromises both endoscopy and arteriography, it is now seldom used as the initial investigation of acute gastro-intestinal haemorrhage.

Endoscopy is now preferred as the first investigation. Using an end-viewing instrument, the bleeding site will be detected in 80–90% of cases. Even if the actual site of bleeding is not detected, oesophageal varices, gastric ulcer and gastric erosions are readily ruled out.

Arteriography detects bleeding into the gastro-intestinal tract when this exceeds 1–2 ml/minute. It is not used as a primary investigation but is indicated when the site of bleeding has not been detected on endoscopy and recurrent or continued bleeding demands surgical intervention. Should the arteriogram demonstrate the bleeding vessel, embolisation may be successful and avoid operation.

## TREATMENT

The majority of patients admitted with massive upper gastro-intestinal haemorrhage stop bleeding spontaneously. In such cases, the patient gradually and steadily improves and within 24–48 hours is able to take a light diet. Although cimetidine has not proved helpful in the control of acute haemorrhage from an ulcer, patients with peptic ulceration should be prescribed full therapeutic doses so that their ulcers heal.

If the continued need for blood replacement (> 5 units) indicates continuous bleeding, or if there is overt recurrent bleeding, surgery is likely to be required to control haemorrhage. Patients with chronic peptic ulceration are more likely to continue to bleed than those with erosive gastritis and patients past middle age are more prone to further haemorrhage. The elderly are at particular risk in that they are least able to contend with the physical demands of repeated or recurrent major haemorrhage. Certain endoscopic appearances also denote an increased risk of further bleeding from peptic ulcer; they include a visible artery in the ulcer base and adherent fresh clot or black slough.

## MANAGEMENT OF SPECIFIC LESIONS

### Erosive gastritis

If endoscopy reveals that bleeding is due to gastritis or erosions, intensive antacid therapy and/or cimetidine is instituted. If bleeding persists, the erosion can be coagulated endoscopically using a laser or diathermy. On rare occasions bleeding persists and surgery is required. There is debate regarding the optimal surgical procedure but truncal vagotomy is an essential part due to its effect on the gastric blood flow. It may be combined with partial gastrectomy or a drainage procedure.

### Chronic peptic ulceration

If conservative measures fail to arrest haemorrhage, surgery is required. On opening the abdomen, the presence of a chronic ulcer is first sought by inspection and palpation of the entire stomach and proximal duodenum. If no lesion is detected, a gastrotomy is performed, incising the front wall of the stomach longitudinally mid-way between the greater and lesser curvature. Clot is evacuated and the gastric mucosa palpated and inspected. If no lesion is found, the incision is closed and a longitudinal incision made through the pylorus so that the proximal duodenum can be inspected (pylorotomy).

A bleeding duodenal ulcer is treated by underrunning the bleeding vessel with non-absorbable sutures. The pylorotomy is sutured transversely as a pyloroplasty and the operation is completed by truncal vagotomy.

A chronic gastric ulcer is best treated by gastric resection with a gastro-duodenal (Billroth I) anastomosis. If the gastric ulcer is located high on the lesser curvature, it may be preferable to underrun it with non-absorbable sutures and then perform a vagotomy and pyloroplasty. In this event an adequate biopsy (with frozen section examination if possible) must be taken. Excision of the ulcer is the best form of biopsy but this is not always possible.

In all cases in which a peptic ulcer remains in situ, the patient must be carefully observed during the post-operative period for possible recurrence of haemorrhage. In this event further surgery may be required, usually with partial gastrectomy.

Trials in progress with endoscopic coagulation of bleeding peptic ulcer (by laser or diathermy) suggests that this mode of therapy may prove to be a useful alternative to emergency surgery.

### Oesophageal varices

See page 478.

### Carcinoma of the stomach

This is a rare cause of acute gastro-intestinal haemorrhage. If severe and exsanguinating an emergency operation may be required. Gastrectomy is the only feasible method of controlling the haemorrhage.

### Anastomotic ulcer

Massive haemorrhage from an anastomotic ulcer may require surgery. Primary control of the haemorrhage may be achieved by direct suture but it may be necessary also to modify the stoma depending on the extent of local deformity and the nature of the previous operation. If definitive surgery is required vagotomy (if not previously performed) combined with antrectomy is ideal.

Haemorrhage from an anastomotic ulcer following gastrectomy is treated by oversewing and vagotomy, resection of additional stomach, or both.

In all cases of anastomotic ulcer the possibility of the Zollinger-Ellison syndrome should be remembered.

The pancreas should be palpated at operation, and suspicious lymph nodes biopsied and serial serum gastrin levels arranged in the postoperative periods.

## MISCELLANEOUS DISORDERS OF THE STOMACH

### Gastric diverticula

These are rare but may be mistaken radiologically for ulceration or neoplasia. Endoscopy resolves the diagnosis.

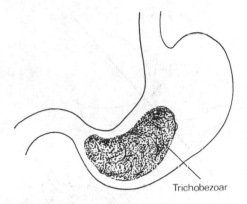

Trichobezoar

**Fig. 27.29** Bezoar

### Bezoars

A bezoar is a concretion formed in the fundus of the stomach (Fig. 27.29). Trichobezoars consist of hair and are seen in young girls or demented patients who chew and swallow their hair. Phytobezoars are less common and consist of aggregations of vegetable material such as orange pith, fruit skin and seeds. Patients after gastric surgery are particularly at risk due to reduced levels of gastric secretion and gastric motor activity. Rare forms of bezoar include semisolid bezoars of *Candida albicans* and shellac bezoars in painters or furniture makers.

Bezoars are rarely of clinical significance but if they attain large size they can cause symptoms due to obstruction, gastritis and bleeding. The diagnosis is made by barium meal examination and surgical removal is advisable.

### Swallowed foreign bodies

Accidental or deliberate ingestion of foreign bodies is common. The majority are radio-opaque and their progress can be followed radiologically. Most foreign bodies will pass through the alimentary tract without incident but operation is indicated if the object is deemed too large to leave the stomach, if signs of peritonitis develop, or if obstruction occurs.

### Gastric volvulus

Volvulus is usually a sequel to development of a para-oesophageal hiatus hernia (p. 356) or eventration of the diaphragm, the stomach rotating

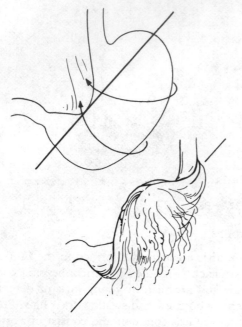

upwards around its longitudinal axis. The patient develops localised epigastric pain, severe nausea but inability to vomit, and epigastric distension. It proves impossible to pass a nasogastric tube into the stomach, and the diagnosis is confirmed by plain films of chest and abdomen followed by a gastrografin meal (Fig. 27.30). Immediate laparotomy is advisable to avoid gastric necrosis with perforation and haemorrhage. The volvulus is reduced and the oesophageal hiatus in the diaphragm is repaired. Resection is indicated if the stomach has undergone necrosis.

## MISCELLANEOUS DISORDERS OF THE DUODENUM

### Duodenal obstruction

Pyloric stenosis (p. 379) is the commonest cause of duodenal obstruction. Neoplastic obstruction due

**Fig. 27.30** Gastric volvulus

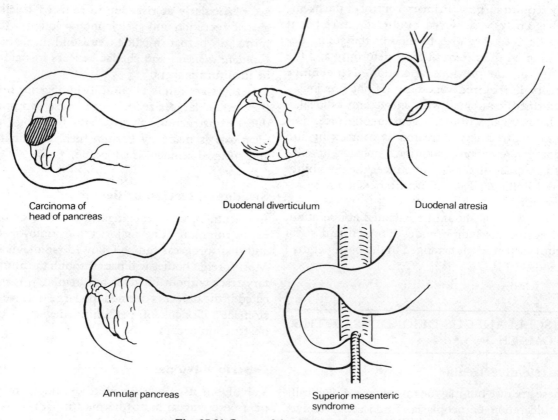

Carcinoma of head of pancreas

Duodenal diverticulum

Duodenal atresia

Annular pancreas

Superior mesenteric syndrome

**Fig. 27.31** Causes of duodenal obstruction

to carcinoma of the pancreas (p. 512), or mesenteric lymph nodes is relatively uncommon. Rare causes of duodenal obstruction include duodenal diverticula, duodenal atresia, annular pancreas, and chronic duodenal ileus (Fig. 27.31).

Symptomatic diverticula are excised, while obstruction due to atresia or annular pancreas is usually bypassed by duodeno-jejunal or gastro-jejunal anastomosis. Chronic duodenal ileus denotes recurrent duodenal obstruction in the absence of an anatomical or pathological cause, and often affects visceroptotic females in the fourth and fifth decade or rapidly growing, thin children around puberty. Epigastric and right hypochondrial pain are accompanied by vomiting, and adoption of the knee-elbow position sometimes brings relief. The explanation for the condition is uncertain but some believe that the superior mesenteric vessels may cause obstruction as they cross the third part of the duodenum (Fig. 27.31). Bypass using duodeno-jejunal anastomosis is indicated if ileus persists. In children the condition is usually self-limiting.

**Duodenal diverticula**

The duodenum is the second commonest site for diverticula formation in the gastro-intestinal tract. They are rare before the age of 40 years, usually affect the second part of the duodenum, and are often adjacent to the entry of the common bile duct (Fig. 27.31). They are usually discovered as an incidental finding on barium meal, but can cause obstruction and bleeding or become inflamed (diverticulitis). Symptomatic diverticula are excised.

**Duodenal trauma** (see p. 123)

# 28. The Small Intestine

## FUNCTIONAL ANATOMY

The small bowel extends from the pylorus to the ileo-caecal valve. Disorders of the duodenum are discussed elsewhere (p. 364). The remainder of this chapter is devoted to the 500 cm of small intestine distal to the ligament of Treitz. The upper two-fifths of this section of the intestine constitute the jejunum, the lower three-fifths the ileum; there is no clear demarcation between them.

The jejunum and ileum are completely invested by peritoneum with the exception of the narrow strip between the layers of the mesentery. The intestinal wall consists of an outer layer of longitudinal muscle, an inner layer of circular muscle, a strong fibro-elastic submucosa, and the mucosa.

The mucosa consists of a single layer of columnar cells interspersed with mucous cells, Paneth cells and APUD cells. The columnar cells are renewed constantly by proliferation of cells in the crypts of Lieberkuhn which take some 4–7 days to migrate to the tips of the villi.

The root of the small bowel mesentery extends from the left side of the body of L2 to the right sacro-iliac joint.

The mesentery contains fat, blood vessels, lymphatics, lymph nodes and nerves. The superior mesenteric artery supplies the jejunum and ileum by a series of straight arteries which originate from arterial arcades in the mesentery. These vessels enter the mesenteric border of the gut. The antimesenteric border has a less profuse arterial supply and is more susceptible to ischaemia. Venous blood from the jejunum and ileum drains to the superior mesenteric vein and from there to the portal vein.

Lymphoid aggregates in the submucosa (Peyers patches) are more numerous in the ileum than the jejunum. Lymph from the small intestine drains to regional nodes in the root of the mesentery before passing to the cisterna chyli. The mesentery contains both parasympathetic and sympathetic nerve fibres, but intestinal pain is mediated only by sensory afferents which follow the course of the sympathetic nerves.

### Function of the small intestine

While the principal function of the small intestine is absorption, it also has important secretory and digestive functions which supplement those of the stomach, duodenum, liver and pancreas. The total area for absorption is 200–500 m². To achieve this absorptive area, the mucosa is thrown into circular mucosal folds (plicae semilunaris) and surface villi (Fig. 28.1). In addition microvilli form finger-like projections on the surface of the epithelial cells.

Ingested fluid and the secretions of the salivary, gastric, pancreatic, biliary and intestine present the jejunum with some 5–8 litres of water each day. Under normal circumstances only 1–2 litres pass on into the colon (Fig. 28.2).

## DIVERTICULA OF THE SMALL INTESTINE

### MECKEL'S DIVERTICULUM

Meckel's diverticulum is the commonest congenital abnormality of the gastro-intestinal tract and results from persistence of the intestinal end of the

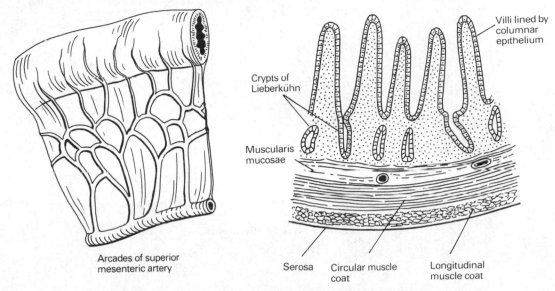

Villi lined by columnar epithelium

Crypts of Lieberkühn

Muscularis mucosae

Serosa   Circular muscle coat   Longitudinal muscle coat

**Fig. 28.1** Anatomy of the small intestine

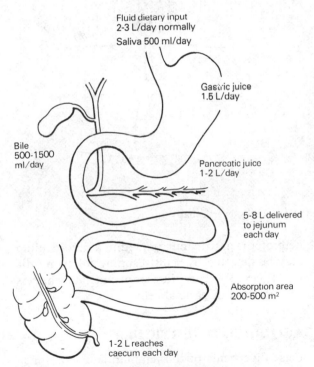

Fluid dietary input 2-3 L/day normally

Saliva 500 ml/day

Gastric juice 1.5 L/day

Bile 500-1500 ml/day

Pancreatic juice 1-2 L/day

5-8 L delivered to jejunum each day

Absorption area 200-500 m$^2$

1-2 L reaches caecum each day

**Fig. 28.2** Fluid shift in the small intestine

vitello-intestinal duct (Fig. 28.3). The diverticulum arises from the anti-mesenteric border of the ileum some 2 feet from the ileo-caecal valve, is 5 cm long (range 1–12 cm), and is present in about 2% of the population. As it contains all layers of the bowel wall it is a true diverticulum. The tip of the diverticulum is usually free but in 10% of cases it is connected to the umbilicus by a fibrous cord representing the remaining portion of the vitello-intestinal duct. Heterotopic tissue is found in 50% of symptomatic diverticula. Most often this is gastric mucosa containing parietal (acid secreting) cells. Other heterotopic tissues include pancreatic, colonic and duodenal mucosa.

## Clinical features

Only 5% of Meckel's diverticula cause symptoms. The patients are usually infants, children or young adults. *Bleeding* from a Meckel's diverticulum is the commonest cause of severe gastro-intestinal bleeding in childhood. This is due to acid secreted by heterotopic gastric mucosa causing peptic ulceration within the diverticulum or, more commonly, of the neighbouring small bowel.

*Intestinal obstruction* may be caused by intussusception of the diverticulum, volvulus around a band extending to the umbilicus, or a loop of bowel becoming trapped beneath such a band to form a 'closed loop'. Strangulation usually follows before operation can be performed.

*Acute diverticulitis* may give rise to abdominal pain and tenderness, pyrexia and leucocytosis. This cannot usually be distinguished clinically

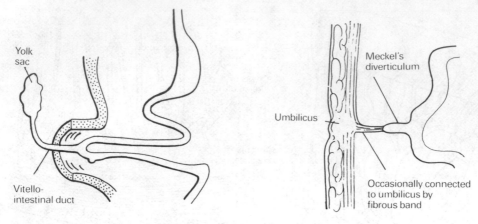

**Fig. 28.3** Meckel's diverticulum

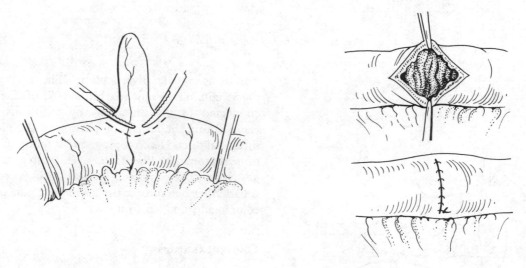

**Fig. 28.4** Method of excision of a Meckel's diverticulum

from acute appendicitis. Perforation is a common complication.

## Management

Symptomatic Meckel's diverticula should be excised (Fig. 28.4). Asymptomatic diverticula discovered as an incidental finding at laparotomy for unrelated disease need not be excised unless they have a narrow neck and are therefore liable to obstruction, or if nodularity indicates that abnormal mucosa is present. In patients with gastro-intestinal haemorrhage from a Meckel's diverticulum it is unusual to demonstrate the diverticulum by barium studies. However, heterotopic gastric mucosa within a diverticulum may be detected by scintiscanning following the injection of $^{99m}$Tc-sodium pertechnetate which is concentrated in parietal cells.

## ACQUIRED DIVERTICULA

False diverticula of the jejunum and ileum may develop with advancing age. The diverticula are usually multiple wide-mouthed sacs caused by herniation of mucosa between the layers of the mesentery at the sites of vessel penetration of the gut wall (Fig. 28.5). The diverticula may cause bleeding, diverticulitis or, if extensive, malabsorption due to accumulation of intestinal organ-

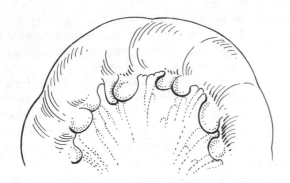

**Fig. 28.5** Jejunal diverticulosis

isms within them. They can be demonstrated by barium studies. If symptoms develop the affected segment of bowel should be excised.

## CROHN'S DISEASE

Crohn's disease was described in 1932 by Crohn and his colleagues at the Mount Sinai Hospital, New York, as a disease which affected the terminal ileum, hence the alternative name of 'regional ileitis'. With recognition that the jejunum could also be affected, the disease became known as 'regional enteritis'. When convincing evidence was presented that it also could affect the colon as an entity distinct from ulcerative colitis, it was realised that any part of the gastro-intestinal tract could be involved. The title of the disease then reverted to 'Crohn's'. The first description of the disease, however, was by a Scottish surgeon, Dalziel.

Crohn's disease is rare: less than one new case per 100 000 per annum.

### Pathological features

The diagnosis of Crohn's disease rests in recognition of its characteristic features on gross and microscopic examination. These include a 'cobblestone' appearance of the mucosa due to intercommunicating crevices or fissures surrounding islands of mucous membrane which become raised through underlying inflammation and oedema. Serpiginous ulceration may also occur. Fibrosis leads to the formation of strictures which may be single or multiple, short or long.

Multiple lesions within the intestinal tract are common and are classically discontinuous with intervening segments of normal bowel. Because of the penetrating nature of the disease process, the serosa may be inflamed or studded with small tubercle-like lesions.

In approximately one-quarter of patients with small bowel disease and three-quarters of those with disease of the large bowel, anal lesions occur at some time. These include chronic fissure, ulceration, oedematous anal tags and anal fistulas. These skin lesions may spread on to the perineum or occasionally may occur at other sites.

Microscopically, the most valuable diagnostic feature is the presence of non-caseating granulomas similar to those found in sarcoidosis which are distinguishable in 50% of all cases. Other microscopic features include fissures or clefts passing deeply into the bowel wall, transmural inflammation with oedema and infiltration of inflammatory cells and foci of lymphocytes.

### Clinical features

The clinical presentation of Crohn's disease is varied. Continuous or episodic diarrhoea, associated with recurrent abdominal pain, lassitude and fever, are common. Declining general health, malabsorption, weight loss and, in children, retardation of growth, may develop. Specific features may be associated with the following complications:

*Intestinal obstruction.* Excessive fibrosis results from chronic granulomatous inflammation and lymphoedema. All layers of the bowel wall become thickened, leading to stenosis and partial intestinal obstruction. The tendency to obstruction is increased by adhesions between the inflamed bowel and neighbouring structures. The clinical presentation is often one of intermittent bouts of incomplete intestinal obstruction, on which complete obstruction may supervene.

*Fistula formation.* Adhesions between inflamed loops of bowel predispose to fistula formation. Internal fistulae may form between loops of small or large intestine, and between bowel and non-alimentary viscera such as bladder. External fistulae are often a consequence of surgical intervention and most often involve the anterior abdominal wall or perineum.

*Abscess formation.* Free perforation is uncommon but sub-clinical bowel perforation often leads to abscess formation. The usual clinical and laboratory evidence of an abscess may be masked by steroid therapy, and considerable clinical judgment is needed to detect these complications and institute prompt management.

*Anal complications.* Anal fissures and fistulas are a common complications of Crohn's disease. The fistulae are frequently multiple and indolent. They commonly open in the perianal region but may involve any part of the perineum including the vagina or scrotum.

*Radiology* plays an essential role in the diagnosis of Crohn's disease. Proliferative changes with thickening of the bowel wall, narrowing of the lumen and separation of bowel loops, coincide with evidence of tissue destruction with ulceration, spike-like fissures and a cobblestone appearance of the mucosa. With developing fibrosis, short and long strictures can be demonstrated and account for the typical 'string sign' in the terminal ileum (Fig. 28.6).

## Management

Uncomplicated Crohn's disease should be managed conservatively. Rest, high protein, low-residue diet, medium-chain triglycerides and vitamins improve nutritional state. Hydrophilic colloid preparations and codeine phosphate may help diarrhoea. Cholestyramine has been used to bind bile salts and this may reduce diarrhoea.

Steroids are used in the acute phase and may reduce inflammatory manifestations. Long-term steroid therapy is not indicated. Sulphasalazine is also used in the acute phase and some believe it has a place in long-term treatment. Azathioprine has been used with limited success.

Ninety per cent of patients with Crohn's disease require surgery at some stage. In that surgery is not curative, it is usually reserved for complications but may be indicated for patients with intractable disease causing severe systemic problems.

The best surgical procedure is resection of the responsible segment or segments of intestine with restoration of continuity if feasible. Extended radical operations are no longer indicated. The recurrence rate after resection is determined more by the natural history of the individual's disease than by the extent of surgery. Bypass of an affected segment is no longer recommended as the majority of patients continue to experience major recurrent problems and come ultimately to resection.

The overall recurrence rate after resection for Crohn's disease involving ileum is around 33%. This is compared to less than 20% when the disease is confined to the colon. Fistulas are uncommon when all involved bowel is resected. They are a frequent complication of laparotomy alone or bypass. In view of the high recurrence rate multiple operations may be necessary.

*Mortality of surgery.* The immediate post-operative mortality is 3–4% in Crohn's disease. Late deaths related to operation bring the overall mortality to around 10%.

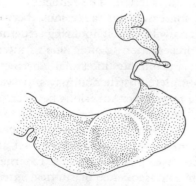

**Fig. 28.6** Radiological appearance of a typical case of Crohn's disease. The 'string sign' of Kantor.

## SMALL INTESTINAL FISTULAS

A fistula is an abnormal communication between two surfaces lined by epithelium (Fig. 28.7). Fistulas involving the small intestine are among the most difficult to manage. However, the principles underlying management of all fistulas arising from the digestive tract are the same.

### Clinical features

External small bowel fistulas are a complication of surgery in over 90% of cases but can arise sponta-

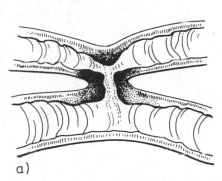
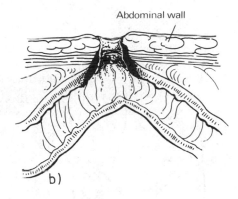

**Fig. 28.7** Intestinal fistulae. (a) Internal. (b) External.

neously, notably in patients with Crohn's disease. Development of a fistula following gastro-intestinal surgery is usually heralded by unexplained pyrexia and tachycardia in the early post-operative period. Abdominal pain and tenderness follow, and are associated with signs suggesting a simple wound infection or abscess. On rupture, frank discharge of intestinal content occurs through the wound or drain track. The escaping intestinal fluid can cause severe excoriation of the surrounding skin, particularly when the fistula originates from the upper small bowel and the fluid contains activated pancreatic secretion. Fistulas are classified as 'high output' and 'low output' according to the amount of fluid lost. 'High output' fistulas develop from the upper small intestine and 'low output' from the lower small intestine and colon.

## Management

The management of intestinal fistulas is as follows:

*Maintain fluid and electrolyte balance.* An accurate fluid balance chart is established with daily measurement of serum urea and electrolyte concentrations. Intravenous fluids are essential. High intestinal fistulas may be associated with loss of 3–4 litres of fluid each day leading to rapid dehydration and serious electrolyte deficits.

*Ensure adequate external drainage.* Material escaping from the intestine must have free egress from the abdomen. Otherwise intra-abdominal abscess formation or disseminated peritonitis with septicaemia will occur. Surgery may be required to establish drainage but at this stage does not include an attempt to close the internal site of leakage. When there is doubt about the formation of an abscess, a small amount of water-soluble contrast should be injected into the external opening during radiological screening.

*Provide nutritional support.* Parenteral nutrition has made a major impact on mortality rates following fistula formation. In patients with low-output fistula it may be possible to maintain nutrition by oral elemental diets, but for patients with high output fistulas it is advisable to stop all oral nutrition until closure has been achieved.

*Exclude distal obstruction.* The majority of alimentary fistulas close on conservative management provided there is no distal intestinal obstruction. Contrast radiology is used to investigate the distal intestine but is usually deferred until the patient's condition has been stabilised in terms of fluid and electrolyte balance, sepsis and nutritional support.

Fistulas associated with Crohn's disease or neoplasia are exceptions in that they are unlikely to close until the affected segment of bowel has been resected.

*Skin care.* Effective suction drainage minimises skin excoriation in high-output intestinal fistulas. Stomahesive and karaya gum are particularly useful in preventing damage to the skin around the external opening, and an ileostomy appliance is often useful (Fig. 28.8).

*Role of surgery.* Definitive surgery (other than that to establish adequate external drainage) is required when there is distal obstruction preventing spontaneous closure, persisting underlying

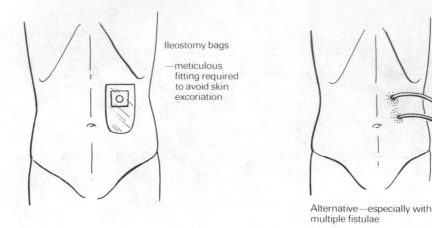

**Fig. 28.8** Skin care of an external fistula

intestinal disease (e.g. Crohn's disease), or when healing fails to take place despite adequate conservative therapy for a number of weeks.

*Fistula units.* In many modern hospitals 'fistula' and 'nutritional support' units have been developed for the specialised care of patients with intestinal fistulas and other complex problems of the intestinal tract which require treatment by long-term parenteral nutrition. As a result methods have been developed to provide 'home-nutrition' which may be continued for months or even years.

## SHORT BOWEL SYNDROME

### Pathophysiology of massive intestinal resection

The considerable functional reserve of the small bowel may be exceeded following massive resection for diseases such as trauma, mesenteric vascular disease, Crohn's disease, radiation enteritis, or neoplasia. The consequences of resection are determined in part by the length and position of the segment removed, the nature of the underlying cause, whether the ileo-caecal valve is intact or has been removed, and the ability of the remaining bowel to increase its absorptive capacity by the compensatory process known as adaptation. The problem of loss of absorptive surface area is compounded by rapid intestinal transit, disturbances in the normal neuro-hormonal regu-

lation of pancreatic and biliary secretion, continued loss of bile salts from the body's bile salt pool, and reflux of bacteria from the colon with overgrowth in the remaining small bowel. Nutritional consequences are usually severe when more than 75% of the small bowel is lost. Loss of the jejunum impairs absorption of fat, carbohydrate and protein although the ileum can compensate to some extent. Loss of the terminal ileum results in permanently impaired absorption of bile salts and vitamin $B_{12}$.

Some patients develop massive gastric hypersecretion, due possibly to loss of intestinal hormones capable of inhibiting gastric secretion. The problem improves with time but can compound malabsorption in that pH is lowered in the intestinal lumen with inactivation of lipase and trypsin.

The characteristic clinical course after massive small bowel resection is one of rapid development of profound fluid and electrolyte loss from severe diarrhoea. The severity usually diminishes after a few weeks, during which time adaptation of the remaining bowel takes place. The mucosa becomes hyperplastic, the villi increase in length, the crypts of Lieberkühn deepen, and the entire wall of the bowel becomes thickened.

Patients who undergo massive ileal resection but retain the colon are at risk of developing calcium oxalate calculi in the urinary tract because of excessive oxalate absorption from the colon. Resection of the terminal ileum also increases the risk of developing gall stones due to depletion of the bile salt pool.

## Management

Immediate post-operative management is directed at intravenous replacement of fluid and electrolyte loss, and provision of parenteral nutrition. Diarrhoea can be combated with codeine phosphate. Oral feeding should not be attempted while severe diarrhoea persists. Cimetidine is useful if gastric hypersecretion is present.

As diarrhoea abates, oral isotonic fluids are commenced cautiously. Elemental diets are used in dilute form and are best given at controlled rates by an infusion pump connected to a fine-bore nasogastric or nasoenteric tube. Such tubes are usually well-tolerated and their use avoids problems caused by lack of palatability of elemental diets. The rate and concentration of the alimentary intake is gradually increased bearing in mind that adaptation may continue for 12-24 months.

Parenteral nutrition is discontinued once an adequate oral intake can be tolerated but long-term parenteral nutrition may be unavoidable in some patients. Vitamins A, D and K are prescribed routinely in patients with persisting malabsorption. Vitamin $B_{12}$ is prescribed for life after extensive ileal resection.

As indicated above the development of nutritional support units and programmes of home-nutrition have greatly improved the care of such patients. An indwelling venous catheter is inserted through which the patient 'feeds himself' during sleep from a 3-litre bag containing all essential nutrients (Fig. 28.9) (see Chapter 10).

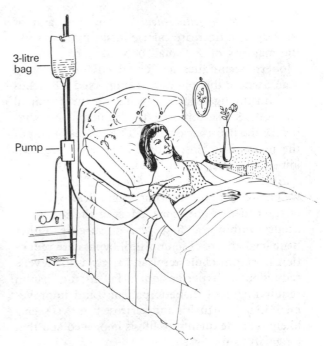

**Fig. 28.9** 'Home nutrition'

by about half following bypass and the reduction is enhanced if diet is modified to reduce cholesterol intake. Xanthelasma and xanthoma generally decrease in size or disappear and angina pectoris often becomes less troublesome. Diarrhoea is an almost inevitable complication of surgery but tends to improve with time. Vitamin $B_{12}$ supplements are advisable but malabsorption of other essential nutrients is seldom a problem and body weight is usually unaffected.

## INTESTINAL BYPASS PROCEDURES

### Partial ileal bypass for hyperlipidaemia

Hyperlipidaemia (hypercholesterolaemia and hypertriglyceridaemia) increases the risk of developing atherosclerosis and its complications. Hyperlipidaemia may be reduced by dietary modifications, drugs (e.g. clofibrate, cholestyramine) and/or partial ileal bypass. Bypass reduces cholesterol absorption and by depleting the bile acid pool further reduces hyperlipidaemia as cholesterol is converted increasingly to bile acids to maintain pool size. Serum cholesterol is reduced

### Jejuno-ileal bypass for morbid obesity

Morbid obesity is defined as a weight increase of at least 45 kg (100 lbs) or 100% relative to ideal weight as determined by age, height and sex. Jejuno-ileal bypass has been used for some 20 years to manage this condition, notably in the United States. It is usually reserved for morbidly obese patients who fail to maintain weight reduction with supervised dietary modification for at least 5 years, and is not undertaken until correctable metabolic or endocrine causes for obesity have been excluded. It is now recognised that morbidly obese female patients have an increased risk of cancer of the breast and uterus.

*Technique of jejuno-ileal bypass.* The aim of surgery is to decrease caloric intake by bypassing the majority of the small bowel absorptive area. Modern techniques are based on the '14 + 4 plan', where the jejunum is transected 14 inches beyond the ligament of Treitz and the proximal jejunum is anastomosed to the ileum 4 inches before the ileo-caecal valve. The cut distal end of the jejunum is closed, or the bypassed segment joined separately to the colon (Fig. 28.10).

*Effects of jejuno-ileal bypass.* The average weight reduction following jejuno-ileal bypass is of the order of one-third. Most of the reduction occurs within the first year of surgery. Other beneficial effects of jejuno-ileal bypass are reduction in serum cholesterol and triglyceride levels, reduction in hypertension, a fall in the insulin requirements of diabetic patients, and improvement in osteoarthritis and varicose veins. It seems likely that the quality of life is improved and that longevity is increased.

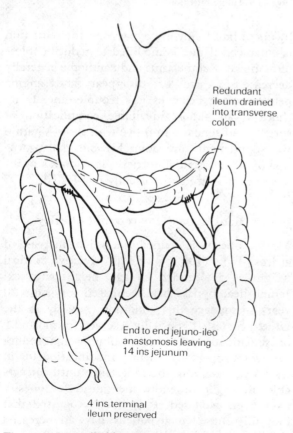

Redundant ileum drained into transverse colon

End to end jejuno-ileo anastomosis leaving 14 ins jejunum

4 ins terminal ileum preserved

**Fig. 28.10** Jejuno-ileal bypass

*Complications of jejuno-ileal bypass.* The operative mortality is generally around 1%, although late deaths related to jejuno-ileal bypass are reported in some 5% of patients. Diarrhoea is invariably troublesome but improves with time and codeine phosphate can be used if necessary. A fall in serum calcium, magnesium and potassium is common in the early months after operation, particularly when diarrhoea is troublesome. Supplements of these elements are advisable for 6 months to a year.

Transient protein malabsorption is common after bypass and serum albumin levels may fall. Some degree of fat malabsorption is inevitable and steatorrhoea is induced readily if fat intake is high. However, not all of the weight loss after jejuno-ileal bypass can be ascribed to malabsorption, and both appetite and food intake are reduced markedly in the early post-operative period. Transient hair loss is attributed to diffuse protein deficiency.

More perturbing complications include migratory polyarthralgia, nephrocalcinosis, and fatty degeneration of the liver. Fatty infiltration and hepatic cirrhosis are recognised complications of morbid obesity and at least some of the changes reported after bypass may be a legacy of the pre-operative state. However, 75% of patients have some degree of fatty change after bypass and a few develop frank hepatic failure and require restoration of intestinal continuity.

Because of these complications methods of reducing the size of the stomach by plication are being studied as an alternative to jejunal bypass which is now rarely performed. An ingenious method recently described is to insert an intragastric balloon which is inflated and acts as a 'bezoar' to reduce the capacity of the stomach and lower food intake.

## INTESTINAL ISCHAEMIA

### ACUTE INTESTINAL ISCHAEMIA

#### Superior mesenteric artery occlusion

Thrombotic or embolic occlusion of the superior mesenteric artery is an acute abdominal emergency with a high mortality. In most patients, thrombosis is the final event in atheromatous narrowing of the vessel. Emboli account for occlusion in one-third of cases and usually originate from intracardiac thrombus in patients with atrial fibrillation or recent myocardial infarction.

Occlusion occurs most commonly in elderly patients affected by cardiac failure. Delay in diagnosis remains a problem, and most patients do not come to surgery until necrosis of the bowel is advanced and peritonitis is established.

It is important to appreciate that abdominal pain and vomiting *in the absence of abdominal signs* may precede peritonitis and collapse for several hours or even some days. Bowel ischaemia proceeds from mucosa to serosa and peritonitis does not develop until all layers are involved. The majority of infarctions affect ileum alone.

*Management.* Successful management requires early diagnosis and operation to restore blood flow before irreversible changes occur in the bowel wall. Plain abdominal films usually show no intestinal abnormality in the critical early period. Aortography or selective superior mesenteric arteriography can be used to confirm the diagnosis of occlusion but must be carried out promptly.

For superior mesenteric artery thrombosis, an aorto-mesenteric bypass graft using autogenous vein can be used if the bowel is viable. Gangrenous bowel requires resection. Segments of bowel of doubtful viability should also be resected. A 'second look' operation 24-48 hours later to confirm viability of remaining bowel is now routine practice in many clinics. Antibiotics, oxygen, peritoneal lavage and adequate fluid replacement are essential parts of management.

Should the occlusion be due to an embolus, embolectomy and the closure of the arteriotomy with a vein patch graft may restore the mesenteric circulation and avoid or minimise the extent of gut resection.

### Mesenteric venous occlusion

Mesenteric venous occlusion is much less common than arterial occlusion but equally devastating. Any disease predisposing to intravascular coagulation can cause venous occlusion and sporadic cases have been reported in pregnancy, in the puerperium, and in young women taking oral contraceptives. The arterial supply to the mid-gut is normal but there is thrombosis of the mesenteric veins and venous gangrene of the bowel follows. Treatment consists of anti-coagulation and bowel resection as required. Only occasionally is venous thrombectomy helpful. The mortality from this condition is high.

### Non-occlusive infarction

Intestinal infarction may occur without demonstrable occlusion of major vessels, as for example, low flow states in severe shock. Conservatism is recommended and resection is only undertaken when there is obviously necrotic bowel.

## CHRONIC INTESTINAL (MESENTERIC) ISCHAEMIA

*Chronic* mid-gut ischaemia is a rare condition which gives rise to pain in the mid-abdomen after eating, diarrhoea due to malabsorption, and weight loss. A bruit in the para-umbilical region is occasionally present and supports the diagnosis. Occult blood is present in the faeces. Arterial narrowing revealed at angiography may be dealt with by surgical reconstruction.

## NEOPLASMS OF THE SMALL INTESTINE

Small bowel neoplasms are rare and comprise less than 5% of gastro-intestinal neoplasms. Benign lesions are 10 times as common as malignant lesions.

### BENIGN TUMOURS

Solitary small bowel tumours include adenomatous or villous polyps, hamartomas, lipomas, haemangiomas and leiomyomas. Multiple hamartomatas occur in the familial Peutz-Jeghers syndrome in association with mucocutaneous pigmentation and diffuse gastro-intestinal polyposis. Operation is indicated if any benign small bowel neoplasm causes symptoms such as bleeding or intussusception.

# MALIGNANT TUMOURS

## Adenocarcinoma

Small bowel adenocarcinomas are extremely rare when one considers the length of the small intestine. Yet they are still the commonest malignant tumour of the small bowel. Symptoms are usually due to obstruction but, by the time they occur, the disease is usually advanced. Treatment is by laparotomy and resection. They are frequently advanced by the time symptoms occur and laparotomy is undertaken.

## Lymphoma

Lymphoma may originate in the small intestine. Resection of a single involved segment is indicated if obstruction or bleeding develops, but the disease should be regarded in the same light as lymphoma arising elsewhere and dealt with by staging laparotomy (p. 552) to plan further treatment. Small deposits of lymphoma can cause perforation of the bowel wall, the patient being admitted to hospital with peritonitis. At operation a small punched-out hole is discovered in the small gut. In such cases *biopsy* by excision of the perforation must precede closure.

## Carcinoid tumours

Carcinoid tumours most frequently arise in the appendix. The small intestine is the second-commonest site of carcinoid formation and one-third of tumours have metastasised by the time of presentation. Symptoms may be produced by obstruction or bleeding, and some 10% of patients present with the carcinoid syndrome. Biologically active tumour products are normally inactivated by the liver, but once hepatic metastases develop these substances are secreted directly into the systemic circulation. The syndrome comprises periodic flushing attacks, diarrhoea, bronchoconstriction, and right-sided heart disease, notably pulmonary stenosis. Urinary levels of 5-hydroxyindoleacetic acid (5-HIAA) are elevated in the majority of patients with the syndrome. Treatment of carcinoid tumours consists of excising all accessible tumour in the small bowel and its mesentery. Hepatic metastases have been treated by hepatic lobectomy in some patients but the role of such radical surgery and of chemotherapy is as yet uncertain.

# 29. The Appendix

## SURGICAL ANATOMY

The appendix normally develops as a conical true diverticulum from the dependent pole of the caecum. Agenesis is rare. As a result of differential caecal growth during infancy the origin of the appendix is pushed medially until it eventually originates from the medial wall of the caecum some 2 cm below the ileo-caecal junction (Fig. 29.1). The taeniae coli converge on the root of the appendix and so aid in its localisation at laparotomy.

Despite its constant point of origin from the caecum, the position of the appendix varies greatly. In most individuals it lies behind the caecum or hangs down over the pelvic brim (Fig. 29.2). In 1–2% of subjects, the appendix lies in front of or behind the terminal ileum. Malrotation of the colon and complete situs inversus are uncommon developmental abnormalities in which the appendix is found in the upper abdomen or left iliac fossa. The position of the appendix has an important influence on the clinical picture of appendicitis.

The appendix is lined by colonic epithelium and has no known function in man. The development of lymphoid tissue in its wall during childhood suggests that it then may have an immunological function. The lymphoid tissue regresses in adolescence. The appendix lumen is frequently obliterated by fibrosis in older patients.

## ACUTE APPENDICITIS

### Incidence

Acute appendicitis is predominantly a disease of Western civilisation and is uncommon in Africa and Asia. The condition may be becoming more common in developing countries due to their adoption of low-residue Western-type diets. The incidence in Britain has fallen dramatically over the past 30 years.

Acute appendicitis remains the most common abdominal surgical emergency in childhood, adolescence and early adult life. Less than 2% of cases occur in infants under 2 years; the peak incidence is during the second and third decades

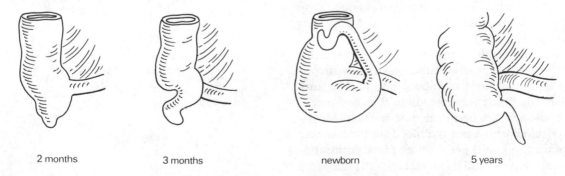

2 months     3 months     newborn     5 years

**Fig. 29.1** The stages in the development of the appendix

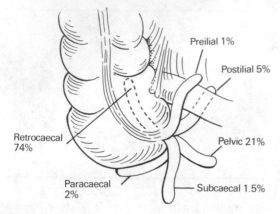

**Fig. 29.2** The positions of the appendix

of life. Thereafter it declines and less than 5% of cases occur in patients over 60 years.

## Aetiology

A combination of stasis and infection is required to produce experimental appendicitis. The typical onset with abdominal colic suggests that obstruction is a major factor. Obstruction causes accumulation of secretion and distension, leading to pressure necrosis of the mucosa and invasion of the wall by bacteria. The peak age incidence of appendicitis parallels that of maximal development of lymphoid tissue. Lymphoid hyperplasia within the wall predisposes to obstruction in younger patients and may also account for the frequency of mesenteric adenitis at that age. In older patients inspissated faeces forming faecoliths are a major cause of obstruction. Less common causes of obstruction include kinks, adhesions and neoplasia. Appendicitis is not caused by specific bacteria. The majority of organisms concerned are normal gut inhabitants. Threadworms can produce signs and symptoms resembling mild appendicitis but are incriminated in only a few cases.

The inflammatory process may resolve. More commonly, progressive infection and obstruction lead to impairment of blood supply. The anti-mesenteric border is most vulnerable, and patchy gangrene appears first in its mid-portion. Morbidity rises sharply once the blood supply has been compromised, and even before frank perforation occurs, bacteria migrate through the damaged wall into the peritoneal cavity. The increased morbidity of appendicitis in the elderly is partly explained by the more rapid development of gangrene and perforation.

Once perforation has occurred, the outcome depends on the ability of the omentum to contain the infection. If adequate an appendix mass or abscess results; if not there is generalised peritonitis. The omentum is not fully developed in infants, and localisation of infection is less effective than in older children and adults. However, in all age groups, *delay* in diagnosis and treatment remains the most important factor which worsens prognosis.

## Clinical features

Many of the so-called 'typical' signs and symptoms of acute appendicitis may be absent, or may appear only in the late stages of the disease. These vary according to the position of the appendix.

## Symptoms (Fig. 29.3)

*Pain* is usually the first and most impressive symptom. In the 'typical' case, pain begins as

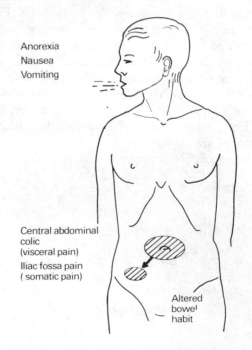

**Fig. 29.3** The main symptoms in acute appendicitis

peri-umbilical colic which may be severe or amount to no more than an aching discomfort. The colic is a true *visceral* pain due to appendiceal obstruction. In children there may appear to be little wrong between the bouts of pain.

Classically, the pain remains peri-umbilical for several hours before shifting to the right iliac fossa. This shift denotes the development of *somatic* pain due to parietal peritonitis. This somatic pain is sharply localised, causing discomfort on moving or coughing. In one-third to one-half of cases, the pain commences in and remains in the right iliac fossa without preceding visceral pain. When the appendix is retrocaecal in position, somatic pain is perceived in the flank and loin rather than in the right iliac fossa. A pelvic appendix may not be associated with any somatic pain.

*Anorexia* is almost invariable. Hunger usually indicates that the patient does not have appendicitis. Nausea occurs in most patients and precedes *vomiting* which is seldom a prominent feature. *Alteration of bowel habit* may be noted. Some patients complain of a sense of fullness and may have taken aperients in an attempt to gain relief; others have constipation which precedes the attack. Diarrhoea may occur in younger children and is a feature of pelvic appendicitis which irritates the neighbouring rectum.

## Signs

*Fever* and *tachycardia* are *not* early signs of appendicitis. Pulse and temperature may not rise significantly until perforation occurs. *Foetor* often accompanies appendicitis, but is not invariable and occurs in many other acute abdominal conditions.

The abdominal signs vary according to the position of the appendix. *Tenderness* and muscle *guarding* localised to the right iliac fossa are the most consistent findings. Tenderness is often maximal over McBurney's point (i.e. one-third of the way along a line drawn between the right anterior superior iliac spine and the umbilicus) (Fig. 29.4) and is associated with rebound tenderness and hyperaesthesia. Other signs include Rovsing's sign (pressure on the left iliac fossa produces right sided pain) (Fig. 29.5) and the

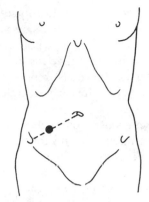

**Fig. 29.4** McBurneys's point

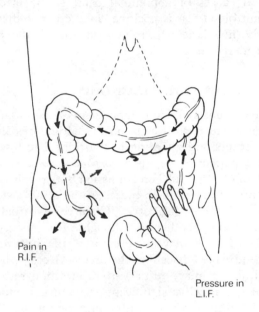

Pain in R.I.F.

Pressure in L.I.F.

**Fig. 29.5** Rovsing's sign

psoas sign (pain during passive extension of the right hip) but these are of variable value (Chapter 16; Fig. 16.7).

Retrocaecal appendicitis is notoriously difficult to diagnose in its early stages. Nausea, vomiting and diarrhoea may be the only symptoms. Perforation, abscess formation or the development of a mass may occur before diagnosis. Tenderness, if present, is maximal in the right flank or loin.

Pelvic appendicitis often produces little tenderness or guarding on abdominal examination, but tenderness is always present on digital rectal examination.

*Perforated appendicitis* with diffuse peritonitis leads to generalised tenderness, guarding and rigidity. Even at this stage, tenderness is often still maximal in the right iliac fossa.

*Bowel sounds* are normal or only slightly reduced in frequency in the early stages of appendicitis.

In some cases a *mass* is palpable in the abdomen or on rectal examination. This inflammatory mass consists of omentum and neighbouring viscera which have adhered to the inflamed appendix.

*Digital rectal examination* reveals tenderness in approximately one-third of patients with appendicitis. It is a valuable means of detecting gynaecological causes of abdominal pain. If the faecal occult blood test is positive, an alternative diagnosis (neoplasia or Crohn's disease) should be considered.

## DIFFERENTIAL DIAGNOSIS

The diagnosis of acute appendicitis is essentially clinical and rests heavily on the finding of pain, tenderness and guarding in the right iliac fossa. Many patients have a *polymorphonuclear leucocytosis* of $10–15 \times 10^9/l$ on admission but, as this is a feature of many other causes of the acute abdomen, it is not diagnostic. *Urinalysis* is usually normal in appendicitis, although a few pus cells and red cells may be present if the inflamed appendix lies adjacent to the ureter. Gross pyuria indicates primary urinary tract infection rather than appendicitis; significant haematuria is more likely to be associated with a ureteric calculus.

The range of differential diagnosis is wider in women than in men. Females especially in the age group 15–20 years are more likely to have a normal appendix removed.

*Plain abdominal X-rays* are of value in diagnosis, primarily as a means of excluding other causes of abdominal pain such as perforated peptic ulcer, ureteric calculi and intestinal obstruction. There are no pathognomic features of acute appendicitis but some patients have fluid levels in the right iliac fossa, a radio-opaque appendiceal faecolith (10% of cases), increased soft tissue density in the right iliac fossa with obliteration of the psoas border, or gas bubbles in the region of the appendix (indicating perforation) (Fig. 29.6).

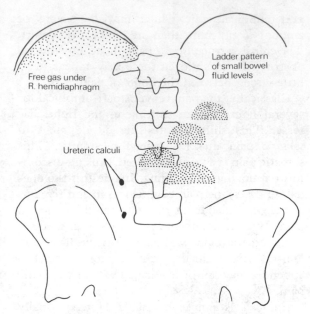

Free gas under R. hemidiaphragm

Ladder pattern of small bowel fluid levels

Ureteric calculi

**Fig. 29.6** Points to watch for on plain abdominal X-ray in the differential diagnosis of acute appendicitis

Acute appendicitis is seldom absent from the differential diagnosis of acute abdominal pain, unless it has been previously removed. Fortunately the majority of conditions which are confused with appendicitis also require laparotomy. However, 'medical' causes of abdominal pain such as basal pneumonia and diabetic ketosis, for which laparotomy is positively contra-indicated, must be excluded. The diagnosis of acute appendicitis is notoriously difficult in the very young and the elderly and this undoubtedly contributes to the high incidence of gangrene and perforation in these age groups.

### Special points in diagnosis

The following should be noted:

1. *Central abdominal colic* in the early stages of appendicitis may suggest *gastroenteritis* or mechanical *intestinal obstruction*. The key to the diagnosis of *gastroenteritis* is that nausea, vomiting and diarrhoea usually precede or accompany pain. Tenderness is seldom localised to the right iliac fossa, and the patient may have symptoms of a viral illness, such as headache, myalgia and photophobia.

2. The clinical features of *intestinal obstruction* depend on the level of the obstructing lesion.

High intestinal obstruction is characterised by profuse vomiting and relatively little abdominal distension, whereas low obstruction causes marked distension and late onset of vomiting. Regardless of the level of the lesion, tenderness is seldom localised to the right iliac fossa.

3. While right iliac fossa pain and tenderness are the most consistent clinical features they can be produced by a large number of conditions including *mittelschmerz, acute mesenteric adenitis, acute terminal ileitis* and inflammation of a *Meckel's diverticulum*. Although the presence of these conditions may be suspected clinically, all can mimic appendicitis closely, and laparotomy is usually indicated if pain and tenderness persist.

4. *Acute salpingitis* can produce right iliac fossa tenderness. The condition is often bilateral and causes suprapubic or diffuse lower abdominal tenderness. Fever is usually higher in salpingitis than appendicitis and the systemic upset is less marked than from a comparable fever in the late stages of appendicitis. Vaginal examination reveals a hot, tender cervix and a vaginal discharge is present in most cases of salpingitis.

5. *Ureteric colic* can be associated with pain and tenderness on deep palpation over the ureter, but the severity and radiation of the pain in the presence of haematuria usually indicate the true diagnosis. Abdominal X-rays and an intravenous urogram are likely to show the calculus.

6. Pelvic appendicitis may be simulated by *salpingitis, diverticular disease*, and perforation of a *colonic carcinoma*. Differentiation between these colonic diseases and appendicitis may be difficult, especially when the sigmoid colon is redundant and lies in the right iliac fossa. As a general rule, tenderness is more diffuse and the involved colon may give rise to a palpable mass.

7. *Retrocaecal* appendicitis causes pain and tenderness which is higher and situated more posteriorly than usual, and may mimic *perinephric abscess, acute pyelonephritis, perforated colon cancer* or *acute cholecystitis*. High fever and chills are more typical of the first two of these conditions than of appendicitis, and pyuria and costovertebral angle tenderness are usually present. Cholecystitis is associated with gallbladder tenderness and a positive Murphy's sign in most cases. Mild icterus and a palpable mass in the region of the gallbladder also suggest cholecystitis.

8. *The presence of a mass* in the right iliac fossa raises the question of *intussusception* in young children; *acute terminal ileitis* and *Crohn's disease* in older children and adults; *ovarian cysts* in women; and *neoplasia of the bowel* in older patients.

9. Should *diffuse peritonitis* develop from appendicitis, the original site of infection may be difficult to define. However, tenderness may still be maximal in the right iliac fossa.

10. *Perforated peptic ulcer* can simulate appendicitis, particularly when escaping gastric and duodenal contents run down the right paracolic gutter and give rise to pain and tenderness in the right iliac fossa. Free perforation of the appendix rarely produces radiological evidence of gas under the liver or diaphragm, in contrast to perforation of a peptic ulcer or perforated *diverticular disease*.

11. Acute *pancreatitis* can mimic appendicitis at all stages, but upper abdominal or diffuse pain in pancreatitis is associated with copious vomiting and retching, back pain, and hyperamylasaemia.

12. *Ruptured ectopic pregnancy* can also simulate all stages of appendicitis, beginning with cramping pain in the iliac fossa, and proceeding to spreading pain and tenderness as blood disseminates throughout the peritoneal cavity. The true diagnosis may be suggested by a history of menstrual irregularity, vaginal bleeding, and shoulder-tip pain which may be induced by elevation of the foot of the bed.

## PROBLEM AREAS IN DIAGNOSIS

### Appendicitis in infancy

This is uncommon, diagnosis is difficult, and the average delay between onset and definitive diagnosis is around 4 days. This delay is reflected in a high incidence of positive radiological signs, and of abscess formation or generalised peritonitis at the time of surgery. Appendicitis is more common in children with Hirschsprung's disease.

In infants and young children, early appendicitis causes irritability and anorexia. Vomiting, pain, fever and loose bowel movements may develop as the disease progresses.

Clinical examination is difficult and tenderness cannot be localised readily. The development of fever in an infant, associated with any abdominal tenderness should always raise the suspicion of acute appendicitis.

## Appendicitis during pregnancy

Acute appendicitis is as common in pregnant as in non-pregnant women (it complicates 1 in 2000 pregnancies) and should always be borne in mind when acute abdominal pain develops during pregnancy.

Early diagnosis is vital but difficult, especially in the third trimester. Then the appendix is displaced upwards by the gravid uterus so that pain and tenderness are higher than expected. Rectal or vaginal signs are absent. The white cell count is normally elevated in pregnancy and abdominal X-rays are contra-indicated.

Delay is so harmful to mother and unborn child that provided urinary tract infection has been excluded, one should operate early. Maternal and fetal deaths do not result from appendicectomy but from peritonitis. The fetal mortality in un-complicated appendicitis is 3%, that following perforation 30%. The incidence of appendicitis is uniform throughout pregnancy, although the risk of maternal mortality increases as pregnancy progresses.

Difficulty in diagnosis, reluctance to operate on pregnant women and avoidable delay account for the high risks of appendicitis in pregnancy.

## Appendicitis in the elderly

Appendicitis has a more rapid course in the elderly. Gangrene and perforation are five times as common in patients over 60 years of age, this due to delay in diagnosis. The 'classical picture' of appendicitis is often lacking, pain being a less prominent feature. Appendicitis may not even be considered as a cause of the patient's symptoms. Awareness of the rising incidence of appendicitis in the elderly, its atypical presentation and a willingness to undertake laparotomy promptly are the keys to successful management.

## Appendicitis developing in hospital

Hospitalised patients are not immune to appendicitis and may develop the condition while undergoing investigation and treatment for unrelated medical conditions, or while recovering from other forms of surgery. Lack of awareness may cause avoidable delay in treatment.

## TREATMENT OF UNCOMPLICATED APPENDICITIS

The aim of treatment is to remove the appendix before gangrene and perforation occur. Pre-operative resuscitation is not generally required unless there is generalised peritonitis.

Appendicectomy is carried out under general anaesthesia. The abdomen is entered through a small transverse incision centred over McBurney's point in the right iliac fossa (Fig. 29.7). A right paramedian incision does not give as good access for appendicectomy, but is used if the diagnosis is in doubt.

The muscles of the anterior abdominal wall are split in the line of their fibres as each layer is encountered: the 'grid-iron' incision. The peritoneal cavity is entered and the caecum is identified and delivered through the wound. The appendix often emerges with the caecum, but may require mobilisation if adherent to neighbouring structures. If the organ cannot be identified readily, the taeniae coli should be traced to its base.

The meso-appendix is divided and its contained appendicular artery ligated (Fig. 29.8). The appendix is ligated at its base and removed. The appendix stump is invaginated into the caecum using a purse-string suture.

The appendix is sent for histological examination to confirm the diagnosis and to exclude the presence of a carcinoid tumour. A bacteriology swab is taken from the peritoneal cavity in all cases.

The wound is closed in layers. Local antiseptic agents such as povidone-iodine reduce the incidence of subsequent wound infection. Many surgeons now prefer to use metronidazole (500 mg IV or 1 g as a suppository with premedication) as a means of reducing the incidence of wound infection. Drainage of the peritoneal cavity or wound is indicated only if there is a localised abscess.

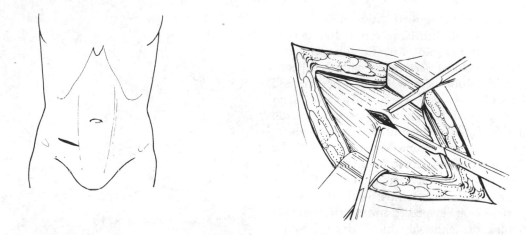

**Fig. 29.7** The gridiron incision

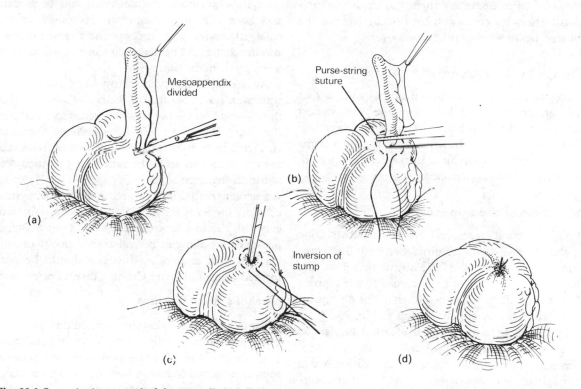

**Fig. 29.8** Stages in the removal of the appendix. (a) division of blood supply, (b) ligation of base and insertion purse-string suture, (c) removal appendix and inversion of stump, (d) purse-string suture tied.

# PROBLEMS DURING APPENDICECTOMY

## The normal appendix

Depending on the policy of the surgeon, an apparently normal appendix will be removed in up to 20% of emergency appendicectomies. At-tempts to improve diagnostic accuracy by delaying operation may be hazardous and lead to an unacceptable increase in morbidity and mortality from gangrene and perforation.

If the appendix is seen not to be acutely inflamed, other pathology must always be excluded. If peritoneal fluid is present it may give a clue to the correct diagnosis. Mesenteric adenitis may be associated with clear yellow free peritoneal fluid, perforation of a peptic ulcer with bile stained fluid, colonic perforation with faecal content, and infarction of bowel with blood-stained fluid. Free blood suggests rupture of a vessel, or an ectopic pregnancy. If there is any uncertainty, the wound is extended or an additional incision made.

If no pathology is immediately apparent, the distal ileum is withdrawn and examined to exclude a Meckel's diverticulum, terminal ileitis, Crohn's disease or mesenteric adenitis. Both ovaries and Fallopian tubes are inspected and an attempt made to visualise the sigmoid colon. Even if other pathology is present, a normal appendix should be removed when operating through a grid-iron incision, otherwise confusion may occur later as the patient bears an appendicectomy scar.

## Lumps in the appendix

At operation there may be a mass palpable within the appendix. *Faecoliths* are the commonest cause. In obstructive appendicitis they may lose their mobility and be mistaken for neoplasms until the removed organ is incised and inspected. Neoplasms are rare (page 416).

## Mucocele of the appendix

This rare condition results from chronic obstruction of the appendix with accumulation of mucin, producing cystic dilatation. The obstruction is usually due to fibrous tissue but sometimes to a malignant mucous papillary adenocarcinoma. Simple mucoceles are cured by appendicectomy (Fig. 29.9).

Pseudomyxoma peritonei is a rare complication of mucocele of the appendix (or ovarian neoplasm). Mucin-producing cells are disseminated throughout the peritoneal cavity. Extreme care should be taken to avoid rupture during removal.

## Acute terminal ileitis and appendicectomy

Acute terminal ileitis used to be regarded as a manifestation of Crohn's disease. It is now realised that it is due to a self-limiting infection with *Yersinia enterocolitica* or *Y. pseudotuberculosis*. Acute ileitis mimics appendicitis clinically, but at laparotomy the terminal ileum is red and thick-

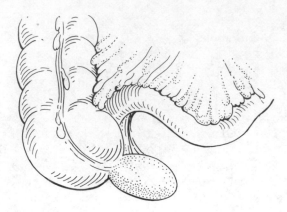

**Fig. 29.9** Mucocele of the appendix

ened, mesenteric adenitis is obvious, and the caecum and appendix appear normal. Histology of the enlarged nodes and the appendix reveals nonspecific changes. The diagnosis can be confirmed by serology or node culture.

At one time appendicectomy was thought to be contra-indicated because of the risk of a fistula from the inflamed bowel but it is now recommended that the ileum should be left alone and the appendix removed. Even in true Crohn's disease of the ileum, the appendix can safely be removed, provided it is not itself involved.

Further treatment is not required after appendicectomy for acute terminal ileitis, except in the rare event of *Yersinia* septicaemia, when tetracycline is prescribed. Following convalescence an out-patient barium meal and follow-through should be performed to exclude true Crohn's disease elsewhere.

## Meckel's diverticulum

Inflammation in a Meckel's diverticulum cannot be distinguished clinically from acute appendicitis. Laparotomy is required for both conditions and an acutely inflamed Meckel's diverticulum is resected.

A diverticulum is sought routinely if the appendix is not inflamed, but this is best avoided in the presence of an inflamed appendix. Meckel's diverticula discovered incidentally need not be removed as a routine (Chapter 17).

## Post-operative complications

Complications are uncommon following early removal of an inflamed appendix. The incidence and severity of complications rises with gangrene and perforation.

*Bleeding* in the immediate post-operative period is rare, and usually due to technical error, and results from slipping of ligatures on the meso-appendix or within the layers of the wound. Reoperation may be required.

*Urinary retention* may be a problem and require catheterisation.

*Wound infection* used to occur in approximately one-third of appendicectomy wounds. The incidence was higher following removal of a gangrenous or perforated appendix. The use of topical antiseptics and systemic metronidazole have reduced this risk (see p. 61).

Contamination of the wound with purulent material during surgery is an indication for delayed primary suture. Only the deeper layers of the wound are closed. The skin and subcutaneous tissues are left open for some 4–5 days. Once it is clear that the wound is healthy and uninfected, it is closed.

The development of pyrexia with erythema, pain and tenderness, around a closed appendicectomy wound is an indication to remove skin sutures to allow free drainage.

*Intraperitoneal abscesses* can occur at any site in the peritoneal cavity following perforation of the appendix. An abscess is especially common in the pelvis. This may take some days to develop, when there is swinging pyrexia with tachycardia, deep seated pelvic pain, and diarrhoea. A tender boggy mass is palpable rectally and may discharge pus spontaneously. Surgical drainage may be required if the patient becomes increasingly toxic or the mass becomes palpable suprapubically. At this stage the abscess can usually be drained through the rectum.

*Post-appendicectomy fistula.* Leakage from the appendix stump rarely follows an uncomplicated appendicectomy. It may cause spreading peritonitis when reoperation is urgently indicated. Alternatively it may discharge through the wound to form a chronic faecal fistula. This is likely to close spontaneously. If it persists one should suspect disease of the caecum, e.g. chronic inflammation (tuberculosis or actinomycosis), Crohn's disease or cancer.

*Intestinal obstruction* may follow laparotomy for acute appendicitis. If it occurs early in the post-operative period, conservative management with nasogastric secretion and intravenous fluids is justifiable, at least initially.

Obstruction later in the post-operative course usually requires operation.

## PROGNOSIS IN ACUTE APPENDICITIS

Uncomplicated appendicitis has an overall mortality of less than 0.1%. Gangrene and perforation increase both morbidity and mortality.

The very young and the very old are at particular risk, but in these as in all age groups, these dangerous complications can largely be avoided by earlier diagnosis and treatment.

## COMPLICATIONS OF ACUTE APPENDICITIS

The complications of appendicitis are avoided by prompt diagnosis and early appendicectomy (Fig. 29.10).

### Perforation

It is unusual for the appendix to perforate within 12 hours of onset of inflammation. Gangrene and perforation occur more rapidly in the elderly, and are hastened in all age groups by ill-advised use of aperients or enemas in the early stages of the

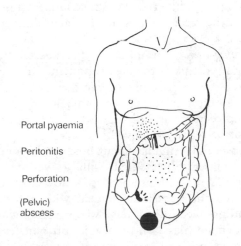

Portal pyaemia

Peritonitis

Perforation

(Pelvic) abscess

**Fig. 29.10** Complications of acute appendicitis (portal pyaemia is now *very* rare)

disease. Pain sometimes eases *temporarily* after perforation, but diffuse pain and tenderness with increasing pyrexia, tachycardia and clinical deterioration follow.

*Management.* Prompt appendicectomy is essential to prevent further spread of infection and deterioration in the general condition. Pre-operative resuscitation may be needed in some cases and must be vigorous so that further delay is avoided. A nasogastric tube is inserted, intravenous fluids are commenced, and systemic antibiotics (metronidazole and gentamicin) are administered. The technique of appendicectomy remains identical to that described for uncomplicated appendicitis. It is particularly important to take a swab for bacteriological culture, to avoid leaving portions of necrotic appendix behind, and to use lavage to aspirate all infected free fluid and pus from the peritoneal cavity. Many surgeons drain the peritoneal cavity after removing a perforated appendix, and all take precautions to reduce the incidence of wound infection (see above).

### Appendix abscess formation

The development of an abscess usually is associated with increasing pyrexia, pain and the presence of a mass. The general condition remains good. The mass is tender and when situated in the right iliac fossa, it is palpable on abdominal examination. A pelvic abscess produces few abdominal signs but is detectable as a tender swelling on digital rectal examination. An abscess behind the caecum or terminal ileum is difficult to detect.

*Management.* Drainage of the abscess with appendicectomy is the best treatment. Great care is taken not to disseminate infection by unnecessary mobilisation. Drainage with delayed interval appendicectomy is practised when the appendix cannot be readily removed.

Conservative management used to be popular when patients presented with a well-defined abdominal mass. This approach is now only practised for the occasional patient with a history extending over several days who presents with a well-defined mass, an otherwise soft non-tender abdomen and no evidence of toxaemia. The patient is confined to bed, given parenteral fluids,

and nothing by mouth. Progress is monitored by regular recording of vital signs and twice daily measurement of the mass.

The aim is to allow inflammation to settle and to permit easy interval appendicectomy. Conservative treatment is abandoned if the mass increases in size, the general condition deteriorates, or there is evidence of dissemination of infection. Under these circumstances adequate drainage is the main object of surgery but the appendix is removed whenever possible. Conservative treatment is inadvisable in young children, the elderly, and pregnant women.

### Portal pyaemia

This is now rare. Suppurative thrombo-phlebitis of the portal vein produces recurring chills, drenching sweats, high swinging pyrexia, and icterus and there are multiple hepatic abscesses. Gas within the portal system is produced by anaerobic organisms, and may be detected radiologically.

*Management.* Vigorous antibiotic treatment plus appendectomy offers the only hope of survival.

## CHRONIC APPENDICITIS

It is conceivable that some cases of intermittent 'grumbling' pain in the right iliac fossa are due to recurring bouts of low-grade appendicitis. The condition remains something of a diagnostic scapegoat, but such patients may be cured of their symptoms by elective appendicectomy. This should be advised only when other investigations prove negative.

## TUMOURS OF THE APPENDIX

### Carcinoid

The appendix is the commonest site of a carcinoid tumour of the gastro-intestinal tract which arises from the argentaffin cells (APUD cells). A carcinoid accounts for 85% of appendix neoplasms;

and is found in 0.5% of removed appendices. It forms a sub-mucosal tumour of distinct yellow colour usually near to the tip of the appendix. Most are benign in nature and an incidental finding at appendicectomy. A malignant carcinoid tumour may infiltrate through the muscle wall, spread to the meso-appendix and metastasise to regional lymph nodes. Liver metastases are very rare; the carcinoid syndrome virtually unknown.

Treatment is by appendicectomy although, if the tumour is large (>2.0 cm), involves the caecal wall or is associated with lymph node involvement, a right hemicolectomy may be necessary.

## Adenocarcinoma

An adenocarcinoma of the appendix is a highly malignant form of colonic neoplasm, doubtless because of its rapid spread to regional lymph nodes. It presents with development of acute appendicitis or an appendix abscess.

Right hemicolectomy is indicated.

# 30. The Large Intestine

## SURGICAL ANATOMY

The large intestine extends from the ileocaecal valve to the anorectal junction. Embryologically it is derived from the distal part of the midgut, the entire hindgut, and portions of the cloaca. It is supplied by branches of the superior and inferior mesenteric artery (Fig. 30.1). The rectum receives an additional supply from branches of the median sacral artery, and middle and inferior rectal branches of the internal iliac artery.

The *ileocaecal valve* is on the medial wall of the caecum. It has two pouting lips and functions as a one-way valve preventing reflux of caecal content into the terminal ileum.

The *caecum* is a blind pouch in the right iliac fossa which overlies the iliacus and psoas muscles and the femoral nerve. It is covered by peritoneum on both sides and anterior surface. However, a peritoneal reflection may also cover the posterior surface creating a retrocaecal space. The *appendix* opens at the base of the caecum in the embryo, but due to differential rates of growth of the caecal wall, it comes to open on the posteromedial wall in the adult.

The *ascending colon* extends upwards from the ileocaecal valve for approximately 15 cm to the *hepatic flexure*. It is covered by peritoneum on its anterior and lateral surfaces and lies lateral to the right ureter. The hepatic flexure usually overlies the lower pole of the right kidney. The *transverse colon* is suspended by mesentery and is approximately 45 cm long. The antimesenteric surface is attached to the greater omentum. The descending colon passes from the *splenic flexure* to the pelvic brim, is covered by peritoneum on its anterior and lateral surfaces, and lies lateral to the left ureter. The superior mesenteric artery supplies the colon almost as far as the splenic flexure, while the distal colon is supplied from the inferior mesenteric artery.

The *sigmoid colon* varies greatly in length, but is usually less than 50 cm. Like the transverse colon, the sigmoid is invested by peritoneum on all sides and has a mesentery. This sigmoid mesocolon forms an inverted V attached to the pelvic brim overlying the left ureter as it crosses the bifurcation of the left common iliac artery.

The *rectum* commences as the colon loses its mesentery. It is approximately 15 cm long and passes downwards in the hollow of the sacrum to end at the anorectal junction. The upper third of the rectum is covered on the front and on both sides by peritoneum, the middle third is peritonealised only in front, and the lower third lies beneath the peritoneal floor of the pelvis. The posterior aspect of the rectum is bound loosely to the sacrum by a condensation of connective tissue, (the fascia of Waldeyer) behind which lies the pelvic plexus of autonomic nerves. Laterally the rectum is attached to the side walls of the pelvis by lateral ligaments which contain the middle rectal arteries.

The wall of the large bowel consists of an outer longitudinal layer and inner circular layer of smooth muscle. In the colon, the longitudinal muscle is condensed into three bands (taeniae) which lie anterior, posteromedial and posterolateral and which meet at the base of the appendix. Over the rectum these bands coalesce to form a continuous investment of longitudinal muscle. The inner circular layer is continuous throughout, but is thickened in the anorectal canal to

*mesentry.*

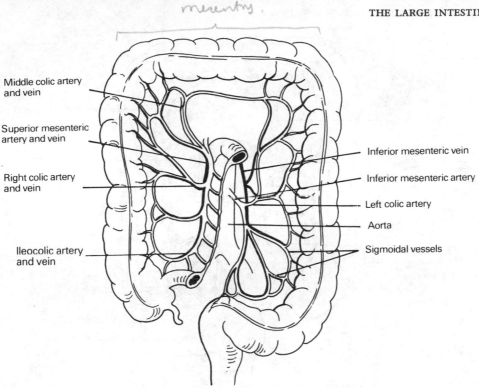

Middle colic artery and vein

Superior mesenteric artery and vein

Right colic artery and vein

Ileocolic artery and vein

Inferior mesenteric vein

Inferior mesenteric artery

Left colic artery

Aorta

Sigmoidal vessels

**Fig. 30.1** The blood supply of the large intestine

form the internal sphincter. The *appendices epi-ploica* are small pedunculated fat pads attached to the bowel wall between the taeniae.

The *mucosa* consists of columnar epithelium with crypts passing down to muscularis mucosa, and numerous goblet cells which secrete mucus. Beneath the muscularis mucosa is a submucosa of fibrous connective tissue. The arteries supplying the large bowel anastomose in the mesentery close to the bowel to form a continuous *marginal artery*, from which vessels pass to encircle the bowel. These circumferential arteries give off numerous small branches which pierce the muscle coat (Fig. 30.2). The mucosal protrusions of diverticular disease lie immediately adjacent to the points of vessel penetration. The venous drainage of the large bowel accompanies the arterial supply.

*Lymph* drains from the colon to epicolic nodes in the bowel wall, and then to paracolic nodes between the marginal artery and the bowel (Fig. 30.3). Lymph then drains to intermediate nodes on the main vessels, and to principal nodes alongside the origin of the superior and inferior mesen-

teric vessels. Lymph from the rectum drains upwards to superior and inferior mesenteric nodes, or laterally along the middle rectal vessels

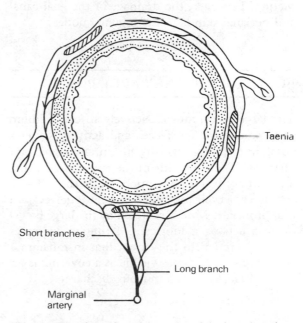

Taenia

Short branches

Long branch

Marginal artery

**Fig. 30.2** The circumferential arteries of the large bowel

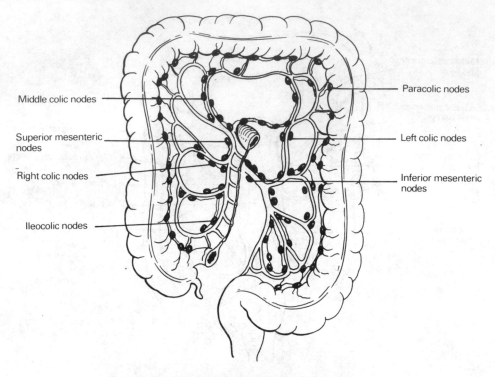

**Fig. 30.3** Lymphatic drainage of large gut

to the internal iliac nodes. Downward spread to inguinal lymph nodes is exceptional from the rectum. However, the drainage of the anal canal and perianal skin is to the inguinal nodes.

## FUNCTION OF THE LARGE BOWEL

The large bowel mucosa actively absorbs sodium and water from the faeces and actively secretes potassium, though usually not in any significant quantity. The right side of the large bowel is the main site of water absorption, while the left side acts as a reservoir for solid faeces until defaecation is appropriate. Mucus secreted by the large bowel mucosa acts as a lubricant. Irritation increases mucus secretion to the extent that in inflammatory disease it becomes visible as a covering layer on solid faeces or as a mucous discharge.

## INVESTIGATION OF LARGE BOWEL DISEASE

### Presentation

Diseases of the large bowel may present with abdominal pain, alteration in bowel habit (which may consist of constipation, diarrhoea or alternating bouts of each) and the passage of blood or mucus *per rectum*. Abdominal pain may be accompanied by nausea. In patients with obstruction it is often associated with abdominal distension and later, vomiting. Weight loss, malaise and anaemia are important non-specific symptoms. A detailed case history is combined with a thorough physical examination. Examination of the abdomen may reveal distension, an obvious mass or visible peristalsis. The caecum is often palpable in thin subjects and the descending colon and sigmoid colon may be palpable when loaded with faeces. The lower two-thirds of the rectum is palpable on rectal examination. Other parts of the large bowel are not normally palpable.

Differentiation between faeces and solid tumour may be difficult. Faeces can sometimes be indented by the examining fingers, whereas a solid tumour can not. Impacted faeces often constitute a large part of the palpable mass in patients with obstructing large bowel cancer. Abdominal auscultation will determine the presence and quality of bowel sounds, and may detect arterial bruits.

Hepatomegaly may be due to hepatic metastases in cancer patients.

Digital rectal examination is mandatory. Seventy-five per cent of rectal carcinomas and up to a third of all colonic carcinomas can be felt rectally. The finding of an empty rectum in a patient with palpable faecal masses in the pelvic colon raises the suspicion of recto-sigmoid obstruction. A tumour in this region may more readily be palpated through the rectal wall if the patient turns onto his *right* side.

The withdrawn finger is always inspected to determine the colour of faeces and detect blood or mucus. A specimen of faeces is tested for the presence of occult blood if blood staining is not obvious.

### Investigation

*Proctoscopy and sigmoidoscopy* are undertaken routinely when large bowel pathology is suspected or when there is a history of bleeding *per rectum*. The sigmoidoscope can usually be passed painlessly up to the level of the recto-sigmoid flexure without special preparation and allows visualisation of the whole of the rectum at the patients' first attendance. A small diameter short instrument (20 cm) is preferred by some. To examine the sigmoid colon the flexible sigmoidoscope may now be used but meticulous bowel preparation is required. A rectal biopsy taken by punch forceps is painless and furnishes material for histological diagnosis.

*Barium enema* is the routine method for detecting gross abnormalities in the bowel lumen. *Double contrast barium enema* allows better mucosal definition in detection of polyps and ulcers. Gas or air is insufflated into the bowel as the second contrast medium. Barium enema should not be carried out within 5 days of rectal biopsy so as to avoid perforation of the bowel at the weakened

biopsy site. As the rectum is not easily visualised by a barium enema, sigmoidoscopy is complementary.

*Fibreoptic colonoscopy* is used to observe and biopsy specific areas of any part of the large bowel. Polyps can be removed by diathermy snare.

*Examination of the stool* by direct microscopy is used to detect parasites and their ova, and culture is used to isolate bacteria. *Clostridium difficile*, one of the causal agents of pseudomembranous colitis or its toxin, may also be detected.

## PRINCIPLES OF LARGE BOWEL SURGERY

Certain principles of pre-operative preparation and management are common to all operations on the large intestine. These may have to be modified if operation is required urgently.

### PRE-OPERATIVE PREPARATION

#### Patient counselling

The type of operation to be undertaken must be discussed as fully as possible with the patient. Particular efforts must be made to explain the need for a temporary or permanent artificial stoma. If a stoma is planned, the site is chosen pre-operatively by trial-fitting of an appliance. A stoma-care nurse is invaluable in pre-operative preparation and subsequent care, and a visit from a member of a local Ileostomy or Colostomy Association can provide valuable reassurance.

#### Nutritional status

Patients with inflammatory or malignant disease of the large bowel are often malnourished and anaemic. Anaemia is readily corrected by transfusion, but malnourishment may take weeks to correct by high calorie-high protein diet. The dangers of delaying operation have to be balanced against the potential benefits of improved nutritional status. In such patients the timing of surgery requires experienced clinical judgement.

## Bowel preparation

The risks and dangers of anastomotic leakage and wound sepsis are reduced if the large bowel is empty at the time of resection. Antimicrobial prophylaxis is of secondary value.

*Mechanical bowel preparation.* The large bowel can be emptied by a combination of purgatives and enemas during the 2–3 days prior to operation. Mannitol 100 g in 1000 ml can be used as an osmotic aperient.

Alternatively, the bowel can be emptied by whole gut irrigation on the day before operation. A nasogastric tube is inserted and 2–4 litres of balanced crystalloid fluid are instilled each hour until the effluent from the anus is clear. A padded commode or flush-toilet is an advantage (Fig. 30.4). Metoclopramide (10 mg IM) and frusemide (20 mg IM) are given on commencement to accelerate gastric emptying and reduce the risk of pulmonary oedema. This technique is contra-indicated in patients with known cardiac or renal disease, and in those with obstructing lesions.

*Low residue diet.* Some surgeons place patients on an elemental low residue diet such as Vivonex or Flexical for 5 days before elective bowel surgery. A large bowel enema is given on the day before operation. Elemental diets are absorbed entirely in the small bowel and reduce bacterial density in the large bowel. Their unpleasant taste may be hidden by flavouring, or they can be given through a nasogastric tube.

*Antibiotic prophylaxis.* Mechanical cleansing of the large bowel is usually combined with attempts to reduce the density of bacteria. A 5-day oral course of non-absorbable sulphonamide in combination with a final 48-hour course of neomycin or kanamycin was the standard method to reduce the bacterial flora. These regimes do not reduce the number of anaerobic organisms (notably *bacteroides*), and it is now customary to include metronidazole (Flagyl) in pre-operative antibiotic prophylaxis.

The use of oral antibiotics in prophylaxis is associated with an increased incidence of post-operative enterocolitis due to overgrowth of resistant organisms. Many surgeons now prefer to use antibiotics parenterally, commencing a 24-hour course with administration of the premedication. A cephelosporin plus metronidazole 500 mg are administered intravenously each 8 hours for three doses, the first being given at the time of induction of anaesthesia. Although expensive, such regimes reduce the incidence of post-operative infection without the risk of enterocolitis.

Metronidazole may also be given, less expensively, by suppository.

## Urinary tract preparation

Ureteric damage is one of the hazards of large bowel surgery and large bowel cancer may invade and obstruct the ureter. An excretion urogram should be carried out before elective operation to detect ureteric obstruction and confirm the presence of two functioning kidneys. A decision at operation to sacrifice an involved ureter and kidney can then be made on rational grounds.

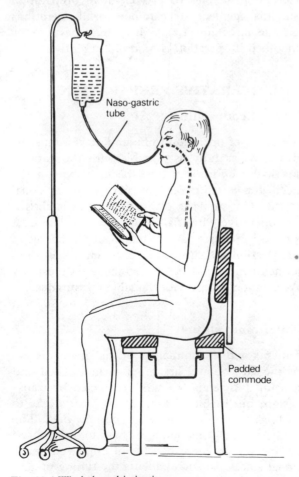

Naso-gastric tube

Padded commode

**Fig. 30.4** Whole bowel irrigation

A urinary catheter is inserted prior to operation to ensure that the bladder does not impede access to the pelvis. Post-operatively the catheter is left in place to prevent urinary retention. Measurement of hourly urine output provides a valuable guide to fluid replacement.

## Emergency large bowel surgery

In patients presenting with obstruction, perforation, toxic dilatation or with massive bleeding from the large bowel, emergency surgery may be required. Adequate resuscitation is essential before anaesthesia. Fluid loss is not a major problem in large bowel obstruction until late, but perforation results in escape of fluid into the peritoneal cavity and associated ileus results in fluid loss into the lumen of the small bowel. In such cases fluid replacement is essential using 0.9% saline with added potassium to replace crystalloid loss. Loss

from massive bleeding is best replaced by blood, although colloids or plasma can be used until blood becomes available (Chapter 9).

Severe bleeding from the large bowel is difficult to localise. If time permits, mesenteric arteriography may localise the source. Otherwise one may have to rely on per-operative colonoscopy to inspect the bowel lumen. This has significant morbidity and may not define the source of bleeding, and many surgeons prefer to perform subtotal colectomy.

## OPERATIVE TECHNIQUE

The extent of resection in both elective and emergency surgery is governed by the arterial blood supply and disease process. In malignant disease, it is essential to remove as much of the draining lymphatic system as possible (Fig. 30.5)

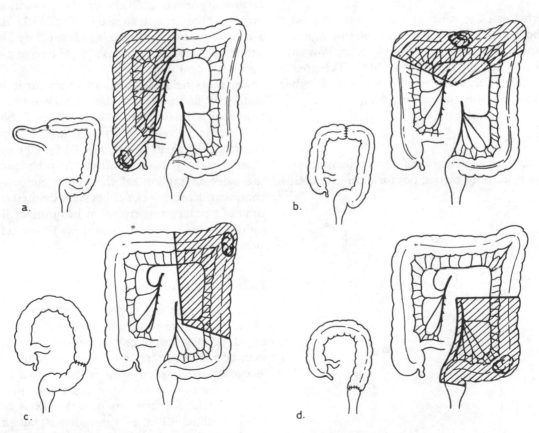

**Fig. 30.5** Principles of surgery in malignant disease of the large bowel. (a) Right hemicolectomy. (b) Transverse colectomy. (c) Left hemicolectomy. (d) Sigmoid colectomy.

and division of peritoneal attachments allows adequate mobilisation of the bowel on its mesentery. Preliminary high ligation of the main vessels supplying the involved segment is desirable to prevent embolisation of tumour cells during handling of the bowel. Similarly, it is wise to place occluding tapes on either side of the growth to avoid luminal dissemination of tumour cells.

Anastomoses must be made without tension. Stapling may be used as an alternative to hand suture.

It is customary to place a soft tube drain down to colonic anastomoses so that any bowel content that may leak from the anastomosis can escape directly to the surface without contaminating the peritoneal cavity or abdominal wound. Leakage is usually manifest by the 5th post-operative day. Drains should be left *in situ* until at least that time.

## INTESTINAL STOMA

A permanent intestinal stoma is best sited on a line between the umbilicus and anterior superior iliac spine, sufficiently far from both to allow easy fixation of an appliance (Fig. 30.6). Temporary colostomies may have to be positioned at other sites to allow subsequent resection.

### Ileostomy

The most common reason for an ileostomy is procto-colectomy carried out for ulcerative colitis

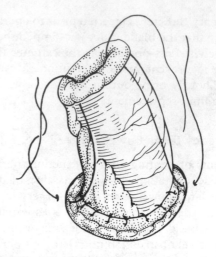

Fig. 30.7 Ileostomy being fashioned

or Crohn's disease. The stoma is fashioned so that a nipple of small bowel protrudes from the skin, facilitating direct delivery of the irritant small bowel content into an appliance (Fig. 30.7). Excoriation of surrounding skin is prevented by a well-fitting appliance and the use of protective agents such as karaya gum.

Conventional ileostomies are incontinent, but a continent ileostomy can be manufactured if a reservoir is made from a loop of small bowel, constructing a valve by artificial intussusception of a length of small bowel (Fig. 30.8). The pouch is emptied by passing a soft plastic tube through the valve to syphon off the pouch contents. A continent ileostomy can either be fashioned at the time of primary surgery or an incontinent ileostomy can be converted into a continent one at subsequent surgery.

### Colostomy (Fig. 30.9)

A *colostomy* may be (1) permanent after removal of the distal large bowel and rectum or (2) temporary following partial colonic resection when the intention is to restore intestinal continuity. If an anastomosis was performed at the time of resection, a temporary proximal colostomy may be used to deflate and defunction the distal bowel until healing of the anastomosis has been confirmed by subsequent radiological examination. This has particular application in resections

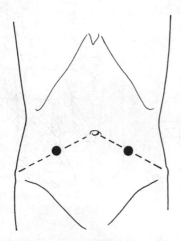

**Fig. 30.6** Sites for intestinal stomas

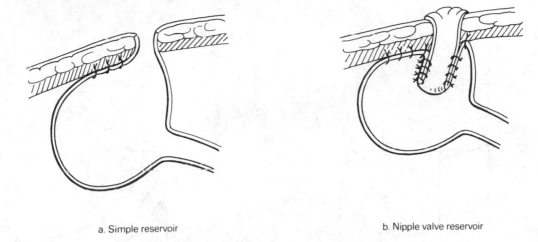

a. Simple reservoir                                    b. Nipple valve reservoir

**Fig. 30.8** Ileostomy with Kock's reservoir

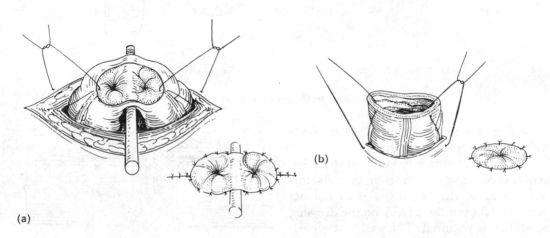

(a)

(b)

**Fig. 30.9** Colostomy. (a) Loop colostomy. (b) End colostomy.

of the rectosigmoid region when the anastomosis may be low down in the pelvis.

A *caecostomy* is used occasionally for temporary decompression of the large bowel. Either the caecum is brought up to the anterior abdominal wall and anastomosed to skin or more commonly, a tube is passed through the anterior abdominal wall into the lumen of the caecum (see p. 452). Caecostomy produces only limited decompression of the large bowel and does not completely divert the fluid faecal stream to the surface. Regular flushing of the tube caecostomy with water is needed to promote continued drainage of faeces.

*Care of colostomy.* Two methods are used to cope with a colostomy which forms an 'incontinent anus' on the abdominal wall (Fig. 30.10). Most commonly patients accept that spontaneous colon movements will occur, and catch the motions in a suitable colostomy bag. A series of disposable adherent appliances are available which can be kept in position for several days at a time and emptied when required. These are either manufactured in one piece, consisting of an adherent fenestrated patch incorporated in the back of a plastic bag; or in two pieces, these being an adherent moulded flange which has a groove onto which a bag can be fixed. An air vent is incorpo-

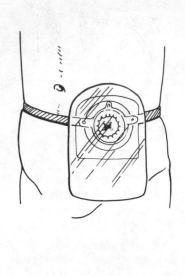

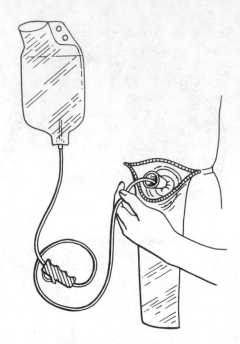

a. Spontaneous type of care          b. Wash out type of care

**Fig. 30.10** Care of colostomy

rated. Neither is perfect, and the skin surrounding the stoma is prone to irritation.

The alternative regime is to wash out the colon through the colostomy each 24 hours. As this empties the colon the colostomy does not act spontaneously during the day. A simple dressing is then all that is required. The wash out regime involves the patient in a fairly troublesome routine requiring the availability of a douch can, tubing and catheters. In this country it is generally advised only if a colostomy appliance proves unsatisfactory.

With both types of colostomy care, the patient will require to regulate his diet so that he can avoid those foods which are known to cause upset. Fruit, vegetables, beers and wines are particularly liable to cause looseness, and are avoided in other than small quantities. Certain specific items of diet, e.g. onions, spices, curries cause excess flatus and are also best avoided.

Attempts have been made to create continent colostomies by the implantation of a magnetic ring around the emerging bowel which holds in place a close-fitting plastic covered metal plug

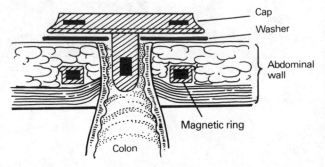

**Fig. 30.11** Continent colostomy

(Fig. 30.11). A carbon filter allows the escape of gas. This method has had varying success and is not in common use.

## COMPLICATIONS OF LARGE BOWEL SURGERY

### Shock

Unrecognised or undertreated pre-operative hypovolaemia will favour the development of hypovolaemic shock during operation. Most anaesthetic agents encourage peripheral pooling of blood and compound the problem. The splanchnic vascular bed is a 'low-priority area' in shock and, by impairing local blood flow, hypovolaemia may have a critical effect on anastomotic healing. Adequate pre-operative volume replacement is essential. *Septicaemic shock* is a potential consequence of spillage of bowel contents at operation. Spillage is more likely to occur in poorly prepared or obstructed patients. Lavage of the peritoneal cavity with saline is indicated. Treatment consists of crystalloid and colloid replacement, oxygen administration and systemic antibiotic therapy.

## Anastomotic leakage

Minor degrees of anastomotic leakage can be demonstrated radiologically from almost 50% of *distal* colonic anastomoses. In only 5% of patients are these leaks of clinical significance. Leakage may result in intra-abdominal collection of faecal material, septicaemia and shock. Treatment consists of surgical drainage after appropriate resuscitation, with formation of a defunctioning colostomy or exteriorisation of both ends of the leaking anastomosis. Anastomotic leaks can also give rise to a faecal fistula with escape of faeces along the drain track or through abdominal and perineal wounds. If there is no distal obstruction and the patient is otherwise well, the fistula may be treated conservatively in the expectation that it will close spontaneously. Closure is hastened by creation of a proximal diverting colostomy or institution of an elemental or parenteral diet to reduce fistula output and maintain adequate nutrition.

## Wound infection

Despite antibiotic prophylaxis, wound infection rates of 15% are common. Endogenous gut bacteria are almost always responsible. Infection delays healing, may cause secondary bleeding, and favours wound dehiscence and incisional hernia.

## Genito-urinary damage

The commonest post-operative urinary problem is retention of urine. This may be due to pre-existing prostatic disease in males or development of partial prolapse in females.

Damage to the parasympathetic nerves (nervi erigentes) as they pass through the pelvis results in loss of bladder motor activity, post-operative retention, and overflow incontinence. Following resection of the lower sigmoid colon or rectum a catheter should be left in the bladder for four or five days. If retention is evident on removal it should be replaced. If the prostate is not the seat of the trouble cystometric studies should be arranged. Prostatic enlargement may require transurethral resection whereas neurogenic bladder dysfunction can usually be managed by parasympathomimetic drugs and teaching the patient to empty the bladder by straining plus bladder neck resection on occasion.

The ureters may be damaged during mobilisation of the colon while the prostatic and membranous urethra may be damaged during excision of the ano-rectum.

After rectal excision, almost one-third of males become impotent due to division of the nervi erigentes. A further third are unable to ejaculate due to division of sympathetic nerves in the pelvic plexus. It is important that male patients are warned of these complications before consenting to this operation.

# DIVERTICULAR DISEASE

With the exception of solitary diverticula of the caecum (see p. 431) diverticula of the large bowel are rare before the age of 35 years. By the age of 65 years at least 30% of the general population are affected. There is a slight male preponderance.

The diverticula, of pulsion type, emerge between the mesenteric and antimesenteric taenia,  and are most common in the sigmoid colon (Fig. 30.12). They result from herniation of the large bowel mucosa through the circular muscle at the site of small penetrating blood vessels. Their wall consists of only mucosa and serosa.

Diverticular disease is associated with increased intraluminal pressure in the large bowel and with hypertrophy of both circular and longitudinal muscle layers. Muscle hypertrophy pre-

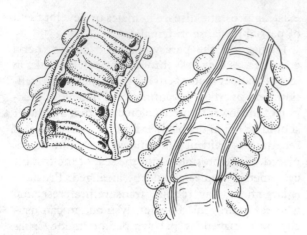

**Fig. 30.12** Diverticular disease

dates the development of diverticula and this 'prediverticular state' may be detected radiologically. In general, the disease is uncommon in those societies eating a high fibre diet.

## CLINICAL FEATURES OF UNCOMPLICATED DIVERTICULAR DISEASE

Diverticular disease may be asymptomatic or may produce central or left iliac fossa pain, alteration in bowel habit and occasional bleeding from the rectum. The diagnosis is confirmed by a barium enema which shows evidence of muscle thickening and multiple diverticula.

### Medical treatment

Medical treatment consists of a high fibre diet (with added bran or hydrophilic colloids) and antispasmodics (e.g. propantheline bromide 15 mg qds) if spasm is thought to be a major feature. Codeine phosphate (30 mg) occasionally may be necessary to control diarrhoea.

### Elective surgery

Elective surgery is indicated only if the patient experiences repeated attacks of acute diverticular disease despite a high-residue and bulk laxative therapy. Sigmoid colectomy is usually performed

with immediate end-to-end anastomosis to restore intestinal continuity. A temporary loop colostomy can be used to protect the anastomosis if bowel preparation has been inadequate.

Sigmoid myotomy was proposed as an alternative to sigmoid colectomy in the elective surgery of diverticular disease. The circular muscle of the affected segment was divided to reduce intraluminal pressure (Fig. 30.13). The myotomy was made longitudinally through one of the antimesenteric taenia until mucosa bulged through the incision. Good results were reported initially but the operation may be complicated by leakage and has not become popular.

## COMPLICATIONS OF DIVERTICULAR DISEASE

### Inflammation

Patients with diverticular disease may develop peri-diverticulitis due to inflammation of a diverticulum and spread of infecion through its wall. This results in severe localised abdominal pain, nausea, vomiting, pyrexia and leucocytosis. There is evidence of local peritonitis with tenderness and guarding in the left iliac fossa. Treatment consists of bed rest, intravenous fluids, and antibiotics. The condition usually settles on this regime after a few days. If not, one should suspect the development of a pericolic abscess, which may become palpable and require drainage. Forty per cent of patients have no further attacks following resolution of inflammation and less than 10% eventually require some form of surgery.

### Perforation

Diffuse peritonitis may complicate peri-diverticulitis from rupture of a pericolic abscess. The peritoneal contents are then purulent. Alternatively faecal peritonitis may occur from free perforation of the colon at the site of a diverticulum, a complication associated with a 50% mortality rate.

Treatment consists of emergency resection of the affected segment of bowel. Immediate anastomosis of the large intestine is usually contraindicated and both ends of the cut bowel are

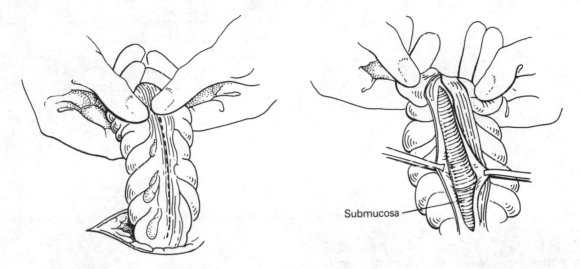

**Fig. 30.13** Sigmoid myotomy

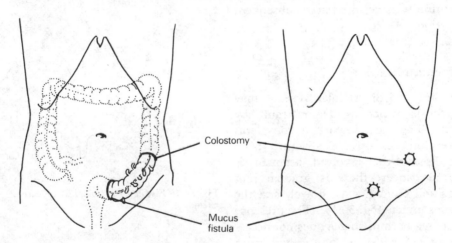

**Fig. 30.14** Principles of resection for perforated diverticular disease

exteriorised to await restoration of intestinal continuity under elective circumstances (Fig. 30.14). Alternatively only the proximal end is exteriorised as a colostomy and the distal end is closed and allowed to drop back into the abdomen (Hartmann's procedure). Continuity is restored at a later date. The peritoneal cavity should be irrigated before closure with 2.5% noxythiolin in saline, tetracycline in saline, or saline alone.

## Obstruction

An acute attack of diverticular disease may present with intestinal obstruction. This may be due to oedema or fibrosis of the large bowel, or to small bowel loops adhering to the inflamed colon. At operation it may be difficult to differentiate the lesion from carcinoma of the colon, and the true diagnosis may not be apparent until histology is available following resection.

In the first instance the obstruction is overcome by fashioning a temporary proximal loop colostomy. Resection of the affected segment of bowel with end-to-end anastomosis is carried out at a second elective operation, and colostomy closure is deferred for a further 4–6 weeks to allow anastomotic healing. Experienced surgeons may be able to avoid this three-step approach by a

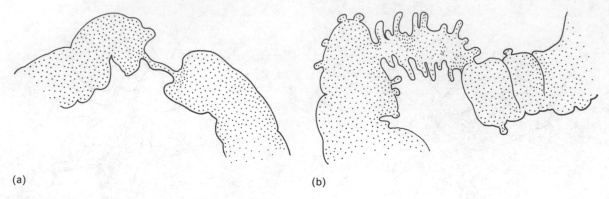

(a)                                                      (b)

**Fig. 30.15** The radiological appearances on barium enema of (a) a carcinoma; (b) diverticular disease of the sigmoid colon

two-stage procedure; the affected segment of colon is resected at emergency operation and intestinal continuity is restored at a subsequent elective operation.

## Stricture formation

Recurrent attacks of diverticular disease may result in stenosis which is demonstrable by barium enema. The most important consideration is to exclude cancer; in stricture from diverticular disease the involved segment is longer than in cancer, there is gradual (not abrupt) transition from normal bowel, and the mucosa remains intact (Fig. 30.15). The presence of diverticula on a barium enema does not necessarily indicate that stenosis is due to diverticular disease. Cancer and diverticular disease frequently co-exist as both conditions are common in older patients.

## Fistula

Diverticular disease may give rise to fistulae between the sigmoid colon and bladder, small bowel or vagina (Fig. 30.16). The disease is the commonest cause of a colovesical fistula, a complication commoner in males than females, in whom the uterus is interposed between the sigmoid colon and bladder

The patient usually gives a history of intractable cystitis with pneumaturia or the passage of faeces per urethram. The diagnosis is confirmed

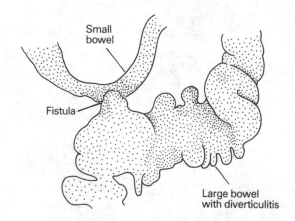

**Fig. 30.16** Fistula — radiological appearance on barium enema

by barium enema or cystography. The fistula is treated surgically. After removal of the affected bowel the bladder usually closes spontaneously if adequate urinary drainage is provided temporarily with a urinary catheter.

## Bleeding

Until recently it was believed that massive rectal bleeding was most likely to be due to diverticular disease. Angiographic investigations have now shown that in two-thirds of such cases the bleeding is due to other causes. Even if diverticula are known to be present in the sigmoid colon it is equally likely that the bleeding has arisen from another lesion. Angiomatous malformations, polyps and diverticula of the right colon are likely causes.

Pre-operative angiography is now advisable in all cases of massive rectal bleeding so that the lesion can be localised and then resected. If no lesion is seen and bleeding continues, 'blind' total colectomy with ileorectal anastomosis is advised.

## DIVERTICULUM OF THE CAECUM

A solitary diverticulum of the caecum is a congenital lesion. It arises from the medial wall of the caecum close to the ileocaecal junction and may extend upwards retroperitoneally. If obstructed by a faecolith it may become acutely inflamed, producing a clinical syndrome similar to acute appendicitis. Repeated attacks of inflammation may lead to fibrosis of the diverticulum leaving a residual ulcer (solitary ulcer) of the caecal mucosa. The condition is often difficult to distinguish from carcinoma at operation but right hemicolectomy is required in either case.

## ULCERATIVE COLITIS

This disease, the aetiology of which is unknown, has an incidence of five new cases per 100 000 population per annum. It most commonly affects adolescents and young adults, particularly women (male:female ratio, 1:1.5). Although more common in first degree relatives, 90% of cases have no family history.

It is primarily a disease of the large bowel. Systemic manifestations (iritis, arthritis, hepatitis, pyoderma gagrenosum) are described but these disappear completely when all of the affected bowel has been removed. In 95% of cases ulcerative colitis is a diffuse disease, starting in the rectum and extending proximally for a variable length. The whole of the colon may become involved, and so-called 'backwash' through the ileocaecal valve can cause ileitis. In 5% the disease is segmental and the rectum is spared. Because of the frequency of rectal involvement, sigmoidoscopy is the key to diagnosis.

The characteristic histological feature is the formation of crypt abscesses in the depths of the glandular tubules with a surrounding inflammatory infiltrate. The abscesses coalesce to form ulcers which undermine the mucosa and penetrate as far as the muscularis mucosa. The intervening mucosa becomes oedematous and swollen and, in severe cases, forms inflammatory pseudo-polyps. The bowel wall loses its haustrations, and becomes thickened and rigid due to muscle hypertrophy. During an acute attack the bowel may become paper-thin and grossly dilated — so called *toxic megacolon* or *toxic dilatation*. This complication is believed to be due to destruction of the myenteric nerve plexus.

Other complications include perforation, massive bleeding, anorectal suppuration, and carcinoma of the colon. These are considered further below.

### Clinical features

Ulcerative colitis usually presents with attacks of diarrhoea and the passage of blood and mucus per rectum. With extensive disease these symptoms are severe, the patient passing up to 10–15 motions daily. Urgency to defaecate can be incapacitating. Severe attacks may be associated with abdominal pain, tenderness and pyrexia.

Most attacks are mild and patients with rectal bleeding may present to the surgeon with a request to assess and treat haemorrhoids. The importance of sigmoidoscopy in the assessment of such patients cannot be overemphasised. Rectal examination should include careful inspection for the anal complications of fissure and fistula. The rectal mucosa may feel thickened and boggy. On sigmoidoscopy the mucosa is red, matt and granular with punctate haemorrhages or spontaneous bleeding. Contact bleeding, produced by gently rubbing the mucosa with a gauze pledget, is a typical feature.

Plain films of the abdomen are of value in the acute attack. Pseudopolyps may be seen in the gas-filled colon, strongly supporting the diagnosis, and averting the need for barium enema at this stage. Attention may be alerted to the possibility of developing toxic dilatation, and in such patients, daily plain films should be taken to monitor progress, and give a much more accurate assessment than measurements of abdominal girth.

A barium enema is of value in assessing the extent of the disease but is contra-indicated in the acute phase because of the danger of perforation. Typical changes include loss of haustration and reduction in the calibre of the bowel, irregular fluffy outline of the mucosa, pseudopolyps and rarely strictures (Fig. 30.17). Widening of the retrorectal space is a regular feature of chronic disease. The disease must be differentiated from amoebic colitis, Crohn's disease and, in the elderly, ischaemic colitis.

The course of ulcerative colitis is almost invariably one of relapse and remission but a chronic continuous form of the disease is also described. In some patients the initial attack is fulminating, and toxic dilatation of the colon with exacerbation of systemic and abdominal symptoms may occur at any time.

## Management

The initial treatment of an attack of ulcerative colitis is medical. With fluid replacement, correction of anaemia, adequate nutrition and steroid therapy, 97% of patients survive their initial attack but 70% are destined to have further attacks. Sulphasalazine (0.5–1 g 6-hourly) given orally as maintenance therapy reduces the incidence of relapse. Local steroid therapy, using suppositories or prednisone retention enemas, will usually control mild attacks, but systemic steroids (prednisone 10–15 mg given orally 6-hourly) are used when there is an acute relapse.

Some 15% of patients eventually require surgery, which may be elective or emergency. It has been calculated that 1:50 patients with proctitis, 1:20 with moderate colitis and 1:3 with extensive disease will come to surgery.

## Indications for elective surgery

*Failure to thrive* despite adequate medical management. This is reflected in retardation of growth and sexual development in children, and by malnourishment and anaemia in adults.

*Anorectal complications.* These occur in almost 20% of cases and include recurrent abscesses and fistulae. They usually remit following removal of the affected colon.

*Benign strictures.* These occur in less than 10% of cases; half are found in the rectum. The stricture is due to submucosal fibrosis and causes acute or subacute obstruction. Strictures are more common in Crohn's disease and that diagnosis must be considered. Carcinoma must also be excluded. Colonoscopy may be useful in clarifying the diagnosis when the stricture is outwith the reach of the sigmoidoscope.

*Polyp formation.* Severe polyp formation with the typical 'sea-wrack' appearance indicates that the bowel is likely to be permanently and severely involved.

*Carcinoma.* The risk of developing carcinoma of the large bowel is greatly increased by ulcerative colitis. At least 10% of patients who have had colitis for 10 years and 20% who have had it 20 years develop this complication. Malignant change is more likely in patients with extensive disease and those with early onset colitis. The average age of development of cancer in colitis patients is 43 years, compared with 63 years in the general population.

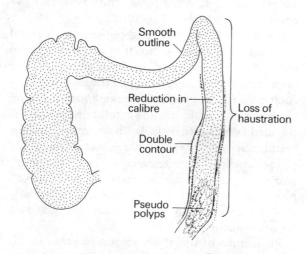

**Fig. 30.17** Ulcerative colitis — radiological appearance on barium enema

The detection of malignant change is difficult as the symptoms remain those of colitis. Patients with long-standing disease should be screened annually by sigmoidoscopy and biopsy of any suspicious lesion, and by regular barium enemas to detect development of stenotic areas.

*Systemic complications.* A variety of systemic complications occur in ulcerative colitis. These include erythema nodosum, pyoderma granulosum, eye lesions, hepatitis and cirrhosis of the liver, sclerosing cholangitis, and ankylosing spondylitis. Provided permanent changes have not occurred, removal of the colon leads to resolution.

## Nature of elective surgery

Elective cases are prepared as outlined (p. 422) except that mechanical bowel cleansing with enemas is usually avoided. The operation of choice is to remove the large bowel including the rectum (panproctocolectomy) and create an ileostomy. Great care is taken to protect the parasympathetic and sympathetic nerves in the sacral plexus by dissecting as close as possible to the rectum. In the rare cases shown to have only segmental disease on barium enema and a histologically normal rectum, the rectum may be left *in situ* and an ileorectal anastomosis performed. However, even in such cases it is safer to perform an ileostomy and bring the proximal end of the rectal stump to the surface as a mucous fistula. If subsequent sigmoidoscopy shows no evidence of continuing rectal disease, an ileorectal anastomosis can be used to restore continuity and continence. Sigmoidoscopy is still carried out regularly to check that the rectal stump does not become involved.

If surgery is undertaken in patients with malignant change, the resection should be more extensive in that regional lymph nodes are also removed.

## Indications for urgent and emergency surgery

*Acute fulminating ulcerative colitis.* This refers to a florid initial attack during which there is marked deterioration in the patient's symptoms associated

**Table 30.1** Oxford regime for acute fulminating colitis and/or toxic megacolon

| |
|---|
| Prednisolone sodium phosphate 40–60 mg daily in divided doses |
| Tetracycline 1.0 g daily in divided doses |
| Hydrocortisone sodium succinate 100 mg t.i.d. by rectal drip for 5 days |

with pyrexia and toxaemia. Medical treatment should always be used first (Table 30.1); but if aggressive therapy fails to control the disease or there is no significant improvement within 5 days, urgent surgery is indicated.

*Toxic megacolon.* Acute dilatation of the colon affects 5% of patients with ulcerative colitis. It may occur during any attack and is associated with abdominal distension, local or diffuse tenderness, feeble or absent bowel sounds and cramping abdominal pain. A plain X-ray shows dilatation of the colon, usually most evident in the transverse colon.

Treatment is initially medical with intensive steroid therapy (Table 30.1) and is usually followed by improvement. Should colonic dilatation persist or should there be any suspicion of peritonitis operation is urgent. Metronidazole has recently been used in treatment.

*Perforation.* This complication also occurs in 5% of patients. It is most commonly associated with toxic dilatation of the colon, complicating one third of such cases. Perforation is notoriously difficult to diagnose but should be suspected when there is rapid deterioration on medical treatment. Abdominal pain and guarding may be present. Free gas on a plain abdominal X-ray is diagnostic. Surgery is indicated should suspicion of perforation arise.

*Massive bleeding.* This is a rare indication for emergency surgery.

**Technique.** Emergency total proctocolectomy carries a high operative mortality (20%). It is usual to leave the rectal stump as a mucous fistula, and remove it subsequently should active disease persist. In severely ill patients with toxic megacolon a double-barrelled ileostomy may be made, allowing diversion of the faecal stream and irrigation of the colon with steroids.

# CROHN'S DISEASE OF COLON

Originally believed to affect the terminal ileum predominantly, it is now recognised that Crohn's disease can occur in any part of the gastro-intestinal tract. Both small and large bowel are affected in half the cases and in a further quarter the large bowel alone is affected. The large bowel is usually affected segmentally, with thickening of the bowel wall and fissuring of the mucosa to produce a cobblestone appearance.

Histologically the most reliable feature is the occurrence of granulomas, although these are not invariable. In 50% of cases the rectum is involved by the disease and 70% of these patients have anal lesions. Fistula-in-ano, abscesses and fissures are commoner in Crohn's disease than in ulcerative colitis. Anal ulceration appears to be specific for Crohn's disease with rectal involvement. There is evidence that carcinoma is more frequent in a colon affected by Crohn's disease.

## Clinical features

The clinical features of Crohn's disease are similar to those of ulcerative colitis. However, diarrhoea is usually less severe, abdominal pain is more common, and tenderness, an abdominal mass or internal or external fistulas are more frequent. If the rectum is involved, sigmoidoscopy may reveal the typical cobblestone appearance or patchy ulceration. On barium enema the lesions may be separated by normal bowel — 'skip lesions' — and show irregularity of the mucosa, rigidity of the bowel and fine radiating spikes due to fissuring. Internal fistulae are common in Crohn's disease.

As in half of all cases the small bowel is also affected, a small bowel enema or barium meal and follow-through examination should also be carried out. Rectal biopsy may not be diagnostic and biopsy during colonoscopy is helpful in assessing the extent of the disease.

Although less common than in ulcerative colitis, toxic dilatation is a recognised complication of Crohn's disease.

## Medical treatment

All efforts are made to correct anaemia and malnourishment. There are no specific therapeutic agents available for the treatment of Crohn's disease. Recent controlled trials confirm that the response of active symptomatic disease to prednisone (20–60 mg daily by mouth) or sulphasalazine (3–4 g daily by mouth) is significantly better than to placebo. In general, patients with large bowel Crohn's disease are especially liable to respond to sulphasalazine (the compound is metabolised by colonic bacteria to its active principles sulphapyridine and 5-aminosalicylate), whereas those with small bowel disease are more liable to respond to steroids. Combination of the two drugs does not appear to confer benefit, and neither agent is capable of preventing relapse or recurrence once the disease has become quiescent or has been treated surgically.

## Indications for surgery

*Failure to thrive*. In some cases chronic ill-health with intractable symptoms demands operation. In others a severe exacerbation of the disease may fail to respond to medical treatment, and surgery offers the only hope of inducing remission. The incidence of cancer in the colon affected by Crohn's disease is not sufficiently high to merit surgery as a prophylactic measure.

*Obstruction*. This is due to cicatricial stenosis. It usually develops insidiously, presenting as subacute or intermittent obstruction.

*Perforation*. Perforation occurs in about 20% of patients with large bowel Crohn's disease, but preceding fibrosis and adhesions limit spread and result in a walled-off abscess, the patient presenting with swinging temperature, toxaemia, local tenderness, and sometimes a palpable mass. Free perforation of the colon resulting in faecal peritonitis is rare, but an abscess may secondarily rupture into the peritoneal cavity to produce purulent peritonitis.

Alternatively, an abscess may perforate into a neighbouring viscus to form an internal fistula. The presence of fistula between loops of intestine is almost diagnostic of Crohn's disease and sudden development of diarrhoea strongly suggests such fistula formation.

While an abscess may resolve with antibiotic therapy, surgical drainage may be required. This results in an entero-cutaneous fistula unless the affected segment of bowel is also resected.

*Fistula.* Formation of a fistula, either enterocutaneous or entero-enteral, occurs in 20% of patients with small and large bowel Crohn's disease and in 10% of those with large bowel disease alone.

Most fistulas eventually require surgery. Preoperative parenteral nutrition is a valuable means of restoring nutritional status before surgery. Patients with colonic fistula can be fed an elemental diet that is completely absorbed in the upper gastro-intestinal tract. The management of colovesical fistula has been discussed on page 430. Early surgery is indicated to avoid urinary tract infection and impairment of renal function.

## Nature of surgery in Crohn's disease

The main principle of the surgical treatment of Crohn's disease is conservation. In elective cases affected bowel is excised with a margin of a few cm of normal bowel at each end, and continuity is restored by an anastomosis. If there is any doubt about the safety of an anastomosis, the ends of the bowel should be exteriorised.

The surgical treatment of Crohn's disease of the colon is similar to that of ulcerative colitis except that the ileum is more commonly resected and the rectum spared. Ileorectal anastomosis has a high incidence of breakdown and leakage, and it may be advisable to perform a temporary ileostomy. In patients with obstruction, ileostomy is advised.

Should only a small segment of colon be involved it may be reasonable to resect this locally, with a margin of approximately 10 cm of normal bowel. A primary anastomosis may be performed, but if there is any doubt about involvement of the ends by the disease, they are better exteriorised. Bowel which has perforated or fistulated must be excised. The extent of the resection depends on the site and the extent of involvement.

It was believed that in resecting Crohn's lesions, it was important to get beyond the involved bowel so that normal bowel was anastomosed. This is no longer the case. Conservation of all normal looking bowel is now preferred.

## PSEUDOMEMBRANOUS COLITIS

This condition was once believed to be due to superinfection of the bowel with staphylococci, but now it is apparent that *Clostridium difficile* is more commonly the organism responsible.

Pseudomembranous colitis is associated with the use of oral antibiotics, particularly clindamycin and lincomycin. There is necrosis of the mucous membrane of the colon associated with profuse watery diarrhoea, toxaemia, shock and collapse. The stools are watery green, foul-smelling, often blood-stained and contain fragments of pseudomembrane (mucosal sloughs). The pseudomembrane is usually evident on sigmoidoscopy and has characterstic histological features. The diagnosis is confirmed by the demonstration of *Cl.difficile* or its toxin in the stool or pseudomembrane obtained by rectal biopsy. Treatment consists of intravenous fluid replacement and vancomycin. Both staphylococci and clostridia are sensitive to vancomycin.

## OTHER INFLAMMATORY CONDITIONS OF THE LARGE BOWEL

## HYPERTROPHIC TUBERCULOUS COLITIS

This condition is rare except in the tropics and Asia. The wall of the colon becomes thickened due to granulomatous infiltration, fibrosis and caseation. Stricturing may occur and the mucosa may appear cobblestoned and ulcerated (Fig. 30.18).

The patient presents with abdominal pain, alteration in bowel habit and occasional passage of blood and mucus. A mass may be palpable in the right iliac fossa. The disease must be differentiated from Crohn's disease and from carcinoma. The treatment of choice is antituberculous chemotherapy, but resection is often the only way of excluding carcinoma. Antituberculous chemo-

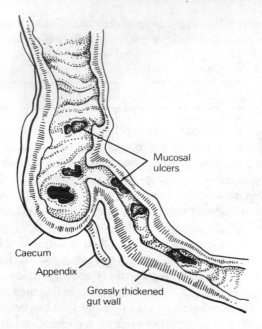

Mucosal ulcers

Caecum

Appendix

Grossly thickened gut wall

**Fig. 30.18** Hypertrophic ileocaecal tuberculosis

therapy is commenced if tuberculosis is confirmed histologically.

Infection of the large bowel by *Schistosomiasis mansoni* (bilharzia), *Entamoeba histolytica* and *Lymphogranuloma venereum* all result in inflammation which may progress to stricture formation and require surgical resection.

## IRRADIATION PROCTITIS

External and internal radiation for the treatment of cancer of the cervix or bladder can result in proctocolitis. An acute granular proctitis occurs as an early reaction and can lead to delayed ulceration, stricture formation and a recto-vaginal fistula. Loose stools, tenesmus, urgency, pain and bleeding are typical clinical features.

On sigmoidoscopy the changes are most prominent on the anterior wall of the rectum and may be confined to this area. In early cases topical steroids may give symptomatic relief, but resection of the rectum may be indicated if stricture or fistula formation have occurred. More commonly colostomy is preferred.

## VOLVULUS

Volvulus denotes rotation of a loop of bowel and its mesentery around a fixed point. It results in closed loop obstruction of the rotated loop and also obstruction of the proximal bowel. The circulation to the involved loop is impaired, and strangulation with gangrene may follow. The sigmoid colon is the commonest part of the intestinal tract to be affected by volvulus but unusual mobility of the right colon may allow volvulus of the caecum and terminal ileum.

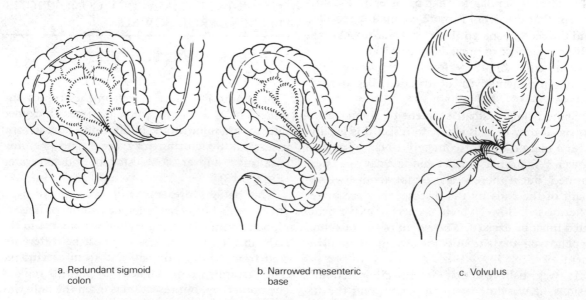

a. Redundant sigmoid colon

b. Narrowed mesenteric base

c. Volvulus

**Fig. 30.19** Sigmoid volvulus

Sigmoid volvulus is common because of the proximity of the limbs of the sigmoid loop at their point of fixation to the pelvic brim, and because of the solid and relatively heavy contents of this part of the gut. The condition is particularly common in countries where diets rich in roughage are consumed, e.g. Africa, Eastern Europe, Russia. The bowel usually rotates in an anti-clockwise direction (Fig. 30.19).

The patient presents with symptoms of large bowel obstruction, i.e. colicky pain, constipation and distension. Distension is asymmetrical and the outline of the distended colon may be visible. A plain X-ray shows a grossly distended sigmoid loop rising out of the pelvis to occupy the whole of the abdominal cavity. Multiple fluid levels may also be present in the distended proximal large and small bowel.

Deflation of the twisted sigmoid colon is attempted by sigmoidoscopy and passage of a soft, well-lubricated rectal tube. Successful passage of the tube through the twist results in rapid decompression. The tube is left in situ for 48 hours, and is gently irrigated to prevent its blockage.

If the tube cannot be passed or if there are signs suggesting strangulation, laparotomy is performed. If the loop is necrotic it is resected and the ends of the colon are exteriorised for later reconstruction. If the bowel is not strangulated, the decision to resect depends on the general condition of the patient. Guiding the rectal tube into the distended loop may be all that is required in patients unfit for more major surgery.

As volvulus of the sigmoid colon has a 40% recurrence rate, definitive treatment by *elective* sigmoid colectomy should be performed wherever possible.

## MEGACOLON

### HIRSCHSPRUNG'S DISEASE

This congenital condition affects 1 in 5000 babies. The disease is due to an absence of ganglion cells in Auerbach's and Meissner's plexus of the large bowel so that there is loss of peristalsis in the affected segment. Usually, the distal large bowel is affected over a short segment of 5–20 cm, but occasionally longer segments and even the whole large bowel may be involved. Bowel proximal to the affected segment becomes grossly distended.

Hirschsprung's disease may present as neonatal large bowel obstruction which must be differentiated from meconium ileus. Digital examination of the rectum may result in initial apparent 'cure', but the condition recurs either immediately or later in childhood and causes constipation with gross gaseous distension. Ischaemic colitis may complicate the disease and must be differentiated from ulcerative colitis.

In the child, Hirschsprung's disease must be differentiated from chronic constipation (Fig. 30.20). Barium enema which is performed without preparation shows a dilated segment above the narrowed aganglionic distal segment. Histological confirmation and assessment of the limit of the abnormal area can be made by a full thickness mucosal biopsy. It should be noted that ganglia are normally absent for about 1.5 cm above the anal verge.

In neonates, treatment consists of saline irrigation of the bowel followed by an operation designed to bring ganglionated bowel down to the anal verge. This is carried out at about the age of 6 weeks. In older children presenting with obstruction, a preliminary colostomy is carried out followed by definitive operation some three months later.

## ACQUIRED MEGACOLON

Chronic constipation in childhood may result in *acquired megacolon* and *megarectum*. The initial complaint may be of faecal soiling. On abdominal examination, the large bowel is full of palpable faeces and on rectal examination faeces are present in a dilated rectum. Although it may be associated with enuresis, psychological or psychiatric upset, chronic constipation is more commonly the result of bad toilet training or the presence of an anal fissure.

The aim of treatment is to maintain an empty large bowel and rectum so that normal muscular tone can be regained. This requires faecal disimpaction under general anaesthesia and regular colonic washouts.

Megacolon due to neurotoxicity may complicate vincristine therapy.

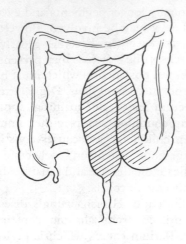

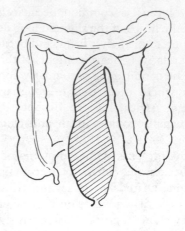

a. Hirschsprung's Disease

b. Acquired megacolon

**Fig. 30.20** Megacolon

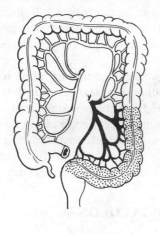

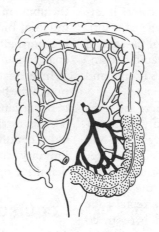

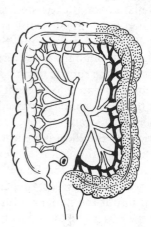

a. Operative division
   of main vessel

b. Spontaneous occlusion
   by embolus or thrombus
   of main vessel

c. Occlusion of small
   mesenteric vessels

**Fig. 30.21** Causes of ischaemic colitis

## ISCHAEMIC COLITIS

Impairment of the vascular supply to the large intestine occurs as a result of division of its main vessels (Fig. 30.21). This occurs with:

1. Operative division of its main feeding vessels, e.g. of the inferior mesenteric artery during resection of an abdominal aortic aneurysm or the middle colic artery during resection of the stomach or pancreas.

2. Spontaneous occlusion of a main artery by atherosclerosis or embolic disease.

3. Occlusion, of the small mesenteric vessels due to distal arterial disease or to an episode of hypotension with associated diminished perfusion.

Provided the arterial system is healthy, occlusion of one main vessel is unlikely to have any untoward effects. However, should the circulation already be compromised by atherosclerosis, ischaemic changes may occur. These may be either permanent or transient.

If permanent, the large bowel becomes gangrenous and this will lead to perforation and peritonitis, necessitating urgent operation.

Transient ischaemia results in abdominal pain, diarrhoea and bleeding. Sigmoidoscopy may show friable, oedematous and granular mucosa starting above the level reached by the rectal blood supply, i.e. 12–15 cm from the anal verge.

Alternatively, barium enema will demonstrate a narrowed segment with an irregular contour, sacculation and 'thumb-printing' due to polypoidal change in the mucosa. This is most commonly situated at the junction between superior and inferior mesenteric blood supplies close to the splenic flexure (Fig. 30.22).

These changes usually resolve on supportive treatment but may proceed to the formation of a fibrous stricture, which may cause delayed obstruction and require resection.

## POLYPS

Polyps of the large intestine are common and take several forms. They may be inflammatory (as in ulcerative colitis), hamartomatous (as in Peutz-Jeghers syndrome) or neoplastic (adenomas or papillomas). While single polyps do occur, most are multiple.

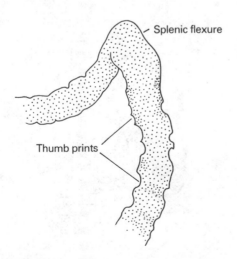

**Fig. 30.22** Ischaemic colitis — radiological appearance on barium enema

### JUVENILE POLYPS

These hamartomas are found in children usually under the age of 10 years and are usually single. They are most common in the rectum and sigmoid colon. The polyps are pedunculated, consisting of a vascular core with an inflammatory cell infiltrate and covered by normal mucosa. Symptoms arise because of bleeding due to torsion of the pedicle or surface trauma, and because of prolapse of the polyp through the anus. The polyps should be removed by snaring and dividing the pedicle at colonoscopy. Recurrence occurs in 10% but there is no risk of malignancy.

### PEUTZ-JEGHER SYNDROME

This is a congenital abnormality characterised by brown or blue pigmented spots on the lip, buccal mucosa, fingers and toes, and multiple hamartomatous polyps mainly in the small bowel, but throughout the whole of the gastrointestinal tract. The polyps may be sessile or pedunculated, and the abnormal muscularis mucosa forms a tree-like structure covered by normal epithelium. As the polyps are not true neoplasms, there is no potential for malignant change. They may cause symptoms through bleeding or intussusception, and local resection may then be required.

### ADENOMATOUS POLYPS

These are true neoplasms, accounting for 90% of neoplastic polyps of the colon. They vary from small sessile seed-like excrescences to large pedunculated masses several centimetres in diameter. They are most commonly pedunculated. Histologically they are formed by a mass of glandular tubules fed by a central fibrovascular core and covered by mucous membrane showing varying degrees of differentiation. In approximately one-third of cases the polyps are multiple. Their distribution is similar to that of carcinoma: 80% are found in the sigmoid colon or rectum (Fig. 30.23).

It is estimated that adenomatous polyps are present in the colon of at least 5% of the normal population. Most are symptomless, but rectal bleeding, intussusception and prolapse through

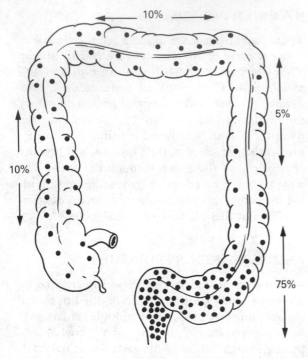

**Fig. 30.23** Distribution of polyps in the large bowel

the anus occur. Over one-third of polyps can be seen at sigmoidoscopy. Double-contrast barium enema will reveal others, provided they are over 0.5 cm in size. Colonoscopy is used both for diagnosis and to remove the polyp by diathermy snare.

The risk of malignant change is proportional to polyp size. Polyps over 1 cm in diameter have a 5% incidence of malignancy; in those less than 1 cm the frequency of carcinoma is less than 1%. Thus all polyps over 1 cm in size should be removed. Histological examination includes a search for malignant change and for invasion of the stalk. Polyp formation signals that the mucosa is liable to develop further polyps or carcinoma and patients must be followed by regular double contrast barium enema or colonoscopy for the rest of their lives.

In view of the distribution of adenomatous polyps and their propensity for malignant change, it has been suggested that most cases of carcinoma of the colon develop from pre-existing polyps. Satellite polyps are present in one-third of cases of carcinoma of the large bowel. It is for this reason that, in some cancer centres, colonoscopy with prophylactic removal of polyps is performed on asymptomatic patients.

## VILLOUS ADENOMA

This tumour accounts for 10% of neoplastic polyps of the large bowel. It is most commonly found in the rectum and sigmoid colon and only rarely affects the caecum and ascending colon. It forms a soft shaggy sessile growth which spreads to involve a considerable area of mucosa (Fig. 30.24). The central connective tissue core bears numerous frond-like branches covered with colonic mucosa. It is generally accepted that this is a pre-malignant lesion; invasive cancer is found in at least 30% of cases.

Rectal bleeding is a late symptom and suggests malignant change. Typically there is excessive mucus secretion and a troublesome mucous discharge. Some patients present with dehydration, hypokalaemia, weakness, oliguria and alkalosis due to excess loss of mucus. If in the rectum, the villous adenoma will be palpable and is seen through the sigmoidoscope as a coarsely granular or shaggy plum-coloured area of mucosa. Areas of induration should raise the suspicion of malignant change. Villous adenomas of the colon are diagnosed by barium enema and colonoscopy. Biopsy is undertaken to confirm the diagnosis, but a report of benign tumour does not exclude cancer as malignant change is usually focal. For this reason all villous adenomas should be excised.

Rectal adenomas can be removed through the anus surgically or with diathermy provided they

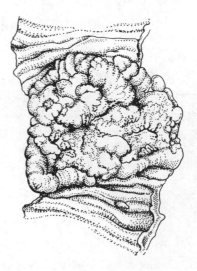

**Fig. 30.24** Villous adenoma

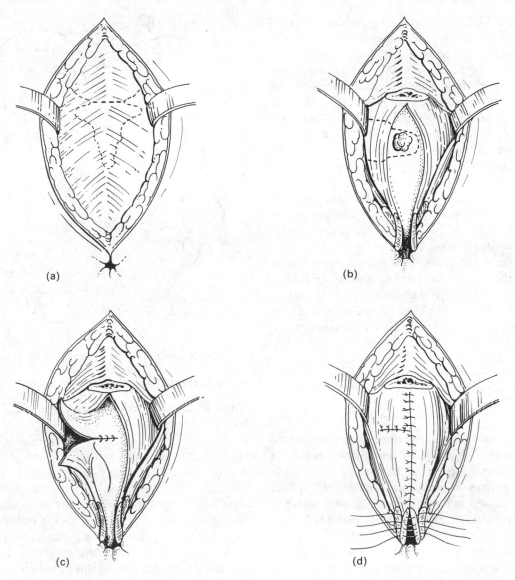

**Fig. 30.25** Posterior approach to the rectum (York-Mason). (a) Exposure. (b) Anal sphincters divided (dotted line shows extent of tumour excision). (c) Defect in rectal wall closed. (d) Individual layers of sphincter mechanism carefully rejoined.

are not too large. For large tumours, a formal posterior approach to the rectum is required; the rectal wall is split and the tumour is excised with surrounding mucosa (Fig. 30.25). The finding of invasive cancer is an indication for formal resection of the affected portion of bowel.

## FAMILIAL POLYPOSIS

This rare hereditary disease is transmitted by an autosomal dominant gene. Thus males and fe-

males are at equal risk, and the chances are that half the children of a given family will be affected. The genetic abnormality is always expressed, so that the disease is transmitted only by those who suffer from it. Sessile and pedunculated adenomas develop during childhood in the large bowel. There may be a few scattered lesions or many hundreds of adenomas. The rectum is almost always involved. Symptoms usually develop between the ages of 10–15 years, and consist principally of rectal bleeding, diarrhoea and mucus discharge. Malignant change is inevitable in individuals who develop polyposis but is virtually unknown before the age of 20 years.

Familial polyposis is treated by total colectomy. At one time most surgeons also removed the rectum and established an ileostomy, but the current trend is to preserve the rectum and perform an ileorectal anastomosis. The rectum is freed from polyps by diathermy, and kept under permanent surveillance by sigmoidoscopy as the risk of malignancy remains. It is essential to examine all other members of the family so that those with polyposis can be treated before cancer supervenes. The ideal time for operation is around school-leaving age.

Gardner's syndrome is a related condition in which sebaceous cysts, dermoid cysts, bony exostosis and connective tissue tumours are found in association with multiple adenomatosis. It accounts for only one in every ten cases of familial polyposis.

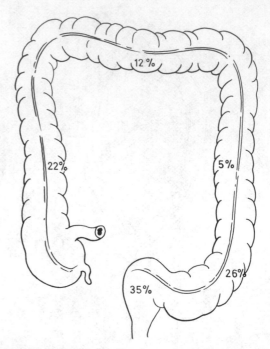

**Fig. 30.26** Cancer of the colon — pattern of distribution

## CARCINOMA OF THE COLON AND RECTUM

Carcinoma of the colon and rectum is second only to lung cancer as a cause of death from cancer in Western society. Scotland has one of the highest incidence rates of colorectal cancer. Within its population of 5 million there are 39 new cases per 100 000 persons per year and 1800 deaths each year.

It is predominantly a disease of older people and is uncommon before the age of 40, though the young are not immune. Overall, males and females have an equal chance of developing the disease. However, there is a sex difference in its distribution. Cancer of the rectum is more common in males while cancer of the colon is more common in females. This suggests that the aetiology of these two conditions is different.

Over 70% of large bowel cancer originates in the rectum and sigmoid colon, 10% occur in the caecum, and the remainder are distributed through the rest of the large bowel (Fig. 30.26). It is a multifocal disease; 3% of cases have synchronous tumours elsewhere while 1% of patients will develop a further tumour of the colon with each 10 years of follow-up.

## AETIOLOGY

Cancer of the large bowel is rare in Africa, in the Orient and in South America. Its incidence parallels that of coronary artery disease and breast cancer. Environmental factors are considered to be important. It is suggested that diets low in fibre and bulk are associated with a higher incidence of the disease. High dietary fibre increases the speed of intestinal transit and it follows that any carcinogen in the diet and faeces will be in contact with the mucosa for a shorter time. The high incidence of cancer of the sigmoid colon and rectum also supports the theory that a contact carcinogen is involved. Bile salts are also thought to be implicated and clostridia and coliform organisms with dehydrogenating activity can convert bile salts to carcinogenic sterols.

Other factors associated with large bowel cancer include ulcerative colitis, adenomatous polyps, familial polyposis and villous adenoma (see above).

## PATHOLOGY

Three gross types of tumour are described: polypoidal, ulcerating and infiltrating (Fig. 30.27).

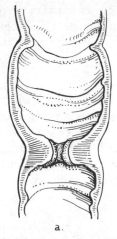 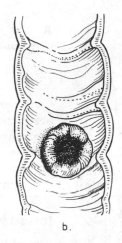 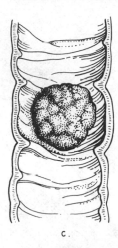

a.  b.  c.

**Fig. 30.27** Pathological types of large bowel cancer. (a) Stenosing. (b) Ulcerating. (c) Papilliferous.

Infiltrating tumours spread circumferentially to cause an annular 'napkin ring' or 'string' stricture. The lesions are adenocarcinomas derived from the columnar epithelium of the bowel and show a wide spectrum of differentiation. A small proportion have a colloid or gelatinous structure; these lesions tend to occur in younger patients and are associated with a poor prognosis.

The cancer may spread by following routes:

1. *Direct* spread occurs circumferentially and radially in the bowel wall. The muscle coats are penetrated and perforation may occur.

2. *Transperitoneal* spread occurs when tumour cells liberated into the peritoneal cavity form seedling deposits in the peritoneum.

3. *Lymphatic* spread leads to nodal involvement in 40% of all cases coming to operation. The affected nodes lie in the mesocolon and paraortic region.

4. *Blood stream* spread gives rise to overt liver metastases in 10–20% of patients at operation.

## Stages

Carcinoma of the large bowel can be classified into four categories by a modification of Dukes classification. These categories are:

A  Growth confined to bowel wall
B  Spread through bowel wall
C  Involvement of regional lymph nodes

$C_1$  Few nodes involved near primary growth but some glands in chain free from metastases below the ligature on the main regional vessels

$C_2$  Continuous string of nodes containing metastases right up to ligature on main regional vessels

D  Distant metastases

More intricate classifications have been developed, e.g. the TNM system, but these are not commonly used.

As might be expected, tumours of category A have the best prognosis. However, neither this classification nor the histological features provide an accurate prognosis for individual patients. Tumour resectability is also an important prognostic indicator and is determined by the degree of extension and local fixation.

## Clinical features

The key clinical features of carcinoma of the colon are alteration of bowel habit and bleeding from the rectum. The nature and degree of these complaints depends on the site of the tumour (Fig. 30.28).

*Right colon.* As the contents of the caecum and ascending colon are fluid, altered bowel function or obstructive symptoms are associated only with large tumours. In most patients, there is at most, mild diarrhoea. Chronic blood loss, although

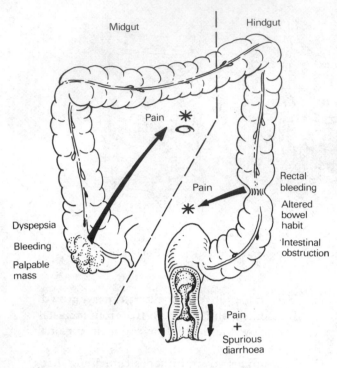

**Fig. 30.28** Clinical features of the large bowel cancer

unrecognised by the patient, causes anaemia and there is deterioration in general health and loss of weight. Vague right iliac fossa pain may be present and a mass may be palpable.

*Left colon.* As the left colon is narrower and has more solid contents, obstruction is relatively common. Increasing constipation requiring progressively larger doses of aperients and alternating bouts of diarrhoea are characteristic. Distension, audible borborygmi and colicky pain are common, and blood and mucus are often passed per rectum. The patient may feel unwell and lose weight.

*Rectum.* Bleeding is a prominent feature of rectal carcinoma. The patient often believes that he has piles and it is only on complete examination that the cause of the bleeding is found to lie higher in the rectum. The presence of a tumour in the rectum causes persistent bowel symptoms. Classically these consist of early morning diarrhoea. This is spurious diarrhoea in that the patient experiences the desire to defaecate but passes only a little slime and blood. This may be repeated several times before a motion is passed and some relief obtained. Urgency, tenesmus and

a feeling of incomplete evacuation of the bowel are also common symptoms. The general health may remain good.

### Complications

Cancer of the colon may present with intestinal obstruction (20% of cases), perforation (10%), formation of entero-colic or vesico-colic fistula, or massive bleeding (rare). Although chronic bleeding from a carcinoma is the rule, serious and life-threatening haemorrhage rarely occurs.

### Investigation

Almost half the patients will have a palpable mass on presentation, either on abdominal or rectal examination. One-third of colorectal cancers lie within reach of a finger on rectal examination. As half of all colorectal tumours lie in the rectum, sigmoidoscopy is an essential investigation in all patients who complain of altered bowel function or rectal bleeding, and is mandatory in patients who complain of piles.

Barium enema is complementary to sigmoidoscopy. The tumour is demonstrated as a short irregular filling defect with shouldering where it meets normal bowel. Even if a rectal cancer is discovered on direct examination it is important to perform a barium enema to exclude a second tumour situated more proximally.

Liver function tests, liver scan and chest X-ray are performed to exclude overt metastases. If the site of the growth is likely to be related to the ureter, an intravenous urogram is advisable.

All tumours within reach of the sigmoidoscope are biopsied. For others, a colonoscopic biopsy is performed if the diagnosis is in doubt.

### Treatment

Intra-abdominal spread and resectability can only be assessed adequately at laparotomy. This is required in all cases except those unfit for general anaesthesia in whom there is no obstruction. The operation performed depends on the site of the cancer. If in the caecum, ascending or transverse colon, a right hemicolectomy or extended right hemicolectomy with ileocolic anastomosis is carried out (Fig. 30.29). More distal colonic lesions

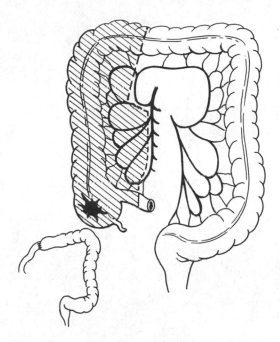

**Fig. 30.29** Right hemicolectomy

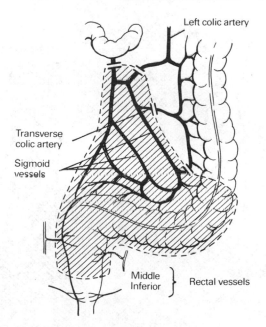

**Fig. 30.30** Anterior resection of rectum

are resected by left hemicolectomy or sigmoid colectomy, removing as much of the regional lymphatic supply as is practicable.

Cancers of the upper third of the rectum are treated by resection of the sigmoid colon and upper rectum with anastomosis between the colon and rectal stump. Carcinoma of the middle third of the rectum can usually be sufficiently mobilised to allow resection and a primary anastomosis between the proximal sigmoid colon and lower rectum (anterior resection) (Fig. 30.30). If the preparation of the bowel is inadequate or the integrity of the anastomosis is in doubt, a temporary proximal colostomy may be performed to minimise leakage.

Carcinomas of the lower third of the rectum are usually treated by a combined abdominal and perineal approach so that the rectum including the anal canal is completely removed (abdomino-perineal resection; Fig. 30.31). The pelvic colon is then brought to the surface as a permanent colostomy. In females the posterior vaginal wall may be removed with the rectum. In males, care must be taken not to damage the urethra or prostate. Damage to autonomic nerves in the presacral nerves or pelvic plexus is unavoidable in many cases.

At one time carcinomas lower than 12 cm from the anal verge were treated routinely by abdomino-perineal resection. The availability of stapling guns now allows an anastomosis even when the growth is as low as 7 cm from the anus. There may also be a place for the treatment of some well differentiated rectal cancers by local resection (see p. 441), diathermy or radiotherapy avoiding the need for either an extensive operation or permanent colostomy.

## MORBIDITY AND MORTALITY

The overall operative mortality in patients with large bowel cancer is around 10% but better results can be achieved in specialist centres. Elective procedures carry an overall operative mortality of 5% whereas the operative mortality of emergency surgery is 20%.

The overall 5-year survival rates for large bowel cancer barely reaches 25%. Approximately 50% of patients have resectable lesions and half of these patients will be alive 5 years after operation. Survival is related to the Dukes stage of the tumour, and varies from 80% at 5 years in those without lymph node involvement (Dukes A and B) to 30% in those with metastases in lymph nodes. If distant metastases are present, survival rarely exceeds 1–2 years.

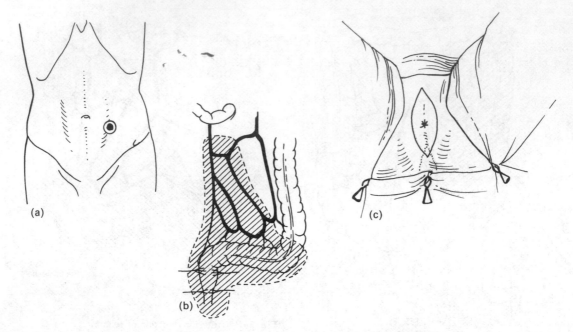

**Fig. 30.31** Abdomino-perineal resection of rectum. (a) Site for colostomy. (b) Extent of resection. (c) Perineal incision.

Pre- and post-operative radiotherapy have been employed in attempts to improve the results of surgery for rectal cancer, and the value of this approach is being assessed by controlled studies.

Radiation can also be used in the palliation of large bowel cancer. Chemotherapy, using 5-fluorouracil and nitrosoureas has proved to be disappointing, both in the treatment of advanced metastatic disease and as adjuvant systemic therapy in patients undergoing resection.

## PRESYMPTOMATIC DIAGNOSIS OF LARGE BOWEL CANCER

Improved survival rates have followed the increased public awareness of the potential significance of altered bowel habit and rectal bleeding. Measures used to detect the disease in asymptomatic patients are under study and include:

1. The use of the haemoccult test to detect occult blood in the faeces. The patient is given three cards impregnated with guaiac on which on successive mornings, they place a smear of faeces. The cards are posted to the laboratory where an oxidising agent is added, producing a blue colour if blood is present. Patients with positive tests are investigated further, initially to determine whether the tests are truly positive and thereafter by full sigmoidoscopic and barium examination of the colon. More specific and sensitive tests are under investigation.

2. In some American screening centres routine sigmoidoscopy, barium enema and colonoscopy are used to examine asymptomatic patients. Such investigations are costly, and not generally available.

3. Carcino-embryonic antigen (CEA) is found in most adenomas and large bowel carcinomas, and serum concentrations are raised in a proportion of patients presenting with large bowel cancer. However CEA has proved disappointing as a tumour marker for diagnostic purposes, being associated with high false positive rates. Serial estimates may be used to detect recurrence following apparently curative bowel resection.

# 31. Intestinal Obstruction

*[handwritten annotations:]*
- Level of obstruction.
- Rate of progression
- base of Pathology

Intestinal obstruction can be classified: (1) according to the level of obstruction of the gastro-intestinal tract (high or low small-bowel, colonic), (2) according to the rate of progression of the obstruction (acute, subacute, chronic or acute-on-chronic), or (3) on the basis of the pathological process responsible (intraluminal, mural, extra-mural).

It is important to differentiate causes which may impair the blood supply and cause strangulation from those which only cause simple occlusion of the lumen. Should strangulation of a segment of bowel occur, urgent surgical intervention is mandatory and the prognosis is more serious. For example, prompt operation on an inguinal hernia causing simple mechanical occlusion of the intestine carries little hazard to life. If operation is delayed and strangulation supervenes, significant mortality results.

It is important also to recognise that obstruction may be associated with perforation of the bowel wall in the absence of devascularisation from strangulation. This can be due to the causative lesion penetrating the bowel wall, or simply from over-distension of bowel proximal to the obstruction. Thus, obstruction of the colon from carcinoma may be complicated by perforation at the site of the tumour. Rupture of a grossly distended caecum can occur but is believed to have an ischaemic basis.

An obstruction may also affect both ends of a loop of bowel. In this event the contents of the loop cannot get out in either direction so that distension of the loop is rapid and the chances of strangulation much higher than in a simple obstruction. This is called 'closed loop' obstruction (Fig. 31.1). Examples are obstructed external or

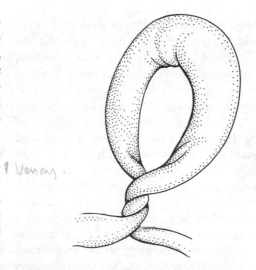

*[handwritten annotation:]* ↑ Venous.

**Fig. 31.1** Volvulus — an example of closed loop obstruction

internal hernia, volvulus of the small or large intestine, or a colonic obstruction in association with competence of the ileocaecal valve. In the latter event small gut material may continue to enter the loop but cannot leave it.

Several factors determine the frequency of the various causes of intestinal obstruction. Atresia of the bowel and other congenital defects are found mainly in infancy; hernias and adhesions occur at any age; carcinoma of the colon is a disease of the elderly. Geographic and racial factors are also determinants of cause. In Britain, approximately one third of intestinal obstructions are each due to hernias; to large bowel cancer and to bands and adhesions. Volvulus is a rare cause whereas in parts of Africa and Russia, sigmoid volvulus is common and second only to hernia as a cause of acute intestinal obstruction. Obstruction due to tuberculous disease is common only in developing countries and that due to amoebiasis in the Tropics.

# PATHOPHYSIOLOGY OF INTESTINAL OBSTRUCTION

## Simple mechanical obstruction

The bowel above the obstructing lesion becomes distended with fluid and gas and this stimulates excessive peristalsis and colic. The gas which accumulates is mainly swallowed air with a small and variable contribution from putrefaction within the bowel lumen. As distension increases, the blood vessels in the bowel wall become stretched and their diameter narrowed, so that blood flow is impaired. The mucosa is the first part of the bowel wall to show the effects of ischaemia, leading to a net excretion of water and electrolytes into the lumen, with depletion of extracellular fluid and hypovolaemia. Some of the ECF passing into the gut lumen will be lost by vomiting. Substantial 'hidden' losses are also inevitable as fluid accumulates in the gut. As a rough guide, a loss of 2 litres of ECF can be assumed prior to vomiting. With established vomiting and dehydration, the loss approximates 4 litres. If there is circulatory collapse with hypovolaemic shock, the deficit is of the order of 6 litres.

The fluid lost is isotonic with ECF but has a relatively high potassium concentration. If the obstruction is at or near the pylorus, there is a preponderant loss of acid and metabolic alkalosis develops. If the obstruction is lower in the intestine, the lost fluid is slightly alkaline and there is no significant acid-base imbalance unless there is gross hypokalaemia (metabolic alkalosis) or shock (metabolic acidosis).

In simple mechanical obstruction, shock occurs late and is due to progressive depletion of ECF. The patient becomes increasingly dehydrated with tachycardia, falling central venous pressure and hypotension. Hypoxia may occur and will be exacerbated by intestinal distension elevating the diaphragm and embarrassing ventilation.

Bacteraemia is not an important factor in the causation of shock associated with simple intestinal obstruction. Although there is an increase in luminal bacterial content, the peritoneal fluid remains sterile unless the bowel wall becomes ischaemic.

## Strangulation obstruction

The initial stage of strangulation is venous occlusion with the development of oedema in the bowel wall. Arterial blood continues to enter the bowel until prevented from doing so by increasing back pressure. The bowel then becomes infarcted. Losses of plasma and blood are substantial and usually overshadow such loss of ECF as is due to preceding mechanical obstruction. Blood and plasma losses are particularly marked in strangulated sigmoid volvulus when up to 70% of the blood volume can be sequestered in the infarcted segment. The development of shock is accelerated by bacteraemia. Bacteria and their toxins pass through the ischaemic bowel wall into the peritoneum and are absorbed into the blood stream.

# CLINICAL FEATURES OF INTESTINAL OBSTRUCTION

## Symptoms

*Abdominal colic* is the cardinal symptom of obstruction. Its distribution reflects the region of the gut which has been obstructed. With small bowel obstruction, the bouts of colic are felt in the centre of the abdomen around the umbilicus and become more frequent and more severe with time. Unlike acute peritonitis, when the patient is afraid to move for fear of exacerbating the pain, the patient with abdominal colic is restless and moves around during an attack. The development of steady and more localised pain associated with tenderness heralds the onset of strangulation and is an indication for urgent operation.

In large bowel obstruction the patient complains of vague lower abdominal pain with periodic exacerbations.

*Vomiting* occurs early in a 'high' intestinal obstruction but may be absent with low small-gut or colon obstructions. Initially, the vomitus contains food but later it becomes fluid and bilious and then brown in colour. This is due to the reflux of small bowel contents and not, as at one time believed, to the vomiting of faecal matter. As the obstructed small gut may be contaminated with faecal organisms, the smell of the vomitus can be offensive.

*Absolute constipation* is the rule with complete obstruction but this symptom may be late, particularly in high obstructions. Even in colonic obstruction, bowel movements or the passing of flatus may continue until the distal bowel is empty of faeces and gas. In low small-bowel or colon obstructions the patient may complain of increasing girth due to intestinal distension.

## Examination of the abdomen

Abdominal distension is described as a cardinal feature of intestinal obstruction. However it may be absent in a high obstruction. In a low small intestinal or colon obstruction visible loops of small intestine may form a 'ladder pattern' across the abdomen. Occasionally, peristalsis may be visible.

Ascites and gross obesity can confuse the picture but gaseous distension of the bowel gives a resonant note on percussion of the abdomen.

Auscultation during an attack of colic reveals a run of exaggerated bowel sounds. When the bowel becomes distended with fluid and gas, bowel sounds become high-pitched and tinkling.

Examination of the abdomen may reveal the cause of obstruction. An abdominal scar raises the possibility of adhesion obstruction or may indicate previous surgery for a disease which can cause recurrent obstruction (e.g. Crohn's disease). The hernial orifices must always be carefully examined. The danger of overlooking a small groin hernia, particularly a femoral hernia, cannot be over-emphasised. There may be little local pain or tenderness, central abdominal colic tends to focus attention away from the causal lesion and if the patient is obese, he or she may be unaware of its presence.

## Digital rectal examination

Digital rectal examination is essential. Faecal impaction is a frequent cause of obstruction in the elderly; and an obstructing cancer of the rectum may be palpable. A mass in the recto-vesical pouch suggests widespread abdominal neoplasia.

## Proctoscopy and sigmoidoscopy

Proctoscopy and sigmoidoscopy should be performed when large intestinal obstruction is suspected. In some cases of sigmoid volvulus, sigmoidoscopy may also allow relief of obstruction.

## Strangulation

Strangulation is notoriously difficult to detect clinically in its early stages. It can never be excluded confidently without laparotomy and, except in a few specific instances (see below), urgent surgical intervention is advised in all patients with mechanical intestinal obstruction. The development of severe constant localised pain with tenderness and guarding suggests local peritonitis due to strangulation. This suspicion is increased if the patient appears more ill than might be expected from the length of history, particularly when there is associated pallor or circulatory collapse.

## RADIOLOGY IN INTESTINAL OBSTRUCTION

Plain films of the abdomen will reveal gaseous distension of the bowel with 'fluid levels' in the erect or lateral decubitus views. Exceptions are high intestinal obstruction when little or no gas is seen other than in the stomach and a gastric fluid level may be detected.

The site of obstruction may be deduced from the plain abdominal film. Obstructed small bowel occupies the centre of the abdomen, has markings which extend across the whole diameter of the bowel (valvulae conniventes) and does not become as grossly distended as the colon. Obstructed large bowel occupies a peripheral position, has haustral indentations and may become grossly distended, particularly when the obstruction is of closed loop type. In some cases, the level at which obstruction has occurred, can be seen by a 'cut-off' in the pattern of gaseous distension.

## Contrast radiology

Contrast radiology is seldom indicated in acute intestinal obstruction unless there is doubt whether this is present. As undiluted barium can compound obstruction, only gastrografin or dilute (half strength) barium should be used. Barium must never be used when perforation is suspected.

# MANAGEMENT OF INTESTINAL OBSTRUCTION

Prompt diagnosis and operation are essential to reduce the risk of strangulation. Specific indications for conservative treatment of intestinal obstruction are given on pp 452 and 453.

## Resuscitation

It is essential to precede operation by adequate resuscitation. In the presence of strangulation it may be impossible to restore the circulatory state and fluid and electrolyte balance to normal and the benefits of delaying operation to allow resuscitation must be balanced against the risk of progressive circulatory impairment in the obstructed bowel. The decision when best to operate may thus be difficult.

## Principles of surgery

*Small bowel obstruction.* Extrinsic lesions, e.g. hernias, bands, adhesions, are the most common cause of small bowel obstruction. The constriction is divided. Lesions within the bowel wall are less common and require resection of the involved segment. Obstruction due to an intraluminal mass, e.g. a bolus of food, is rare. It is managed by milking the obturating agent into the large bowel if possible. Otherwise enterotomy is needed to remove the obstructing agent. A bypass operation is sometimes required to deal with an unremoveable obstruction (Fig. 31.2). Strangulated gut is blue-black in colour, lacking in sheen, papery in consistency and does not show peristalsis when flicked or squeezed. If it is suspected that the bowel is non-viable, warm moist packs should be applied to the bowel for 5 minutes. Failure to improve in appearance is an indication for resection.

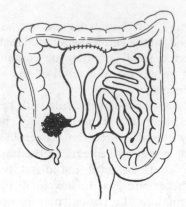

**Fig. 31.2** A bypass procedure (ileo-transverse anastomosis) for an irresectable lesion at the ileo-caecal junction

*Large bowel obstruction.* Obstructing lesions of the right side of the colon can usually be managed by right hemicolectomy with immediate ileo-colic anastomosis. Bypass without resection with an ileo-colic anastomosis may be considered as a palliative measure if the patient has non-resectable carcinoma. It may also be performed as a preliminary to later resection · if the patient's general condition is poor.

The management of obstructing lesions of the left side of the large bowel is more difficult. Emergency resection with immediate anastomosis carries a high risk of anastomotic leakage and is generally not advised. The classical three-stage approach is usually employed (Fig. 31.3). This consists of (1) an emergency transverse colostomy to relieve obstruction; (2) following preparation an elective resection of the affected segment of bowel is usually carried out some weeks later. The transverse colostomy is retained to divert the faecal stream until anastomotic healing has been confirmed by the installation of barium through the distal loop; (3) the transverse colostomy is closed, usually about 4–6 weeks after the second stage.

Several alternatives to this classical policy have been introduced to allow completion of the operative treatment in two stages (Fig. 31.4). These are:

1. The initial decompressing colostomy is placed close to the tumour so that at a second and final stage, radical resection can be performed which includes removal of the tumour and the colostomy with reconstitution by end-to-end anastomosis.

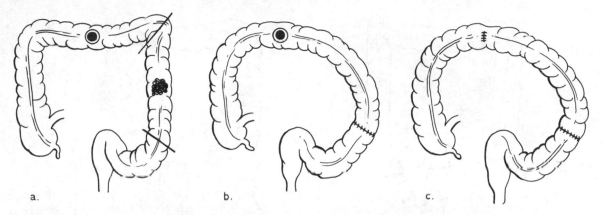

**Fig. 31.3** Three stage resection of large bowel. (a) Transverse colostomy (site of resection marked). (b) Following resection of diseased large bowel. (c) Following closure of colostomy.

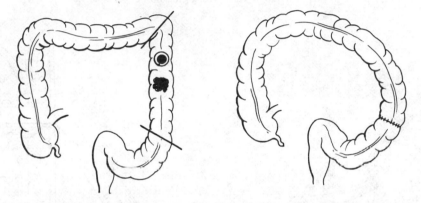

**Fig. 31.4** Two stage resection of large bowel, with defunctioning colostomy adjacent to lesion and subsequent resection and colostomy

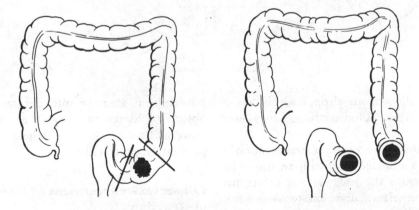

**Fig. 31.5** Resection of large bowel with exteriorisation of both ends

2. Resection of the segment of bowel containing the tumour at the initial operation with exteriorisation of proximal and distal ends of the bowel (Fig. 31.5). At a later, second operation continuity is restored.

3. The *Hartmann procedure* is a variation used when the tumour is in the lower pelvic colon or rectum. Following primary resection only the proximal cut end is brought to the surface as a colostomy, the distal limb of the bowel being

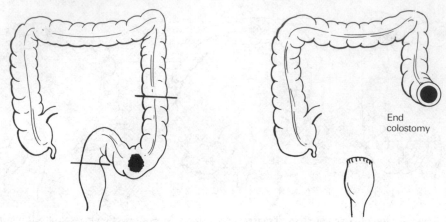

**Fig. 31.6** Resection of large bowel with end colostomy and oversewing of rectal stump — Hartmann's procedure

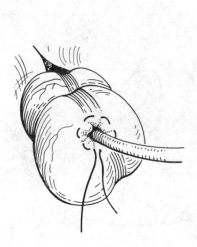

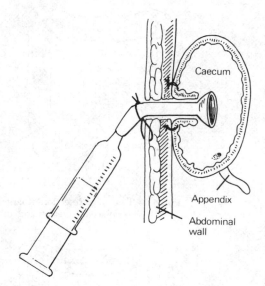

**Fig. 31.7** Caecostomy

oversewn and allowed to drop back into the abdomen (Fig. 31.6). Colon continuity may later be restored.

Resection is always necessary if strangulation is present. Right hemicolectomy with an ileo-colic anastomosis remains the procedure of choice for right-sided lesions. Immediate anastomosis is not recommended following resection of strangulated segments of the left colon or rectum and either both ends of the bowel should be exteriorised or a Hartmann's procedure performed.

Rarely, a patient with large bowel obstruction is unfit for laparotomy. A blind caecostomy may be performed under local anaesthesia. A large

bore tube is inserted into the caecum with the object of decompressing the proximal large bowel. The tube has to be irrigated at intervals to prevent blockage (Fig. 31.7).

## Conservative treatment of intestinal obstruction

Non-operative treatment of mechanical intestinal obstruction is indicated in the following circumstances.

*Adhesion obstruction.* If a patient has already undergone multiple operations for episodes of obstruction due to peritoneal adhesions, further surgery carries little prospect of long-term success and may be hazardous owing to inadvertent entry into the bowel lumen. Conservative treatment with fluid replacement and nasogastric suction is preferred but must be abandoned if there are signs suggesting strangulation or if obstruction persists.

*Widespread intra-abdominal malignancy.* If a patient is known to have carcinomatosis, intestinal obstruction is treated by operation only if the surgeon in consultation with the patient and relatives believes that this is in the patient's best interests. Usually, it is not.

*Crohn's disease.* When it affects the small intestine this inflammatory disease is often complicated by bouts of subacute obstruction. These usually resolve on conservative management but, if not, operation is required.

*Postoperative obstruction.* While abdominal distension, vomiting, failure to pass flatus and other changes during the post-operative phase, are generally attributed to paralytic ileus, mechanical problems can follow any intra-abdominal operation. These are due to adhesions or to the bowel becoming trapped in peritoneal or mesenteric defects. If a post-operative patient has signs of mechanical intestinal obstruction persisting for more than 2–3 days, laparotomy is undertaken.

*Sigmoid volvulus.* Initially, this is usually treated conservatively by the insertion of a soft lubricated rubber tube through a sigmoidoscope into the twisted loop to allow decompression. If this fails or if strangulation is suspected, laparotomy should be performed Resection of the sigmoid colon is usually indicated and is mandatory in the presence of ischaemia. Either both ends of the bowel are exteriorised or a Hartmann procedure performed, with a view to later restoration of colonic continuity. A caecal volvulus is rare; right hemicolectomy is the best treatment.

## PARALYTIC ILEUS

Paralytic ileus may complicate mechanical obstruction or may arise as a result of peritonitis, retroperitoneal bleeding or acute pancreatitis. It is due to interference with splanchnic nerve function or a direct toxic effect on the bowel wall (e.g. in peritonitis). Gross electrolyte depletion, notably of potassium and magnesium, hypoxia and shock can also cause ileus.

In contrast to a mechanical obstruction, intestinal colic is not a feature. The abdomen is distended, there is little tenderness and no guarding on palpation. Bowel sounds are absent. Vomiting or nasogastric aspirations are often copious. Plain films show gaseous distension with multiple fluid levels throughout the whole length of the gut.

Treatment is conservative and consists of nasogastric aspiration and the intravenous replacement of fluid and electrolytes. Parasympathomimetic drugs have been used but are not generally advised. Surgery is contra-indicated but the patient must be reviewed twice daily so that a positive decision can be made to persist with conservative therapy. Any suggestion of mechanical intestinal obstruction or strangulation demands operation.

## PSEUDO-OBSTRUCTION

Pseudo-obstruction is a condition in which gross gaseous distension of the abdomen, obstructive bowel sounds and fluid levels on X-ray, suggest mechanical obstruction of the large intestine. The condition occurs in patients with respiratory or renal disease or may occur after major trauma or following a major operation, not necessarily on the gastro-intestinal tract.

In some cases, gas may be seen extending into the rectum on the plain abdominal X-ray but if not, an enema with dilute barium confirms the absence of an obstructing lesion. Treatment is conservative and laparotomy is advised only if the diagnosis is in doubt or if the distension is so gross as to raise fear of caecal perforation.

Colonoscopic decompression of the distended bowel has been used successfully in a few patients.

# 32. Anorectal Conditions

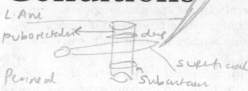
## ANATOMY OF THE ANORECTAL REGION

### MUSCULATURE

The anal canal is three to four centimetres long and consists of two muscular tubes; the inner tube is a continuation of the smooth muscle of the gut, while the outer tube consists of a sheath of striated muscle (Fig. 32.1).

*The inner tube.* The internal sphincter is the final condensation of the circular layer of gut muscle, and as such is controlled by the autonomic nervous system. The longitudinal muscle of the gut becomes fibrous as it passes between the internal and external sphincters, ending as a series of bands which radiate to the peri-anal skin (Fig. 32.1).

*The outer tube.* The *puborectalis* fibres of levator ani originate from the back of the pubic symphysis, and form a U-shaped loop which blends with the outer layer of the bowel as it passes through

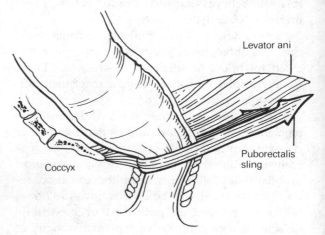

**Fig. 32.2** Puborectalis sling, establishing 'perineal angle'

the pelvic floor. This loop helps to maintain the 80° angle between the axis of the rectum and anal canal (Fig. 32.2) and also compresses the anal canal into an anteroposterior slit.

The lower border of puborectalis is in continuity with the external sphincter (Fig. 32.1), both muscles being striated and under voluntary control. The *anorectal ring* is the condensed ring of muscle formed by puborectalis and upper edges of the internal and external sphincters. The ring can be felt rectally and is vital to continence.

### THE LINING OF THE ANAL CANAL

The anal valves are crescentic mucosal folds which form a serrated or "pectinate" line around the lumen some two centimetres from the anal verge (Fig. 32.3). The pectinate line corresponds to the line of fusion between endoderm of the embryonic hindgut, and ectoderm of the anal pit. The canal above this line has a mucosal lining

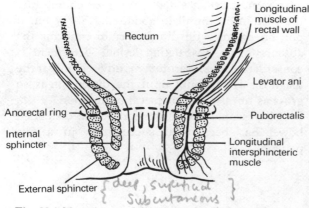

**Fig. 32.1** Musculature of the anorectal region

Rectum

Longitudinal muscle of rectal wall

Levator ani

Anorectal ring

Puborectalis

Internal sphincter

Longitudinal intersphincteric muscle

External sphincter { deep, superficial, subcutaneous }

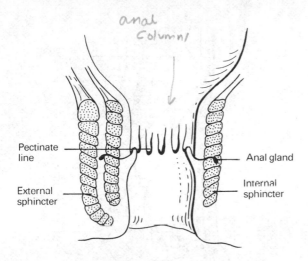

anal
columns

Fig. 32.3 Lining of the anal canal

Pectinate line · External sphincter · Anal gland · Internal sphincter

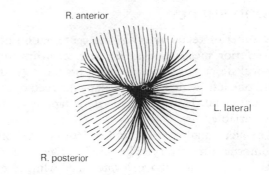

R. anterior
L. lateral
R. posterior

**Fig. 32.4** Anal cushions — the position for internal haemorrhoids

innervated by the autonomic nervous system, whereas beneath the pectinate line, it is lined by modified skin innervated by the peripheral nervous system. Histologically there is a gradual transition from mucus-secreting columnar mucosa to stratified squamous epithelium. Keratinisation and epidermal appendages appear only beyond the anal verge.

The mucosa above the pectinate line is thrown into vertical folds or anal columns, the distal ends of which fuse to form the anal valves. Each valve encloses an anal crypt, and an anal gland opens into the floor of some of the crypts. These glands ramify in the submucosa to reach the internal sphincter, some of them penetrating to the inter-sphincteric plane (Fig. 32.3). The glands are important in the spread of anorectal infection.

The submucosa of the anal canal forms three pads of vascular connective tissue or anal cushions. These lie in the left lateral, right posterior and right anterior positions, and impart a Y-shaped configuration to the lumen (Fig. 32.4).

## TISSUE SPACES IN RELATION TO THE ANORECTAL REGION

*The ischiorectal fossa* is the pyramidal space bounded laterally by the side wall of the pelvis, medially by the external anal sphincter and superiorly by the levator ani (Fig. 32.5). The fossa contains fatty connective tissue and is crossed by

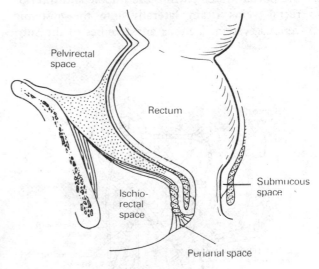

Pelvirectal space · Rectum · Ischio-rectal space · Submucous space · Perianal space

**Fig. 32.5** Tissue spaces in relation to the anorectal region

the inferior rectal vessels. The two fossae communicate behind the anal canal.

*The peri-anal space* lies below the inferior margins of the anal sphincters and is loculated by fibrous septae.

*The submucous space* lies between the internal sphincter and the muco-cutaneous lining of the upper two-thirds of the anal canal, and contains the internal haemorrhoidal venous plexus.

*The pelvirectal space* is a potential space between the upper surface of the levator ani and the pelvic peritoneum, and contains the lateral ligaments of the rectum.

## BLOOD SUPPLY

The superior rectal artery is the continuation of the inferior mesenteric artery and according to classical descriptions forms three branches (two right, one left) which descend along the rectum to the anal canal. However, the arterial anatomy is very variable.

The anal canal is also supplied by branches of the internal iliac artery. The middle rectal artery enters the rectum above levator ani, while the inferior rectal artery transverses the ischiorectal fossa. There is a profuse anastomosis between the three rectal arteries (Fig. 32.6).

The superior rectal vein drains upwards into the portal system, while the middle and inferior rectal veins drain laterally into the systemic venous system. Venous anastomoses in the sub-

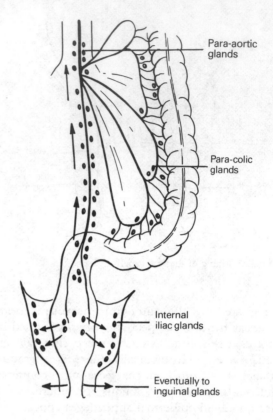

Fig. 32.7 Lymphatic drainage of the rectum

mucosa form the internal haemorrhoidal plexus above the pectinate line, and the external haemorrhoidal plexus below.

## LYMPHATIC DRAINAGE

Carcinoma of the rectum spreads upwards along the superior rectal lymphatic vessels, although lesions in the lower extra-peritoneal rectum occasionally spread laterally to the internal iliac glands. Metastasis to inguinal glands occurs only when carcinoma involves the skin of the lower anal canal or peri-anal region (Fig. 32.7).

## ANAL CONTINENCE

The internal sphincter provides resting anal tone, but relaxes following distention of the rectum by flatus or faeces. The external sphincter is contracted voluntarily if defaecation has to be post-

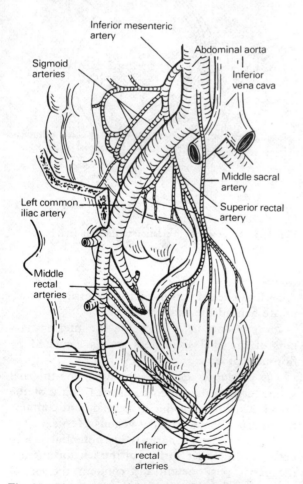

Fig. 32.6 Blood supply of the rectum (from behind)

poned, and although contraction can only be maintained for a minute or so, the rise in rectal pressure usually abates if the call to stool is resisted.

Continence depends upon (i) intact *rectal and pelvic floor innervation* to appreciate rectal distention; (ii) intact *anal sensation* to determine the nature of the rectal contents; and (iii) intact *innervated anal sphincters* and *levator ani*. Division of the lower portion of one or both anal sphincters only produces minor defects in continence, but division of the anorectal ring causes disastrous loss of control.

The following mechanical factors may contribute to continence:

(1) The 80° angle of the perineal flexure results in increases in intra-abdominal pressure pressing the anterior rectal wall down on to the anal canal. This prevents inadvertent escape of flatus or faeces when intra-abdominal pressure rises during coughing and exercise (Fig. 32.2).

(2) The anal canal has been likened to a flutter valve as it passes through the pelvic diaphragm. The canal walls are kept in apposition by the internal sphincter and the puborectalis sling so that continence is maintained without conscious effort during rises in intra-abdominal pressure (Fig. 32.8). When pressure rises *within* the rectum, the valve opens and contraction of the external sphincter is needed to preserve continence.

(3) The striated muscle of the external sphincter and puborectalis is maintained in a state of tonic contraction. This is important in maintaining (1) and (2).

(4) The bulk of the anal cushions may contribute to closure. Minor defects in continence occur in about a quarter of patients following haemorrhoidectomy.

## CONTROL OF DEFAECATION

An increase in intrarectal pressure is followed over a few minutes by relaxation or 'accommodation' of the rectum. During this period there is a feeling of fullness if the rectum is sufficiently distended. At the same time, the internal anal sphincter partly relaxes thus allowing rectal contents to reach the upper part of the somatic sensory epithelium. Gas can be detected by a voluntary slight increase in intra-abdominal pressure which allows a small amount of gas to escape. However, if stool is present, the external sphincter is rapidly contracted until accommodation in the rectum has been completed. During defaecation there is a release of cortical inhibition and a voluntary increase in intra-abdominal pressure. The angle between rectum and anal canal is straightened and the sphincters and pelvic floor relax. There is reflex contraction of pelvic colon and rectum.

## ANAL INCONTINENCE

Anal incontinence may result from the following causes:

*Congenital abnormalities.* Incontinence is a feature of some congenital abnormalities such as anorectal agenesis with recto-cloacal fistula.

*Trauma.* Division of the sphincters and anorectal ring may follow accidental injury, obstetric tears or operative trauma.

*Neurological and psychological disease.* Various diseases affecting the nervous system, eg, spina bifida, spinal trauma, spinal tumours, multiple sclerosis and tabes dorsalis may all give rise to anal incontinence. Incontinence of faeces is a common manifestation of behavioural problems in children, senile dementia, and all other forms of psychotic illness.

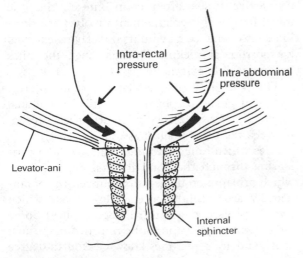

Fig. 32.8 Mechanism of continence

*Anorectal disease.* Rectal prolapse, third degree piles, chronic inflammatory bowel disease, and anorectal cancer may cause incontinence by stretching, infiltrating or destroying the sphincter mechanism.

*Faecal impaction.* Impaction of faeces leads first to constipation and then to overflow incontinence of faeces with a feeling of incomplete evacuation of the bowel. Faecal impaction in elderly and bedbound patients is the commonest cause of incontinence in surgical practice.

## Treatment of anal incontinence

There is no satisfactory treatment for many causes of incontinence. The management of congenital abnormalities is outwith the scope of this book. Traumatic division of the sphincter mechanism can be repaired surgically under cover of a temporary defunctioning colostomy. If there is gross contamination at the time of injury it is advisable to carry out wound toilet with colostomy and defer definitive repair until the acute inflammation has subsided. Obstetric tears can often be dealt with by primary suture, or by subsequent repair of the perineum.

Laxity of the anal sphincters may be reduced by suture if the sphincter muscle has been partially or completely divided. A preliminary defunctioning colostomy is advisable. Sphincteroplasty operations are also available to tighten the sphincters and puborectalis muscle. Insertion of an encircling Thiersch wire or nylon tape may be considered in elderly unfit patients.

Faecal impaction demands manual or instrumental disimpaction followed by enemas and aperients to restore normal bowel action.

These various surgical manoeuvres often fail. A permanent colostomy is then required.

---

# HAEMORRHOIDS

---

# AETIOLOGY

Haemorrhoids (piles) remain one of the commonest ailments of Western society, although their aetiology remains uncertain. Piles commonly develop or increase in size during pregnancy and are associated with constipation and straining at stool. There are no valves in the portal venous system, and it may be that increases in intra-abdominal pressure could dilate unsupported anal canal veins. Refined low-residue Western diets with a consequent need to strain at stool may be a factor.

However, there are a number of facts which do not support the varicose vein theory of origin. The development of piles in pregnancy could equally be due to increased laxity and vascularity of the pelvic tissues; piles are not more common in patients with portal hypertension. Rectal cancer is said to predispose to pile formation by obstructing venous drainage, but it is just as likely that these two common conditions co-exist fortuitously.

Alternative explanations for haemorrhoidal formation include hyperplasia of a submucosal vascular network, straining at stool with attenuation of the supporting framework of the anal cushions, and the development of constricting fibrous bands within the anal canal.

# CLASSIFICATION

## Internal piles

These originate as bulges in the upper anal canal and lower rectum. The piles contain the internal haemorrhoidal plexus but thickened mucosa and connective tissue often contribute to the pile mass. Progressive enlargement involves the skin-lined lower anal canal with its underlying external haemorrhoidal plexus. At this stage the piles become visible externally.

The piles lie in the left lateral, right anterior and right posterior positions relative to the anal canal. Smaller accessory piles are often present between the three main masses (Fig. 32.4).

Piles which bulge into the lumen without prolapsing through the anus are first degree, those which prolapse on defaecation but return spontaneously are second degree, while those which remain prolapsed are third degree piles. Some long-standing piles cannot be returned to the anal canal, and are sometimes known as fourth degree piles.

*Thrombosed internal haemorrhoids.* This acute painful condition is often described by patients as 'an attack of piles'. It occurs when the anal sphincters contract around prolapsed piles to prevent their return to the anal canal and obstruct venous return. Congestion and thrombosis follow and the piles become hard and tender, in contrast to uncomplicated third degree piles. Necrosis may follow. The skin-covered part of the piles and the peri-anal skin become oedematous, overhanging and hiding the swollen mucosal component. Proctoscopy is usually impossible because of discomfort, and is not needed to establish the diagnosis. The term 'strangulated piles' is commonly used to describe this sequence of events.

### External piles

These originate outside the anal canal and are quite distinct from the internal haemorrhoids described above. The term is used to describe anal haematomas (which may also be acutely painful) and skin tags, but is confusing and best avoided.

## CLINICAL FEATURES

*Bleeding* is traditionally the first symptom. While this remains true for first degree piles, many patients with prolapsing piles consider prolapse to occur first. Bleeding is usually noted first as a bright red streak on the stool surface or on the toilet paper, but increases in frequency and severity until a steady drip or squirting of blood accompanies defaecation. Severe secondary anaemia is uncommon.

*Prolapse* produces symptoms in the majority of patients. It is at first a transient feature on defaecation, but occurs with increasing frequency until third degree piles result.

*Mucous discharge* occurs when there is exposure of anal mucosa. Associated *skin tags* are common and may cause excoriation and pruritus.

*Pain* is rare in uncomplicated piles. Many patients experience discomfort and some consider this to be their main complaint.

*Thrombosed piles* can cause severe pain in relation to the pile bearing areas.

## ASSESSMENT AND DIAGNOSIS

A careful history and abdominal examination precede anorectal examination. Anal bleeding cannot be attributed to piles until other anorectal pathology, particularly a neoplasm, has been excluded.

Inspection of the peri-anal area is carried out with the patient in the left lateral position. First degree piles produce no outward abnormality. Separation of the buttocks often reveals the skin-covered component of second degree piles, and the piles may prolapse when the patient is asked to strain. In prolapsed third degree piles, the red anal mucosa is usually visible, separated by a furrow from the skin-lined component.

Digital rectal examination may reveal no abnormality, unless the piles are long-standing and thickened. Proctoscopy is the key diagnostic investigation, the piles bulging into the lumen as the instrument is withdrawn. The patient is asked to strain during withdrawal so that vascular engorgement is produced and the degree of prolapse can be determined. Sigmoidoscopy is essential to exclude co-existing rectal pathology which might mimic bleeding from piles. Barium enema is indicated only when symptoms cannot be explained by proctoscopic and sigmoidoscopic findings.

With thrombosed piles the skin around the anus is swollen and oedematous in relation to the pile-bearing areas. Gentle separation of these allows a glimpse of the thrombosed pile masses which may be red, blue or, if necrotic, black.

## TREATMENT

### Conservative treatment

Small asymptomatic first degree piles which are discovered as an incidental finding should be left alone. Symptomatic piles merit treatment but there is little place for 'medical' treatment by local ointment or suppositories. A high residue diet or bulk laxative should be advised to combat habitual constipation, and this may be all that is necessary to cure the condition.

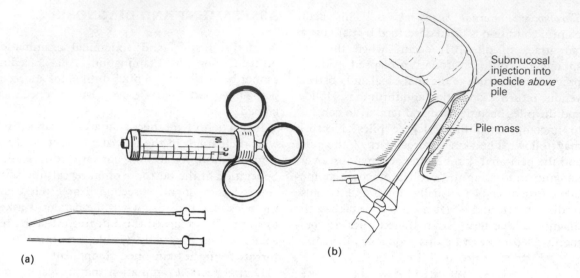

**Fig. 32.9** a) Gabriel syringe, b) Injection of haemorrhoid through proctoscope

## Specific treatment

*Injection*. First degree piles are ideal for injection. A trial of injection is also worthwhile in second degree piles but not in those of third degree which cannot be cured by this means. However, when operation is contra-indicated in such prolapsing piles, injections may give some relief.

The object of injection therapy is to produce submucosal fibrosis in the upper anal canal and lower rectum, constricting vascular spaces within the pile, and decreasing mucosal mobility. A Gabriel syringe (Fig. 32.9) is filled with sclerosant (5% phenol in almond oil), and using a proctoscope, 3–5 ml is injected into each pile pedicle at or just above the anorectal ring. Transient deep-seated aching sometimes follows injection of sclerosant but the technique is usually painless when performed correctly.

Complications such as ulceration and necrosis at the injection site, submucosal abscess, haematuria and prostatic abscess, oleogranuloma, and transient inflammatory anal canal narrowing are all rare.

Bleeding should cease within 24–48 hours of successful injection. Injection may be repeated if symptoms recur but then operation is usually advised.

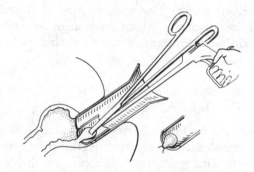

**Fig. 32.10** Rubber band ligation of haemorrhoids

*Rubber-band ligation*. This technique provides an alternative to injection. The pile mass is pulled down through a proctoscope, and a rubber band applied around the mucosally-covered pedicle (Fig. 32.10). One pile is ligated at each visit, further banding being carried out at 3-week intervals. Approximately one-third of patients require medication for discomfort. Banding is not applicable to the skin-lined component of piles or associated skin tags.

*Cryodestruction*. Cryosurgery has been used to treat second and third degree piles without anaesthesia. A profuse offensive discharge persists for about 10 days but the patient can usually return to work on the day after treatment.

*CO₂ laser.* This technique has not been applied widely but recent reports of the use of the $CO_2$-laser suggest that this may be an acceptable alternative.

*Manual anal dilatation under general anaesthesia.* (Lord's technique) Manual dilatation of the anal canal and lower rectum to '4-fingers' is used to treat piles of any degree. A moist sponge is inserted for one hour to prevent haematoma formation, and the patient is allowed home after recovery from anaesthesia. He is provided with a bulk laxative and an anal dilator to prevent recurrent anal constriction. Mild incontinence of flatus may occur after dilatation, but faecal incontinence is rare. The technique has become popular as an alternative to formal haemorrhoidectomy.

## Inpatient haemorrhoidectomy

Several operations are described to treat internal piles. Most commonly practised is ligation and excision of each pile mass following its dissection from the anal canal.

The plane of dissection passes just within the internal sphincter which is carefully preserved (Fig. 32.11). Each vascular pedicle is transfixed and ligated, and the piles excised to leave three raw areas separated by bridges of skin and mucosa. Epithelialisation of the raw areas takes place in 3–4 weeks and prevents excessive fibrosis or anal narrowing. Modification of this technique, including submucosal dissection, makes little difference to the overall results.

*Complications.* Postoperative pain is the commonest problem, and considerable discomfort accompanies the first bowel motion. It is advised that stools should be kept soft, e.g., by methyl cellulose for 3–4 weeks while epithelialisation takes place. Male patients occasionally have difficulty in micturition but catheterisation is rarely needed. Reactionary haemorrhage occurs in less than 2% of patients, and secondary haemorrhage 7–10 days after operation occurs in just over 1% of cases. Anal stenosis, fissure, abscess and fistula are rare complications. The late results show that while only 5% of patients have recurrent symptoms, two-thirds will have first degree piles on proctoscopy. On careful questioning some patients admit to intermittent flatus incontinence or soiling of underwear, but significant faecal incontinence is rare.

*Thrombosed internal haemorrhoids.* In the early stages it may still be possible to return prolapsed piles to the anal canal and allow the congestion to settle. This is seldom feasible by the time the majority of patients present although anal dilatation performed under general anaesthetic may promote reduction. Conservative treatment includes bed rest, local application of dressings soaked in hypertonic saline, analgesic and mild aperients.

Resolution takes about 10 days. Although haemorrhoidectomy is usually required at future date, in some cases the attack of thrombosis will cure the piles. Immediate haemorrhoidectomy is now seldom advised.

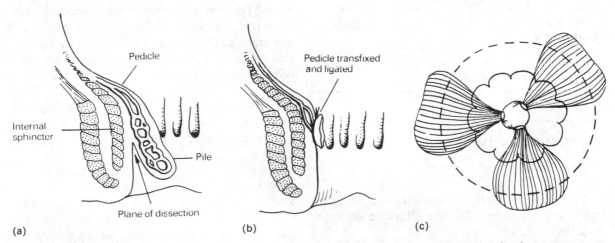

(a)  (b)  (c)

**Fig. 32.11** Haemorrhoidectomy. a) Anatomy, b) Haemorrhoid excised, c) Anus at end of operation showing raw areas.

## Conclusions regarding the treatment of haemorrhoids

Injection or banding are the mainstays of treatment for symptomatic first degree and early second degree piles. Ligature and excision are still practised widely for third degree piles and those second degree piles which are unsuitable for injection or fail to respond. Manual dilatation avoids in-patient treatment, is less painful for the patient, and has increased in popularity. Haemorrhoidectomy may best be reserved for those cases in which dilatation fails. Thrombosed piles are best treated conservatively at first.

## PERI-ANAL HAEMATOMA

This common condition (*syn.* thrombosed external pile) follows rupture of a vein at the anal verge with haematoma formation. A small painful lump develops rapidly, often appearing after an episode of straining at stool. The lump is tense, blue, well-circumscribed and exquisitely tender. The haematoma is readily distinguished from thrombosed internal haemorrhoids by its restricted size, and from peri-anal abscess by its colour.

Spontaneous resolution takes some days and often leaves a skin tag at the site. Occasionally the haematoma ruptures or becomes secondarily infected.

Operation is generally advisable to relieve pain and tenderness and speed recovery. The haematoma is evacuated under local anaesthesia and the wound is left to granulate.

---

## RECTAL PROLAPSE

---

## CLASSIFICATION

Two main types of prolapse of the rectum are described:

1. *Incomplete, partial* or *minimal* prolapse, when the mucous membrane lining the anal canal is lax and protrudes through the anus.

2. *Complete* prolapse in which the whole thickness of the bowel protrudes through the anus. In effect this is a sliding hernia of the pouch of Douglas. If there is associated vaginal prolapse, the term *procidentia* is applied.

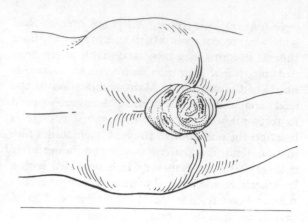

**Fig. 32.12** Complete rectal prolapse

Any type of prolapse can occur at any time of life. However, *incomplete* prolapse is common in young children whereas *complete* prolapse is commoner in adults. Eighty-five per cent of affected adults are women, and older females are particularly at risk.

## AETIOLOGY

*Partial prolapse.* Prolapse in childhood is favoured if the sacral curve of the rectum is lacking so that rectum and anus form a vertical tube. Excessive straining at stool is a major factor, and malnourishment contributes by reducing the amount of fat within the supporting ischiorectal and pararectal tissues. There is an association with cystic fibrosis of the pancreas.

Partial prolapse in adults may complicate haemorrhoid formation or may follow damage to the anal sphincters during labour or anal surgery.

*Complete prolapse.* Additional factors concerned with complete prolapse include deficient tone in the pelvic floor muscles and anal canal, lack of fixation of the rectum to its sacral bed, intussusception of the rectum, and an abnormally deep recto-vaginal or recto-vesical pouch.

## CLINICAL FEATURES

Prolapse is first noted during defaecation. For a time it will reduce spontaneously once straining ceases. Discomfort during defaecation is common, and there may be bleeding and mucus discharge from the engorged mucosa. The prolapse recurs with increasing ease and may even be caused by mild exertion such as coughing and walking. The bowel habit becomes irregular, and laxity of musculature coupled with impaired rectal sensation lead to incontinence of both flatus and faeces. Such incontinence is the main reason for many patients seeking help. Associated uterine prolapse compounds the problem by causing incontinence of urine.

The prolapse may not be apparent until the patient is asked to bear down and strain. The anus is usually patulous and can be opened widely simply by drawing the buttocks apart. Digital rectal examination reveals poor sphincter tone and two or more fingers can be inserted without apparent discomfort. The prolapse appears progressively on straining but seldom protrudes for more than 10 cm. The mucosa is thickened, engorged and corrugated but mucosal folds may be ironed out as the prolapse emerges. The thickness of the prolapse is judged between finger and thumb in order to decide whether it is partial or complete. Partial prolapse seldom protrudes for more than 5 cm. The mucosa is smooth.

The complications of rectal prolapse include irreducibility with ulceration, bleeding and gangrene, and rarely rupture of the prolapsed bowel.

The diagnosis of rectal prolapse is usually straightforward. The appearance can be confused with large third degree piles, and on occasions with prolapse of a rectal neoplasm.

## TREATMENT

### Children

Operation is rarely required. Prolapse responds to conservative measures in most cases and rarely persists beyond the age of 5 years. Constipation and straining at stool are avoided, and the buttocks may be strapped together to discourage prolapse during defaecation. If non-operative measures fail, the submucosal injection of phenol may be used to fix lax mucosa to underlying tissues.

### Adults

*Partial prolapse.* Provided sphincter tone is satisfactory, partial prolapse in adults can be treated by excising prolapsing mucosa by a technique similar to that used for the dissection and ligature of haemorrhoids. Patients with poor sphincter tone are seldom improved in this way. Their main complaint is incontinence rather than the prolapse. Various methods of improving sphincter tone have been described although none are entirely satisfactory. These methods include voluntary exercises of sphincter muscle, electrical stimulation, and perineorrhaphy to tighten puborectalis. Education of bowel habit is an important part of treatment, and insertion of a Thiersch wire (see below) may be considered in the frail elderly patient.

*Complete prolapse.* Various methods are available for the treatment of complete prolapse; none are ideal.

*Narrowing of the anus.* The simplest form of surgery consists of inserting a Thiersch wire of stainless steel or synthetic monofilament material around the anal canal, but this procedure rarely is successful in complete prolapse (Fig. 32.13). The incidence of faecal impaction is high so that regular stool softeners require to be taken indefinitely. Although some surgeons advise this procedure for elderly patients, they can tolerate an abdominal repair surprisingly well.

*Repair of pelvic structures and fixation of the rectum.* A variety of repairs can be carried out through the abdomen. These are successful in an anatomical sense of preventing further prolapse, but some degree of incontinence persists in about 30% of patients. Most methods include thorough mobilisation of the rectum, fixing of the rectum to the sacrum, suture of the levator ani muscles in front of the rectum, and obliteration of the deep pouch of Douglas. Mobilisation of the rectum favours extensive adhesion formation and prevents further prolapse by fixing the rectum to the

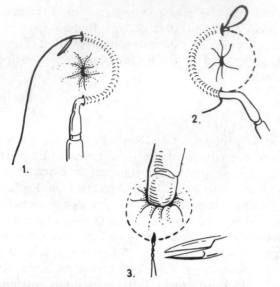

**Fig. 32.13** Thiersch wire treatment of rectal prolapse, showing insertion of wire using aneurysm needle (The wire is tightened around one finger)

sacrum. Additional fixation can be achieved by fixing a sheet of Ivalon sponge to the front of the sacrum and wrapping this sheet around the mobilised rectum or by placing non-absorbable sutures between the rectum and periosteum of the sacrum. Repair without bowel resection is advised whenever possible, but anterior restorative resection may be required. Abdomino-perineal resection of the rectum is a last resort in patients with gross incontinence who fail to respond to less radical measures. In the very frail colostomy alone may suffice.

# PRURITIS ANI

## AETIOLOGY

This is a common condition which occurs more frequently in men, especially between the ages of 30–60 years. Causal factors can be identified in only 50% of patients. It is assumed that psychogenic problems, chemical irritation by some constituent of faeces, or food allergy are responsible in the remainder. Defined causes of pruritus ani include the following:

*Skin disease*. Skin lesions may be localised to the peri-anal area or, as in the case of psoriasis and lichen planus, there may be lesions elsewhere. Contact eczema can be caused by local application of steroid, antibiotic, local anaesthetic or lanoline ointment or creams. Premalignant keratosis is a rare cause of peri-anal itching.

*Infective conditions*. Candidiasis must be considered in diabetics and those who have received prolonged courses of corticosteroid or broad spectrum antibiotics. Fungal infections occur occasionally. Threadworms are common in children but not in adults. Anal warts are commonly complicated by pruritus. Skin tags may predispose to infection

*Gastrointestinal conditions*. Pruritus may be a feature of many anorectal disorders which cause a rectal discharge. Such disorders include piles, fissure, fistula, proctitis, polyps and rectal cancer. Frequent bowel movements in the irritable bowel syndrome, ulcerative colitis or malabsorptive disorders predispose to pruritus.

*Miscellaneous conditions*. Some drugs such as quinidine and colchicine cause pruritus when taken for prolonged periods. Obesity increases the risk of pruritus.

## CLINICAL FEATURES

The itching varies from a minor nuisance to a source of overwhelming misery. The urge to scratch is often irresistible so that the skin is damaged with local discomfort or pain. Symptoms are worst after defaecation and at night, regardless of the cause of pruritus.

The peri-anal skin may show no abnormality on examination, but more often appears raw and excoriated with linear cracks, ulcers and lichenification. Psoriasis and fungal infection often have a well-defined border.

Investigation is aimed at establishing the underlying cause. The entire skin surface is inspected, and proctoscopy and sigmoidoscopy are performed. The urine is examined for glucose. Candidiasis and fungal infection can be confirmed on skin scrapings.

## TREATMENT

Underlying causes such as psoriasis, diabetes and infections are treated in the usual manner. Abnormalities of the anal region such as skin tags, fissures and fistulae should be surgically corrected.

In the large number of patients where no cause can be defined, a number of useful symptomatic measures can be introduced. First, all local applications are discontinued. Attention to anal hygiene is essential as there may be primary or secondary sensitivity to faeces or rectal mucus. The region should be washed with lukewarm water in the morning and evening, and immediately after defaecation. Medicated soaps are avoided as their contained antiseptic may irritate. Excessive use of any form of soap is discouraged. After washing, the area is patted dry with a soft towel. It must not be rubbed vigorously. Application of talcum powder may be useful in warm weather to combat excessive sweating, and shaving of the peri-anal skin may be worthwhile. Woollen and nylon underwear favour sweating and should be replaced by cotton mesh garments.

It may be possible to identify certain items of diet which exacerbate pruritus, e.g. beer, red wine, coffee, curries, fruit and milk. Ingestion of mineral oil may favour pruritus by causing anal leakage, but advice on laxatives is essential. Bulk laxatives are preferred as a means of achieving a regular soft motion.

Considerable will-power is needed to stop scratching during waking hours. Involuntary scratching during sleep can be reduced by sedation with phenothiazines. Post-menopausal women may benefit from oestrogen therapy, particularly if there is associated genital pruritus.

Continuing support is essential. Regular review ensures that the prescribed measures are being carried out.

Surgical treatment by denervation of the peri-anal skin through two curved incisions, one on either side of the peri-anal verge, has been described. The results are variable.

## ANORECTAL ABSCESS

### AETIOLOGY

Anorectal abscesses are a common cause of admission to hospital. They are two to three times more common in males, the highest incidence being in the third and fourth decades.

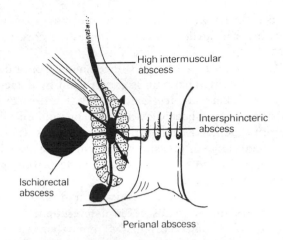

**Fig. 32.14** Development and sites of anorectal abscesses

There is no apparent cause for abscess formation in the majority of patients. It has been suggested that infection arises in an anal gland, passes to the intersphincteric space (Fig. 32.14), and can then track downwards to present as a peri-anal abscess, outwards to form an ischiorectal abscess, or upwards to produce a high intermuscular abscess. Intersphincteric abscesses undoubtedly occur, but are less common than this concept suggests.

Associated underlying diseases such as Crohn's disease, ulcerative colitis, rectal cancer and active tuberculosis are present in a minority of patients and should always be considered in patients with recurrent anorectal infection.

Anorectal abscess may lead to the development of a fistula-in-ano or, conversely, may complicate the presence of a fistula. In all recurrent abscesses an underlying fistula should be kept in mind.

## CLINICAL FEATURES OF ANORECTAL ABSCESS

*Peri-anal abscess* is common and presents as an acute painful tender swelling at the anal verge. Systemic upset is minimal but pain on defecation leads to constipation.

*Ischiorectal abscess* is also common and produces a brawny diffuse induration lateral to the anus. The swelling is painful and tender but fluctuation occurs late. Systemic upset is pronounced. The swelling may be palpable on digital rectal examination and infection may extend behind the anal canal as a 'horseshoe abscess' involving both ischiorectal fossae.

*Intersphincteric abscess* is uncommon. Continuous throbbing anal pain is exacerbated by defaecation. There are few external signs unless the abscess is complicated by peri-anal or ischiorectal suppuration. Discharge into the anal canal leads to the passage of pus and blood. On digital rectal examination there is a boggy, tender swelling under the mucosa.

*High intermuscular abscess* is rare and resembles an intersphincteric abscess in its presentation.

*Pelvirectal abscess* originates from pelvic sepsis.

## TREATMENT

Peri-anal and ischiorectal abscesses are incised and drained under general anaesthesia. A specimen of pus is taken for bacteriological examination. The cavity walls are probed gently to detect any communication with the anal lumen. Fistulous connections can be demonstrated in up to one-third of the patients but many such 'fistulae' are caused by injudicious probing. Assuming that no communication is detected, the abscess is deroofed by making a cruciate incision and excising the four triangles of skin (Fig. 32.15). The excised skin and a biopsy of the abscess wall are sent routinely for histological examination. A minority of surgeons suture the wound under antibiotic cover.

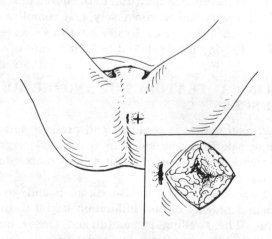

**Fig. 32.15** Ischiorectal abscess — cruciate incision and drainage

## PROBLEMS IN THE TREATMENT OF ANORECTAL ABSCESS

*Fistula-in-ano.* If the internal opening of a fistula-in-ano is demonstrated on exploration and is below the pectinate line, the fistula should be laid open. This should only be performed by an experienced surgeon. If there is doubt about the level of the fistula, treatment should be deferred.

*Recurrence.* About one quarter of patients presenting with an anorectal abscess develop recurrent abscess or a fistula, those with ischiorectal abscesses being most at risk. The rate of recurrence is not influenced by the primary treatment, ie, whether primary suture is carried out, or the wound left to drain and heal by granulation.

*Inflammatory bowel disease.* Anorectal abscess may be the first manifestation of Crohn's disease, ulcerative colitis or much less commonly, tuberculosis. These abscesses are characteristically indolent and lined by pale grey granulation tissue. They should be incised and drained. Bacteriological and histological confirmation of the diagnosis is essential. Incision is frequently followed by fistula formation. Radical treatment should always be avoided in the first instance.

## FISSURE-IN-ANO    [Very painful]

An anal fissure is a tear in the sensitive skin-lined lower anal canal which produces pain on defaecation. The fissure commonly presents as an isolated primary problem, but can be associated with other gastrointestinal diseases.

## CLASSIFICATION

### Primary fissure-in-ano (Fig. 32.16)

The aetiology is uncertain but many patients first notice symptoms after passage of a hard constipated stool. The superficial fibres of the external sphincter are deficient posteriorly, and this may explain the frequency with which anal fissures occur in the posterior midline.

### Secondary fissure-in-ano

Fissures are common in Crohn's disease and ulcerative colitis. Such secondary fissures are

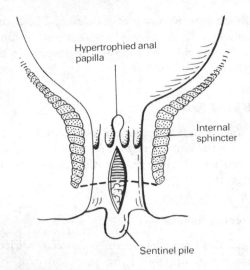

**Fig. 32.16** Fissure-in-ano

frequently multiple, occur at any point on the canal circumference, are broad based and characteristically indolent. Fissures are a rare complication of anorectal operations such as hae-morrhoidectomy.

## PATHOLOGY OF PRIMARY FISSURE

The typical primary fissure is a longitudinal tear extending from the anal verge to the pectinate line in the posterior midline. In 15% of female patients and in 1% of males, the tear is in the midline anteriorly. The tear becomes a canoe-shaped ulcer, the floor of which contains the lower third of the internal sphincter (Fig. 32.16). Inflammation causes swelling of the margins of the fissure, and an oedematous skin tag develops at the anal verge and is known as a sentinel pile. The swollen anal valve at the upper extent of the fissure is called a 'hypertrophied anal papilla'. Infection may produce a peri-anal abscess, incision of which results in a low anal fistula.

Anal fissures may heal spontaneously if un-treated, or become chronic with fibrosis of the spastic internal sphincter.

## CLINICAL FEATURES

The principal feature of a fissure is severe burn-ing pain on defaecation which may persist for several hours. The pain may be so intense that

defaecation is avoided. Bleeding sometimes oc-curs on defaecation, but is seldom profuse. The sentinel pile and associated serous discharge may cause excoriation and pruritus. Peri-anal ab-scesses and anal fistulae can complicate the fissure.

Recurrent or indolent fissures or those in unu-sual sites suggest the possibility of Crohn's dis-ease or ulcerative colitis.

The diagnosis can usually be made on the history alone. Inspection reveals the sentinel pile, and traction on the anal skin may bring the lower part of the fissure into view. Digital rectal exami-nation is painful and not often practicable. If the finger can be inserted, sphincter spasm is confirmed and the indurated margins of the fissure are apparent. Maximal tenderness is elicited when the base of the fissure is palpated. Proctoscopy and sigmoidoscopy are essential to exclude other anorectal disease, but require to be carried out under anaesthesia.

## TREATMENT

### Conservative treatment

Anal fissures can heal spontaneously. Conserva-tive treatment with local anaesthetic ointments and suppositories has usually been tried without success by the time the patient is referred to hospital. Operative treatment allows a full anorec-tal examination, provides a rapid, more certain cure, and is generally advocated. Chronic fissures are unlikely to heal without operation.

### Operative treatment

General anaesthesia is essential. The patient is placed in the lithotomy position, and the anal canal and rectum are examined thoroughly.

*Anal dilatation.* The majority of acute fissures respond to dilatation with dramatic relief of pain and spasm and subsequent healing. Transient impairment of anal control occurs in about one in four patients.

*Lateral subcutaneous internal sphincterotomy.* This operation gives a better guarantee of success as a first-line measure for both acute and chronic fissures. A tenotomy knife is introduced through

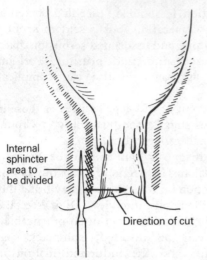

Internal
sphincter
area to
be divided

Direction of cut

**Fig. 32.17** Lateral subcutaneous internal sphincterotomy —
diagram of operation

the peri-anal skin on one side of the anal canal, and
the internal sphincter is divided from the pectinate
line downwards without entering the canal lumen
(Fig. 32.17). The procedure gives immediate relief
of pain. Open internal sphincterotomy and excision
of the fissure is no longer practised.

## FISTULA-IN-ANO

### AETIOLOGY

The aetiology of fistula-in-ano is uncertain. It
may be that infection commences in an anal
gland, spreads to produce an intersphincteric
abscess and then tracks into the peri-anal or
ischiorectal region (Fig. 32.18). Surgical incision
or spontaneous discharge completes the fistula
which is kept open by continuing infection from
the anal lumen.

Anal fistulas have a well-recognised association
with Crohn's disease, ulcerative colitis, tuberculosis, colloid carcinoma of the rectum and lymphogranuloma venereum.

### CLASSIFICATION

#### Low anal fistula

This is the commonest anal fistula. The track
does not extend higher than the anal crypts and

usually enters the bowel at this level. The fistula
may traverse both internal and external sphincters as it passes to the exterior, or descend in the
intersphincteric plane.

### High anal fistula

The track extends above the pectinate line, but
not above the anorectal ring. As with low fistulas,
the track may traverse both sphincters or descend
between them.

### Anorectal fistula

These fistulas are rare. In the *ischiorectal* variety,
the track extends above the anorectal ring, but
does not pass through the levator ani to enter the
rectum.

### Pelvi-rectal fistula

The rarer *pelvi-rectal* fistula does penetrate the
levator, entering the rectum above the anorectal
ring.

### Goodsall's rule

Fistulas with an external opening in front of a
transverse line through the anus generally open
into the anal canal at the nearest point on its
circumference. Fistulas with external openings
behind this line tend to open internally in the
posterior midline, and may extend behind the
anal canal on both sides forming a horseshoe
fistula (Fig. 32.19).

### CLINICAL FEATURES

Fistulas commonly present as abscesses, surgical
incision of which completes the fistula. Alternatively, the patient notices a small discharging
sinus with excoriation and pruritus. Once the
fistula has formed it is generally painless unless
blockage leads to abscess formation. Carcinoma is
a very rare complication of long-standing fistulas.

Examination reveals the external opening or
openings. Digital rectal examination may detect
induration along the fistula track, while pressure
on the indurated area expresses pus from the

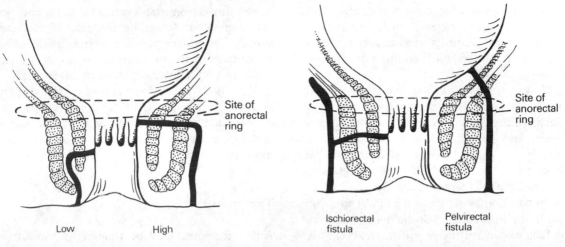

Fig. 32.18 Types of fistula-in-ano

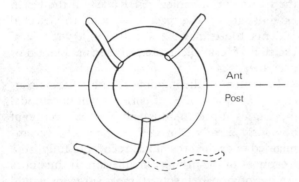

GOODSALL'S RULE

Fig. 32.19 Goodsall's rule

external opening. The internal opening may occasionally be seen on proctoscopy, and a malleable probe can be passed carefully along the fistula to define its course. Sigmoidoscopy is performed to exclude associated rectal disease.

## TREATMENT

Fistulas associated with other anorectal disease are usually treated conservatively in the first instance. Fistulas arising *de novo* rarely close spontaneously and operation is generally advised. The course of the fistula must be determined before embarking on surgery and the anorectal ring must be preserved. Disastrous permanent incontinence follows its inadvertent division.

Low anal fistulae are laid open along their entire length and allowed to heal by granulation and epithelialisation. High anal fistulas and the ischiorectal type of anorectal fistulas are treated in the same way provided that the surgeon is certain that laying open the fistulas will not entail division of the anorectal ring. A two-stage procedure is sometimes used, passing a suture along the track and leaving it as a 'seton' to allow fibrosis to occur before dividing sphincteric muscle.

The rare pelvi-rectal fistula cannot be laid open without producing incontinence. The alternatives to a difficult formal repair are conservative treatment, long-term defunctioning colostomy, or excision of the rectum with permanent iliac colostomy.

## ANAL NEOPLASIA

### BENIGN NEOPLASMS

The skin of the lower anal canal and peri-anal region may be affected by those benign neoplasms which affect the skin elsewhere.

### Anal papillomas (syn. anal warts, condylomata acuminata)

These deserve special mention. They arise from the anus or peri-anal skin, are often multiple, and often completely surround the anal region. Individual papillomas may be sessile or pedunculated, are often friable and bleed readily, and are usually associated with an offensive irritating discharge. The lesions are due to a viral infection and may present a serious problem in immunosuppressed patients.

Although they are particularly common in male homosexuals, these papillomas must not be confused with the flatter, smoother condylomata lata of secondary syphilis. Dark ground illumination of the discharge fluid will reveal large numbers of spirochaetes and establish the diagnosis of syphilis if there is any uncertainty.

Anal papillomas are treated by local application of podophyllin. Excision or diathermy is needed if this fails to control the problem. In severe infections interferon has been used with success.

## SQUAMOUS CELL CARCINOMA

This lesion accounts for at least 50% of malignant growths arising in the region of the anus and anal canal, but is rare when compared with carcinoma of the rectum which is about 50 times more common. Squamous carcinoma of the anus is more common in males. The aetiology of anal carcinoma is unknown but chronic irritation or infection may be predisposing factors.

### Clinical features

The patient usually presents with a localised ulcer or raised warty growth with an irregular ulcerated surface. A history of bleeding may give rise to an erroneous diagnosis of haemorrhoids. A profuse discharge results from ulceration and some patients develop incontinence due to involvement of the anal sphincter. Female patients may experience a vaginal discharge due to development of a fistulous communication with the vagina.

The lesion is usually indurated, may spread around the anus, and is often fixed to underlying tissues by the time of presentation. Digital rectal examination may prove impossible because of stenosis or discomfort, but it is important to make certain that the lesion arises from the anus or anal canal, and is not a prolapsing or spreading adeno-carcinoma of the lower rectum. The inguinal lymph nodes are examined carefully as they receive lymph from the lower anal canal and peri-anal region, and may be the seat of metastatic spread. Secondary sepsis produces nodes which are soft or firm, in contrast to the stony hard nodes of secondary neoplastic involvement.

The differential diagnosis of anal carcinoma includes anal papillomas, condylomata lata, primary syphilitic chancre, anal fissure, thrombosed piles, and Crohn's disease. The diagnosis must always be confirmed by biopsy.

### Treatment

Anal carcinoma may be treated by radium implantation or X-ray therapy, but surgical excision is usually preferred if possible. Abdomino-perineal excision of the anus, anal canal and rectum is the treatment of choice, particularly if the lesion extends above the pectinate line. In selected patients there may be a case for a wide local excision of lesions confined to the anal margin or peri-anal area.

Treatment of the inguinal lymph nodes is controversial. Some 40% of patients will have nodal metastases at presentation and block dissection of obviously involved nodes is generally recommended once the patient has recovered fully from treatment of the primary anal lesion. If the nodes are not obviously involved, most surgeons would adopt a watching policy rather than carry out an unnecessary 'prophylactic' block dissection with its attendant hazards of sepsis, skin necrosis and lymphoedema. Radiotherapy offers an alternative method of treating involved inguinal nodes but many surgeons reserve its use for patients with fixed inoperable nodes.

### Results

The prognosis for patients with anal carcinoma is influenced by the extent of spread at the time of presentation, but in general the outlook is less good than that reported for carcinoma of the rectum. Five-year survival rates of around 50% can be achieved if excision is feasible, but few patients with obvious nodal metastases at presentation survive for more than 5 years.

## RARE MALIGNANT TUMOURS

### Adenocarcinoma

Primary adenocarcinoma of the anal region is exceptionally rare but the neoplasm may arise in a long-standing fistula-in-ano, in the anal glands, or in the apocrine glands of the skin around the anal margin. Adenocarcinoma of the rectum may extend into the anal region and malignant cells from a colo-rectal cancer may implant in the raw wound following haemorrhoidectomy.

Primary anal adenocarcinoma is treated in the same way as squamous carcinoma but, in general, the prognosis is poor.

### Basal-cell carcinoma

Basal-cell carcinoma arising in the anal region is rare. The lesion has the same characteristic as basal-cell carcinoma elsewhere and is treated by surgery or radiotherapy.

### Malignant melanoma

Malignant melanoma of the anal region may occasionally be seen.

---

## PILONIDAL SINUS

A pilonidal sinus occurs predominately in the natal cleft of young adults. Pilonidal sinuses are also described in the hands of barbers and occasionally as a cause of umbilical sepsis.

Typically a postanal pilonidal sinus starts at an opening situated 2 cm posterior to the anus and extends subcutaneously in a headward direction for 2–5 cm, expanding into a cavity. Secondary sinuses may arise from this and open onto the surface about 2 cm above the primary opening.

The opening of the sinus is lined by squamous epithelium but only for a few mm. Most of its wall is composed of granulation tissue. A typical feature of the sinus is its content of hairs. These are drawn into the sinus, tips first, and held in its depth by the direction of their scales.

Various theories have been presented to explain the origin of a pilonidal sinus. These include congenital and traction dermoid cysts, remnants of vestigial glands, penetration by hairs due to the rolling action of the buttocks, infection of hair follicles. They were common in US Army personnel during World War II: hence the name 'Jeep disease'.

## CLINICAL FEATURES

A pilonidal sinus does not usually become evident until infected. Then an acute or chronic abscess forms, either forming a red tender hot swelling or a chronic discharge from the sinus. If seen in a quiescent phase the site of the external orifice is diagnostic.

## TREATMENT    Roof Removed and left open.

A pilonidal abscess is drained under general anaesthesia. The abscess cavity is deroofed and thoroughly cleaned out removing hair, granulation tissue and debris at the time. It is left open to granulate and will heal over several weeks.

In a quiescent case, the sinus track is either excised or laid open. Excision of the sinus and its ramifications requires wide removal of tissue (Fig. 32.20). Primary suture is preferable but can be difficult without 'tenting' the skin over the underlying cavity. Rotation flaps have been used to facilitate primary healing.

When primary suture is not feasible or has failed, it is necessary to leave the wound open to granulate. Healing may then take many months. For this reason, marsupialization of the sinuses by laying them open and 'guttering' them by excising the skin edges is preferred by many surgeons. The wound is left open, the skin edges being held apart by a pack or 'stent' of silicone foam so that they cannot reunite.

Recently destruction of granulations by the injection of phenol into the sinus track has been reported to control symptoms.

## AFTER-CARE

Treated pilonidal sinuses are prone to recur. It is important that following any operative procedure for a pilonidal sinus the postanal area is kept clean. In the hirsute, regular shaving is advised.

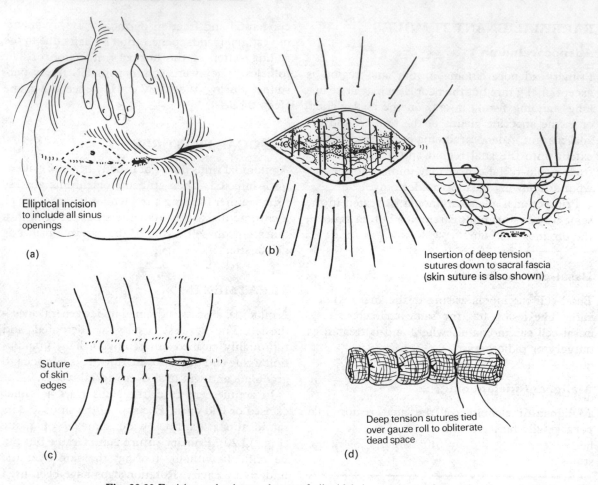

Elliptical incision to include all sinus openings

(a)

(b)

Insertion of deep tension sutures down to sacral fascia (skin suture is also shown)

Suture of skin edges

(c)

Deep tension sutures tied over gauze roll to obliterate dead space

(d)

**Fig. 32.20** Excision and primary closure of pilonidal sinus — steps of operation

# 33. Liver and Biliary System

## LIVER

### ANATOMY

The liver is the largest abdominal organ, weighing approximately 1500 g. It extends from the 5th intercostal space to the right costal margin. It is triangular in shape, its apex reaching the left midclavicular line in the 5th space.

The liver is attached to the undersurface of the diaphragm by suspensory ligaments which enclose a 'bare area', the only part of its surface without a peritoneal covering. Its inferior or visceral surface lies on the right kidney, duodenum, colon and stomach.

Topographically the liver is divided by the attachment of the falciform ligament into right and left lobes; fissures on its visceral surface demarcate two further lobes, the quadrate and caudate. These divisions are of little surgical import. From a practical standpoint it is the segmental anatomy of the liver, as defined by the distribution of its blood supply, which is important to the surgeon.

### Vascular segmental anatomy

The portal vein and hepatic artery divide into right and left branches in the porta hepatis. Occluding the right or left branch produces an easily visible line of demarcation which runs from the gall bladder bed to the inferior vena cava fossa and which separates the surgical lobes. The right surgical lobe is further divided into anterior and posterior segments and the left lobe into medial and lateral segments corresponding to the main branches of the hepatic artery and portal vein (Fig. 33.1).

### Blood supply

The liver has a dual blood supply; 80% from the portal vein and 20% from the hepatic artery. Because of its better oxygenation the hepatic artery supplies 30% of the oxygen requirements.

The venous drainage of the liver is by the right and left hepatic veins, which leave the two surgical lobes of the liver to enter the vena cava. Communications between the portal and systemic venous systems occur at certain defined points, the most important of which from a clinical standpoint lies at the oesophago-gastric junction (Fig. 33.2).

The functional unit of the liver is the hepatic lobule. Sheets of liver cells (hepatocytes) one cell thick are separated by interlacing sinusoids through which blood flows from the portal tract to the central branches of the hepatic venous system. The lobule forms a many sided structure at each angle of which is a portal space containing a branch of the portal vein, hepatic artery and bile duct. Bile is secreted by the liver cells into small canaliculi which pass centrifugally through the lobule to drain into bile ductules leading to the right and left hepatic ducts (Fig. 33.3).

### JAUNDICE

Jaundice is a yellow discolouration of the tissues, most obvious in those containing elastica, e.g.

473

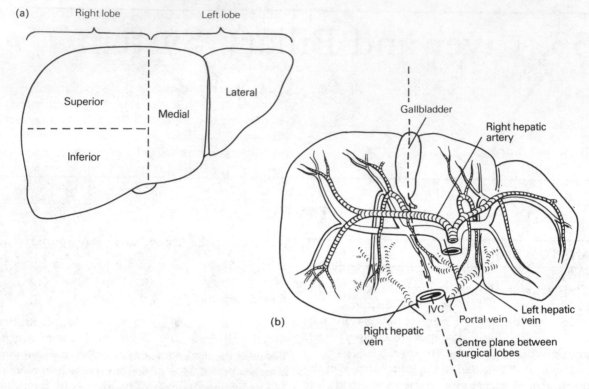

(a)

Right lobe | Left lobe

Superior

Medial | Lateral

Inferior

(b)

Gallbladder

Right hepatic artery

Right hepatic vein

IVC

Portal vein

Left hepatic vein

Centre plane between surgical lobes

**Fig. 33.1** Surgical anatomy of the liver. (a) Lobes. (b) Vasculature.

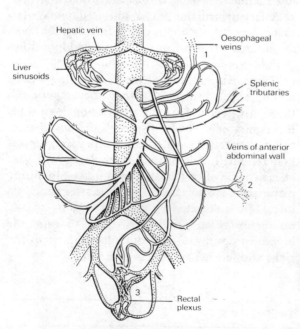

Hepatic vein

Liver sinusoids

Oesophageal veins

Splenic tributaries

Veins of anterior abdominal wall

Rectal plexus

**Fig. 33.2** Portal venous system — the porto-systemic anastomoses are marked 1–3. Retroperitoneal communications also exist

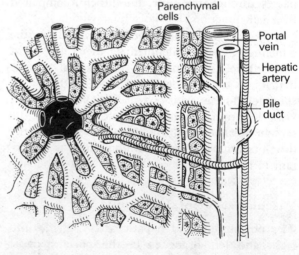

Parenchymal cells

Portal vein

Hepatic artery

Bile duct

**Fig. 33.3** Hepatic lobule

skin and sclera. It is produced by an increase in the amount of circulating bilirubin. Except in the neonatal period and in certain types of liver disease bilirubin does not cross the blood-brain barrier. Increased bilirubin levels may result

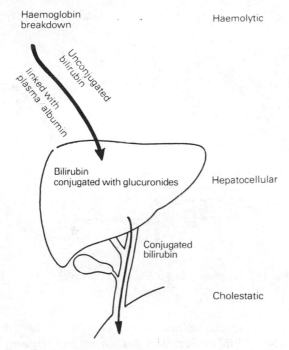

Haemoglobin breakdown

Haemolytic

Unconjugated bilirubin linked with plasma albumin

Bilirubin conjugated with glucuronides

Hepatocellular

Conjugated bilirubin

Cholestatic

**Fig. 33.4** Types of jaundice

from excessive destruction of red blood corpuscles (haemolytic jaundice) or from failure to remove bilirubin from the circulating blood as it passes through the liver due either to impaired liver cell function (hepatocellular jaundice) or to obstruction to the flow of bile from the liver (cholestatic jaundice) (Fig. 33.4).

To the surgeon the most important type of haemolytic jaundice is that caused by hereditary spherocytosis, in which splenectomy may be advised for treatment (see Chapter 37). Haemolytic jaundice may also occur after any operative procedure or trauma, where haematoma formation may give rise to a pigment load which exceeds hepatic excretory capacity.

Hepatocellular jaundice is rarely a surgical problem, but damage to liver cells can follow a general anaesthetic, e.g. with halothane. Cholestatic jaundice due to intrahepatic obstruction of bile canaliculi must be differentiated from extrahepatic biliary obstruction, the cause of jaundice which is of greatest surgical relevance.

Jaundice produced by obstruction to the extrahepatic biliary tract most commonly results from gallstones; other common causes are cancer of the head of the pancreas or major bile ducts, strictures within a duct, or extrinsic compression of the bile ducts, most commonly by metastatic tumour.

## Diagnosis

An accurate diagnosis of the cause of jaundice must be made as soon as possible so that appropriate therapy may be promptly instituted. The age, sex, occupation, social habits, drug and alcohol intake and general demeanour of the patient must all be considered. Detailed enquiry is made concerning abdominal pain, the presence of pruritus, and passage of pale stools or dark urine. The abdomen must be carefully examined for evidence of hepatomegaly, splenomegaly and gallbladder distension, for ascites, and for collateral veins in the abdominal wall. Other stigmata of chronic liver disease such as liver palms, spider naevi, testicular atrophy and gynaecomastia should be sought.

## Biochemical investigations

Liver function tests are of value in determining whether the cause of jaundice is obstructive or not. However, when swelling of the liver cells has both compromised their function and caused biliary obstruction the results may be difficult to interpret.

Biliary obstruction is characterised by circulating bilirubin of conjugated type, which being water soluble, is excreted by the kidneys and therefore is detectable in the urine. As bile cannot pass into the gastro-intestinal tract, urobilinogen is absent from the urine. Blood levels of bilirubin may exceed 500 $\mu$mol/l. Raised serum transaminases and lactic dehydrogenase indicate hepatocellular damage, but these enzymes may still rise in obstructive jaundice. Biliary obstruction increases the formation of alkaline phosphatase by the bile-duct cells and produces raised serum levels. In extrahepatic biliary obstruction the rise in alkaline phosphatase precedes that of bilirubin. When the obstruction is relieved the fall in alkaline phosphatase is more gradual than that of bilirubin.

Serum hepatitis B-surface-antigen status should be tested in all cases of jaundice.

## Imaging investigations

The diagnosis of jaundice has been revolutionised by the development of new imaging techniques.

These include ultrasonic scanning and percutaneous transhepatic cholangiography, using the 'skinny' flexible Chiba needle developed in Japan.

(1) *Ultrasonic scanning* is primarily of value in detecting gallstones, a distended gallbladder, and dilated intra- and extra-hepatic ducts. Liver metastases and a mass in the head of the pancreas may also be detectable.

(2) If duct dilatation is shown by the ultrasonic scan a *percutaneous transhepatic cholangiogram* is used to define the site, nature and in some cases, extent of the obstructing lesion.

(3) If the biliary tract is completely obstructed, the lower extent of the obstruction can be outlined with contrast medium injected through a cannula inserted endoscopically into the bile duct (ERCP — endoscopic retrograde cholangiopancreatography).

(4) An *isotopic liver-scan* using $^{99m}$Tc-sulphur colloid may be helpful in demonstrating liver metastases or other space occupying lesions.

(5) Other radiological investigations, e.g. plain abdominal X-ray, barium swallow and meal, or hypotonic duodenogram (air contrast study of the duodenum which is relaxed by an anticholinergic drug) are of limited value in defining the cause of jaundice and are now seldom employed. Computerised axial tomography (CT-scans) may be useful to identify space-occupying lesions within the liver substance.

## Other investigations

Liver biopsy is a valuable diagnostic procedure in patients with unexplained jaundice in whom an obstructing lesion has been excluded by ultrasonic scanning and/or percutaneous cholangiography. It may be preceded by an isotope (or CT) scan to determine the likelihood of metastatic disease. If metastases are suspected the diagnostic yield is increased if the biopsy is performed under direct vision through a laparoscope (Fig. 33.5). Alternatively a 'target' liver biopsy can be carried out under ultrasound or CT-scanning control, eliminating the need for laparoscopy. Needle aspiration cytology is preferred by some.

The patient's prothrombin time, platelet count and hepatitis B-surface-antigen status must

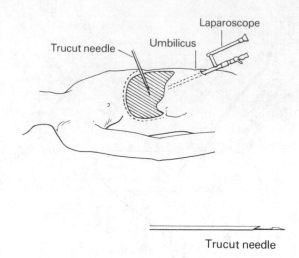

**Fig. 33.5** Laparoscopic needle biopsy of the liver

always be determined and if possible corrected before biopsy. Facilities for emergency laparotomy should be available.

If a tumour of the liver or biliary tract is suspected, a pre-operative arteriogram to demonstrate the vascular anatomy of the liver is advisable. This is performed by selective cannulation of the coeliac and superior mesenteric arteries and injection of contrast medium.

Laparotomy is now seldom necessary to *establish* the cause of jaundice, and with the availability of sophisticated investigations, the modern objective of laparotomy is to *treat* the causative lesion and/or relieve obstruction. Appropriate pre-operative preparation is of particular importance in jaundiced patients (see Chapter 3).

# CONGENITAL ABNORMALITIES

Structural abnormalities of surgical import are rare. Polycystic disease is a cause of liver enlargement and may be associated with polycystic kidneys. Cavernous haemangiomas may cause space-filling defects.

Anatomical abnormalities of the extrahepatic bile ducts are common. These are discussed on page 487.

## LIVER TRAUMA

After the spleen the liver is the solid organ most commonly damaged as a result of abdominal trauma, particularly following road traffic accidents. Stab injuries and gunshot wounds of the liver are also increasing in incidence. These are considered in Chapter 11.

## INFECTIONS AND INFESTATIONS

Acute infections and infestations of the liver may be bacterial, parasitic or viral in origin. The route of infection may be: 1. biliary as a result of ascending cholangitis 2. through the portal venous system from sepsis within the abdomen 3. by the hepatic artery, e.g. from a septic focus elsewhere 4. by direct spread from adjacent sepsis, e.g. empyema of the gallbladder or a subhepatic abscess 5. following direct injury, e.g. stab wounds

The commonest surgical cause of infection is calculous obstruction of the biliary tree with cholangitis. Infection via the portal route (portal pyaemia) used to occur from appendicitis or diverticulitis, but is now rare. Amoebic hepatitis, actinomycosis and hydatid disease of the liver arise by portal venous spread of the causal agent.

### Pyogenic liver abscess

This is a rare condition. The symptoms are typically insidious and the abscess may present as pyrexia of unknown origin. A history of sepsis elsewhere, particularly within the abdomen, may then be helpful. Other cases present with pyrexia, rigors, toxicity and jaundice.

The liver may be enlarged and tender. A plain X-ray may show an elevated diaphragm, right pleural effusion or basal lobe collapse. Leucocytosis (over $15 \times 10^9/l$) is usually present and the serum alkaline phosphatase may be raised. Repeated blood cultures should be performed. Ultrasonic, radioisotope ($^{99m}$Tc-sulphur colloid) liver scan, or CT-scan will demonstrate a space occupying lesion, while ultrasonic or CT-scan will differentiate abscess from tumour.

If left untreated, spread within the liver produces multiple abscesses with progressive parenchymal damage. Fatal septicaemia may occur.

Treatment consists of adequate surgical drainage under antibiotic cover. This is performed by a transperitoneal approach, a large tube being inserted into the abscess cavity and brought out through the abdominal wall. The tube is left *in situ* until serial X-rays following injection of contrast material have shown that the abscess cavity has collapsed around it. Appropriate antibiotic therapy depends upon the organism responsible. If this is not known pre-operatively, a broad-spectrum antibiotic combined with metronidazole should be used. If the position of the abscess is suitable a drain may be inserted percutaneously under ultrasonic guidance. Multiple small abscesses may resolve on antibiotic treatment alone.

### Amoebic hepatitis and abscess

*Entamoeba histolytica* is a protozoal parasite which infests the large intestine. The amoebae may spread through the portal system to the liver to produce amoebic hepatitis and an amoebic abscess. Usually solitary and situated in the right lobe, the abscess is large and thin-walled and contains brownish sterile pus resembling anchovy sauce. Amoebae may be demonstrated in its wall.

Pain in the right upper quadrant is the most striking symptom. This is accompanied by anorexia, nausea, weight loss and night sweats. Over 90% of patients have tender enlargement of the liver. Other signs include basal pulmonary collapse, pleural effusion and leucocytosis. Ultrasonic and radio-isotope liver scans are helpful to demonstrate the site and size of the abscess.

The stool should be examined for amoebae or cysts. Direct and indirect serological tests to detect amoebic protein are available.

If untreated an amoebic abscess may rupture into the peritoneal cavity or into a bronchus. Metastatic brain abscesses have been reported. Treatment consists of administration of an amoebicide (metronidazole) and usually results in rapid resolution. If there is no clinical response within 72 hours the abscess should be aspirated by needle puncture. Drainage by open operation is indicated only when there is secondary infection.

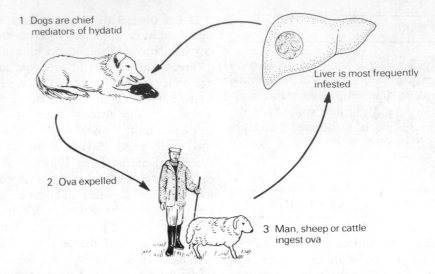

1 Dogs are chief
mediators of hydatid

Liver is most frequently
infested

2 Ova expelled

3 Man, sheep or cattle
ingest ova

**Fig. 33.6** Life cycle of *Echinococcus granulosus*

## Hydatid disease

This is most commonly caused by the tapeworm of the dog *(Echinococcus granulosus)*; sheep or man serve as the intermediate host (Fig. 33.6). The condition is common in sheep- rearing areas, e.g. Greece or Australia where dogs, sheep and men live in close contact. In Britain it is most common in South Wales. The tapeworm normally inhabits the dog intestine. Its ova are passed in the faeces which may contaminate the food or fingers and so be ingested by man. They hatch in the duodenum and the embryos enter the portal venous system and pass to the liver where they form a hydatid cyst. The cyst wall is surrounded by an adventitial layer of fibrous tissue and consists of a laminated membrane lined by germinal epithelium on which brood capsules containing scoleces develop.

The disease may be symptomless, but chronic right upper quadrant pain and enlargement of the liver are common presenting features. The cyst may rupture into the biliary tree or peritoneal cavity, the latter sometimes causing an acute anaphylactic reaction from absorption of foreign hydatid protein. Other complications include secondary infection and biliary obstruction with jaundice.

Eosinophilia is common and serological tests are available to detect the foreign protein.

Hydatid cysts commonly calcify and may be seen on a plain film of the abdomen. Alternatively they can be detected by ultrasonic, radioisotope, or CT-scans of the liver.

Treatment consists of shelling out the cyst or resecting it in its entirety with surrounding liver tissue. To prevent seeding of brood capsules it is customary first to inject the cyst with 3% sodium chloride, 0.5% formalin or 0.5% sodium hypochlorite to kill the scoleces. During operation, care is taken not to spill the contents into the peritoneal cavity or anaphylaxis may result.

## PORTAL HYPERTENSION

Portal hypertension is usually caused by increased resistance to portal venous blood flow, the obstruction being either pre-hepatic, hepatic or post-hepatic. Rarely it results primarily from an increase in portal blood flow. The normal pressure in the portal vein varies from 5–15 cm water (5–10 mm Hg). When the portal venous pressure is consistently raised above 25 cm of water (20 mmHg) there may be serious clinical consequences.

The causes of portal hypertension are shown in Table 33.1.

Portal vein thrombosis is a rare cause. It is most commonly due to neonatal umbilical sepsis, though the effects may not be manifest for many years.

By far the commonest cause of portal hyperten-

**Table 33.1** Causes of portal hypertension

1. Pre-hepatic
   a. Congenital atresia of the portal vein
   b. Portal vein thrombosis — neonatal sepsis
                              — pyelophlebitis
                              — trauma
                              — tumour
   c. Extrinsic compression — pancreatic disease
      of portal vein        — lymphadenopathy
                            — biliary tract tumours

2. Intrahepatic
   a. Cirrhosis
   b. Schistosomiasis

3. Post-hepatic
   a. Budd-Chiari syndrome
   b. Inferior vena caval webs
   c. Constrictive pericarditis
4. Increased portal blood flow
   a. Arteriovenous fistula
   b. Increased splenic blood flow

sion is cirrhosis of the liver. This results from chronic liver disease and is characterised by liver cell damage, fibrosis and nodular regeneration. Micronodular and macronodular types are described. In micronodular cirrhosis there is an even distribution of nodules a few mm in diameter in contrast to those of macronodular cirrhosis which are uneven in size and sometimes very large. Macronodules are usually found in end-stage cirrhosis, irrespective of its aetiology. The fibrosis obstructs portal venous return and portal hypertension develops. Arterio-venous shunts within the liver also contribute to the hypertension.

Alcohol is the commonest aetiological factor in Western countries and is increasing in prevalence. In North Africa, the Middle East and China schistosomiasis due to *Bilharzia mansonii* is a common cause. Chronic active hepatitis, primary and secondary biliary cirrhosis are relatively rare causes in this country. In a large number of patients the cause of cirrhosis remains obscure (cryptogenic cirrhosis).

Obstruction of hepatic venous blood flow is the most frequent cause of post-hepatic portal hypertension. It is most frequently a consequence of spontaneous thrombosis of the hepatic veins and has been associated with neoplasia, oral contraceptive agents and polycythaemia. The resulting Budd-Chiari syndrome is characterised by portal hypertension, liver failure and gross ascites.

## EFFECTS OF PORTAL HYPERTENSION

As a result of gradual or chronic occlusion of the portal venous system, collateral pathways develop between portal and systemic venous circulations. Eventually a large proportion of portal venous blood enters the systemic circulation directly, and may give rise to hepatic encephalopathy. Porta-systemic shunting occurs at the junction of oesophagus and fundus of the stomach, in retroperitoneal and peri-umbilical collaterals, and in anastomotic veins in the anal region (Fig. 33.2).

The most important consequence of shunting is the development of oesophageal varices. The submucosal plexus of veins in the lower oesophagus and gastric fundus becomes variceal: oesophageal varices may then rupture to cause acute massive gastrointestinal tract bleeding. Such bleeding occurs in about 40% of cirrhotics. The initial episode of variceal haemorrhage may be fatal.

Progressive enlargement of the spleen occurs from vascular engorgement and associated hypertrophy. Haematological consequences are anaemia, thrombocytopenia and leucopenia (hypersplenism: see Chapter 37). Ascites may develop and is due to an increased formation of hepatic and splanchnic lymph, hypoalbuminaemia, and salt and water retention. Increased aldosterone and antidiuretic hormone levels may contribute.

*Porta-systemic encephalopathy* is due to the increasing levels of toxins such as ammonia in the systemic circulation. This is particularly likely to develop where there are large spontaneous or surgically created porta-systemic shunts. Gastrointestinal haemorrhage increases the absorption of nitrogenous products and predisposes to encephalopathy.

## CLINICAL PRESENTATION

Patients with portal hypertension usually present to a surgeon (1) because of active and sometimes massive bleeding from oesophageal varices, (2) for consideration of elective surgical treatment after recovery from an episode of acute haemorrhage and (3) because of the discovery of varices which have not yet bled. Patients in this third group are usually only kept under supervision, but they remain a cause for concern.

## ACUTE BLEEDING

Patients presenting with acute upper gastro-intestinal bleeding are carefully examined for evidence of chronic liver disease. The liver may be palpably enlarged, firm or nodular, the spleen may be enlarged, and ascites may be present. Jaundice, spider naevi, liver palms, opaque nails and finger clubbing are also sought. Distended collateral veins may be visible, particularly around the umbilicus where they give rise to a 'caput medusa'. Slurring of speech, a flapping tremor or dysarthria may point to encephalo-pathy, and this may be precipitated or intensified by accumulation of blood in the gastrointestinal tract. Liver function tests and a coagulation screen are arranged.

While a barium swallow and meal will detect oesophageal and gastric varices, the key investiga-tion during an episode of active bleeding is endo-scopy. This allows recognition of varices and defines whether they are or have been the actual site of bleeding. It is important to remember that peptic ulcer and gastritis are common complaints which occur in 20% of patients with varices. Even although a patient is known to have chronic liver disease and varices, bleeding cannot be assumed to be due to this cause.

## Management

The priorities in the management of bleeding oesophageal varices are as follows (Table 33.2):

*Active resuscitation.* Blood is withdrawn for grouping and cross-matching, a free-flowing intra-venous line is established, a urinary catheter is inserted to measure hourly urine output, pulse rate and blood pressure are monitored, and a central venous line is inserted to monitor central venous pressure. Large volumes of blood may be lost rapidly in these patients and the aim should be to replace blood loss quickly with a view to urgent endoscopy. Many patients bleeding from varices will have coagulation defects from the outset and thrombocytopenia is common as a manifestation of hypersplenism. Fresh blood is preferred for transfusion purposes and the advice of a haematologist may be sought regarding the use of fresh frozen plasma or platelet transfusion.

*Urgent endoscopy* is performed at the earliest opportunity and in patients threatened by mas-sive bleeding, active resuscitation is instituted and continued in the endoscopy suite. If varices are confirmed as the site of blood loss, measures are instituted to control bleeding.

*Control of bleeding.* Balloon tamponade is most commonly used. The four lumen Minnesota tube

**Table 33.2** Priorities in management of bleeding oesophageal varices

*Active resuscitation*
  group and cross match blood
  establish IV infusion line(s)
  monitor pulse
    blood pressure
    hourly urine output
    central venous pressure
*Measure coagulation*
  thrombin time
  kaolin cephalin clotting time
  prothrombin time
  platelet count
*Urgent endoscopy*
*Arrest haemorrhage*
  tamponade (Minnesota tube)
  pharmacological measures (e.g. vasopressin)
*Treat hepatocellular decompensation*
*Treat/prevent portasystemic encephalopathy*
*Prevent further bleeding from varices*
  Injection sclerotherapy
  Staple oesophago-gastric junction
  Portasystemic shunting

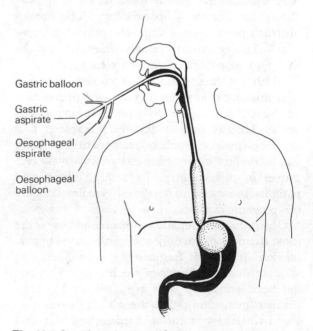

Gastric balloon

Gastric aspirate

Oesophageal aspirate

Oesophageal balloon

**Fig. 33.7** Oesophageal tamponade

(Fig. 33.7) has replaced the three lumen Sengstaken-Blakemore tube. The four lumina allow: 1. aspiration of gastric contents 2. inflation of a gastric balloon with 150 ml of water to which a radio-opaque dye (Hypaque) has been added so that balloon position can be checked radiologically. This balloon compresses the gastric fundus and oesophago-gastric junction, so reducing the flow of blood into the oesophageal varices. 3. inflation of an oesophageal balloon with air to a pressure of 40 mmHg using a sphygmomanometer. This balloon applies direct pressure to the oesophageal varices. 4. aspiration of the oesophagus and pharynx above the oesophageal balloon, so reducing the risk of aspiration pneumonitis and pneumonia.

Traction is applied to the Minnesota tube by pulling the gastric balloon up against the oesophago-gastric junction and then taping a spatula to the tube as it emerges from the angle of the mouth. A trained nurse should be in constant attendance and the pharynx and stomach are aspirated at 15–30 minute intervals. Balloon tamponade will arrest bleeding from varices in over 90% of patients but the tube should not be left in place for more than 24–36 hours for fear of causing oesophageal necrosis. Tamponade should be regarded as a 'holding measure' which allows further resuscitation and treatment of hepatic decompensation. Unless more definitive measures are used to prevent further variceal bleeding (see below), two-thirds of individuals will rebleed while still in hospital and 90% will rebleed within a year.

Some physicians advocate *vasopressin* as the first-line measure to arrest variceal haemorrhage. The agent is administered intravenously, and infusion (20 units in 200 ml saline over 20 minutes) is now generally preferred to bolus injection. Vasopressin constricts splanchnic arterioles, thus reducing mesenteric blood flow and portal venous pressure. The dose may be repeated after 3–4 hours but the compound is usually less effective when used repeatedly. Vasopressin constricts coronary arterioles and is contra-indicated in the elderly and those known to have myocardial ischaemia.

The $\beta$-adrenergic blocking drug propanolol is now under trial.

*Further resuscitation and treatment of hepatocellular decompensation.* Control of variceal bleeding allows blood loss to be made good and permits full assessment of coagulopathy. Cimetidine (400 mg i.v. 6-hourly) is prescribed to reduce the risk of bleeding from gastritis or peptic ulceration, and may be combined with instillation of antacids down the gastric lumen of the Minnesota tube. A daily bowel washout is used to evacuate blood from the gut and reduce the risk of porta-systemic encephalopathy. This endeavour can be assisted by prescribing aperients such as magnesium sulphate. Alternatively, magnesium trisilicate (30 ml 4-hourly) can be used for both its antacid and aperient properties. Oral neomycin (0.5 g 6-hourly) and lactulose (15–30 ml t.d.s.) are prescribed to reduce bacterial degradation of blood in the gut lumen and further reduce the risk of encephalopathy. Patients with oesophageal varices due to liver disease frequently have major defects in both the intrinsic and extrinsic clotting systems which may prove refractory to therapy. Vitamin $K_1$ is prescribed to aid restoration of the extrinsic system, but fresh frozen plasma, factor concentrates and platelet transfusion may all be required to cover specific procedures such as sclerotherapy or surgery. It should be stressed that these transfusion measures have transient effects on blood coagulation and that the ultimate coagulation status depends upon restoration of hepatic function.

*Prevention of further bleeding.* A number of methods are now available to reduce the risk of further variceal bleeding. It is as yet uncertain which method or methods offer the safest most effective form of management. Alternatives are:

1. *Injection sclerotherapy.* The varices may be closed by direct injection of sclerosant (e.g. ethanolamine) using a rigid or fibre-optic oesophagoscope. The rigid oesophagoscope has the disadvantage that general anaesthesia is required and carries a higher risk of oesophageal trauma with perforation. On the other hand, bleeding during injection can be controlled more readily by direct pressure from the oesophagoscope, and more powerful suction can be used to maintain vision throughout the procedure. Multiple or excessive injection may be complicated by oesophageal ulceration and necrosis.

Some surgeons employ injection sclerotherapy as an 'extended holding procedure' to buy time in which to prepare patients for surgery. In some centres the method is being employed on a long-term basis in the hope that surgery can be avoided.

2. *Percutaneous transhepatic embolisation.* Oeso-

phageal varices can be occluded by embolisation with material (e.g. gelfoam, autologous clot) introduced through a catheter passed through the liver and thence via the portal vein into the veins at the oesophago-gastric junction. This method has not been applied widely but may be useful in the acute bleeding phase.

3. *Surgical disconnection.* The flow of blood into oesophageal varices from the portal venous system can be interrupted by direct venous ligation using a trans-thoracic approach to the oesophagus, by transecting and then rejoining the oesophago-gastric junction or cardia, or by stapling the oesophago-gastric junction (Fig. 33.8). Stapling is relatively easy to perform and a stapling device is passed into the oesophago-gastric junction having first opened the stomach at laparotomy. A double row of staples is then inserted through the full thickness of the oesophageal wall to occlude venous flow.

4. *Emergency porta-systemic shunting.* Emergency shunting carries a prohibitive mortality and is no longer advised.

## CHRONIC PORTAL HYPERTENSION

Following the control of bleeding the patient requires assessment to determine whether surgi-cal decompression of the portal venous system by a porta-systemic venous shunt is indicated. This produces an abrupt fall in portal venous pressure, and recurrent variceal bleeding is unlikely. However, postoperative encephalopathy can be a serious problem.

The indications for shunting are therefore strict. In general operation is advised only for patients with venous obstruction (portal vein thrombosis) and those cirrhotics whose condition is not complicated by jaundice, ascites or encephalopathy (Table 33.3).

## Portal venography

This is an essential pre-operative investigation to determine the anatomy of the portal vein. It is performed by injecting contrast material into the splenic pulp and taking serial X-rays. The portal venous pressure can also be measured. Alternatively a coeliac angiogram can be performed and films taken during the venous phase to demonstrate portal venous patency. Ultrasonic and CT-scans may also be used to examine the state of the portal vein.

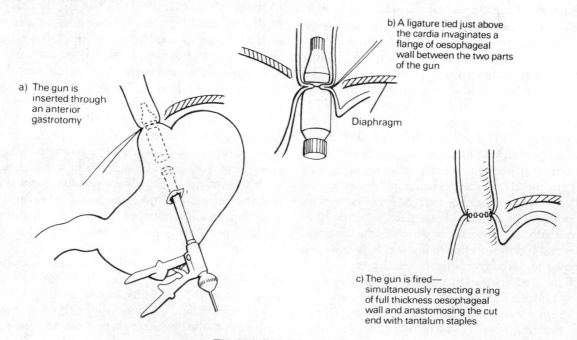

a) The gun is inserted through an anterior gastrotomy

b) A ligature tied just above the cardia invaginates a flange of oesophageal wall between the two parts of the gun

Diaphragm

c) The gun is fired— simultaneously resecting a ring of full thickness oesophageal wall and anastomosing the cut end with tantalum staples

**Fig. 33.8** Oesophageal stapling

## Shunt operations

There are several anatomical sites at which porta-systemic shunts can be performed (Fig. 33.9). In a portacaval shunt the portal vein is anastomosed, either end-to-side or side-to-side to the vena cava. Mesocaval shunts are formed between the superior mesenteric vein and the vena cava using either an autogenous saphenous vein graft or a synthetic H-graft. They are easier to perform but have a high incidence of thrombosis.

Splenorenal shunts, between the splenic and renal veins, are most appropriate when there is portal vein obstruction. Encephalopathy is reported to be less frequent. The distal splenorenal shunt (Warren), which selectively decompresses the lower oesophagus and upper stomach and maintains liver blood flow, is preferred now by many surgeons. The incidence of encephalopathy is reported to be lower than after other shunt procedures.

The results of shunt surgery are very variable.

**Table 33.3** Assessment of patients with portal hypertension by modification of Child's criteria (shunt contraindicated in group C)

| Criterion | Points scored | | |
|---|---|---|---|
| | 1 | 2 | 3 |
| Encephalopathy | none | minimal | marked |
| Ascites | none | slight | moderate |
| Bilirubin ($\mu$mol/l) | <35 | 35–50 | >50 |
| Albumin (g/1) | >35 | 28–35 | <28 |
| Prothrombin ratio | <1.4 | 1.4–2.0 | >2.0 |

Grade A = score   5–6
     B =         7–9
     C =       10–15

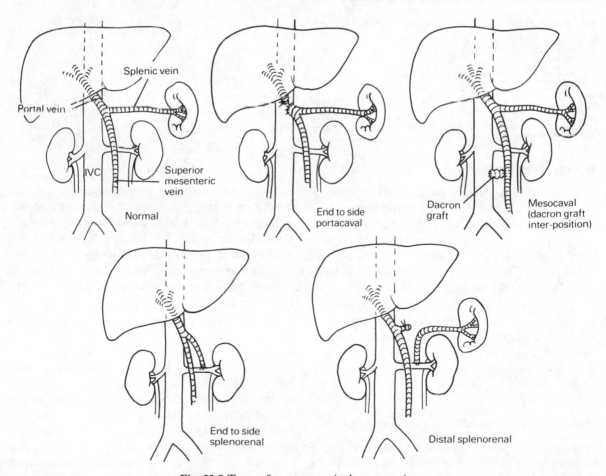

**Fig. 33.9** Types of porta-systemic shunt operations

## ASCITES

Ascites can be controlled with salt and water restriction and a combination of a sodium-losing diuretic (frusemide) and an aldosterone inhibitor (spironolactone). If refractory, ascites can be treated by inserting a peritoneojugular shunt (LeVeen) which allows one-way flow between the peritoneum and jugular vein (Fig. 33.10).

## ENCEPHALOPATHY

Encephalopathy is treated by a low-protein diet, oral neomycin and, should these fail, lactulose, the objective being to reduce the bacterial decomposition of protein in the intestine.

## TUMOURS OF THE LIVER

Hepatic tumours are either benign or malignant, primary or secondary.

## PRIMARY TUMOURS

Primary tumours may arise from the parenchymal cells, the epithelium of the bile ducts or supporting tissues.

### Benign hepatic tumours

The *cavernous haemangioma* is the most common benign liver tumour. Most are asymptomatic and are found incidentally at laparotomy. Occasionally they reach a large size and patients present with pain, an abdominal mass, or haemorrhage. Heart failure may develop if there is a large arteriovenous communication.

*Liver-cell adenomas* have increased markedly in incidence over the last decade. It has been suggested that oral contraceptive agents are responsible. Focal nodular hyperplasia of the liver has also been associated with oral contraceptive agents.

### Hepatocellular carcinoma (hepatoma)

Hepatocellular carcinoma (hepatoma) is relatively uncommon in the Western world while in Africa and the Far East it is common. Environmental

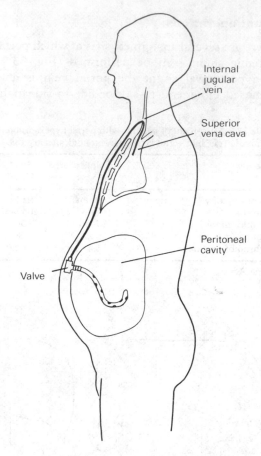

**Fig. 33.10** LeVeen shunt

factors are probably of great importance; in the American negro the incidence is the same as that in the white American population. The tumour is commoner in males than females. In the Western world about two-thirds of patients have pre-existing cirrhosis; many others have hepatitis B-surface-antigen in their blood. In Africa and the East, 'aflatoxin' derived from the fungus *Aspergillus flavus*, which contaminates maize and nuts, is an important hepatocarcinogen. Viral hepatitis is also now regarded as an aetiological factor.

*Clinical features.* The diagnosis is usually made late in the course of the disease. Common presenting features include abdominal pain, weight loss, abdominal distension, fever and intraperitoneal haemorrhage. In Westerners, rapid increase in symptoms in a cirrhotic patient should lead to suspicion of tumour. Jaundice is uncommon unless the tumour is associated with advanced cirrhosis. On examination the liver is usually grossly enlarged.

Serum alpha-fetoprotein (an oncofetal antigen) is present in the serum of 80% of African patients with hepatocellular carcinoma. It is present in only 30% of the white population with this disease. A filling defect is apparent on scintiscanning with $^{99m}$Tc sulphur colloid, while the same area shows an increased uptake when $^{75}$Se selenomethionine is used. Plain X-ray may show calcification or detect pulmonary or other metastases. Ultrasonic scan, CT-scans and selective coeliac arteriography are valuable to determine the extent of the tumour and assess the feasibility of resection.

*Treatment.* The only chance of cure lies in complete surgical resection of the tumour. This is only feasible when one lobe or segment of the liver is completely free of disease. As there is a tendency for satellite lesions to surround a primary central tumour, this is unusual. For advanced tumours either hepatic artery ligation or chemotherapy using doxorubicin (Adriamycin), methotrexate or 5-fluorouracil may have palliative value. The disease is usually advanced at the time of presentation and the 5-year survival rate is less than 10%.

### Cholangiocarcinoma

This is an adenocarcinoma arising from the bile duct system. It may arise anywhere in the biliary tree including the intrahepatic radicles. It accounts for about 20% of malignant primary neoplasms of the liver in Western medicine. In the Orient it is most commonly associated with chronic parasitic infestation of the biliary tree.

Jaundice is the common presenting feature, and the diagnosis is usually made by percutaneous transhepatic cholangiography which defines the site of the tumour. An ERCP may be necessary to outline its extent. Treatment consists of resection when possible. Palliative intubation with a 'stent' or U-tube may relieve jaundice even when the tumour is within the liver.

### Angiosarcoma

This is a rare tumour of the liver which arises after industrial exposure to vinyl chloride. It is a late complication of exposure to the radiological contrast medium Thorotrast or to arsenicals.

The prognosis in patients with malignant liver tumours is extremely poor but improved techniques of liver resection and transplantation may influence this picture.

## METASTATIC TUMOURS

The liver is a common site for metastatic disease. Secondary liver tumours are 20 times more common than primary ones. In one half of cases the original tumour is in the intestinal tract; other common sites are the breast, ovaries, bronchus and kidney. Almost 90% of patients with hepatic metastases have tumour deposits in other organs.

Hepatomegaly and tenderness are distinctive features, and individual deposits may be palpable. The patient is often cachectic and ascites or jaundice may be present. Pyrexia occurs in 10–20% of patients with metastatic tumours of the liver, and may initially be regarded as pyrexia of unknown origin. Liver function tests are abnormal, particularly the alkaline phosphatase, LDH and gamma-glutamyl transpeptidase which are raised. Ultrasonic scans, scintiscans and CT-scans may demonstrate multiple filling defects. The diagnosis is confirmed by aspiration cytology or needle biopsy, best performed through a laparoscope.

There is no effective treatment for most patients with hepatic metastases. Both lobes of the liver are usually involved making surgical resection impossible. Hepatic artery ligation, radiotherapy and chemotherapy have all been used but the results have been disappointing.

Palpation of the liver for metastases should be carried out at all laparotomies. As benign cysts and adenomas may lead to confusion with small surface metastases, suspicious lesions should be visualised if at all possible. In some tumours, e.g. colon, an apparently solitary metastases may be resected, and reasonable survival periods have been reported.

## LIVER RESECTION

The techniques of liver resection are complicated and in general such operations as hepatic lobectomy should be performed only by those with experience. Basically the vascular supply to the involved area of the liver is ligated and divided following which the devascularised lobe or segment can be separated by 'finger-fracture' of the parenchyma along the border with fully vascularised tissue. Intervening biliary and vascular channels can be felt, defined and ligated.

Adequate drainage of the area is essential following resection.

## LIVER TRANSPLANTATION

This is considered on page 153.

# THE GALL BLADDER AND BILE DUCTS

## ANATOMY OF THE BILIARY SYSTEM

The biliary 'tree' consists of fine intrahepatic biliary radicles, the right and left hepatic ducts, the common hepatic duct and the common bile duct. The right and left hepatic ducts converge to form the common hepatic duct which is 3–4 cm in length. It is joined at a variable position by the cystic duct to form the common bile duct which ends at the papilla of Vater, usually in the second part of the duodenum (Fig. 33.11).

The common bile duct is approximately 8 cm in length and 6 mm in diameter. It lies in the free edge of the lesser omentum before passing behind the first part of the duodenum and into the head of the pancreas. The bile duct is usually joined by the pancreatic duct just before entering the duodenum.

The gallbladder lies in its bed on the undersurface of the liver between the right and left lobes. It is a muscular pyriform structure which has four portions: fundus, corpus, infundibulum and the neck which tapers into the cystic duct. Hartmann's pouch is a dilatation of the gallbladder outlet adjacent to the origin of the cystic duct in which gallstones frequently become impacted. The gallbladder is supplied by the cystic artery, a branch of the right hepatic.

## PHYSIOLOGY OF BILE AND THE GALLBLADDER

### BILE ACIDS AND THE ENTEROHEPATIC CIRCULATION

Bile acids are sterols synthesised by the liver from cholesterol. The primary bile acids are *chenodeoxy-*

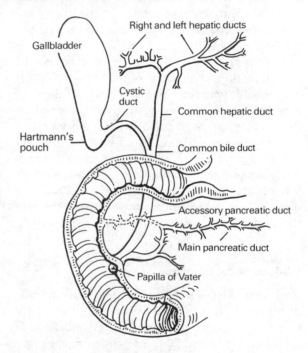

Fig. 33.11 The anatomy of the biliary tree

*cholic* acid and *cholic acid*; these are conjugated with either glycine or taurine to enhance water solubility. The action of intestinal bacteria on these compounds produces the secondary bile acids, *deoxycholic acid* and *lithocholic acid*.

Bile acids are detergents. They increase the solubility of lipids to facilitate their absorption. In aqueous solutions bile acids aggregate in groups of 8–10 molecules to form *micelles* (Fig. 33.12). *Lecithin* and *cholesterol* which comprise 90% of the solid constituents of bile are transported within these micelles. On reaching the distal ileum 95% of the bile acids excreted into the intestine are reabsorbed and recirculated

MICELLE

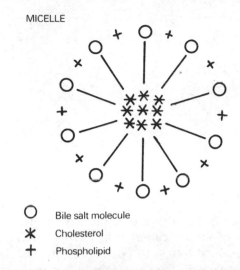

○  Bile salt molecule
✱  Cholesterol
╈  Phospholipid

**Fig. 33.12** Cholesterol micelle

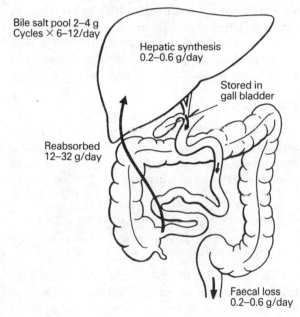

Bile salt pool 2–4 g
Cycles × 6–12/day

Hepatic synthesis
0.2–0.6 g/day

Stored in
gall bladder

Reabsorbed
12–32 g/day

Faecal loss
0.2–0.6 g/day

**Fig. 33.13** The enterohepatic circulation

through the liver — the *enterohepatic circulation* (Fig. 33.13).

The normal bile acid pool is between 3–5 g. The gallbladder has a capacity of about 50 ml and is capable of concentrating bile by a factor of 10. Bile pigments and cholesterol are not absorbed in the gallbladder. Consequently their concentration in the bile is increased. The gallbladder contracts in response to cholecystokinin which is released from the duodenal mucosa following a meal, and

to a lesser extent on vagal stimulation. Contraction is accompanied by reciprocal relaxation of the sphincter of Oddi.

## CONGENITAL ABNORMALITIES

Congenital abnormalities of the gallbladder and bile ducts are of some surgical importance. The gallbladder may be absent (agenesis), double, partitioned with a fundic fold (Phrygian cap), or multiseptate. Anomalies of the bile ducts and extrahepatic biliary vessels are common. The cystic duct is absent in 1.5% while accessory ducts are present in 10% of persons. The cystic artery may be duplicated or may arise from the common hepatic or left hepatic artery.

### Biliary atresia

Biliary atresia is a failure of the duct system to develop. It occurs once in every 20 000 to 30 000 births and may be familial. Overall, biliary atresia affects the sexes equally. When confined to the extra-hepatic biliary radicles (which occurs in two-thirds of patients) there is a male preponderance of 2:1.

In some cases a slight icteric tinge is present at birth; more often jaundice begins in the first few weeks of life and thereafter progresses rapidly. The urine is dark, the stools clay-coloured, and the liver and spleen enlarge. The alkaline phosphatase and bilirubin are markedly elevated. There is a moderate rise in serum transaminases.

Treatment consists of surgical exploration and, where possible, anastomosis of the dilated hepatic ducts to the jejunum. Delays cause cirrhosis and liver failure. Intrahepatic duct atresia is rarely amenable to surgical reconstruction, and liver transplant may be considered.

### Choledochal cysts

Cystic transformation of the common bile duct, (choledochal cyst) is a rare condition which is usually associated with an anatomical abnormality of the lower end of the common bile duct. Although the cyst may not become evident clinically for many years, the majority are congenital. Some

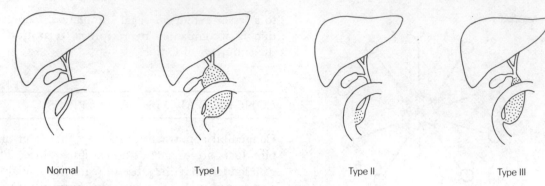

**Fig. 33.14** Choledochal cysts

develop during pregnancy as a result of connective tissue relaxation.

There are three major varieties (Fig. 33.14):

1. cystic dilatation involving the entire common bile duct and common hepatic duct system, the cystic duct entering the choledochal cyst

2. a small cyst usually localised to the distal common bile duct, and

3. diffuse fusiform dilatation of the common bile duct.

Congenital multicystic saccular transformation of the biliary tree (Caroli's disease) is a rare abnormality affecting the whole biliary system.

Choledochal cysts present with attacks of obstructive jaundice, usually accompanied by upper abdominal pain and pyrexia. A mass may be palpable in the right hypochondrium. Ultrasonic scans and cholangiography establish the diagnosis. The treatment of choice is excision of the cyst with choledocho-jejunostomy (Roux-en-Y, Fig. 33.15). Alternatively the cyst may be drained into the duodenum or jejunum. Malignant change may complicate long-standing untreated choledochal cysts.

## GALLSTONES

### PATHOGENESIS OF GALLSTONES

Gallstones are crystalline structures formed from the constituents of bile. There are two main types — cholesterol and calcium bilirubinate (pigment) stones, and both are composed of substances insoluble in water. 'Mixed' stones contain appreciable amounts of cholesterol and bile pigment, but usually contain at least 50% cholesterol, and

are regarded as a type of cholesterol stone.

Gallstones are common in Europe and North America and less so throughout Africa and Asia. In 'developed' countries they occur in at least 20% of women over the age of 40; the incidence in males is approximately one third that in females. The disease is increasing in frequency, so that the number of cholecystectomies performed over the past 10 years in Britain, France and Canada has doubled.

### Cholesterol stones

Cholesterol stones occur in both sexes from the late teens onwards but predominate in middle aged, obese, multiparous females. There are three phases in gallstone formation:

1. formation of saturated bile
2. nucleation, or initiation of stone formation, and
3. growth of the stone.

The solubility of cholesterol in bile is determined by the amount of bile and lecithin present, and by water content. Cholesterol precipitates when there is too much cholesterol to be solubilised in micelles or when there is too little bile acid and lecithin. Factors responsible for cholesterol supersaturation are: enzymatic changes in the bile, reduction in the bile salt pool and a relative increase in cholesterol concentration during fasting. Not all subjects with supersaturated bile develop gallstones and other factors must be implicated.

No matter how saturated the bile, stones form only if cholesterol crystals are present. Formation of cholesterol crystals is called 'nucleation' and

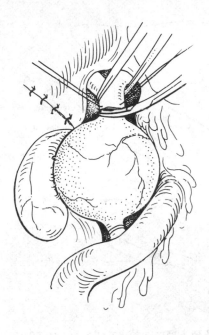

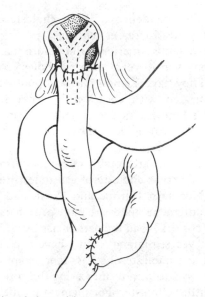

**Fig. 33.15** Treatment of choledochal cyst using cholecyst-jejunostomy

occurs either from random coalescence of cholesterol molecules, or from precipitation around
some other particles of mucus, calcium bilirubinate, cells from the gallbladder mucosa, and bacteria. Pure cholesterol stones are yellowish-green
with a regular shape but rough surface.

Cholesterol stone formation is associated with:

1. *Obesity*. This is accompanied by highly supersaturated gallbladder bile, predisposing to cholesterol cholelithiasis.

2. *Diet*. Obesity apart, a high-calorie diet promotes gallstone formation through an increase in
hepatic cholesterol secretion. Low-calorie diets
producing drastic weight reduction lead to mobilisation of cholesterol from adipose tissue. As initially this cholesterol is secreted into a smaller bile-
acid pool, supersaturation of bile results. Diets
high in cholesterol and polyunsaturated fat and
possibly those low in dietary fibre, also predispose
to gallstone formation.

3. *Gastrointestinal disorders*. Disease, resection or
bypass of the terminal ileum interrupts the enterohepatic circulation of bile acids. The bile-acid pool
shrinks and gallstone formation is enhanced.

4. *Drugs*. An increased frequency of gallstones
occurs in patients taking clofibrate.

5. *Female sex hormones*. Women taking oral
contraceptive agents and postmenopausal oestrogen replacement are more prone to develop gallstones.

In humans hypercholesterolaemia is not associated with an increase in gallstone formation.

## Pigment stones

Pigment stones consist of calcium bilirubinate.
They are small, black, shiny and amorphous and
vary in size from 5 mm to sludge particles.

Pigment stones account for 30% of gallstones.
They are more commonly found in older patients.
The sex-ratio is equal and affected patients are
often lean. Factors influencing pigment stone
formation are:

1. *Haemolysis*. Conditions that shorten the life-
span of red cells, including haemolysis from prosthetic heart valves, malaria, haemoglobinopathies
and hereditary spherocytosis.

2. *Alcoholic cirrhosis*. The mechanism is unknown.

3. *Infected bile*. Escherichia coli produces $\beta$-
glucuronidase which hydrolyses bilirubin glucuronide to the unconjugated water insoluble form.

## Other factors predisposing to gallstone formation

*Age.* The incidence of both cholesterol and pigment stones increases with age.

*Race.* In some American tribes more than 75% of women over 40 years develop cholesterol gallstones. They have a small bile-acid pool which is supersaturated with cholesterol. Conversely, in Chile, the high incidence of gallstones in young women is due to cholesterol hypersecretion into a normal bile-acid pool.

Pigment stones are notably rare among American Indians. Whereas cholesterol gallstones predominate in Northern Europe and North and South America, pigment stones are more prevalent in the rural Orient. In Japan the pattern has been shifting in recent years; pigment stones have become less frequent and cholesterol stones more common.

*Stasis.* In addition to increasing the concentration of either cholesterol or pigment in bile, stasis predisposes to gallstone formation. Stasis due to muscular relaxation in the later months of pregnancy may predispose multiparous patients to gallstone formation. Infection as a secondary phenomenon may alter the physicochemical constitution of the bile, or infective debris may form a nidus around which gallstones develop. After vagotomy the gallbladder becomes flaccid and increases in volume. The resulting stasis may predispose to gallstone formation.

## PATHOLOGICAL EFFECTS OF GALLSTONES (Fig. 33.16)

### Inflammation

Inflammation of the gallbladder may be acute or chronic. Bacteria are cultivated from the bile of approximately one half of patients with gallstones. The common organisms are *Escherichia coli*, *Klebsiella aerogenes* and *Streptococcus faecalis*. Staphylococci, clostridia and salmonella are occasionally present.

### Acute cholecystitis

This is usually produced by obstruction of the neck of the gallbladder or cystic duct by a stone. When prolonged obstruction of the gallbladder

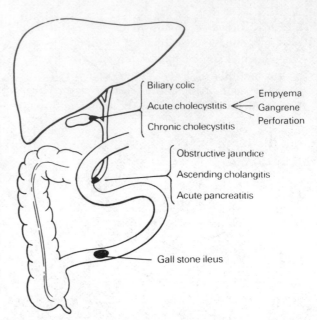

Fig. 33.16 The pathological effects of gallstones

occurs in the presence of infected bile, an *empyema* may ensue. The thickened gallbladder becomes intensely inflamed, oedematous and occasionally gangrenous. The fundus of the distended, inflamed gallbladder may perforate giving rise to localised *abscess formation* or occasionally *biliary peritonitis*.

### Chronic cholecystitis

Infection may reach the gallbladder through the biliary tract or by lymphatic or haematogenous spread. Stasis predisposes to infection. Chronic inflammatory change is commonly present in the gallbladders of typhoid carriers, which often harbour organisms for long periods of time.

### Mucocoele

A mucocoele develops when the outlet of the gallbladder becomes obstructed in the absence of infected bile. The imprisoned bile is absorbed but clear mucus continues to be secreted into the distended gallbladder.

### Choledocholithiasis

When gallstones enter the common bile duct they may pass spontaneously or give rise to *obstructive jaundice*, *ascending cholangitis* or *acute pancreatitis*. Gallstone pancreatitis most commonly occurs when a small stone becomes temporarily arrested at the ampulla of Vater. The exact mechanism whereby acute pancreatitis results is not clear. Reflux of infected bile into the pancreatic ducts may be responsible.

### Carcinoma

The incidence of carcinoma of the gallbladder and bile ducts is increased in patients with long-standing gallstones.

## CLINICAL FEATURES

Approximately 30% of patients with gallstones are asymptomatic or have only vague symptoms of distension and flatulence. Half of such patients will develop severe symptoms or complications of their gallstones within 10 years. Gallstones may give rise to symptoms in several ways:

### Biliary colic

Biliary colic is due to transient obstruction of the gallbladder from an impacted stone. There is severe gripping pain, often developing in the evening, and maximal in the epigastrium and right hypochondrium, radiating to the back. Though continuous, the pain may wax and wane in intensity over several hours. Vomiting and retching occur. Resolution follows when the stone falls back into the gallbladder lumen or occasionally passes into the common bile duct. The following day the patient is vaguely unwell but recovers rapidly. Repeated bouts of colic are common.

### Acute cholecystitis

Acute cholecystitis results in a more prolonged and severe illness. It usually begins with an attack of biliary colic, though its onset may be more gradual. Severe right hypochondrial pain radiating to the back and occasionally to the right shoulder (from diaphragmatic irritation) is present together with tachycardia, pyrexia, nausea, vomiting and leucocytosis. Abdominal tenderness and

rigidity may be generalised but are most marked over the gallbladder. Murphy's sign (a catching of the breath when the gallbladder is palpated on deep inspiration) is present. A right hypochondrial mass may be felt. This is due to omentum 'wrapped around' the inflamed gallbladder.

The attack usually settles within 4–5 days but tenderness may spread and pyrexia and tachycardia persist. If an *empyema* forms there is a tender mass associated with rigors and marked pyrexia. The gallbladder may become gangrenous and perforate giving rise to biliary peritonitis.

Jaundice can develop during the acute attack. Usually, this is associated with stones in the common bile duct but oedema of the bile ducts may be responsible.

Acute cholecystitis must be differentiated from perforated peptic ulcer, high retrocaecal appendicitis, acute pancreatitis, myocardial infarction and basal pneumonia. Acute cholecystitis can develop in the absence of gallstones (acalculous cholecystitis). This is rare.

### Chronic cholecystitis

Chronic cholecystitis is the common form of symptomatic gallbladder disease. It is almost invariably associated with gallstones. Repeated bouts of biliary colic or acute cholecystitis culminate in fibrosis, contraction of the gallbladder and chronic inflammatory change with marked thickening of the wall. The gallbladder ceases to function. Recurrent flatulence, right upper quadrant pain and fatty food intolerance occur. The pain is worse after meals and is often associated with a feeling of distension.

The differential diagnosis includes duodenal ulcer, hiatus hernia, myocardial ischaemia, chronic pancreatitis, and gastro-intestinal neoplasia.

### Mucocoele

A piriform swelling is palpable in the right hypochondrium. It is not tender and there is no pyrexia.

### Choledocholithiasis

Stones are present in the common bile duct of 10–15% of patients with gallstones. There is little muscle in the wall of the bile duct and pain is not a symptom unless the stone impedes flow through the sphincter of Oddi. Then colic occurs. The vast majority of stones in the common bile duct originate in the gallbladder. 'Primary' duct stones are extremely rare.

When a stone impacts at the sphincter, there is obstruction to the flow of bile with jaundice, the passage of pale stools, and dark urine. Obstruction commonly persists for several days but may clear spontaneously, either as a result of passage of the stone or its disimpaction. Small stones may pass through the common bile duct without causing symptoms. Stones over 7mm in diameter are unlikely to pass through the sphincter of Oddi.

In long standing obstruction the bile ducts become markedly dilated. For the common bile duct a diameter of 10 mm is regarded as the upper limit of normal. A totally obstructed duct system becomes filled with clear 'white bile'; back pressure on the hepatocytes prevents clearance of bilirubin and mucus secretion is increased.

Infection of an obstructed biliary tract causes *ascending cholangitis* with pain, pyrexia and jaundice (Charcot's intermittent biliary fever). Long-standing obstruction of the biliary tract with repeated infection leads to *secondary biliary cirrhosis*.

*Acute pancreatitis* may be associated with a stone in the common bile duct. This is difficult to differentiate clinically from other forms of acute pancreatitis. A history of jaundice, or ascending cholangitis suggests that a stone has been in the common bile duct at the time of the attack.

The differential diagnosis of stones in the common bile duct is from other causes of obstructive jaundice. Malignant obstruction of the biliary tract, cholestatic jaundice and acute viral or alcoholic hepatitis must be excluded.

*Courvoisier's Law.* Fibrosed gallbladders which contain stones are incapable of distending in response to increased pressure in the obstructed biliary tree. Courvoisier's Law states that if the gallbladder is palpable in the presence of jaundice, the jaundice is unlikely to be due to stone. This law is not inviolate.

Distended gallbladders are not always easy to feel but can be detected readily by ultrasonic scans.

### Gallstone ileus

This is a rare complication of gallstones. A large impacted stone erodes through the neck of the gallbladder into the duodenum. It is propelled down the gut and usually impacts in its narrowest portion; the terminal ileum.

## ACALCULOUS CONDITIONS OF THE GALLBLADDER

### Cholesterosis

Cholesterosis or 'strawberry gallbladder' is a condition in which the mucous membrane of the gallbladder is infiltrated with lipid and cholesterol. It affects middle aged and elderly patients of either sex. Two types are described:

1. Diffuse infiltration of the entire mucous membrane.
2. A punctate lipid-laden papillomatous type

Cholesterol stones are found in the gallbladders of half of these patients. Macroscopically the mucosa is brick-red, speckled with bright yellow nodules. Symptoms are of acute and chronic cholecystitis.

### Adenomyomatosis

This is a rare condition of the gallbladder characterised by mucosal diverticula (Rokitansky-Aschoff sinuses), particularly in the fundus. There is epithelial proliferation with penetration of the mucosa through the muscular layers to the serosa. Muscular hypertrophy and inflammatory cell infiltrates are present. The gallbladder often contains stones or biliary gravel. The condition is usually apparent on cholecystography.

## INVESTIGATION OF THE PATIENT WITH SUSPECTED GALLSTONES

### Plain abdominal X-ray

Only 15% of gallstones contain calcium in sufficient concentration to be seen on a plain radiograph. Gas is occasionally present in the biliary tree (1) following the recent passage of a stone through the ampulla of Vater, (2) when ascending cholangitis is associated with a gas forming organism; or (3) when a fistula is present between the biliary tree and the duodenum or stomach. Fistulas may result from erosion by a gallstone, or may have been created surgically, e.g. by choledocho-duodenostomy.

## Oral cholecystography

An iodine-containing fat-soluble compound is given by mouth. Following absorption it is conjugated by the liver and excreted in the bile. On passing into the gallbladder it is concentrated, and outlines the viscus. Some 70% of gallstones are identified as filling defects within the gallbladder.

Oral cholecystography will not outline the gallbladder when the serum bilirubin level is higher than 30–40 $\mu$mol/l. Depressed liver function impairs excretion of contrast medium.

Failure to opacify the gallbladder in the presence of normal liver function may be due to (1) obstruction of the cystic duct, (2) diseased mucosa unable to concentrate the dye, and (3) pyloric stenosis, vomiting, diarrhoea or failure to take the tablets.

## Intravenous cholangiography

A water-soluble iodine-containing compound, excreted by the liver in sufficient concentration to display the biliary duct system, is administered intravenously and serial X-rays taken. Absence of gallbladder opacification in the presence of normal biochemical liver function indicates that the cystic duct is obstructed.

## Percutaneous transhepatic cholangiography (PTC)

In the patient who is clinically jaundiced neither oral cholecystography nor intravenous cholangiography will be of any value. Direct injection of radio-opaque mechanism into the intrahepatic ducts using a slim flexible Chiba needle has proved invaluable. Leakage of infected bile is rare but antibiotic cover is essential to prevent septicaemia, and facilities for urgent surgery should be at hand. PTC will outline the duct system and

define the site of obstruction in virtually all patients with obstruction and duct dilatation, and will be successful in two-thirds of patients who do not have dilated ducts.

## Grey-scale ultrasonography

This is of great value in the diagnosis of gallstones both in jaundiced and non-jaundiced patients. It also demonstrates dilated intrahepatic bile ducts in patients with extrahepatic biliary obstruction. The accuracy of the method is observer-variable and experience and skill are required. Ultrasound is now used in many centres as the first investigation of patients with suspected gallstones or with obstructive jaundice.

A suggested plan of investigation of the patient with suspected gallstones is shown in Fig. 33.17.

## Acute cholecystitis

In acute cholecystitis, hepatobiliary scanning and infusion tomography may have diagnostic value. *Hepatobiliary scanning* is performed by a gamma camera scintiscan of the gallbladder region following the injection of $^{99m}$Tc-HIDA (dimethyl acetanilide-imino-diacetic acid). Failure to visualise the gallbladder within 2 hours suggests acute cholecystitis. *Infusion tomography* is performed by taking tomographic 'cuts' through the region of the gallbladder after an intravenous infusion of urografin. A visible circle or crescent of gallblad-

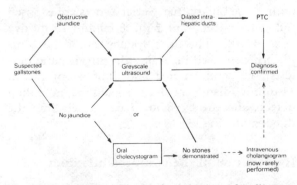

Fig. 33.17 One plan for the investigation of gallstones (IV cholangiography is now rarely used)

der wall suggests hypervascularity from acute inflammation.

## SURGICAL TREATMENT OF GALLSTONES

In general, patients with gallstones require surgical treatment. Patients with *asymptomatic gallstones* diagnosed incidentally should also be advised to undergo surgical treatment unless they are old and frail, or have other medical conditions likely to preclude safe surgery.

### Cholecystectomy

Surgical treatment of gallstones consists of removal of the gallbladder and its contained stones (cholecystectomy). The obese patient is advised to lose weight pre-operatively.

Cholecystectomy is one of the commonest operations performed. The gallbladder is approached either by a vertical paramedian or midline incision or by one parallel to the costal margin (subcostal). Following careful inspection and palpation, the gallbladder is mobilised by ligating and dividing the cystic duct and cystic artery and dissecting it free from its bed. Some surgeons prefer a retrograde approach and divide the cystic artery, mobilise the gallbladder from its bed and only then divide the cystic duct. Haemostasis is secured, a drain is inserted into the subhepatic pouch, and the abdominal wound is closed.

*Peroperative cholangiography* should be carried out routinely. A small cannula is inserted into the cystic duct and 25% urografin is injected to outline the biliary tree. Serial X-rays are exposed following injection of 2 ml, 8 ml and 15 ml dye (Fig. 33.18). The duct system should be completely visualised including the intrahepatic radicles, the common bile duct should not exceed 11mm in diameter, there should be no filling defects and the dye should pass freely into the duodenum (Fig. 33.19).

### Exploration of the common bile duct

Common bile duct stones are suspected when there is a history of jaundice, cholangitis or

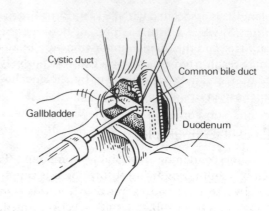

**Fig. 33.18** Operative cholangiography

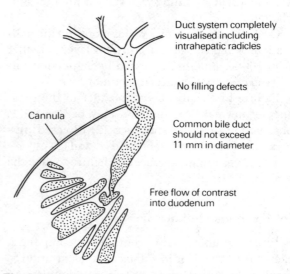

**Fig. 33.19** A normal cholangiogram

pancreatitis, and when at operation the bile ducts are dilated and the gallbladder contains multiple stones. Operative cholangiography is still mandatory as duct stones will be excluded and thus unnecessary exploration of the bile duct avoided in half such patients.

If stones are present within the bile ducts, the duct is opened (choledochotomy) and the stones removed (choledocholithotomy). To explore the common bile duct the anterior wall of the duct is incised longitudinally between stay sutures. Exploration and stone removal is carried out with specially designed forceps (Desjardin forceps) or a balloon catheter. Following exploration of the duct further cholangiogram films are taken to exclude residual stones. This is best performed by inserting a paediatric Foley catheter into the bile duct through which contrast medium is injected (Fig. 33.20).

Following exploration the common bile duct is closed around a T-tube drain, and brought out through a stab incision in the abdominal wall (Fig. 33.21). This allows free bile drainage and permits subsequent X-ray following instillation of iodine-containing dye into the biliary tree (postoperative cholangiogram). This is normally performed 7–9 days after operation.

If at operation a stone is firmly impacted at the lower end of the bile duct, it may have to be removed through the duodenum. The muscle surrounding the lower end of the duct is divided to release the stone (transduodenal sphincterotomy). If the duct is grossly dilated and filled with debris and mud, it may either be anastomosed to the duodenum (choledochoduodenostomy: Fig. 33.22) or its lower end is incised and its mucosa is sutured to that of the duodenum (sphincteroplasty: Fig. 33.23).

## Choledochoscopy

Examination of the biliary tree during operation can be performed with a choledochoscope. These

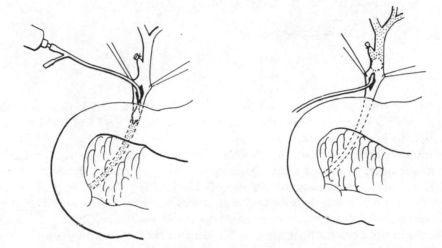

**Fig. 33.20** Post exploration cholangiogram using Foley catheter technique

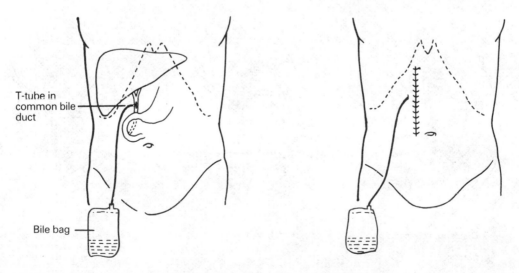

T-tube in common bile duct

Bile bag

**Fig. 33.21** T-tube drainage of common bile duct

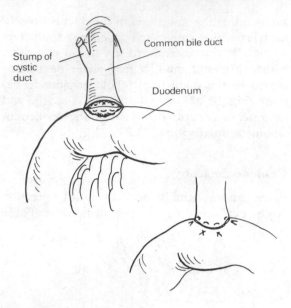

**Fig. 33.22** Choledochoduodenostomy

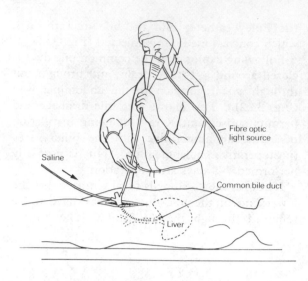

**Fig. 33.24** Choledochoscopy

may be either metallic and rigid or fibre-optic and flexible. The choledochoscope is inserted through the bile duct incision and the upper and lower segments of the bile ducts examined under direct vision (Fig. 33.24). It is necessary to fill the wound with saline so that optical integrity can be preserved. Stone-removing forceps can be passed through a channel in the choledochoscope.

## POST-OPERATIVE COMPLICATIONS OF CHOLECYSTECTOMY

Operative mortality following elective cholecystectomy performed for uncomplicated gallstones is low (0.2%); the presence of common bile duct stones and obstructive jaundice increases morbidity and mortality (2%). The major complications of cholecystectomy are as follows:

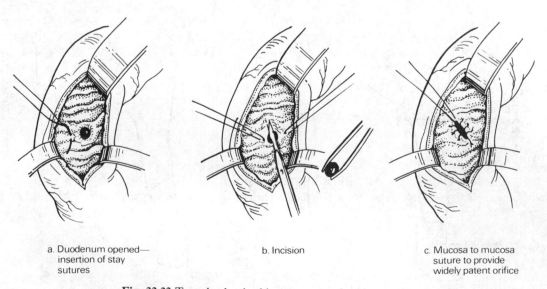

a. Duodenum opened— insertion of stay sutures

b. Incision

c. Mucosa to mucosa suture to provide widely patent orifice

**Fig. 33.23** Transduodenal sphincterotomy and sphincteroplasty

## Haemorrhage

This may occur from the cystic artery or gall-bladder bed. The patient becomes shocked and bright red blood issues from the drain. Re-exploration is mandatory.

## Infective complications

These are usually due to organisms in the bile: *Escherichia coli* (50–60%), *Klebsiella aerogenes* (10–20%) and *Streptococcus faecalis* (10–15%). The incidence of postoperative infection is reduced by short-term antibiotic therapy using either a cephalosporin or cotrimoxazole. This is advised in all 'acute' cholecystectomies.

## Bile leakage

This may be due to division of an accessory cystic duct, to a ligature coming off the cystic duct, to damage of the common bile duct or to a stone left within the common bile duct. If substantial, re-exploration is required.

## Retained common bile duct stones

When postoperative T-tube cholangiography indicates that there is still a stone in the bile duct, the residual stone should be treated initially by irrigation via the T-tube. Solutions of cholic acid, lignocaine, sodium mono-octanoin and heparin have been used for this purpose with some success. Cholic acid is generally preferred. If repeated irrigations fail to clear the common bile duct in 4–6 weeks, stones may be extracted under radiological control. The T-tube is removed and a specially designed hollow tube inserted through its track to enter the bile duct. A Dormia basket is passed through the tube into the duct and the stone or stones extracted (Fig. 33.25).

If a residual stone is diagnosed after the T-tube has been removed, it can be treated by *transendoscopic sphincterotomy* (Fig. 33.26). A diathermy knife is passed through a duodenoscope to widen the papilla and the stones extracted with either a Dormia basket or a balloon catheter. If these methods fail the bile duct will require to be re-explored at open operation.

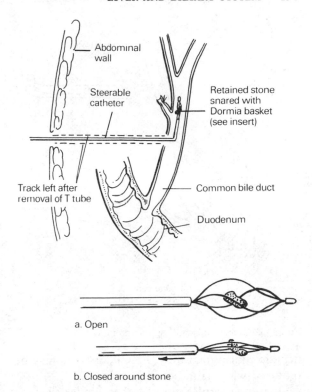

Fig. 33.25 Removal of a retained common bile duct stone

## Biliary strictures

About 90% of benign biliary strictures result from damage during cholecystectomy in which the bile duct is cut or ligated, or devascularised. The remainder result from abdominal trauma or erosion of the bile duct by a gallstone.

*Clinical features.* If the duct is completely occluded severe jaundice develops rapidly. The cardinal features of partial stricture are attacks of cholangitis and jaundice. Bouts of pain, fever, chills and mild jaundice develop, usually within a year of cholecystectomy. The alkaline phosphatase and liver enzymes are elevated in most cases. During the attacks of acute cholangitis blood cultures may be positive. If left untreated persistent cholangitis progresses to hepatic abscess formation, secondary biliary cirrhosis, portal hypertension and liver failure. Reconstructive surgery is essential.

*Management.* The exact position and extent of the stricture should first be determined radiologically. Intravenous cholangiography may suffice when the bilirubin is normal; percutaneous trans-

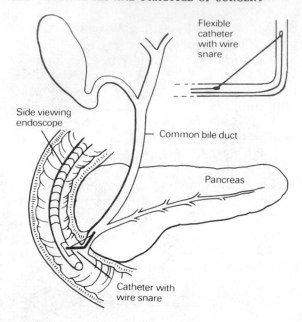

Fig. 33.26 Transendoscopic sphincterotomy

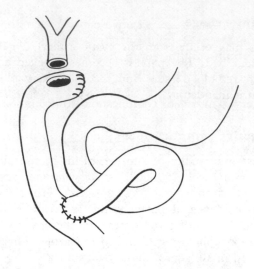

Fig. 33.27 Principle underlying reconstruction of the bile duct by a Roux loop

hepatic cholangiography, ERCP, or both, may be required when jaundice is persistent.

Operative exploration is then undertaken to define the upper end of the bile duct and to anastomose it to a loop of jejunum (Roux-en-Y) (Fig. 33.27). A mucosa-to-mucosa anastomosis is essential to prevent further stricture. The new anastomosis is temporarily splinted with a tube brought out through the jejunal loop.

### Post-cholecystectomy syndrome

This includes a heterogeneous group of complaints which may follow cholecystectomy. These include postprandial flatulence, fat intolerance and other vague dyspeptic symptoms. They are most common when cholecystectomy has been performed in the absence of gallstones.

Retained common bile duct stones and other causes of upper alimentary tract symptoms such as peptic ulceration, gastritis and pancreatic disease must be excluded. In the majority of patients investigations prove negative.

## MANAGEMENT OF ACUTE CHOLECYSTITIS

Patients with acute cholecystitis are admitted to hospital. The pulse is measured hourly; blood pressure and temperature are recorded 4-hourly; and analgesics, intravenous fluid and broad-spectrum antibiotics (either cotrimoxazole, gentamicin or cephalosporin) are prescribed. A nasogastric tube may be inserted, particularly if the patient is vomiting. The majority of patients settle on this regime within a few days. Failure to settle suggests the presence of an empyema.

Many surgeons delay operation for about 6 weeks after the attack in the expectation that the acute inflammatory reaction will have resolved. Others prefer to perform cholecystectomy within 72 hours of the onset of the attack. Provided the operation is carried out by an experienced surgeon and under antibiotic cover, such 'early' cholecystectomies are not associated with an increased incidence of complications. The duration of the illness and hospitalisation are reduced and further attacks of acute cholecystitis during the waiting period for elective surgery are averted. It should be noted that this is a planned procedure carried out with all facilities on a routine elective list. 'Emergency' (through the night) cholecystectomy as soon as the patient is admitted to hospital is not advised other than for empyema of the gallbladder or when there is evidence of spreading peritonitis.

If surrounding inflammation creates difficulties in identifying the relevant anatomical structures, *cholecystostomy*, i.e. drainage of the gallbladder with removal of gallstones, may be performed as an interim measure. Elective cholecystectomy is then performed approximately 2 months later.

High unremitting fever, with marked leucocytosis and the development of generalised peritonitis may indicate free perforation requiring emergency surgery. This major complication is uncommon.

## ACALCULOUS CHOLECYSTITIS

Patients with acalculous cholecystitis, cholesterosis or adenomyomatosis are advised to undergo cholecystectomy with peroperative cholangiography.

## MEDICAL TREATMENT OF GALLSTONES

If a patient is considered unfit for elective cholecystectomy chenodeoxycholic acid (15 mg/kg per day) or ursodeoxycholic acid may be given. This substance expands the bile acid pool to normal, desaturates the bile of cholesterol, and slowly dissolves non-calcified stones in a functioning gallbladder. Patients not suitable for this form of therapy are those with calcified stones, stones greater than 15 mm in diameter, a non-functioning gallbladder, a stone in the common bile duct, and women wishing to bear children.

The treatment may take a year or more to dissolve all the stones during which time the patient remains subject to any of the complications of gallstones. On stopping treatment bile reverts to its supersaturated state in 1–3 weeks. Gallstone formation may then recur.

## ASIATIC CHOLANGIO-HEPATITIS

This condition occurs in the Far East, almost exclusively in Chinese, and most commonly along the coastline of southeast Asia. A suppurative cholangitis develops and multiple pigment stones form within the intrahepatic ducts. *Escherichia coli* and *Streptococcus faecalis* are isolated from the bile and portal blood. The aetiology of the condition is unknown, but deconjugation of bilirubin glucuronide by bacteria may be a factor. The clinical features are those of cholangitis with

attacks of pain, pyrexia and jaundice. If left untreated liver abscesses occur.

The condition is difficult to treat. Decompression of the bile duct by sphincterotomy or choledochoduodenostomy may give temporary relief but recurrence is common. A permanent T-tube through which the bile ducts can be repeatedly flushed out may be required.

Hepatic lobectomy has also been practised.

## TUMOURS OF THE EXTRAHEPATIC BILIARY TRACT

## CARCINOMA OF THE GALLBLADDER

Carcinoma of the gallbladder is rare and almost invariably related to the presence of gallstones. The condition is four times as common in females as males. About 90% of lesions are adenocarcinomas, the remainder squamous.

Direct invasion commonly obstructs the bile duct or porta hepatis. Initial symptoms are indistinguishable from those of gallstones but jaundice is unremitting. A mass is frequently palpable.

Cholecystectomy is possible only in the early stages of tumour growth. Some surgeons recommend en bloc wedge resection of an adjacent 3–5 cm of normal liver and dissection of regional lymph nodes. In most cases the condition is inoperable.

The 5-year survival rate is less than 5%; only patients having well-localised early tumours survive.

## BILE DUCT TUMOURS

Malignant tumours of the bile duct are rare. They grow slowly, usually occur in the elderly, affecting males and females equally. They may be situated intrahepatically involving the major right or left hepatic ducts, in the common hepatic duct or in the common bile duct. Carcinoma of the ampulla of Vater may also occur.

### Clinical features

Patients present with obstructive jaundice of gradual but relentless progression. Intermittent

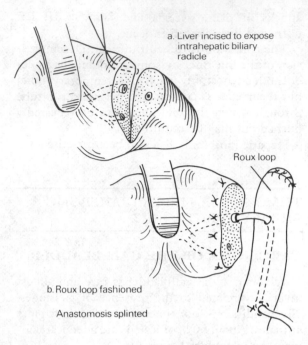

a. Liver incised to expose intrahepatic biliary radicle

Roux loop

b. Roux loop fashioned

Anastomosis splinted

**Fig. 33.28** Intrahepatic cholangio-jejunostomy

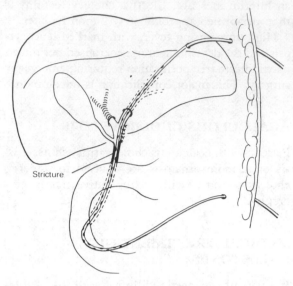

Stricture

**Fig. 33.29** U-tube biliary decompression

bouts of pain and cholangitis may occur. Gall-stones may be present along with the tumour. There is loss of weight but metastases are rare.

## Investigations

Percutaneous transhepatic cholangiography is used to define the lesion. If obstruction is total its distal extent can be defined by ERCP, when specimens for cytological examination may also be obtained. Selective coeliac and superior mesenteric arteriography may be helpful in determining resectability.

## Management

Tumours of the distal common bile duct, when resectable, are treated by pancreaticoduodenec-tomy (Whipple's operation). Where primary re-section is not possible palliation with relief of jaundice may be achieved by cholecystojejun-ostomy. Tumours of the supraduodenal portion of the common bile ducts are resected, if possible, using choledochojejunostomy to re-establish bile flow. Intrahepatic cholangiocarcinomas may be treated, where appropriate, by liver resection; or by palliative by-pass where an intrahepatic biliary radical is anastomosed to a loop of jejunum (intra-hepatic cholangiojejunostomy) or the gallbladder (Fig. 33.28). Palliative decompression has been achieved by dilatation of the malignant stricture and the introduction of a U-tube or 'stent', the ends of which are brought out through the liver and the duodenum, and can be kept free from debris by flushing (Fig. 33.29). Recently percuta-neous insertion of a biliary endoprosthesis under radiological control has become an increasingly popular method of palliation.

# 34. The Pancreas

## SURGICAL ANATOMY

The pancreas develops from a ventral and a dorsal bud. These appear during the fourth week of fetal life, rotate to the right and fuse. With rotation of the duodenum the pancreas shifts to the left and takes up its definitive position. Most of the duct which drains the dorsal bud joins that from the ventral bud to form the main pancreatic duct (of Wirsung); the rest of the dorsal duct becomes the accessory pancreatic duct (of Santorini). This enters the duodenum 2.5 cm proximal to the main duct (Fig. 34.1).

The main pancreatic duct and the common bile duct converge as they enter the second part of the duodenum. The majority of individuals have a short common channel, and only 10% retain an ampulla of Vater into which these two ducts enter separately.

The pancreas lies behind the lesser sac and stomach and is relatively inaccessible for clinical and radiological examination (Fig. 34.2). The head of the gland lies within the C loop of the duodenum with which it shares a common blood supply from superior and inferior pancreatico-duodenal arteries. The superior mesenteric and splenic veins join behind the neck of the pancreas to form the portal vein, while the body and tail of pancreas lie in front of the splenic vein as far as the splenic hilum. The body and tail of pancreas receive arterial blood from the splenic artery as it runs along the upper border of the gland. The pancreas is friable. This and its intimate relationship with major blood vessels explains why bleeding is the main cause of death after pancreatic trauma.

The common bile duct passes through the head of the pancreas and obstructive jaundice is frequently due to neoplasia or inflammation involving this part of the gland.

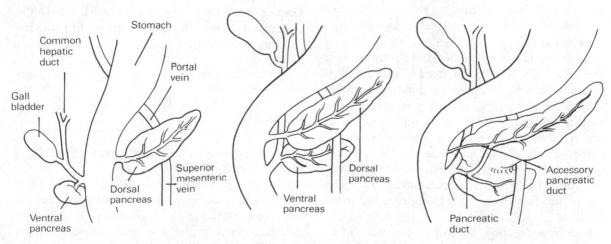

**Fig. 34.1** The development of the pancreas

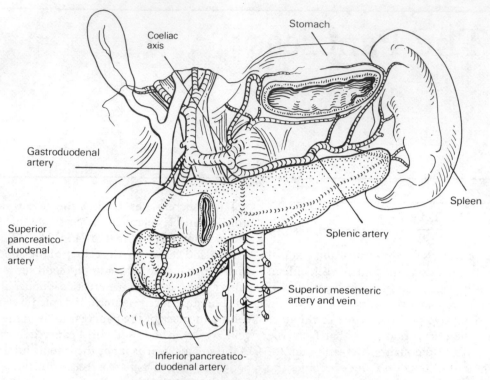

**Fig. 34.2** Relationships of the pancreas

## SURGICAL PHYSIOLOGY

*Exocrine function.* The acinar cells of the pancreas secrete 1–2 litres of alkaline (pH 7.1–8.2) enzyme-rich juice each day. The enzymes are synthesised and stored in zymogen granules in the acinar cells. Lipase and amylase are secreted in an active form. Proteolytic enzymes are secreted as inactive precursors which are activated by duodenal enterokinase.

The exocrine secretion of the pancreas is stimulated by food in the duodenum and proximal jejunum, and by acid in the duodenum. Food-stimulated pancreatic secretion is mediated by cholecystokinin (CCK) while that induced by acid is mediated by secretin. Secretin stimulates watery alkaline secretion whereas CCK stimulates secretion rich in enzymes. The vagus nerve also stimulates pancreatic secretion and hormonal and neural factors interact to regulate pancreatic function.

*Endocrine function.* Endocrine functions of the pancreas are subserved by the cells which form the islets of Langerhans. A variety of cell types are now recognised: type A cells which secrete glucagon, B cells which secrete insulin, D cells which secrete somatostatin, PP cells which secrete pancreatic polypeptide, and $D_1$ cells which may secrete VIP. Only glucagon and insulin have established physiological roles and the significance of the other endocrine cells is uncertain. Gastrin-producing (G) cells are not found in the pancreas except in the rare Zollinger-Ellison syndrome (see p. 385).

## CONGENITAL DISORDERS OF THE PANCREAS

*Annular pancreas.* This is a rare cause of duodenal obstruction (see p. 394).

*Aberrant pancreatic tissue.* Rests of heterotopic pancreas may be found at any point in the gastro-intestinal tract, but are commonest in the duodenum, stomach and proximal jejunum. Many remain asymptomatic but they can cause ulceration, bleeding or obstruction. Further, they may cause confusion in the interpretation of a barium meal.

*Cystic fibrosis (mucoviscidosis)*. Cystic fibrosis affects sweat glands, pancreas and bronchial mucous glands. Meconium ileus may follow and require relief of intestinal obstruction in neonates. Malabsorption becomes a feature as the disease progresses.

## INFLAMMATORY DISORDERS OF THE PANCREAS

Pancreatitis may be acute or chronic. After an attack of acute pancreatitis the gland usually returns to anatomical and functional normality. Chronic pancreatitis is associated with permanent derangement of structure and function. Some patients suffer from recurrent (or relapsing) acute pancreatitis, enjoying normal relatively health between attacks, and may progress to chronic pancreatitis.

### ACUTE PANCREATITIS

In Britain there are 50–100 new cases of acute pancreatitis per million population each year. The incidence is increasing, possibly as a result of increasing alcohol consumption. All age groups are affected. Acute pancreatitis is a serious condition with a mortality around 10%.

### Aetiology

The cause of acute pancreatitis is undefined. Premature activation of pancreatic enzymes with rupture of the duct system leads to autodigestion of the gland. Intraduct activation of enzymes such as trypsinogen, chymotrypsinogen, phospholipase, elastase and catalase unleashes a chain reaction of cell necrosis, further enzyme release and changes in the microcirculation. Reflux of duodenal juice and bile into the pancreatic duct or spasm at the sphincter of Oddi may be important causes of enzyme activation within the duct system.

Conditions associated with the development of acute pancreatitis are listed in Table 34.1. Biliary tract disease and alcohol are of overriding importance.

**Table 34.1** Aetiology of acute pancreatitis

| | |
|---|---|
| *Non-traumatic causes* (75%) | |
| Major factors (70%) | biliary tract disease |
| | alcohol |
| Minor factors (5%) | pancreatic cancer |
| | drugs e.g. steroids |
| | renal transplantation |
| | hyperlipidaemia |
| | hyperparathyroidism |
| | viral infection (mumps, Coxsackie) |
| | scorpion bites (Trinidad) |
| | hypothermia |
| | periarteritis nodosa |
| | pregnancy |
| | previous Polya gastrectomy |
| *Traumatic causes* (5%) | |
| | operative trauma |
| | blunt or penetrating injury |
| | investigation (ERCP or |
| | arteriography) |
| *Idiopathic* (20%) | |

*Biliary tract disease and acute pancreatitis*. Gallstones are present in about 50% of patients who develop acute pancreatitis in Britain. The great majority of these patients have at least a short common channel involving the terminal portion of the common bile duct and pancreatic duct (Fig. 34.3), and it seems likely that stones impacting at the lower end of the bile duct may occlude pancreatic drainage or promote reflux into the pancreatic duct system. In some 5–10% of cases, gallstones are subsequently defined in the distal common bile duct, while in some 80% of patients stones ranging in diameter from 1–12 mm can be recovered from the faeces a few days following the onset of pancreatitis. These stones have the same chemical composition as stones recovered from the gallbladder at subsequent surgery and it is believed that their transient impaction at the sphincter of Oddi is the cause of the attack of pancreatitis. Further support for a causal relationship between gallstones and acute pancreatitis is provided by the observation that further attacks of pancreatitis are exceptional once biliary tract disease has been eradicated.

*Alcohol-associated pancreatitis*. The proportion of cases of acute pancreatitis associated with alcohol varies greatly in different parts of the world. In Scotland the figure is 25%, whereas in North America, South Africa and France the figure may be as high as 50–90%. The mecha-

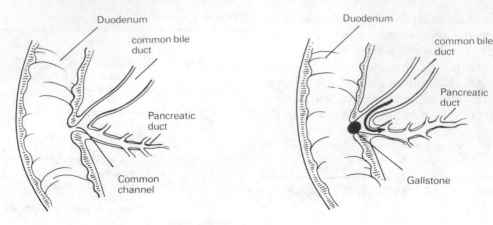

**Fig. 34.3** The common channel shared by the bile duct and the pancreatic duct

nism is uncertain. Suggested causes include a specific toxic effect, pancreatic protein hypersecretion with plug formation, spasm of the sphincter of Oddi and duodenitis.

## Pathophysiology

Pancreatic inflammation ranges in severity from mild oedema to severe necrosis and haemorrhage. Proteolytic enzymes released from the gland are responsible for increased capillary permeability, protein exudation, retroperitoneal oedema and peritoneal exudation. Vasoactive kinins such as bradykinin and kallikrein are also released by proteolytic enzyme activity. Many of the circulatory changes in acute pancreatitis result from fluid, electrolyte and protein loss in oedema and exudate. Additional factors include:

1. development of acute renal failure, possibly due to local intravascular coagulation and release of a vasopressor substance affecting the renal vascular bed,

2. development of ECG changes suggesting ischaemia, possibly due to coronary vasoconstriction by a 'myocardial depressant factor',

3. development of shock lung with atelectasis, left-sided pleural effusion, pulmonary oedema and right-to-left shunting of blood,

4. consumptive coagulopathy.

Liver function may be disturbed in acute pancreatitis by obstruction of the common bile duct, cholangitis or direct hepatocellular depression. This may account for the unreliability of radio-

logical investigation of the biliary tree for 2–3 weeks after the attack.

## Clinical features

Previous attacks of dyspepsia, biliary colic or transient jaundice may be described. Alcohol intake should be documented carefully, bearing in mind that an attack of pancreatitis is often delayed for some 24 hours after ingestion of alcohol or eating a large meal. The rarer causes of acute pancreatitis (Table 34.1) are considered when there is no evidence of gallstones, alcohol intake or trauma. Agonising pain in the epigastrium or right hypochondrium with radiation through to the back is common. Shoulder-tip pain is uncommon. Nausea and vomiting and retching are prominent. Severe pancreatitis is accompanied by shock (see p. 128).

Classically the clinical signs are less impressive than expected from the symptoms and this may prevent consideration of the correct diagnosis. There is little muscle guarding or rigidity and tenderness is relatively slight. Bruising around the umbilicus (Cullen's sign) or in the loin (Grey Turner's sign) are rare late manifestations of pancreatitis which do not contribute to the immediate diagnosis.

## Diagnosis

The key to a diagnosis of acute pancreatitis are a high index of suspicion and measurement of the

**Table 34.2** Non-pancreatic disorders capable of causing hyperamylasaemia

Acute cholecystitis
Perforated duodenal ulcer
High intestinal obstruction
Mesenteric vascular occlusion
Bowel strangulation
Dissection of aortic aneurysm
Rupture of aortic aneurysm
Ruptured ectopic pregnancy

serum amylase levels. With inflammation there is rupture of cells and parts of the ductal system with release of amylase into the circulation. The normal range for serum amylase is 100–300 i.u./l and levels greater than 1000 i.u./l strongly support the diagnosis of acute pancreatitis. False negative results occur in about 5% of patients with pancreatitis. A number of other conditions can give rise to 'false positive' results by causing hyperamylasaemia (Table 34.2).

Persistent hyperamylasaemia in the absence of abnormal urinary amylase levels suggests *macro-amylasaemia*, a rare condition in which amylase is bound to globulin and forms a complex too large to be excreted by the kidney.

In pancreatitis the rise in serum amylase is frequently transient, occurring within 6 hours of the attack and persisting for some 48 hours. Urinary amylase levels are also increased and persist after serum levels have returned to normal.

The amylase-creatinine clearance ratio (ACCR) is elevated above the normal (1–4%) in most patients with acute pancreatitis. This may be a more reliable diagnostic test than serum amylase alone. ACCR is calculated according to the formula: urine amylase/serum amylase × serum creatinine/urine creatinine × 100%.

There are no pathognomic radiological signs of acute pancreatitis but plain films of the chest and abdomen may reveal:

1. left-sided pleural effusion (20% of cases),
2. blurring of the psoas margin by retroperitoneal inflammation,
3. a bowel empty of gas apart from a 'sentinel loop' of jejunum resulting from local ileus in bowel overlying the inflamed gland. Gas may be seen in the hepatic and splenic flexures but not in the transverse colon (the 'colon cut-off' sign),
4. associated gallstones.

Gastrografin studies are not usually indicated but may be of value when perforation cannot be excluded clinically. The C loop of the duodenum may be widened by inflammation in the head of the pancreas, the duodenal folds oedematous and coarse, and the papilla of Vater retracted (the 'reversed-3 sign') from oedema of the medial wall of the duodenum.

Urea and electrolyte determinations reflect dehydration and are useful in the management of fluid and electrolyte balance. Liver function tests sometimes reveal hyperbilirubinaemia and marginal elevation of liver enzymes. Hyperglycaemia and glycosuria may occur transiently.

Arterial blood gas measurement is essential in shocked patients and may reveal severe hypoxia. Moderate polymorphonuclear leucocytosis is common.

The serum calcium should be estimated. Hypocalcaemia in acute pancreatitis is due partly to calcium soap formation as a consequence of fat necrosis, but mostly to a fall in serum albumin concentration and hence a reduction in protein-bound calcium levels. Marked reduction in the level of ionised calcium is unusual and frank tetany is exceptional.

## Treatment

There is no specific treatment for acute pancreatitis. The majority of cases settle on management which includes the following:

*Pain relief.* Severe pain requires the administration of opiates. Morphine and pethidine both cause spasm of the sphincter of Oddi and are contraindicated on theoretical grounds. In practice, pethidine is frequently prescribed and is of benefit.

*Treatment of shock* (see Chapter 12). Large volumes of crystalloid, plasma or dextran may be needed to relieve dehydration and maintain circulating fluid volume. Oxygen therapy is essential.

*Suppression of pancreatic function.* A nasogastric tube is passed. The patient is forbidden to drink or eat. Absence of food and acid from the duodenum prevents liberation of duodenal secretin and CCK and thus avoids stimulation of pancreatic secretion. Propantheline bromide or atropine inhibit vagal activity and relax the sphincter of Oddi, but there is no clear-cut evidence of their value.

*Other medical measures.* Some surgeons prescribe a broad-spectrum antibiotic routinely for patients with pancreatitis. However they are not of proven value and the majority of surgeons now elect to await evidence of infection. If there is associated cholangitis an antibiotic should be given.

Although rare, the development of diabetes may require insulin therapy.

The kallikrein inhibitor, aprotinin (Trasylol), has no proven therapeutic value and is seldom prescribed. Glucagon was once regarded as a useful means of suppressing pancreatic secretion but is now not used. The use of corticosteroids remains controversial. They are not recommended.

Peritoneal lavage with isotonic crystalloid solutions may prove useful as a means of recovering peritoneal fluid when the diagnosis of pancreatitis is uncertain and may have a therapeutic role.

Lavage aims to remove fluid containing enzymes and vasoactive substances and so prevent their absorption into the blood stream. Preliminary results are encouraging (Fig. 34.4).

*Surgical treatment.* There is general agreement that acute pancreatitis should be managed conservatively if possible. Laparotomy is indicated:

1. *When the diagnosis is uncertain.* As shown in Table 34.2, a number of acute abdominal conditions may cause hyperamylasaemia and the majority of these may prove fatal if not treated surgically. Laparotomy is indicated if the diagnosis of acute pancreatitis is in doubt.

If laparotomy reveals mild pancreatitis, the abdomen is closed without drainage. Drainage of the lesser sac with peritoneal lavage is considered if the pancreatitis is severe. Examination of the biliary tree is an essential part of laparotomy. If

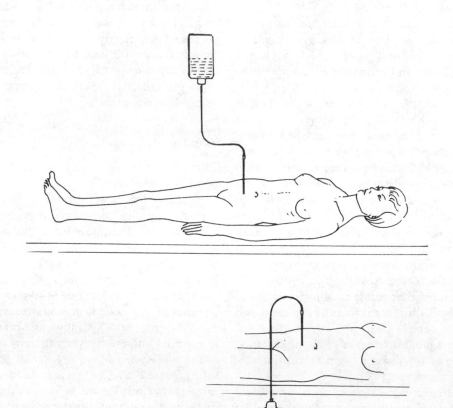

**Fig. 34.4** Principle of peritoneal lavage

gallstones are found most surgeons prefer to delay biliary surgery until the acute attack has settled. However, there is a growing feeling that provided the general condition of the patient is good, cholecystectomy, operative cholangiography, and if necessary, removal of stones from the bile ducts, is the correct procedure. Cholecystostomy with T-tube drainage of the common bile duct may be considered if gallstones are found in a patient whose general condition is poor.

2. *When the patient fails to improve on conservative management.* If the general condition of the patient deteriorates despite intensive medical management laparotomy should be performed. Necrotic pancreatic tissue is removed and the peritoneal cavity is irrigated with saline. Two large peritoneal drains are inserted and postoperative lavage instituted. Resection of the pancreas has been advocated as a 'last ditch' measure in such patients. This is a formidable undertaking, and even in experienced hands has a mortality of at least 50%.

# COMPLICATIONS OF ACUTE PANCREATITIS

## Pancreatic pseudocyst

A pancreatic pseudocyst is a collection of pancreatic secretion and inflammatory exudate, the wall of which is lined by inflammatory tissue rather than epithelium (true cyst). A pseudocyst is usually located in the lesser sac or retroperitoneal tissue around the pancreas.

Pseudocysts develop in about 10% of patients and are most common following alcoholic or traumatic pancreatitis.

Small pseudocysts are often asymptomatic and usually resolve spontaneously. Larger collections displace and compress the stomach or duodenum, and may cause considerable discomfort.

*Clinical features.* Pseudocysts typically do not become manifest for some 2–3 weeks after the episode of pancreatitis. Persistent or intermittent hyperamylasaemia may signal their presence. Ultrasound is of great value in monitoring the progress of pancreatic inflammation and in detecting pseudocyst formation. Some cysts become so large that they are palpable.

*Treatment.* The presence of a pseudocyst is not in itself an indication for surgical treatment. An enlarging cyst is. Ideally, the form of the operation should depend on whether or not the pseudocyst communicates with the duct system. A non-communicating cyst should resolve following drainage to the exterior, whereas one which communicates with the duct system can be by internal drainage of the cyst to the stomach (cystogastrostomy), duodenum (cystoduodenostomy), or to a Roux loop of the jejunum (cystjejunumostomy) or occasionally by parital resection of the pancreas (Fig. 34.5).

Determination of whether or not a cyst communicates with the duct system requires pancreatography. As this is not generally available many surgeons prefer to perform internal drainage in all cases. As the tissues holding the sutures must be firm, it is wise to allow the pseudocyst time to 'mature' (6–8 weeks) before operating.

## Pancreatic abscess

The presentation may resemble that of pancreatic pseudocyst but the patient is usually ill, and has pyrexia and leucocytosis. The presence of an abscess is confirmed by ultrasound. Adequate drainage under antibiotic cover is mandatory.

## Progressive jaundice

Persistent or progressively deepening jaundice may indicate that a gallstone is impacted at the lower end of the biliary tree or that the bile duct is compressed by pancreatic inflammation. Early operation is indicated. Calculous obstruction is treated by cholecystectomy, operative cholangiography, and extraction of the offending gallstone. If radiology fails to reveal a gallstone, the biliary tree is decompressed by insertion of a T-tube until pancreatic inflammation resolves. The finding of a pseudocyst in the head of the pancreas demands appropriate treatment.

## Persistent duodenal ileus

Protracted ileus usually reflects continuing pancreatic inflammation. In the absence of a pseudocyst requiring drainage, persistent duodenal ileus may be bypassed by gastro-enterostomy. Parenteral nutrition or tube feeding (via jejunostomy or naso-enteric tube) is often needed to maintain nutritional status while pancreatitis is resolving.

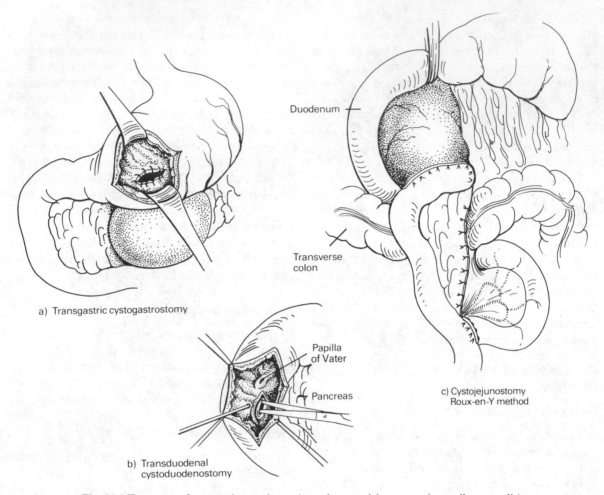

a) Transgastric cystogastrostomy

Duodenum

Transverse colon

c) Cystojejunostomy Roux-en-Y method

Papilla of Vater

Pancreas

b) Transduodenal cystoduodenostomy

**Fig. 34.5** Treatment of pancreatic pseudocyst (note that cystojejunostomy is usually retrocolic)

## Gastro-intestinal bleeding

Severe acute pancreatitis may be complicated by bleeding from gastritis, gastric erosions or acute duodenal ulceration. Prophylactic cimetidine is advisable in patients thought to have severe disease. Should bleeding develop, the guidelines for investigation and management are as outlined on page 390. On rare occasions, laparotomy is required urgently for massive intraperitoneal bleeding due to erosion of blood vessels by the inflammatory process or from microaneurysms in a pseudocyst.

## PROGNOSIS IN ACUTE PANCREATITIS

A number of clinical and laboratory criteria have been defined which have prognostic significance

(Table 34.3). Three or more positive criteria indicate severe disease. Then the patient is more likely to develop complications, and the disease to prove fatal.

**Table 34.3** Factors used to predict severity of acute pancreatitis (Severe disease predicted when three or more factors positive)

| | |
|---|---|
| Age | $> 55$ |
| White cell count | $> 15 \times 10^9/l$ |
| Blood glucose (no diabetic history) | $> 10$ mmol/l |
| Serum urea (no response to IV fluids) | $> 16$ mmol/l |
| $PaO_2$ | $< 60$ mmHg |
| Serum calcium | $< 2.0$ mmol/l |
| Serum albumin | $< 32$ g/l |
| Serum lactate dehydrogenase | $> 600$ u/l |
| Serum aspartate aminotransferase/alanine aminotransferase | $> 100$ u/l |

Following resolution of the acute attack, the subsequent prognosis depends on the aetiological factor concerned. The biliary tree must be investigated in all cases. Gallstone-associated pancreatitis carries an excellent long-term outlook once cholecystectomy has been carried out and gallstones have been cleared from the biliary tree. In the past, it has been customary to delay cholecystectomy for some 6–8 weeks to allow pancreatic inflammation to resolve completely. As many patients develop further attacks of pancreatitis while awaiting readmission, many centres now encourage cholecystectomy during the initial admission.

The prognosis in alcohol-associated pancreatitis is less favourable. Many patients are unable or unwilling to abstain from drinking and suffer further attacks of acute pancreatitis (relapsing pancreatitis) or progress to chronic pancreatitis.

## CHRONIC PANCREATITIS

### Aetiology

Chronic pancreatitis is a relatively rare disease in the United Kingdom. Its incidence may be increasing in association with the growing problem of alcoholism. Although alcoholism is much the commonest aetiological factor, cholelithiasis is present in some 25% of patients and may have a contributory role. In India and Africa where the disease affects younger patients, malnutrition is an important cause. Rarer causes include mucoviscidosis, hyperparathyroidism, haemochromatosis and familial pancreatitis.

### Pathophysiology

Chronic inflammation leads to progressive replacement of the gland by fibrous tissue, destruction of acinar tissue, and eventual destruction of islet tissue. Multiple strictures form in the pancreatic duct, impair drainage and cause further inflammation in the obstructed gland. Protein plugs form in the ducts and later calcify, leading to speckled calcification on plain abdominal X-ray. The exact mechanism whereby alcohol damages the pancreas is uncertain but protein hypersecretion with plug formation may be a factor.

### Clinical features

*Weight loss* is invariable. It may be associated with frank malabsorption and steatorrhoea, the bowel motion being pale, bulky, offensive, floating on water, and difficult to flush. *Pain* is a prominent feature in almost all cases due to alcohol but may be less marked in those patients with a non-alcoholic basis for their disease. The pain may be precipitated by eating and so contribute to weight loss. It is characteristically epigastric and in the back and is eased by bending forward (Fig. 34.6). Delay in diagnosis may lead to drug addiction in some patients. Attacks of pain are usually associated with episodes of inflammation, and denote stricture formation.

*Obstructive jaundice* may be present if the head of pancreas is inflamed. Jaundice is usually incomplete, transient or intermittent.

*Diabetes mellitus* develops in about one-third of patients. It may take several years to become manifest.

Carcinoma of the pancreas was said to be more common in patients with chronic pancreatitis. This may but reflect the difficulty in distinguishing between the two conditions, and the likelihood that cancer blocks the duct system and predisposes to inflammation.

## INVESTIGATION AND DIAGNOSIS

Investigations are performed to define (1) the degree of exocrine and endocrine functional impairment, and (2) the extent of structural damage to the duct system.

*Exocrine function* is assessed by duodenal intubation and collection of pancreatic juice after stimulation by secretin and CCK. Pancreatic insufficiency may not be evident *clinically* until 90% of the functional parenchyma is destroyed but 80–90% of patients with chronic pancreatitis have abnormal function tests with a low secretory volume, low bicarbonate concentration, and low enzyme output. Function tests do not discriminate clearly between chronic pancreatitis and other pancreatic diseases.

Steatorrhoea is assessed by measuring faecal fat excretion over a 3–5 day period while fat intake is controlled at 100 g/day. Normal individuals excrete less than 5 g/day. Alternatively, fat absorp-

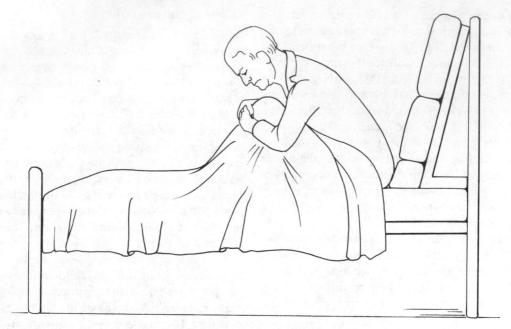

**Fig. 34.6** Common posture of patient with pancreatic pain

tion can be measured by isotopic labelling of dietary fat. Pancreatic scintiscanning using $^{75}$Se-selenomethionine is of little value and is not recommended.

*Endocrine function* is assessed by measurement of fasting glucose concentrations, supplemented if necessary by a glucose tolerance test. The diagnosis of pancreatic insufficiency is virtually certain if steatorrhoea is accompanied by abnormal glucose tolerance.

### Radiology

Abdominal plain films may reveal speckled calcification in patients with chronic pancreatitis. Ultrasound and CT scan may detect pancreatic enlargement. Endoscopic retrograde choledocho-pancreatography (ERCP) is of greater value and should always be performed if operation is contemplated (Fig. 34.7). The architecture of the pancreatic duct is revealed and it may also prove possible to outline the biliary tract and so avoid further biliary radiology. Pure pancreatic juice is obtained for cytological examination to exclude neoplasia.

### Management

The principles of medical management are:

1. to remove the aetiological agent (e.g. alcohol)
2. to deal with functional insufficiency and
3. to relieve pain.

The management of functional deficiency includes the treatment of diabetes and the replacement of deficient exocrine secretion.

A number of commercial enzyme preparations are available (e.g. Cotazym B, Nutrizym) but all are subject to enzymic degradation by gastric acid-pepsin, and steatorrhoea may prove difficult to eradicate. The addition of cimetidine may prove helpful if steatorrhoea remains troublesome.

For the relief of pain opiates are avoided as addiction may result. After removal of the precipitating cause, simple analgesics only should be required. Coeliac plexus block may be successful and is worth trying.

*Surgical treatment.* Operation is indicated if pain persists, if gallstones are present, if inflammation is complicated by pseudocyst or abscess formation, and when pancreatic carcinoma cannot

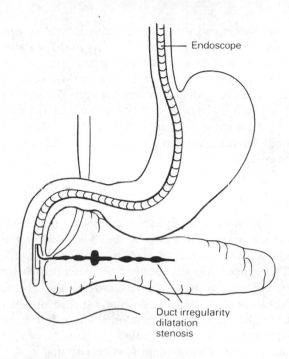

Fig. 34.7 ERCP in chronic pancreatitis

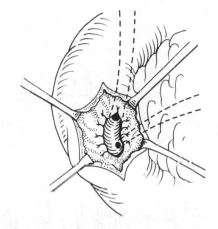

**Fig. 34.8** Sphincteroplasty

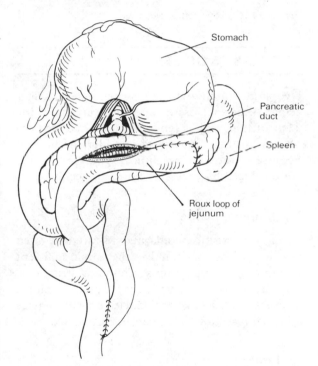

**Fig. 34.9** Pancreatic duct decompression

be excluded. Persisting severe pain is the most common indication for operation.

The object of surgery is to preserve functioning pancreatic tissue by providing adequate drainage, or if this is not possible, to resect the involved portion of the gland. Demonstration of ductal anatomy is essential in selecting the most appropriate operation, and operative pancreatography is mandatory if ERCP has not been successful.

The method of draining the duct system depends on the extent of obstruction. In some cases there is a single area of narrowing close to the sphincter of Oddi but sphincteroplasty rarely suffices (Fig. 34.8). In others there are multiple strictures throughout the length of the duct, which must be slit open by 'filleting' the gland and anastomosing a Roux loop of duodenum to the whole length of the pancreatic duct (Fig. 34.9).

If drainage is not feasible 95% of the gland may be resected leaving only a rim of pancreas attached to the C loop of the duodenum to protect the bile ducts (Fig. 34.10).

Providing the patient ceases to drink alcohol, pain is likely to be relieved following a drainage procedure and pancreatic insufficiency will not worsen or may even improve. Total pancreatec-

tomy is more certain to relieve pain but this is at the expense of permanent diabetes and loss of exocrine pancreatic function. Occasionally chronic pancreatitis is limited to the distal half of the gland, when treatment by distal pancreatectomy is simple and effective.

Unfortunately, many patients will continue to take alcohol and the results of surgery are then disappointing.

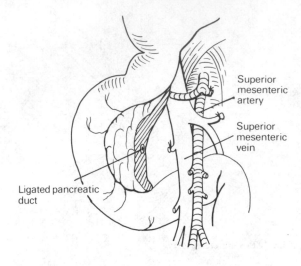

**Fig. 34.10** 95% resection of pancreas

## NEOPLASMS OF THE PANCREAS

Neoplasms of the pancreas arise from ductal or acinar (exocrine) tissue, and those arising in the islets of Langerhans (endocrine). Endocrine neoplasms are rare but are of considerable interest because of the specific clinical syndromes which are produced by excessive hormone secretion.

### Benign neoplasms

Benign pancreatic neoplasms are rare and often remain asymptomatic, unless they attain sufficient size to cause pressure on surrounding structures. Such tumours are usually cystadenomas, unless small, when they may be enucleated, and require a formal resection. This can be formidable.

### Malignant neoplasms

Adenocarcinoma is by far the commonest malignant lesion of the exocrine pancreas. Cystadenocarcinoma and sarcoma are extremely rare.

### ADENOCARCINOMA OF THE PANCREAS

#### Aetiology

The cause of pancreatic cancer is unknown. It is increasing in frequency and is now the fourth commonest cause of cancer death in males, and sixth commonest in females. It accounts for about 10% of all cancers of the alimentary system.

Men are more commonly affected than women, and the peak incidence lies between 55 and 70 years of age. Factors thought to increase the risk of pancreatic cancer include tobacco smoking, a high-fat, high-protein diet and excessive drinking of coffee.

#### Pathology

The great majority of adenocarcinomas arise from ductal rather than acinar tissue. The head of the gland is more often affected than the body or tail. The cancer spreads locally and disseminates by lymphatics to lymph nodes around the gland. Regardless of the site of origin, spread outwith the reach of surgical resection is the rule by the time the disease is diagnosed. Survival for more than 5 years from diagnosis is exceptional.

Cancer arising in the periampullary region, duodenum or distal common bile duct is much more favourable. Biliary obstruction occurs early leading to its discovery at a time when resection offers a much better prospect of cure.

#### Clinical features

*Weight loss* is invariable and may be the first symptom. Cancer of the head of the pancreas was said to cause *painless* obstructive jaundice but this is not true. *Ill-defined upper abdominal pain* is present in most patients and is probably due to ductal obstruction with some degree of pancreatitis. Neoplastic infiltration can cause severe pain in the back.

*Obstructive jaundice* is the best-known feature of cancer of the head of the pancreas. It is usually progressive unlike the fluctuant jaundice common in calculous obstruction. When cancer originates in the body or tail of the pancreas, jaundice may be due to liver metastases or extension of the cancer into the porta hepatis. In keeping with Courvoisier's law (Ch. 33), the gallbladder is palpable in some (but not all) patients with obstructive jaundice due to cancer of the pancreas. A distended gallbladder is felt more laterally than expected from its surface marking.

Signs and symptoms of *pancreatic insufficiency*

are common. *Diabetes mellitus* or impaired glucose tolerance is found in 30% of patients with pancreatic cancer and may rarely be the presenting feature. *Steatorrhoea* due to impaired digestion and absorption of fat may be associated with weight loss.

*Thrombophlebitis migrans* is seen in some patients but is not specific for this form of cancer. It tends to be a late manifestation.

### Investigation and diagnosis

A high index of suspicion is essential for the early diagnosis of cancer of the pancreas. In the vast majority of patients, pancreatic cancer is diagnosed too late for successful surgery.

In patients with jaundice, its obstructive nature is confirmed by examination of the urine, stool and blood (see Ch. 33). Ultrasound scanning will detect obstruction and dilatation of the biliary tree, and exclude gallstones. If biliary tract obstruction is demonstrated, percutaneous trans-hepatic cholangiography can be used to display the site of obstruction. In patients who are deeply jaundiced, a cannula can be left in the biliary tree so that jaundice can be relieved in preparation for surgery.

If the diagnosis remains in doubt or if pancreatic cancer is suspected in a patient who is not jaundiced, endoscopic retrograde cholangiopancreatography (ERCP) is an invaluable investigation. It allows inspection of the stomach and proximal duodenum, and both biliary and pancreatic systems can be radiologically defined. Lesions within the gastro-duodenal lumen can be biopsied and pancreatic juice sampled for cytological examination. ERCP has superseded barium meal and hypotonic duodenography as a means of diagnosing pancreatic cancer.

Pancreatic function tests and pancreatic scintiscanning are of little value but CT-scans and selective angiography are helpful in some cases. CT-scanning has the great advantage that it is non-invasive. Angiography is now usually reserved to display the vascular anatomy in those few patients in whom pancreatic resection is contemplated.

The choice of tests is influenced by the facilities available. Every effort should be made to provide both radiological, cytological or histological confirmation of the diagnosis prior to surgery. Pancreatic tissue can now be obtained for histology by percutaneous fine needle aspiration, the needle being guided into the target area by ultrasonic or CT-scanning.

### Management

*Curative treatment.* Surgical resection offers the only prospect of cure. Cancers of the pancreas are usually too advanced to justify resection but in a few selected cases resection may be justifiable when cancer arises in the head of the gland.

The standard operation of radical pancreaticoduodenectomy (Whipple's procedure) entails enbloc resection of the head of the pancreas, duodenum, distal half of stomach and lower common bile duct with reconstruction of biliary, pancreatic and gastro-intestinal continuity (Fig. 34.11). The operation aims to eradicate the cancer but retain enough pancreatic tissue to ensure adequate endocrine and exocrine function. The operative mortality is high (10–20%) and survival rates differ little from those achieved by palliative bypass surgery.

Leakage from the pancreatico-jejunal anastomosis is a major source of mortality, and total excision of gland may be a safer and more effective operation when radical surgery is contemplated. However, life-long insulin therapy and pancreatic exocrine supplements are then required.

The prospects for patients with cancer of the peri-ampullary region, duodenum or distal common bile duct are less gloomy. Radical pancreatico-duodenectomy is associated with a more acceptable operative mortality rate (2–10%) and a reasonable 5-year survival rate (20–30%).

*Palliative treatment.* Relief of obstructive jaundice and duodenal obstruction are all that can be offered to the majority of patients with pancreatic cancer. Jaundice is usually relieved by cholecysto-jejunostomy (or choledocho-jejunostomy), and duodenal obstruction by gastro-jejunostomy.

Survival following palliative surgery is usually short and seldom 12 months. Survival for longer periods should raise doubt regarding the original diagnosis. The distinction between cancer and chronic pancreatitis is difficult. Biopsy confirmation of the diagnosis is essential and should always be performed before embarking on pancreatectomy.

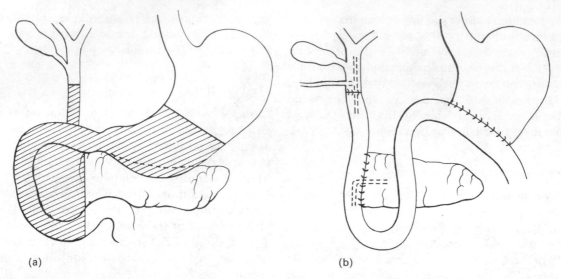

(a)                                              (b)

**Fig. 34.11** Whipple's operation. (a) Area resected. (b) Anastomoses performed. (The gall-bladder is usually removed)

Attempts to treat pancreatic cancer by chemo-therapy or radiotherapy have proved disappointing but continued trials are justified by the poor results of surgery. Pain relief is a vital part of the management of advanced disease, and the aid of a neurosurgeon may be enlisted if pain is not controlled by appropriate analgesic therapy.

## ENDOCRINE TUMOURS OF THE PANCREAS

Tumours arising in the pancreatic islets are un-common but they may be functional and show endocrine activity.

The commonest islet-cell tumour is the insuli-noma; it arises from B-cells and over-secretes insulin producing episodes of hypoglycaemia. Gastrinomas arise from G-cells and secrete gas-trin to give rise to the Zollinger-Ellison syndrome (see p. 385). Tumours of the A-cells secrete glucagon.

A series of non-B-cell tumours also are described which may secrete a variety of amines or polypep-tide hormones. For example, excess secretion of serotonin causes the carcinoid syndrome (see p. 406); ACTH, Cushing's syndrome (see p. 576); vasoactive intestinal peptide (VIP), pancreatic cholera. Such tumours may secrete more than one hormone and a proportion of patients will also have tumours or hyperplasia of endocrine cells at other sites.

The cell types which give rise to these tumours belong to the APUD series, having the capacity to take up and decarboxylate amine precursors (see p. 583). Rarely hyperplasia of islet tissue rather than a tumour can cause similar endocrine syndromes.

## INSULINOMA

This is a functioning endocrine tumour arising from the B-cells of the islands of Langerhans which secrete insulin. Such tumours are generally small (< 3 cm), single and they may be situated in any part of the gland. Multiple insulinomas do occur, usually as part of a multiple endocrine neoplasia syndrome (see p. 583). The great majority of insu-linomas are benign; less than 10% are malignant.

### Clinical features

The clinical features of an insulinoma result from inappropriate circulating levels of insulin. Unlike normal islet cells which secrete in response to glucose concentrations in the blood which perfuses them, an insulinoma secretes autonomously. As a result the glucose pool is inappropriately lowered and the central nervous system starved of glucose. Hypoglycaemic symptoms are usually mild but, over the years, there may be intellectual and motor impairment with insidious personality changes.

More severe attacks of hypoglycaemia may occur during which there are a wide variety of psychoneurological symptoms which include bizarre behaviour, sweating, palpitations and tremulousness. Because of memory lapses, the patient may not recall these events and the diagnosis may be suspected only when the patient is found in a state of hypoglycaemic coma.

Typically, attacks of hypoglycaemia are precipitated by fasting and relieved by taking glucose. Many patients become obese because of the associated hunger. Some patients are regarded as suffering from a psychiatric illness and are admitted to a mental hospital. The diagnosis is difficult and is made within one year of the first symptom in only one-third of patients.

## Diagnosis

The diagnosis of insulinoma depends on the demonstration of two things.

1. Hypoglycaemia (fasting blood sugar < 2.2 mmol/1) after an overnight (12–14 hour) fast.

2. Confirmation that the hypoglycaemia is due to excess insulin secretion. This is made by the finding of inappropriate insulin : glucose levels in the circulating blood. Insulin cannot normally be detected when glucose levels are subnormal but in a patient with an insulinoma, serial plasma insulin assays during a 12–14 hour fast will show persisting insulin levels in the face of falling glucose levels.

Further support for the diagnosis is demonstrated by a reduction of circulating insulin levels by diazoxide (600 mg infused IV over 1 hour) which inhibits insulin synthesis and suppresses insulin secretion. During this test ECG monitoring is necessary as the drug can cause cardiac arrhythmias.

An exaggerated response of insulin secretion to tolbutamide and glucagon has also been described but such provocative tests are potentially dangerous and not now used.

*Definition of tumour.* It is important to exclude other causes of inappropriate insulin secretion such as extrapancreatic tumours (particularly fibrosarcomas) and to localise insulinomas in the pancreas. Methods include ultrasonography, CT-scan and selective angiography but, because of the small size of the tumour, these are successful in only 40% of cases. Selective venous sampling from the splenic and portal vein by a catheter inserted through the liver allows plotting of the concentration of insulin at various sites and may define the point at which excess secretion is entering the venous system. Provided the diagnostic criteria are met, laparotomy is required but there is debate as to whether selective venous sampling should be used in all cases before surgery.

*Treatment.* Surgical removal of the tumour is the treatment of choice. Patients should initally be treated with diazoxide 1 g daily by mouth until they are fully controlled both symptomatically and biochemically. The abdomen is then explored and the pancreas mobilised and carefully palpated. Should the adenoma be found, it is removed.

If no tumour can be palpated, surgeons used to recommend that the body and tail of the pancreas should be removed in the hope that it contains the impalpable lesion. However, as only about half of occult tumours are situated in this region of the pancreas, it is better to leave the gland intact. Selective venous sampling is used post-operatively to localise the lesion which is subsequently removed.

## MALIGNANT TUMOURS

If a malignant tumour is found streptozotocin or nitrosoureas (BiCNU) are useful chemotherapeutic compounds. Symptoms of hyperinsulinism can be controlled by diazoxide although nausea, cardiac arrhythmias, leucopenia, hypertrichosis and postural hypotension may be troublesome.

## GLUCAGONOMA

Tumours producing excess glucagon occasionally arise from A-cells of the pancreatic islets and produce an unusual clinical syndrome predominantly found in middle-aged women. The most prominent feature is a necrotising migratory dermatitis which is associated with painful glossitis, stomatitis, constipation, weight loss, mild diabetes and anaemia. Plasma levels of glucagon are raised and a tumour may be defined on angiography.

Resection of the tumour, which is usually benign, reverses these effects. Streptozotocin may be beneficial in patients with non-resectable tumours.

# VIPOMA

Tumours arising in non-B-cells of the pancreatic islets can secrete a variety of polypeptides of which VIP (vasoactive intestinal peptide) is the most active. Such tumours may be solitary and benign but 50% are malignant. Diffuse hyperplasia of non-B-cells is also described.

## Clinical features

VIPoma causes the syndrome of watery diarrhoea, hypokalaemia and achlorhydria (WDHA syndrome) or 'pancreatic cholera'. As its name suggests, the characteristic feature is of profuse watery diarrhoea with the passage of 5 litres or more of fluid resembling weak tea and rich in potassium (50–60 mmol/1). The daily loss of potassium may be as much as 300 mmol causing severe hypokalaemia and metabolic alkalosis. The patient may be confused and intestinal ileus and abdominal distension may lead to a suspicion of intestinal obstruction. Tetany may occur due to hypomagnesaemia.

These symptoms can be intermittent and diagnosis may be delayed for some years after their onset. For this reason, malignant tumours have usually metastasised by the time of their discovery.

Diagnosis is achieved by the demonstration of hypokalaemia, achlorhydria and increased levels of VIP in the circulating blood. As these tumours are larger than other islet-cell tumours, angiography should always be performed and, in most cases will demonstrate the tumour.

## Treatment

Adequate fluid and electrolyte replacement before surgery is mandatory. Corticosteroids may help to control the diarrhoea. Surgical treatment aims at removing the tumour and, in the case of a solitary tumour, this can be successfully performed. Sub-total or total pancreatectomy is often required.

In unresectable cases or when metastases are present, streptozotocin or embolisation of feeding vessels through arterial catheters may relieve symptoms. Following successful treatment, there may be a rebound of gastric secretion and this should be controlled with cimetidine.

# 35. The Abdominal Wall and Hernia

## UMBILICUS

The umbilicus is the site of attachment of the umbilical cord, the 'life-line' of the developing fetus. Various congenital defects may affect the vitello-intestinal duct and urachus, which connect the umbilical cord to the intestinal and urinary tracts of the fetus.

### VITELLO-INTESTINAL DUCT

In the fetus the vitello-intestinal duct runs from the middle of the mid-gut loop to the umbilicus to connect with the yolk sac. Normally it is obliterated at birth. The duct may remain open for its whole length (vitello-intestinal fistula) causing a faecal fistula at the umbilicus at birth. A Meckel's diverticulum (see p. 396) is due to persistence of its intestinal extremity. Less commonly a portion of the duct may remain patent to form a cyst or mucocoele which hangs from the anti-mesenteric border of the ileum (enterocystoma). Alternatively the umbilical portion of the duct may form a polypoidal raspberry-like tumour on the surface enteroteratoma (Fig. 35.1).

Treatment of symptomatic remnants, e.g., a fistula or an obvious lesion at the umbilicus consists of excision. Asymptomatic remnants, e.g., enterocystoma or a Meckel's diverticulum, may be discovered at laparotomy. These may be excised to prevent complications although a Meckel's diverticulum can safely be left if broad-based.

A vitello-intestinal band (obliterated duct) may cause intestinal obstruction.

## URACHUS

The urachus runs from the apex of the bladder to the umbilicus. Normally obliterated at birth, it may remain patent giving rise to a urinary fistula at the umbilicus. Cysts may form from persistent urachal remnants. Symptomatic remnants of the urachus are best treated by excision.

## UMBILICAL SEPSIS

In new-born children umbilical sepsis may be the cause of portal thrombophlebitis and fatal jaundice or portal hypertension. Tetanus neonatorum due to the application of cow-dung to the umbilicus to promote healing was once common. In adults, umbilical sepsis results from retention of inspissated sebum within the folds of the umbilicus. Pilonidal sinuses of the umbilicus, similar to those in the natal cleft, are also described. Infantile sepsis is treated by frequent cleansing with an antiseptic and the application of an antibacterial powder. Adult lesions are eradicated by excision.

## UMBILICAL TUMOURS

Squamous carcinoma and melanoma may occur within the umbilicus. They may only be discovered when the umbilicus is excised for a persistent discharge. Secondary deposits of carcinoma at the umbilicus arise from the spread of tumour along the ligamentum teres, either from the liver or from lymph nodes in the porta hepatis.

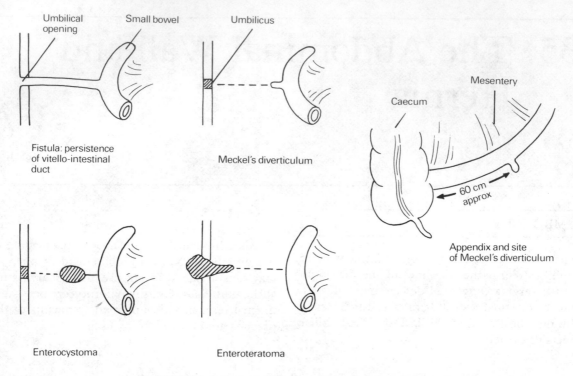

**Fig. 35.1** The vitello-intestinal duct and its clinical syndromes

## AFFLICTIONS OF THE RECTUS MUSCLE

### HAEMATOMA OF THE RECTUS SHEATH

Rupture of the inferior epigastric artery may follow direct trauma or may arise spontaneously following sudden contraction of the rectus. It causes a painful swelling of the rectus sheath associated with muscle rigidity. This condition is rare but can arise during pregnancy. Exploration, with ligature of the offending vessel and evacuation of clot is indicated.

### DESMOID TUMOUR

This rare fibromatous tumour arises from a fibrous intramuscular septum in the lower rectus. It is said to be commoner in women of child-bearing age and may be associated with intestinal polyposis (Gardner's syndrome). As it is prone to recur and give rise to a fibrosarcoma, it must be widely excised.

## HERNIAS

A hernia or rupture is a swelling caused by the protrusion of part of an organ, or other tissue, through an aperture in the walls of its retaining space (Fig. 35.2). Such an aperture may be present normally or may be abnormal in which case it can be congenital or acquired (e.g. following trauma).

A hernia can affect any viscus (e.g., brain, lung, intestine) or tissue (e.g., muscle, tendon) which lies within a cavity or constraining sheath. It may take the name of the organ involved (eg cerebral, small bowel), the aperture through which it has occurred (hiatus hernia), or the region where it presents (lumbar or epigastric hernia).

### ABDOMINAL HERNIA

Hernias of the abdominal wall are common. While, in theory, they can occur at any site, they commonly exploit natural orifices in the abdominal wall through which structures enter and leave the abdominal cavity. These are the inguinal and

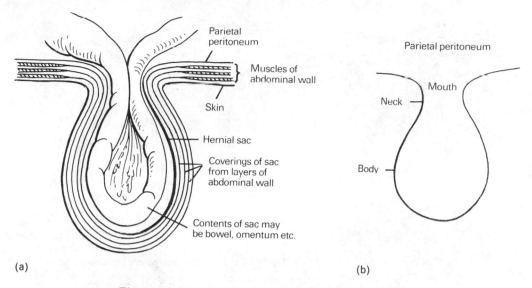

**Fig. 35.2** A hernia. (a) Anatomy. (b) Parts of the hernial sac.

femoral canals, the umbilicus, the obturator canal and the oesophageal hiatus in the diaphragm. Other hernias protrude through an area of weakness in the abdominal wall, either due to stretching of the abdominal muscles (direct inguinal hernia), a gap in a fibrous layer (epigastric hernia) or a surgical incision (incisional hernia).

An abdominal hernia is immediately enclosed by the peritoneal lining of the abdominal cavity. This forms the peritoneal *sac* which is covered by those tissues stretched in front as it protrudes to the surface (the *coverings*). The neck of the sac is that part which corresponds to the orifice through which it protrudes. A hernia may contain any intraperitoneal structure. Most commonly this is bowel or omentum. Should only a segment of the circumference of the bowel wall be included, it is called a 'Richter's hernia' (Fig. 35.3).

A hernia may be reducible (can be returned to the abdominal cavity) or irreducible. If irreducible, its contained bowel may become obstructed (if the lumen is constricted) or strangulated (if the blood supply is impaired). Omentum may also become strangulated. These effects are due to constriction at the neck of the sac.

## GROIN HERNIAS

Hernias in the region of the groin account for 75–80% of all abdominal wall hernias. There are three common types: indirect inguinal (60%), direct inguinal (25%) and femoral (15%). The majority (85%) of all groin hernias occur in males.

In early life an indirect inguinal hernia is by far the commonest groin hernia. After middle age increasing weakness of the abdominal musculature leads to an increase in the incidence of direct hernias, particularly in males. Femoral hernia is relatively more common in females but an indirect inguinal hernia is still the commonest groin hernia in women.

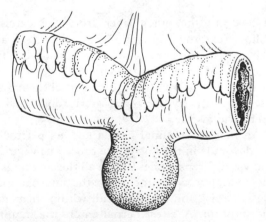

**Fig. 35.3** Richter's hernia

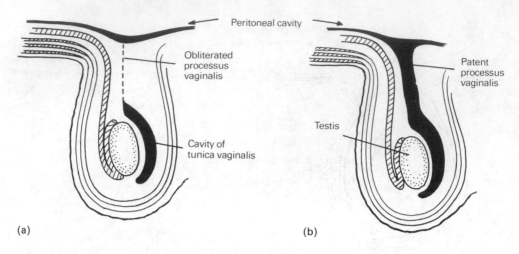

**Fig. 35.4** Processus vaginalis. (a) Normal. (b) Persistence of patent processus.

# INGUINAL HERNIA

## Anatomy of inguinal canal

The inguinal canal is formed by the descent of the testis through the abdominal wall during fetal life. The testis drags with it a tube-like covering of peritoneum, the processus vaginalis. This covering of peritoneum persists as the tunica vaginalis testis in the scrotum; the processus is normally obliterated (Fig. 35.4).

The testis and its peritoneal covering pass obliquely through the three muscles of the anterior abdominal wall on their route to the scrotum. The internal opening lies 1 cm above the mid-inguinal point (internal inguinal ring) while the external opening lies just above and medial to the pubic tubercle (the external inguinal ring). The internal ring is bounded medially by the inferior epigastric artery (Fig. 35.5). At birth the inguinal canal is short and straight so that the internal and external rings lie one on top of the other. The spermatic cord, consisting of vas deferens and the testicular vessels and lymphatics and fascial coverings occupies the inguinal canal, and runs down from the external ring into the scrotum.

As it passes through the abdominal wall the testis and its supporting vessels receive a covering from each layer (Fig. 35.4). The innermost layer is derived from the transversalis fascia (the internal spermatic fascia), the middle layer from the internal oblique muscle (cremasteric muscle and

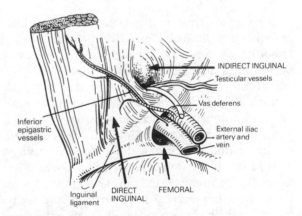

**Fig. 35.5** Anatomy of the internal ring, showing the sites of herniation from within

fascia) and the outer layer from the external oblique (external spermatic fascia). The testis and that part of the cord which lies outside the full thickness of the abdominal wall are covered by all three layers. Within the inguinal canal the cord is covered only by the cremasteric and internal spermatic fasciae.

An *indirect* inguinal hernia and its peritoneal sac descends in the line of the processus vaginalis and vas deferens. It lies within all the coverings of the spermatic cord (including the internal spermatic fascia) and may descend within them into the scrotum. A *direct* hernia enters the inguinal canal through the posterior wall of the canal medial to the internal ring. Its sac lies behind and distinct from the cord and its coverings, and is covered only by transversalis fascia. If it protrudes through the external ring it picks up a covering of external spermatic fascia but does not normally descend into the scrotum.

## INDIRECT INGUINAL HERNIA

The commonest cause of an indirect inguinal hernia is believed to be failure of obliteration of the processus vaginalis, so that the sac of peritoneum still extends for a varying distance down the inguinal canal. If complete the sac extends into the scrotum and is continuous with the tunica vaginalis. The vas deferens is closely adherent to the medial wall of the sac.

It is uncertain that all indirect hernias can be explained on the basis of a persistent processus and preformed sac. However, even if a peritoneal sac is acquired by descent of the hernia, it occupies the same anatomical position as the obliterated processus.

An indirect inguinal hernia usually descends through the external inguinal ring. If it remains within the inguinal canal it forms a localised swelling or bubonocoele. Alternatively, it may enlarge between the muscular layers of the abdominal wall to become an *interstitial hernia*.

The contents of the hernial sac may include omentum, small intestine, the appendix, an ovary or even a Meckel's diverticulum. As these viscera lie free within the peritoneal cavity they can descend freely within the sac.

Should large intestine form the hernia, it may be covered only partially with peritoneum and form a sliding hernia (see p. 524).

The internal and external inguinal rings in themselves seldom constrict the contents of the hernia and an indirect hernia is usually reducible. Irreducibility is usually due to thickening of the neck of the peritoneal sac to form an unyielding fibrous ring.

### Clinical features

An indirect inguinal hernia is commoner in males and on the right side. Herniation may be associated with a sudden pain in the groin or may pass unnoticed. Thereafter there is at most a dragging discomfort in the groin, particularly during lifting or strain. Further pain *in the hernia* will occur only when it is complicated by strangulation.

An indirect hernia forms a swelling in the inguinal canal, at the external ring, in the upper part of the scrotum or in almost the entire side of the scrotum. An inguinal hernia passes through the abdominal wall above and medial to the pubic tubercle, in contrast to a femoral hernia which emerges below and lateral to the tubercle (Fig. 35.6). A cough impulse may be visible or palpable as a thrill. Bowel sounds may be heard on auscultation of the hernia. Adult inguinal hernias are best treated surgically. As hernia repairs can be adequately performed under local anaesthesia, contra-indications to operation are few in number. Should operation be refused or contra-indicated a truss may be prescribed, but this tends to be uncomfortable. As a truss causes pressure atrophy of the muscles subsequent surgery becomes more difficult.

An indirect hernia often reduces spontaneously when the patient lies down, or when gentle pressure is applied in an upward and lateral direction. Then the only sign of a hernia may be thickening of the spermatic cord (due to the sac) or a cough impulse.

Once reduced an indirect hernia can be con-

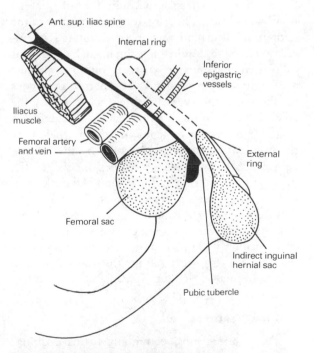

**Fig. 35.6** Exit of femoral and inguinal hernias

trolled by placing a finger over the internal ring. A cough impulse may then be palpated. Alternatively the skin of the upper scrotum can be invaginated by the little finger which is run along the spermatic cord to the external ring; the patient then is asked to cough.

If a patient complains of a bulge or swelling on exercise but no hernia is visible or palpable, he should be asked to stand with his legs apart and a cough impulse sought. If the diagnosis is still in doubt he should be asked to exercise and report when the hernia is down. Exploration is justifiable if the patient gives a clear history of a reducible swelling in the inguinal region.

### Interstitial inguinal hernia

In this type of hernia, the sac extends between the layers of the abdominal wall to form a large diffuse bulge extending upwards and medially from the internal ring. Such an extension is rarely seen in Europeans unless the inguinal canal is obstructed by an undescended testis. However, it is common in some African countries.

## DIRECT INGUINAL HERNIA

Direct inguinal hernias account for 40% of all inguinal hernias. They are due to a weakness of the abdominal wall and may be precipitated by increased intra-abdominal tension in such conditions as obstructive airways disease, obesity, chronic constipation or prostatism. The hernia protrudes through the transversalis fascia as it forms the posterior wall of the inguinal canal. The defect is bounded above by the conjoint tendon, below by the inguinal ligament and laterally by the inferior epigastric artery. This vessel lies medial to the internal inguinal ring and separates the neck of an indirect from that of direct hernial sac (Fig. 35.5). The hernia may protrude through the external ring but the transversalis fascia cannot stretch sufficiently to allow it to proceed down to the scrotum. As the defect is large and the neck of the sac wide, a direct hernia is seldom irreducible and rarely obstructs or strangulates.

### Clinical features

A direct hernia most commonly forms a diffuse bulge over the medial part of the inguinal canal

and is easily reduced by backward pressure. Following reduction the edges of the defect in the posterior wall of the canal may be palpable. Reduction by backward pressure is in contrast to that required in an indirect hernia which reduces obliquely by pressure directed upwards and laterally. Occasionally the sac of a direct hernia is funicular and extends down through the external ring to present just above the pubic tubercle.

Sliding direct inguinal hernias are common (see p. 524). As they are medially placed the urinary bladder may descend in the medial wall of the sac.

## TREATMENT OF UNCOMPLICATED INGUINAL HERNIA

### Conservative treatment

In infants, an indirect inguinal hernia may disappear spontaneously due to fusion of the walls of its sac. A simple pressure pad of wool is inserted in the diaper to maintain reduction and is all that is required as a preliminary measure.

Infantile hernias seldom strangulate, and little risk is incurred by leaving them alone. Operation is indicated if the hernia is still present at 2 years of age.

Adult inguinal hernias can be controlled by a truss but are best treated surgically. Only if operation is refused or contraindicated should a truss be prescribed. Hernia repairs can be adequately performed under local anaesthesia.

A truss consists of a pressure pad which is incorporated in a steel spring clipped around the waist (Fig. 35.7). The pad lies over the internal inguinal ring and the hernia must be reduced before it is applied. A patient will usually apply the truss before getting out of bed each morning and wears it throughout the day. The adequacy of control can be checked by asking the patient to stand with his legs apart and to cough violently. A truss is uncomfortable, causes pressure atrophy of the muscles and makes subsequent surgery more difficult.

### Surgical repair of an inguinal hernia

The first principle of an operation for an *indirect inguinal hernia* is to free the sac and remove it after transfixing its neck with a ligature (Fig. 35.8). In

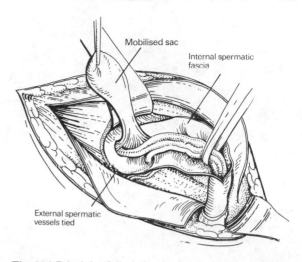

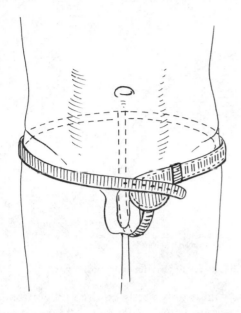

**Fig. 35.7** Inguinal hernia truss

**Fig. 35.8** Principle of dissection in the repair of an inguinal hernia

young children, the abdominal musculature is normal, the internal ring is not dilated and simple excision of the sac (herniotomy) is all that this required.

In older children and young adults the internal ring is dilated. Provided the musculature is normal, narrowing of the ring around the cord with a few non-absorbable sutures will complete the operation. Careful suture of the transversalis fascia around the internal ring is advised.

In older patients the posterior wall of the canal is stretched and weakened and a variety of surgical procedures are used to tighten the deep inguinal ring and strengthen the posterior wall and so prevent recurrence. The simplest method is to plicate the transversalis fascia (Fig. 35.9). More commonly the conjoint tendon and internal oblique muscles are also sutured to the pubic tubercle and under surface of the inguinal ligament using

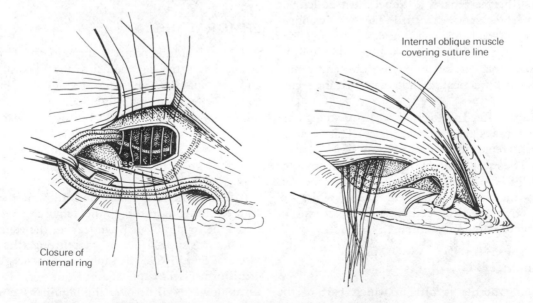

**Fig. 35.9** Plication of transversalis fascia in inguinal hernia repair

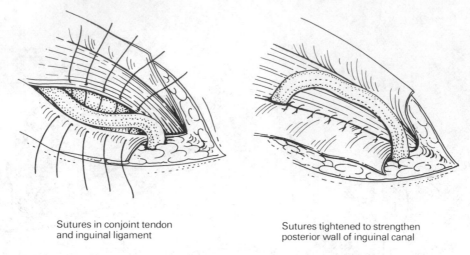

Sutures in conjoint tendon
and inguinal ligament

Sutures tightened to strengthen
posterior wall of inguinal canal

**Fig. 35.10** Posterior wall strengthened in inguinal hernia repair (Bassini-type repair)

non-absorbable interrupted sutures (herniorrhaphy) (Fig. 35.10). Tension can be avoided by incising the anterior rectus sheath (Tanner's slide).

In a *direct hernia*, excision of the sac is not usually required. The sac is simply invaginated by a few sutures placed in the transversalis fascia. If the sac projects through a clearly defined defect in the posterior wall of the canal, it can be excised. Repair of the posterior wall of the canal can be difficult as the tissues are stretched and thinned. In some cases it is necessary to use a mesh of terylene for reinforcement.

In all hernia repairs a tunnel must be left for the emerging spermatic cord. This may compromise the repair of large hernias, and, in older patients, removal of the testis and cord so that the inguinal canal can be completely obliterated may be the most practical method of preventing recurrence.

*Results.* After any form of repair of an inguinal hernia there is a risk of recurrence. This varies in different reported series, but can be as high as 10%. The most common form of recurrence after repair of an indirect hernia is another indirect hernia, this due to incomplete excision of the sac. After repair of a direct hernia, a direct type of recurrence is more common.

### Sliding hernia

A sliding hernia is one in which part of the circumference of the sac is formed by a viscus whose wall is only partly covered by peritoneum, e.g., caecum, colon or bladder. The viscus is part of the hernial sac, but lies outside the peritoneum (Fig. 35.11). A sliding hernia is usually large, and occurs most commonly in elderly patients. Repair can be difficult, and a variety of operative procedures have been described to re-peritonealise the bowel so that it can be returned to the abdomen. This is unnecessary and it is better to excise the sac distal to the bowel which is then gently pushed back into its normal retroperitoneal position before repair is carried out.

### FEMORAL HERNIA [more common in ♀]

A femoral hernia projects through the femoral canal. The canal lies medial to the femoral vein and opens into the abdomen through the femoral ring. The femoral ring is bounded in front by the inguinal ligament, laterally by the femoral vein and medially by the lacunar ligament. Posteriorly the pubic bone has a thickened ridge of periosteum known as the pectineal ligament of Cooper (Fig. 35.12).

A femoral hernia pushes the extraperitoneal fat and peritoneum through the femoral ring and down the femoral canal. On leaving the canal the hernia turns superficially to pass through the deep fascia of the thigh at the saphenous opening. The cribriform fascia is pushed in front of it. It then turns upwards to lie over the inguinal ligament. Because of its many coverings, the size of a

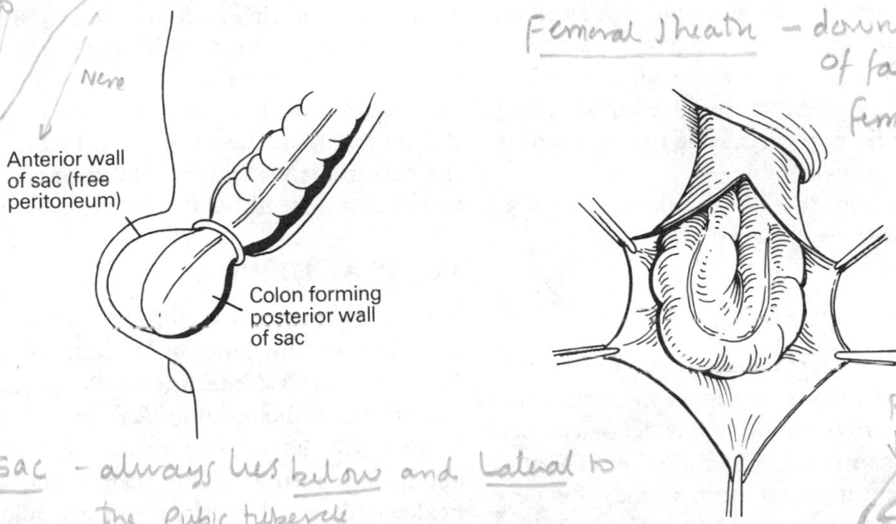

*Femoral Ring*   *Lymphatics*   *(Lateral)*

*Nerve*

*NOTE Femoral nerve outside*
*sheath at Lateral*

*Femoral Sheath — downward prolongation*
*of fascial lining and*
*femoral vessels and*
*Lymphatics*

Anterior wall
of sac (free
peritoneum)

V   A

*Femoral*
*Sheath*

Colon forming
posterior wall
of sac

*pectineal Lig*

*inguinal*
*Lig*

*Lacunar Ligament*

*Femoral Sheath*

*NECK of SAC — always lies below and Lateral to*
*the pubic tubercle*

Fig. 35.11 Sliding hernia

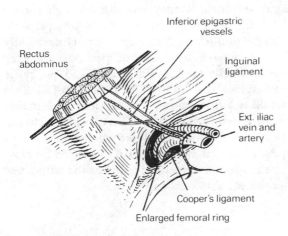

Inferior epigastric
vessels

Rectus
abdominus

Inguinal
ligament

Ext. iliac
vein and
artery

Cooper's ligament

Enlarged femoral ring

Fig. 35.12 Anatomy of the femoral ring

femoral hernia is deceptive. Thus, only a small sac may be present in the middle of a large mass of fatty and fibrous tissue.

A femoral hernia normally contains omentum, small bowel or both. Urinary bladder may be found in the medial wall of the sac.

A femoral hernia accounts for 5% of groin hernias in men and 20% in women. This sex difference is attributable to the stretching of the pelvic ligaments and widening of the femoral ring during pregnancy. Nulliparous females have the same incidence of femoral hernias as males.

## Clinical features

A femoral hernia typically presents as a bulge in the upper inner aspect of the thigh just beneath the inguinal ligament. Once it emerges from the saphenous opening it forms a well defined, soft or firm swelling which is situated below and lateral to the pubic tubercle but which may extend upwards over the inguinal ligament. This type of hernia is particularly difficult to distinguish from an *inguinal hernia* but the diagnosis is suggested by the absence of a cough impulse over the inguinal ring and the fact that a femoral hernia is difficult to reduce along its tortuous J-shaped course.

The relationship of the hernia to the pubic tubercle is the key to the diagnosis. The tubercle is defined by tracing the tendon of adductor longus upwards to its insertion. A femoral hernia emerges below and lateral to the pubic tubercle while inguinal herniae emerge above and medial to it. If there is doubt about the nature of a hernia in the groin it usually proves to be femoral.

A femoral hernia must also be differentiated from:

1. *inguinal lymph nodes* which usually are multiple and occupy the normal distribution of the inguinal nodes. There is no cough impulse and they cannot be reduced.

2. *Saphenous varix* which is a dilated terminal

portion of the saphenous vein. The soft swelling in the upper medial part of the thigh disappears when the patient lies down and the leg is elevated. There is a clearly palpable impulse on coughing (saphenous thrill) or on percussing the long saphenous vein lower down the leg.

3. A *lipoma*, forming a soft lobulated, subcutaneous, irreducible swelling.

## Treatment

A femoral hernia is particularly liable to strangulate. As it cannot readily be reduced and its point of emergence from the abdomen is deep-seated, a truss will not control it. Operation is indicated and, as with an inguinal hernia, may be performed under local or general anaesthesia.

The principles of the operation are complete excision of the sac and the repair of the defect (obliteration of the femoral ring). The femoral canal can be approached (1) from below the inguinal ligament; (2) through the posterior wall of the inguinal canal and (3) from above, by incising the anterior wall of the rectus sheath and dissecting downwards between the transversalis fascia and peritoneum to expose the inner surface of the pubis (Fig. 35.13). The latter approach gives best access to the femoral ring and is preferred if there is any hint of strangulation. Following reduction and excision of the hernial

sac the femoral ring is obliterated by suturing the inner surface of the conjoint tendon to the pectineal ligament of the pubis.

If reduction of the sac from above is difficult, the lower flap of the wound can be elevated from the subcutaneous tissues, allowing the sac to be exposed and freed below the inguinal ligament.

## VENTRAL HERNIAS

Ventral hernias occur through areas of natural weakness in the anterior abdominal wall (Fig. 35.14). These are the linea alba (epigastric hernia), the umbilicus (umbilical and paraumbilical hernia), the lateral border of the rectus sheath (Spigelian hernia). The scar tissue of poorly healed abdominal incisions may also allow herniation (incisional hernias).

### Epigastric hernia

Extraperitoneal fat may protrude through a small defect in the linea alba to form a soft palpable midline swelling in the epigastrium. Occasionally there is also a small sac of peritoneum. This hernia usually occurs in thin men and can cause marked local discomfort. The presence of a hernia should not be regarded as sufficient explanation for a history of dyspepsia. This complaint should always be investigated by orthodox means.

An epigastric hernia is easily repaired by closing the slit-like defect in the linea alba with a few non-absorbable sutures.

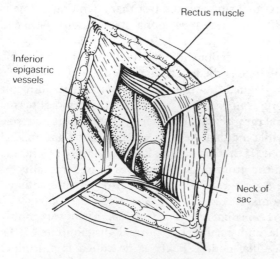

**Fig. 35.13** Surgical approach to a femoral hernia (McEvedy's approach)

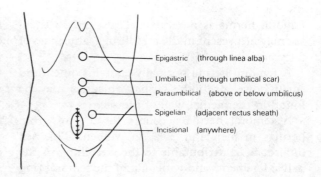

**Fig. 35.14** Sites of ventral hernias

## Umbilical hernia

A true umbilical hernia occurs in infants. A small sac of peritoneum protrudes through the umbilicus everting the skin when the child cries (Fig. 35.15). It is easily reduced, and the edges of the ring-like defect are then clearly palpable. An umbilical pad will maintain reduction.

Although these hernias usually close by puberty, persistence to the age of 2 years is usually an indication for operation. This is a simple procedure. If the neck of the sac is narrow it can be ligated by inserting a subcutaneous suture (Fig. 35.16). If larger, a formal repair may be required. Even then the umbilicus need not be excised.

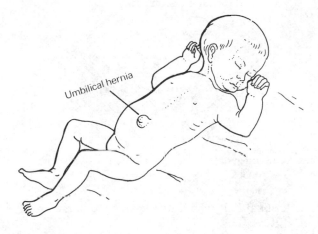

**Fig. 35.15** Clinical picture of an infantile umbilical hernia

## Para-umbilical hernia

This arises from gradual weakening of the tissues around the umbilcus. It predominantly affects obese multiparous women. The hernia passes through the attenuated linea alba and may be situated above or below the umbilicus. It gradually increases in size. The coverings become stretched and thinned and loops of bowel may be visible under parchment-like skin. The skin may become reddened, excoriated and ulcerated, and a faecal fistula can occur.

The sac is multilocular, and contains adherent omentum with loops of large and/or small bowel. These can become entrapped, and obstruction and strangulation are common. Such large hernias are invariably irreducible.

Operation is advised unless the patient is unfit. Strangulation, when it occurs, has a high mortality. The operation consists of excision of the hernia sac and its overlying skin including the umbilicus. An elliptical incision is made above and below the umbilicus and is deepened to define the linea alba and anterior sheath of the recuts. The edges of the defect are defined around its outer circumference and the peritoneum is then divided around the neck of the hernias. The omentum and bowel are separated from the sac, which is then removed with its overlying skin.

The aponeurotic defect in the linea alba is closed by overlapping the layers of the abdominal wall using mattress sutures of non-absorbable

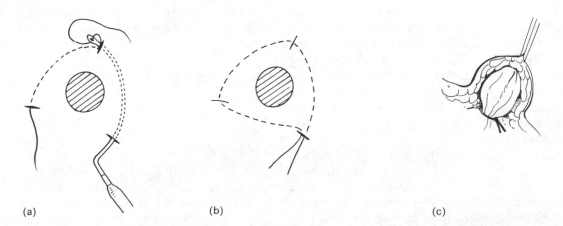

(a)  (b)  (c)

**Fig. 35.16** Repair of an infantile umbilical hernia. (a) & (b) Insertion of a subcutaneous suture using three puncture wounds. (c) Suture tied while sac kept taut and cut short to allow retraction into subcutaneous tissues.

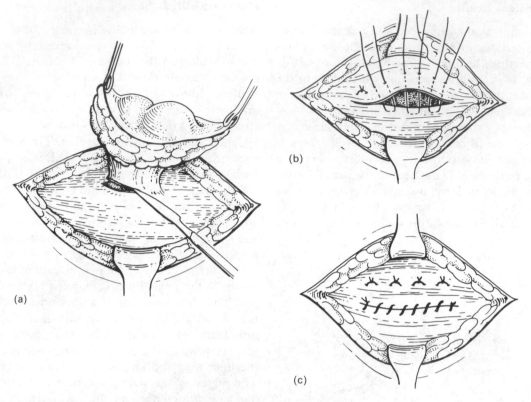

**Fig. 35.17** Mayo repair of umbilical hernia. (a) Excision of sac. (b) Insertion of overlapping sutures into rectus sheath. (c) Final result.

material (Fig. 35.17). Occasionally in large defects a Terylene mesh implant may be required.

## Incisional hernia

There is a diffuse protrusion of peritoneum and abdominal contents through a weakened area in an abdominal scar. Midline vertical incisions are most frequently affected, particularly below the umbilicus. The weakened area is due to non-healing or stretching of the linea alba. Poor suture techniques, wound dehiscence, chest and wound infection, and postoperative distension are precipitating factors.

There is a diffuse bulging of the wound, best seen when the patient is asked to raise his head and shoulders (or straight legs) from the bed and so contracts his abdominal muscles. Herniation may be association with a sensation of weakness.

Strangulation is rare but surgical repair is usually advised. Some patients prefer to wear an abdominal belt which may give adequate control of the hernia.

The skin wound is excised and the flaps elevated to expose normal aponeurosis. The edges of the defect are defined and repaired either by overlapping or by the insertion of a terylene mesh. The sac is either excised or invaginated depending on its size.

## COMPLICATIONS OF HERNIAS

The main complications associated with a hernia are irreducibility, obstruction and strangulation.

### Irreducibility

An irreducible hernia is one which cannot be returned to the abdominal cavity by manipulation. Most commonly this is attributable to narrowing of the neck of the sac by fibrosis, distension of the contained bowel or adhesion of contained omentum to the walls of the peritoneal sac.

## Obstruction

An irreducible hernia is a common cause of intestinal obstruction. Abdominal pain, vomiting and distension may indicate urgent operation. The hernial orifices *must* be inspected in all patients with suspected acute intestinal obstruction. In fact, this is an important step in *any examination of the abdomen.*

## Strangulation

The vessels supplying the loop of bowel contained in the hernia are compressed by the neck of the sac or constricting ring. The veins are affected first, and the bowel becomes cyanosed and oedematous, with an exudation of blood-stained fluid. The arterial supply is then compromised and gangrene follows. Organisms and toxins pass out through the bowel wall causing a local peritonitis of the hernial sac.

The patient complains of pain in the hernia, this being associated with the clinical features of intestinal obstruction. The hernia is tender, the cough impulse is lost and, if the hernia is in the groin, the hip is held in a flexed position. In a Richter's hernia, where only part of the wall of the bowel is strangulated, features of intestinal obstruction may be absent.

## Treatment

Provided there is no suggestion of strangulation an attempt can be made to reduce an irreducible hernia by the administration of analgesics, elevating the foot of the bed, and gentle pressure. Heavy pressure should never be used for fear of rupturing the bowel, or of returning it to the abdomen 'en masse' within the sac, when the obstruction is not relieved. If reduction is not achieved within a few hours, operation is advised. In infants strangulation rarely occurs, and it is reasonable to wait longer.

Except in infants, early operation is indicated for all cases of obstructed hernia. One can never be certain that the hernia is not strangulated and delay may be dangerous. The hernia is explored, the sac opened and the cause of the obstruction ascertained. In the case of an inguinal hernia

this is likely to be narrowing of the neck of the sac; in the case of a femoral hernia constriction of the femoral ring; and in the case of an umbilical hernia adhesions within the sac. The bowel is carefully inspected and preserved only if there is no doubt as to its viability. Devitalised bowel is resected. The contents are returned to the abdomen, the sac excised and the hernia repaired.

## RARE EXTERNAL HERNIAS

### Lumbar hernia

This rare hernia forms a diffuse bulge above the crest of the ileum, between the posterior border of external oblique and anterior border of latissimus dorsi.

### Obturator hernia

Commoner in women, this rare hernia is a protrusion of peritoneum and small bowel into the obturator canal, normally occupied by the obturator nerve and vessels. The diagnosis is normally made only when the hernia has strangulated and then it is discovered at laparotomy. The characteristic clinical feature of pain referred down the inner side of the thigh and knee (in the distribu-

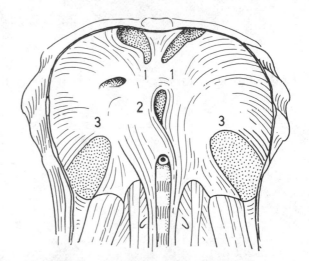

**Fig. 35.18** Sites of diaphragmatic herniation. 1. Between the sternal and costal slips of the diaphragm (Morgagni), 2. The oesophageal hiatus, 3. The pleuroperitoneal canal (Bochdalek).

tion of the geniculate branch of the obturator nerve) is very rare.

## INTERNAL ABDOMINAL HERNIA

A variety of cul-de-sacs and peritoneal gaps resulting from the rotation of the bowel may be responsible for entrapment of bowel and acute intestinal obstruction.

For example, herniation through the foramen of the lesser sac (epiploic foramen of Winslow) into various fossa around the duodenum (paraduodenal) or through a gap at the attachment of the mesocolon of the pelvic colon (intersigmoid fossa).

Iatrogenic hernias may also occur through holes in the mesentery made at operations. Such gaps must always be carefully closed at the primary operation.

### Diaphragmatic hernia

*Congenital* diaphragmatic hernias occur through a persistent pleuro-peritoneal canal or between the central and anterolateral portions of the developing diaphragm (parasternal). (Fig. 35.18) *Acquired* diaphragmatic hernias occur through the oesophageal hiatus (see p. 354). *Traumatic* diaphragmatic hernia occurs from stab and gunshot wounds. Blunt abdominal trauma may also result in unrecognised diaphragmatic rupture or weakness, with immediate eventration, or later development of a large diaphragmatic hernia. Such hernias may also follow operations, e.g. oesophago-gastrectomy, in which the diaphragm is divided.

DDx Femoral hernia

(1) Inguinal canal ?

(2) superficial inguinal L/N — Lymphadenitis
Ca anal canal

(3) Great Saphenous vein — Saphenous Varix. Is there Varicose vein elsewhere

(4) psoas sheath — swelling above and below

(5) aneurysm of femoral artery

# 36. The Peritoneum

## ANATOMY

The abdominal cavity is lined by a thin sheet of endothelium which forms the internal layer of the abdominal wall (parietal peritoneum). During development of the abdominal viscera and organs, the peritoneal sac is invaginated to clothe these viscera with a layer of peritoneum (visceral peritoneum) and to form several pouches and compartments between them. The largest of these are the greater and lesser sacs of peritoneum connected by the epiploic foramen.

The peritoneum is smooth and glistening and secretes a small amount of fluid. Under certain circumstances, this may be increased to an abnormal amount so that it forms obvious free fluid in the abdominal cavity (ascites).

The visceral peritoneum is insensitive to touch, heat or chemical stimuli. The parietal peritoneum is exquisitely sensitive to all of these (Chapter 32).

The peritoneum is relatively resistant to infection but contamination of the peritoneal cavity, e.g. by perforation of a hollow viscus or spread of inflammation from a contained organ, may lead to peritonitis.

The omentum is a double fold of peritoneum connecting the liver to the stomach (lesser omentum) or the stomach to the colon (greater omentum) (Fig. 36.1). As the greater omentum is folded back on itself, it consists of four layers enclosing a continuation of the lesser sac of peritoneum which extends behind the stomach. The omentum contains variable amounts of fat and, in elderly patients, may become grossly adipose.

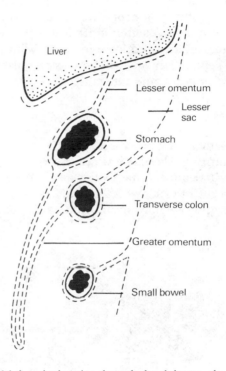

**Fig. 36.1** A sagittal section through the abdomen, showing the arrangement of peritoneal folds which form the lesser omentum and the greater omentum

## PERITONITIS

Peritonitis means inflammation of the peritoneum. The process may be acute or chronic; septic (due to pyogenic organisms) or aseptic (due to chemical irritation); primary (without pre-existing visceral disease) or secondary (caused by pre-existing visceral disease). Aseptic peritonitis usually becomes secondarily infected within 6–12 hours.

## ACUTE SUPPURATIVE PERITONITIS

Acute septic or pyogenic peritonitis may be primary or secondary. The common surgical form of peritonitis is secondary to one of the following: (1) inflammatory disease of the abdominal viscera; (2) perforation of the bowel or biliary tract; (3) infection of the female genital tract; (4) penetrating injury of the abdominal wall; or (5) rupture of an intra-abdominal abscess, e.g. subhepatic or pericolic (Fig. 36.2).

The site and extent of the inflammation depends on the origin of the infection. In acute cholecystitis or acute appendicitis, peritonitis may remain localised for some time. With perforated peptic ulcer or small bowel strangulation, it may rapidly become generalised.

## Pathology

The pathological process is similar to that of acute inflammation elsewhere. Both visceral and parietal peritoneum become acutely inflamed and there is a purulent exudate. Localisation of the inflammatory process may occur as the omentum 'walls off' the primary site of infection. An intra-abdominal abscess may then form.

Alternatively the infection may remain diffuse, when the abdomen is filled with foul-smelling purulent material. The intestine becomes flaccid and dilated and covered with fibrinous plaques which form adhesions between bowel loops.

## Clinical features

The initial symptoms of acute secondary peritonitis may be preceded by those of the primary condition which may cause visceral pain or other symptoms. Once the parietal peritoneum is involved the pain becomes somatic and well localised to the site of infection. As infection spreads within the peritoneal cavity the pain becomes diffuse. Pain in the shoulder indicates involvement of the diaphragmatic peritoneum. Vomiting is common but initially is not severe.

In these initial stages the patient lies still and is afraid to move (Fig. 36.3). Respiration is shallow and the abdomen is scaphoid. The most important single clinical sign is tenderness on direct pressure, the extent of which depends upon the area of involvement. Maximum tenderness occurs over the site of origin and may be defined by percussion or rebound tenderness. Muscular rigidity and/or guarding are present, and are maximal over the site of greatest tenderness. On auscultation the abdomen is silent. The pulse and temperature are usually moderately elevated.

If untreated the clinical picture gradually deteriorates. Pain becomes less prominent and vomiting more profuse. The vomitus consists first of bile and then small bowel content. With dilatation of the bowel from accumulation of fluid and gas and lessening of rigidity from increasing toxicity,

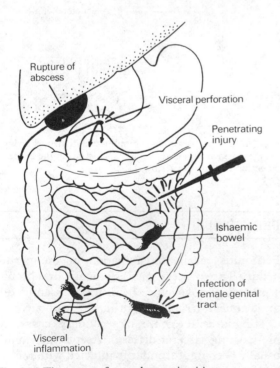

Fig. 36.2 The causes of secondary peritonitis

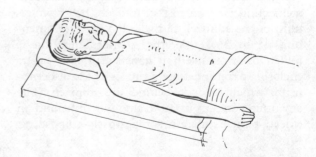

Fig. 36.3 The attitude of a patient with peritonitis

the abdomen becomes distended and the patient becomes obviously toxic and dehydrated. The pulse becomes rapid and weak and hypovolaemia, sepsis and shock supervene.

Plain abdominal X-rays may give a clue to the cause of the peritonitis, but usually do not contribute greatly to the diagnosis unless free gas is present. Biochemical tests are also of limited diagnostic value, although an increase in serum amylase levels suggests acute pancreatitis. In the late stages of peritonitis, estimates of blood gases are required in addition to electrolyte determinations which are routine in all cases.

## Treatment

The most important aspect of treatment of secondary peritonitis is to deal with the cause. For example, repair of a perforated viscus, resection of infarcted bowel, drainage or removal of an infective focus are essential measures. This will require an operation which should be performed with the minimum of delay. The only time which should be spent before operation is that necessary to resuscitate an ill patient. In established pyogenic peritonitis, antibiotic cover is indicated. Peritoneal lavage, with or without additive antibiotics, should be performed during operation, and is a useful procedure to wash out bacteria and infected material.

Peritonitis due to acute pancreatitis is an exception to this general rule. A non-operative policy is usually followed (p. 503).

Chronic ambulatory peritoneal dialysis may allow infection of the peritoneum and is usually controlled successfully by antibiotics.

## PRIMARY PERITONITIS

In paediatric practice, primary acute peritonitis accounts for approximately 15% of acute abdominal emergencies in infants and children.

The condition used to be most common in female children under 10 years of age, when it was due to pneumococcal or haemolytic streptococcal infection spreading to the peritoneal cavity from the genital tract. Nowadays E.coli is the predominant causative organism. It usually gains access to the peritoneal cavity through the wall of the intestine but some cases may be due to blood-borne spread from a septic focus elsewhere.

Primary peritonitis is a recognised complication of cirrhosis of the liver and nephrotic syndrome, particularly when associated with ascites. It is relatively rare in adult practice.

## Clinical features

The onset of primary peritonitis is abrupt. Classically, diffuse peritonitis with generalised abdominal tenderness and rigidity develop within 24 hours of onset. Fever and leucocytosis occur early. A plain abdominal X-ray shows no specific changes.

## Treatment

Appropriate antibiotic therapy is the mainstay of successful treatment. An exploratory laparotomy is usually required to rule out a correctable surgical cause and a specimen of peritoneal exudate is obtained for immediate Gram stain and culture. The appendix is removed and the abdomen closed without drainage. Irrigation of the peritoneal cavity with an anti-bacterial solution is advised by some.

Antibiotic therapy on the basis of the Gram stain is started immediately. This is modified according to the results of culture and sensitivity tests.

## TUBERCULOUS PERITONITIS

Most commonly occurring in females between the ages of 20 and 40 years, tuberculous peritonitis is now rare in this country. It is invariably secondary to tuberculosis elsewhere although the site of the primary infection is frequently unrecognised.

Two types of tuberculous peritonitis are described: (1) 'moist' or ascitic; and (2) 'dry' or plastic.

### Ascitic tuberculous peritonitis

Fever and progressive ascites are the most common clinical features. Abdominal pain is not usually severe. Anorexia, weight loss and night sweats may occur.

Diagnosis is by laparotomy or laparoscopy. Multiple caseating tubercles stud the peritoneum; biopsy establishes the diagnosis.

Percutaneous needle biopsy of the peritoneum

may be used as an alternative means of diagnosis. Culture of the ascitic fluid is unhelpful.

### Plastic tuberculous peritonitis

In this condition there is a dense inflammatory exudate with adhesions which mat the coils of intestine into multiple abdominal masses (Fig. 36.4). Fistulas may follow operation and laparotomy should be avoided unless required to relieve intestinal obstruction.

## ASEPTIC PERITONITIS

Various factors, e.g. foreign body, bile, blood, gastric juice, pancreatic enzymes, produce a peritoneal exudate which is initially sterile. Secondary infection is the rule. The management then is that of secondary peritonitis.

A *foreign body* may gain access to the peritoneal cavity: (1) through the abdominal wall as a result of a penetrating injury, e.g. a gunshot wound; (2) from the alimentary tract by penetration of the gut wall by a swallowed object or one inserted per rectum; or (3) by leaving a swab or instrument behind after operation. A sterile collection or abscess may develop with the later development of a sinus or fistula.

If symptoms are severe the abdomen is explored and the foreign body removed. Surgical swabs and instruments should be removed immediately their misplacement is discovered.

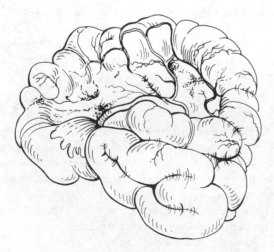

**Fig. 36.4** Plastic tuberculous peritonitis

Although *bile* is only a mild chemical irritant, infected bile causes a virulent peritonitis with severe toxaemia. Leakage of bile may complicate acute cholecystitis but occurs most commonly following biliary surgery. Spontaneous leakage from an apparently intact biliary tract is described.

*Blood* also is only a mild peritoneal irritant but sudden severe haemorrhage into the peritoneal cavity can cause severe abdominal pain and signs of acute abdominal disease. It should be removed, as it may form a nidus for secondary infection.

*Gastric juice* is very irritating to the peritoneum. Following perforation of a peptic ulcer there is an acute chemical peritonitis with severe abdominal pain, rigidity and shock. Sterile *urine* from an intraperitoneal rupture of the bladder behaves similarly. In both cases secondary bacterial infection is the rule. *Pancreatic enzymes* escape into the peritoneum in acute pancreatitis and are also severe irritants.

## GRANULOMATOUS PERITONITIS

Foreign body reactions of a chronic nature occur following contamination of the peritoneum with talc or starch as previously were used to powder surgical gloves. Multiple granulomas form on the peritoneal surfaces leading to the formation of fibrous adhesions.

Leakage of barium into the peritoneal cavity causes a severe plastic peritonitis with multiple dense adhesions.

## POST-OPERATIVE PERITONITIS

Peritonitis may follow any abdominal operation. This may be residual to the primary disease for which the operation was carried out or may occur as a direct complication of the operation, e.g. leaking anastomosis or a strangulated loop of bowel.

The diagnosis is difficult as: (1) the patient is receiving post-operative sedation and may not complain of pain; (2) such pain and tenderness as is present may be attributed to the presence of the wound; (3) normally there is a period of time after all abdominal operations (usually 48 hours) when bowel sounds are absent or diminished and the abdomen distended.

Persistence of abdominal distension for more than a few days after operation or the development of distension or vomiting after an initial return to normality should raise suspicion of peritoneal infection. In some patients the first signs of this development are tachycardia or altered mental state. Plain abdominal X-ray shows dilatation of the intestine; a leaking anastomosis may be demonstrated by gastrografin studies.

The treatment of post-operative peritonitis consists of fluid and electrolyte replacement, nasogastric tube decompression, broad spectrum antibiotic therapy and, if continuing intraperitoneal infection is suspected, laparotomy.

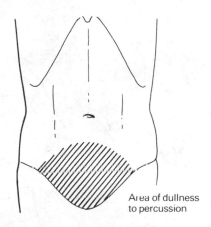

**Fig. 36.5** Suprapubic dullness to percussion due to full bladder or ovarian cyst

## ASCITES

Ascites is the accumulation of free fluid within the peritoneal cavity. Commonly, ascitic fluid is clear and straw coloured and is due to *transudation* across the peritoneal membrane in conditions such as cardiac failure, certain types of chronic renal failure, and portal hypertension. More often in surgical wards, ascites is due to the involvement of the parietal peritoneum by malignant deposits, which irritate the peritoneum, producing an *exudate* with a higher protein content than a transudate. Occasionally, the accumulation of free fluid may be due to blockage of lymph flow through the thoracic duct — the fluid is then milky in appearance due to the high content of absorbed fat in abdominal lymph (chylous ascites).

The clinical signs of ascites consist of:

1. Abdominal distension.

2. Dullness to percussion in the flanks (an ovarian cyst or a full urinary bladder is dull to percussion in the suprapubic region) (Fig. 36.5).

3. 'Shifting dullness' — the level of dullness in the flank alters as the patient rolls onto one or other side (Fig. 36.6).

4. 'Fluid thrill' — an impulse can be detected by a hand placed flat on one flank when the other flank is tapped with the fingers of the other hand. If an impulse is present, transmission through the abdominal wall must be prevented by a third hand (Fig. 36.7).

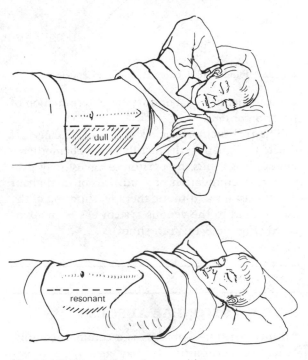

**Fig. 36.6** Shifting dullness due to ascites

5. A plain abdominal X-ray will demonstrate a uniform ground-glass appearance.

If ascites is suspected, a peritoneal tap is performed by inserting a needle at a point half-way between the umbilicus and the anterior superior iliac spine. If fluid is obtained, it should be sent to the cytological laboratory for examination, to the bacteriology laboratory for culture, and to the

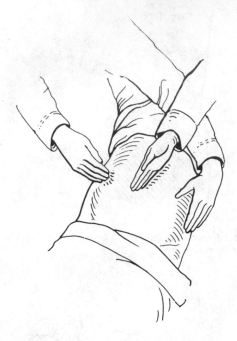

**Fig. 36.7** Fluid thrill due to ascites — clinical detection

clinical chemistry laboratory for determination of protein content.

The treatment of ascites is that of its cause. If due to malignancy, the instillation of chemotherapeutic drugs into the peritoneal cavity may prevent re-accumulation of fluid. In non-malignant cases resistant to diuretic therapy, shunting of the ascitic fluid to the venous system has been advocated (Fig. 36.8 LeVeen shunt).

## ABSCESS

### INTRAPERITONEAL ABSCESS

An intraperitoneal abscess is a common complication of peritonitis. It may also occur postoperatively as a result of contamination of the peritoneal cavity or following a leak from an anastomosis. Common sites of intraperitoneal abscess formation are shown in Figure 36.9.

The main clinical sign of an intra-abdominal abscess is persistent fever but more severe complications can occur. For example, erosion into a large vessel can cause catastrophic haemorrhage or rupture can induce peritonitis. Septicaemia may complicate all abscesses.

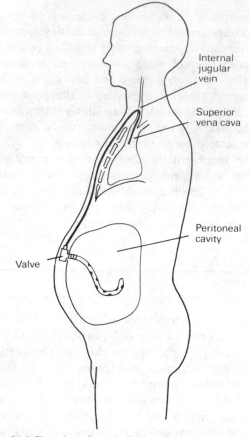

**Fig. 36.8** Shunting of ascitic fluid to the venous system

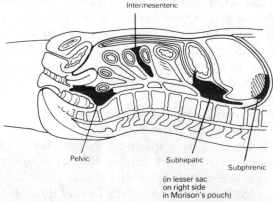

**Fig. 36.9** Common sites for intraperitoneal abscess formation. Note subhepatic abscess shown is on the left and in the lesser sac; on the right it would be in the subhepatic (Morison's) pouch.

The site of the abscess may be suspected from clinical examination but this can prove difficult and ultrasonic, CT and isotope scans (following the injection of [111]Indium labelled leucocytes) are of great value in localisation. Ultrasound may also guide the percutaneous insertion of a needle into the abscess cavity so that a definitive diagnosis can be made and, in some cases, drainage instituted.

Surgical drainage is still the most important treatment. Antibiotic therapy without drainage may confuse the picture by abolishing systemic signs and giving a false sense of security. An undrained intra-abdominal abscess is a potent source of septicaemic shock.

## SUBPHRENIC ABSCESS (Fig. 36.10)

Approximately half of all intra-abdominal abscesses occur in the subphrenic space. Three main separate spaces are described on each side, (Fig. 36.10) but these are of little practical importance.

Because of the relative inaccessability of these spaces, physical signs are notoriously absent in patients with subphrenic infections. Unexplained fever after a peritoneal infection or operation should always raise the suspicion of a subphrenic abscess.

In some cases, the site of the abscess can be suspected from its likely origin. Further, there may be pain and tenderness anteriorly or posteriorly on the affected side, and this may be intensified by compression of the lower ribs. Shoulder pain and oedema over the lower intercostal spaces may also occur and there may be dullness to percussion over the lower chest.

X-ray examination by anterior, lateral and oblique views is necessary in all suspected cases. This may demonstrate a pleural effusion and/or a fluid-gas-filled space below the diaphragm. Screening of the diaphragm or X-rays taken in full inspiration and expiration will demonstrate relative immobility on the affected side. Ultrasonic and CT scans may be diagnostic.

The treatment is by surgical drainage. The route, whether anterior or posterior, intra- or extra-peritoneal, depends upon the site of the abscess (Fig. 36.11). Repeated operations may be necessary. If the position is suitable percutaneous drainage under ultrasonic control may be sufficient.

## PELVIC ABSCESS

A pelvic abscess is a recognised complication of acute appendicitis and may follow appendicectomy. Fever, lower abdominal discomfort and diarrhoea are characteristic. Rectal examination discloses a tender, boggy swelling anteriorly (Fig. 36.12). If large, a pelvic abscess may form a palpable mass in the suprapubic region.

Spontaneous drainage of the abscess into the rectum usually occurs and treatment is normally

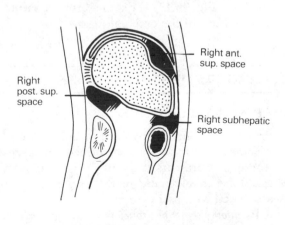
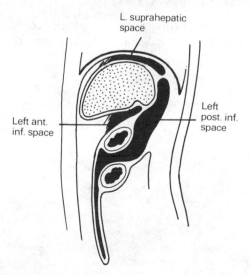

**Fig. 36.10** Sites of subphrenic abscess

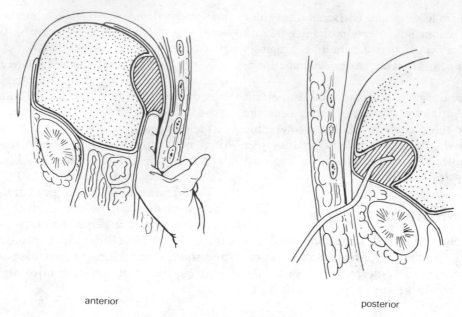

anterior                                    posterior

**Fig. 36.11** Routes of drainage for subphrenic abscess

expectant, with frequent rectal examination to assess progress. If it is clear that spontaneous drainage is unlikely, or the abscess is increasing in size with increased toxicity of the patient, surgical drainage of the abscess is performed either through the rectum or by an extraperitoneal suprapubic approach. Following adequate drainage, the symptoms and signs rapidly resolve.

## MESENTERIC CYST

This is a rare embryonic cyst which occurs in the mesentery of the small intestine and forms a

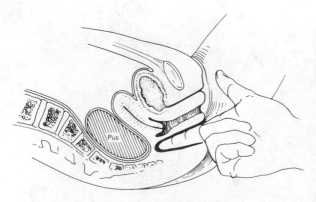

**Fig. 36.12** Rectal examination for pelvic abscess

round tense swelling in the right lower quadrant of the abdomen which classically is mobile in a vertical but not horizontal direction. Similar cysts may form in the omentum. Surgical removal is indicated.

## OMENTAL TORSION

If fixed by an adhesion, the omentum may undergo torsion and give rise to acute abdominal pain associated with a tender palpable central abdominal mass (Fig. 36.13). Treatment is by laparotomy and excision of the omental mass.

## TUMOURS OF THE PERITONEUM

### PRIMARY TUMOURS

Primary tumours of the peritoneum are rare but *mesothelioma* has been described in asbestos workers. It presents as a bulky epigastric mass or as diffuse involvement of the peritoneal surface associated with ascites.

*Pseudomyxoma peritonei* is a low grade malignant tumour which spreads throughout the peritoneal cavity and is usually of ovarian origin. It may also follow mucocoele of the appendix. Lobulated

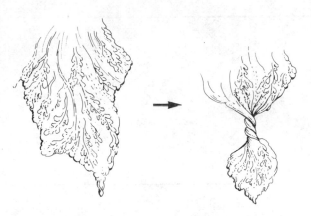

**Fig. 36.13** Omental torsion

deposits form on the peritoneal surfaces and there may be secretion of abundant mucus causing abdominal distension. The condition is commonly associated with intermittent bouts of intestinal obstruction and repeated operations to debulk the abdomen of tumour may be necessary. In view of its low grade malignancy, survival may be prolonged.

## SECONDARY TUMOURS

The peritoneal cavity is a common site of spread of malignant disease. Seedling deposits form on the peritoneal surfaces and ascites follows.

In most cases, a primary site is known and if the diagnosis is confirmed by cytological examination of the ascitic fluid there is little that can be done to palliate. Installation of chemotherapeutic agents may be tried but only temporises. Palpable deposits of tumour may be present in the recto-vesical pouch.

## RETRO-PERITONEAL TUMOURS

A variety of retro-peritoneal tumours, usually of connective tissue origin, present as a retro-peritoneal abdominal mass. Abdominal exploration and biopsy are necessary in all cases but the prognosis is usually hopeless. Occasionally, however, if the tumour is lymphomatous, radiotherapy and/or chemotherapy may cause regression and prolong life.

# 37. Spleen

## ANATOMY

The spleen is a friable blood-filled organ lying in the upper left quadrant of the abdomen and protected by the 9th, 10th and 11th ribs. It weighs 150 g, is ellipsoid or 'coffee bean' in shape and its long axis lies along the line of the 10th rib.

Its convex outer surface lies in contact with the diaphragm above and its lower pole with the splenic flexure of the colon below. Its concave inner surface is related to the fundus of the stomach, the tail of the pancreas and the upper pole of the right kidney. It is surrounded by a fibrous capsule and except at its hilus, covered by peritoneum which is reflected as ligaments running to adjacent organs. These are the lieno-renal, gastrosplenic and lieno-colic ligaments. The phrenico-colic ligament which runs between the splenic flexure of the colon and the undersurface of the diaphragm provides additional support.

About 350 litres of blood flow through the splenic artery each day. This is a branch of the coeliac axis which transmits 40% of the splanchnic blood flow into the spleen which then drains into the portal venous system by the splenic vein (Fig. 37.1). The splenic vessels are closely related to the pancreas and run between the gastrosplenic ligament anteriorly and the lieno-renal ligament posteriorly to reach the splenic hilum, the only part of the spleen without a peritoneal covering. These vessels also supply the uppermost part of the greater curvature of the stomach through the left gastroepiploic and short gastric vessels. Both the gastrosplenic and lieno-renal ligament and their contained vessels must be divided during splenectomy.

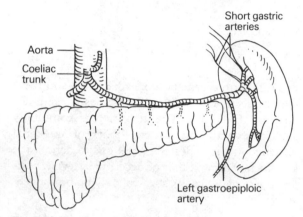

**Fig. 37.1** Blood supply of the spleen

The spleen is composed of white and red pulp. Some 25% of the lymphoid tissue of the body is contained within the spleen and forms the 'white pulp' which consists of lymphoid follicles (Malpighian bodies) and lymphatic tissue, containing lymphocytes, macrophages and plasma cells. These cells migrate to the spleen from the bone marrow; 30–50% are thymus-dependent. The red pulp is a loose honeycomb of reticular tissue which contains the splenic sinusoids. The blood vessels are carried into the pulp along fibrous trabeculae formed from the capsule (Fig. 37.2). The arterioles first traverse white pulp where they are surrounded by lymphoid tissue and then flow into the red pulp and sinusoids. It is controversial whether blood flows through the pulp spaces on its way to the sinusoids, or whether it enters the sinusoids directly and then meanders slowly backwards and forwards through the pulp. Erythrocytes move in and out of the pulp tissue so that 1% of the body red cells and 20–30% of the platelets are sequestrated at any given moment.

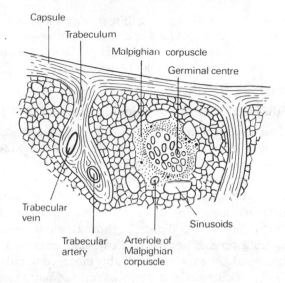

Fig. 37.2 Architecture of the splenic pulp

Normally the spleen is impalpable and cannot be percussed. When enlarged it extends downwards and medially below the costal margin. It is then best palpated bimanually with the patient's left side turned slightly forwards (Fig. 37.3) when the distinctive notch on its antero-inferior border will be felt. On percussion an enlarged spleen results in an area of dullness over the 9th rib in the mid-axillary line. Splenic enlargement can also be detected by soft tissue X-ray, a splenic scintiscan (using $^{99m}$Tc sulphur colloid to label the reticuloendothelial cells), ultrasonic or CT scan.

## FUNCTION OF THE SPLEEN

*Haemopoiesis.* The spleen is a source of red blood cells and granulocytes in fetal life. Thereafter extramedullary haemopoiesis occurs only in the myeloproliferative syndromes.

*Filtration of blood cells.* Normal blood cells pass through the spleen unchanged. Abnormal and ageing cells are trapped. Following splenectomy there is an increased number of misshapen red cells, those containing nuclear remnants (Howell-Jolly bodies) and those containing clumps of iron (siderocytes) in the peripheral blood. It has been estimated that 20 ml of red cells are phagocytosed daily. White cells and platelets, particularly when coated with antibodies, also are removed.

*Immune mechanisms.* The spleen is an important site for effecting both cell-mediated and humoral immunity. Particulate antigens are filtered off and immunoglobulins (particularly IgM) and phago-cytosis-promoting peptides are produced. Following splenectomy immunological responses are impaired.

*Reservoir.* In dogs the spleen acts as a reservoir for blood and in states of shock empties by contraction of its muscular capsule to provide an 'autotransfusion'. This is not a function of the spleen in man.

*Endocrine effects.* There is some evidence that the spleen exerts a humoral effect on the bone marrow, stimulating erythropoiesis and depressing white cell and platelet counts.

## INDICATIONS FOR SPLENECTOMY

While the decision to recommend removal of the spleen is usually in the hands of the haematologist, the surgeon must be aware of the indications for splenectomy and the criteria which should be

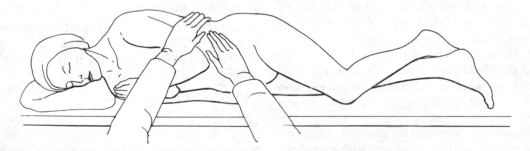

Fig. 37.3 Position for palpation of the spleen

fulfilled before acceptance of a patient for operation. The common indications are as follows:

## TRAUMA

Injury to the spleen is an indication for splenectomy. It is important to remember that spleens involved by pathological conditions such as portal hypertension, polycythaemia and infective mononucleosis are prone to rupture on slight trauma. Also it must be appreciated that following rupture, temporary improvement in the clinical signs may precede sudden deterioration. Awareness and careful observation are critical, particularly in those patients in whom a subcapsular haematoma can cause a 'delayed rupture'. These matters are considered in detail on p. 122.

## HAEMOLYTIC ANAEMIAS

### Hereditary spherocytosis

This autosomal dominant genetic disease affects the red blood cells which are spherical rather than biconcave, unduly fragile and less able to withstand the effects of passing through the splenic pulp than normal cells. Excess haemolysis results in anaemia, jaundice and splenic enlargement. It is a disease of remissions and relapses with 'haemolytic crises' requiring transfusion. Gallstones occur in 30–60% of cases.

Splenectomy is indicated in all cases when health is impaired. However, it should not be performed before the age of 3–4 years. If gallstones are present cholecystectomy should be carried out simultaneously.

### Acquired haemolytic anaemias

Excess haemolysis may be acquired (1) secondary to exposure to chemicals, drugs, infection, physical agents, chronic infections or extensive burns, or (2) as a result of an autoimmune phenomenon. In the latter condition the red cells are coated with an abnormal protein which is associated with the presence of an agglutinating gammaglobulin in the serum. These can be detected by direct and indirect Coomb's tests.

Autoimmune haemolytic anaemia predominantly affects middle-aged women who have severe haemolytic crises superimposed on a background of mild anaemia. Treatment consists of steroids, but if this fails to control the disease and excess sequestration of red cells has been demonstrated, splenectomy may be recommended.

## THE PURPURAS

### Idiopathic thrombocytopenic purpura (ITP)

This disease of unknown aetiology is characterised by low platelet counts and short platelet life-span despite plentiful megakaryocytes in the marrow. Cyclical episodes of bleeding occur from gastro-intestinal and other sites associated with petechiae and ecchymoses. Platelet counts will be below $50 \times 10^9/l$, bleeding time is prolonged, clotting time is normal and capillary fragility is increased. The spleen is palpably enlarged in only 2–3% of patients and dense adhesions may form around it.

There are two types of clinical course:

1. an acute 'short-history' form with a high incidence of spontaneous remission and an excellent response to steroids or splenectomy;

2. a chronic 'long-history' type with repeated relapses over many months or years, a poor response to steroids and a less satisfactory course following splenectomy.

The acute form of the disease is treated initially by steroid therapy. Rapid remission is associated with a good prospect of complete and lasting remission when therapy is stopped. If remission to steroid therapy does not occur rapidly, splenectomy should be advised. Splenectomy is required for the 'long-history' cases; steroids are of use only to provide temporary improvement before surgery.

Because of the high incidence of spontaneous remission splenectomy is not advised for acute ITP in children.

### Secondary thrombocytopenia

Splenectomy is contraindicated in secondary haemorrhagic purpuras, although it may be advised if proven hypersplenism is associated with secondary thrombocytopenia.

## HYPERSPLENISM

This syndrome consists of splenomegaly and pancytopenia in the presence of an apparently normal bone marrow and in the absence of an autoimmune disorder. There is sequestration and destruction of blood cells in the spleen affecting predominantly white cells and platelets.

Hypersplenism may be 'primary' when the spleen has responded by hypertrophy to an increased workload brought about by the need to sequestrate and destroy abnormal cells or secondary, when inappropriate cell destruction is secondary to an abnormality of the spleen which has resulted in its enlargement. Examples are:

1. inflammation, e.g. malaria, Leishmaniasis, sarcoidosis, rheumatoid arthritis (Felty syndrome);

2. congestive splenomegaly in portal hypertension, bilharziasis, portal vein thrombosis; and

3. infiltration, e.g. the mycloproliferative and lympho-proliferative disorders.

The effects of hypersplenism include expansion of the total blood volume, this being necessary to fill the increased vascular spaces of the enlarged spleen and splanchnic bed. There is increased pooling of cells within the enlarged spleen and excess destruction, possibly by metabolic damage due to the packing together in the enlarged spleen. In the peripheral blood there is anaemia, leucopenia, thrombocytopenia, but marrow turnover is increased with reticulocytosis, leucoerythroblastosis and increased urobilinogen in the urine.

Removal of a grossly enlarged spleen carries considerable morbidity and mortality and by eradicating a large mass of lymphoid tissue puts the patient at risk from serious bacterial infection. It must not be undertaken lightly and the haematologist will take into account the degree of cytopenia, the extent of splenic enlargement, the amount of discomfort caused and the incidence of recurrent infections from leucopenia. Isotopic studies of the sequestration of red cells in the liver and spleen will be performed and operation advised only if the spleen to liver index exceeds 2:1 (Fig. 37.4). This is calculated from the 'half-life' of the labelled red cells as measured over the spleen and liver compared to precordial counts.

## PROLIFERATIVE DISORDERS

### Myelofibrosis.

This condition was once believed to be due to obliteration of the blood-forming elements in the bone marrow by fibrosis. The resulting gross

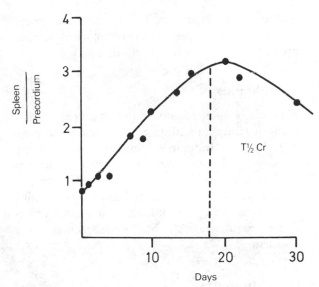

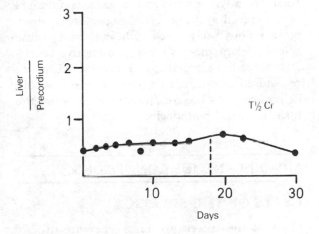

**Fig. 37.4** Measurement of spleen–liver sequestration. In this case, the spleen:liver ratio is 3.2:0.8 i.e. 4.0. Experience has shown that if this ratio is greater than 2.5, splenectomy is likely to alleviate a haemolytic process.

enlargement of the spleen was thought to be a secondary phenomenon to provide a site for extramedullary haemopoiesis. Splenectomy was contraindicated.

It is now recognised that the condition is due to an abnormal proliferation of mesenchymal elements in the bone marrow, spleen, liver and lymph nodes, and that extramedullary haemopoiesis occurs at many sites. Contrary to previous belief, splenectomy does not lead to a lethal aplastic anaemia, but decreases transfusion requirements. By relieving the discomfort of a grossly enlarged spleen, it also improves symptoms. However, careful haematological studies are indicated before it is advised.

### Lymphomas

The role of splenectomy in the staging and treatment of Hodgkin's disease is considered on page 553. In non-Hodgkin's lymphoma splenectomy is only rarely indicated, e.g. when a primary neoplasm is confined to the spleen. However, in both myelo-and lymphoproliferative conditions splenectomy may be indicated to reduce transfusion requirements when hypersplenism is a problem.

### Other tumours

Apart from lymphomas and leukaemias, tumours of the spleen are rare. Haemangiomas (capillary or cavernous) may reach sufficient size to cause splenic enlargement with a consumptive coagulopathy and haemorrhagic tendency. Most are recognised at operation when the spleen should be removed. As the condition may also affect the liver, it should be biopsied.

---

## MISCELLANEOUS CONDITIONS

### CYSTS OF THE SPLEEN

Cysts of the spleen are rare. They are usually single but occasionally multiple (polycystic disease).

Single cysts are classified as:

*Congenital* due to an embryonic defect and resulting in a dermoid-like cyst. They are lined by flattened epithelium and contain thin blood-stained fluid or thick creamy material sometimes with hair and teeth.

*Degenerative* resulting from liquefaction of an infarct or haematoma. The wall is fibrous, often calcified and filled with brownish fluid or paste-like material.

*Parasitic* due to *Echinococcus granulosus* (hydatid disease).

Splenic cysts usually cause no symptoms and are discovered fortuitously by detecting splenic enlargement clinically or finding abnormal calcification on an abdominal X-ray. The diagnosis can be confirmed by ultrasound. Treatment is by splenectomy. As rarely a cyst may be parasitic, transabdominal needle aspiration is not advised.

## ABSCESS OF THE SPLEEN

A splenic abscess is a rare condition. It is suspected when progressive splenic enlargement is associated with bacteraemia and abscess formation at other sites. Splenectomy, although desirable, may not prove feasible. Drainage of the abscess may only be possible.

## SPLENIC ARTERY ANEURYSM

This is a relatively common complication of atherosclerosis in an elderly patient. The calcified wall of the aneurysm is visible on X-ray and is usually associated with obvious calcification of the tortuous splenic artery. The presence of an uncomplicated atherosclerotic aneurysm does not indicate surgical treatment; bleeding can however occur, when operation is mandatory.

Rarely a congenital aneurysm affects the splenic artery. These are more common in women and may rupture during pregnancy. An asymptomatic congenital aneurysm may be discovered by the finding of a thin calcified ring shadow on an abdominal X-ray. Because of the risk of rupture, it should be treated electively.

As most congenital aneurysms lie close to the splenic hilus, splenectomy is usually required. At other sites excision may be possible.

---

## SPLENECTOMY

### Technique

Operations on a normal-sized and non-adherent spleen are carried out by mobilising the spleen medially by division of its lateral peritoneal attachments; identifying, doubly ligating and dividing the splenic artery and vein; and ligating and dividing of the gastro-splenic ligament with the short gastric and gastroepiploic vessels.

When the spleen is enlarged or adherent, preliminary mobilisation may not be possible, and dissection of the vascular pedicle is first performed. In this event the customary approach to the splenic artery and vein is by division of the gastrosplenic ligament between ligatures. The artery is identified at the upper border of the pancreas and doubly ligated and divided. Alternatively, it may first be ligated in continuity so that the spleen shrinks in size. The spleen is then mobilised so that the vessels can be ligated close to the splenic hilum.

When adhesions are present between the spleen and the diaphragm, it is advisable to ligate and divide its vascular supply before interfering with these.

Occasionally a thoraco-abdominal incision is necessary to remove a large spleen but in most cases a long vertical or subcostal abdominal incision is adequate.

## Pre-operative preparation

As the stomach will be handled during splenectomy, a nasogastric tube should always be inserted.

Routine pre-operative preparation is as for any abdominal operation, but particular attention must be paid to the state of the blood. This includes platelet counts. In the presence of any bleeding tendency, pre-operative transfusions of blood or platelets may be required.

If thrombocytopenia is present, platelets should be available to cover the operation and postoperative phase.

The surgeon should know the degree of splenic enlargement before operation. If in doubt he should request a soft tissue X-ray, or CT scan. He should remember that massively enlarged spleens, particularly those due to tropical disease, may give a spurious impression of mobility despite gross adhesion formation. This results from movement of the attenuated diaphragm.

## Post-operative course and complications

Drainage of the abdomen is not normally required after removal of a normal-sized spleen. At most a small suction drain is used.

After removal of an enlarged organ, *postoperative bleeding* from the pedicle should not occur provided the splenic vessels have been doubly ligated, but oozing from multiple adhesions is common and drainage therefore advised.

A *bleeding tendency,* e.g. in a patient with ITP, increases the likelihood of this complication. Hypotension and circulatory collapse within 48 hours of surgery indicates re-exploration of the abdomen.

*Pancreatitis* occasionally follows splenectomy. This is due to handling and bruising of the tail of the pancreas during mobilisation of the spleen.

*Accessory spleens* occur around the splenic hilum, its pedicle, or in the omentum, and may account for relapse of the condition for which the splenectomy was performed. Scintiscanning after the administration of $^{51}$Cr-labelled red cells may be used to detect functioning accessory splenic tissue but it is preferable that accessory spleens should be recognised and removed at the time of primary surgery.

*Local complications* of splenectomy include lower lobe collapse and an abscess in the splenic bed.

Following splenectomy there is a transient increase in the *platelet* and *white cell* count. This predisposes to a risk of venous thrombosis. Low-dose heparin is advised in all patients having splenectomy.

Loss of *lymphoid tissue* reduces immune activity and impairs the response to bacteraemia. There is a deficiency in the production of phagocytosis-promoting peptides and immunoglobulin. While the risks of serious infection are greatest when splenectomy is performed in childhood, an increased incidence of death from pneumonia, complicated by disseminated intravascular coagulation and adrenal failure, has been described in adults.

As most infections occur within 3 years of splenectomy, some surgeons advise prophylactic penicillin for this period of time. This is mandatory in young children. Polyvalent anti-pneumococcal vaccine may also be given.

Splenectomy should be avoided if at all possible in all young children. Lacerations should be sutured and even if the spleen is ruptured a partial splenectomy is preferable to total splenectomy if feasible.

# 38. Lymphatic System

## FUNCTION OF LYMPHATICS

The lymphatic system drains fluid from the interstitial spaces into the venous system. The lymphatic capillaries differ from those of the bloodstream by having little if any basement membrane and no tight junction between endothelial cells, an arrangement which allows macromolecules such as protein to pass through the lymphatic wall. The protein content of lymph varies from 0.5 g/100 ml in the periphery to 4–6 g/100 ml in the thoracic duct and liver.

Flow in the lymphatics is directed centrally by endothelial valves and is increased by muscle contraction. The lymphatics do not remove large amounts of fluid from the tissues. The total daily flow into the venous system is only 2–4 litres.

The lymphatics of the limbs form a plexus within the dermis and within the muscle fascial compartments. Solitary lymph nodes occur along the course of the major lymphatic trunks which then pass through regional nodes at the root of the limb. A lymph node consists of a supporting framework of reticulo-endothelial tissue and contains aggregates of lymphoid tissue. They have filtering, phagocytic and immunological functions (Fig. 38.1).

## LYMPHANGIOGRAPHY

Injection techniques were used to demonstrate lymphatics in the cadaver by 1692, but visualisation did not become practicable in the living subject until 1952. Water-soluble iodine-containing dyes were used initially, but ultra-fluid oily preparations are now available. These opacify nodes as well as lymphatic vessels. For lymph-

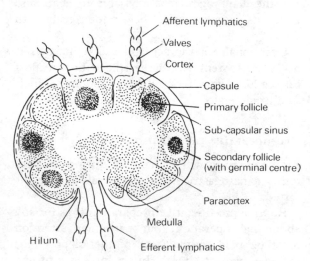

**Fig. 38.1** Lymph node

angiography a subcutaneous lymphatic on the dorsum of the hand or foot is first visualised by injecting 0.5 ml of 2.5% patent blue dye into a web space. On exercise for 5–10 minutes, the lymphatics show clearly through the skin as blue lines. A transverse skin incision is made over one lymphatic which is cannulated. Image-intensification following injection of a small amount of water-soluble contrast confirms that the cannula is correctly placed and 10 ml oily ultrafluid lipiodol is infused slowly from a pump. The dye can be followed by image intensification and permanent records obtained by radiography (Fig. 38.2).

Contrast remains in normal nodes for 6 months, and in pathological nodes for 2 years. Serial radiographs can therefore be used to monitor the progress of node metastases.

The examination takes 2 hours to perform. The patient should be warned that he will pass blue

infiltration. Alternatively, a node which is invaded by tumour may fail to opacify, one cause of a false negative examination.

## ABNORMALITIES OF THE LYMPHATIC VESSELS

### ACUTE LYMPHANGITIS

Inflammation of the dermal lymphatics (superficial lymphangitis) is most commonly due to streptococcal infection. The primary site of infection is often a minor wound or puncture with associated cellulitis. The inflamed lymph trunks cause linear red streaks in the skin and may be palpable and tender. There is usually associated tender enlargement of regional lymph nodes (lymphadenitis).

The affected part is rested and elevated if there is marked swelling. Antibiotic therapy is indicated and large doses of penicillin are prescribed in the first instance. Surgery is required only if there is suppuration or a retained foreign body at the primary site of infection.

### CHRONIC LYMPHANGITIS

This condition is uncommon. Mondor's disease is a form of chronic lymphangitis which gives rise to tense tender 'strings' in the skin or subcutaneous tissues particularly over the female breast or in the cubital fossa.

### LYMPHOEDEMA

Blockage of lymphatic flow upsets the normal balance of forces controlling the passage of fluid across capillary membranes of the bloodstream. Accumulation of protein molecules in the tissue spaces increases the osmotic pressure and hence the volume of interstitial fluid (Fig. 38.3). This increase in protein-rich fluid (protein content 10–50 g/l) is known as lymphoedema. Fluid rich in protein can also accumulate without lymphatic blockage, as for example after burns. Then increased capillary permeability allows more protein to accumulate in the tissue spaces than can be removed by the lymphatics.

Lymphoedema should also be differentiated

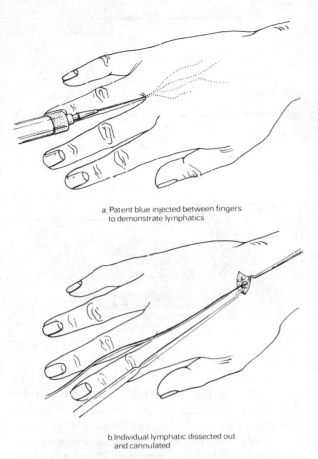

a. Patent blue injected between fingers to demonstrate lymphatics

b. Individual lymphatic dissected out and cannulated

**Fig. 38.2** Lymphangiography

urine for up to 48 hours. Complications are infrequent but include skin sepsis, thrombophlebitis, oil embolus to the lung, and hypersensitivity to the oily medium.

Lymphangiography is used to display the lymphatic vessels in lymphoedema and the nodes in patients with melanoma, seminoma, lymphoma and renal carcinoma. It is used occasionally to investigate obscure abdominal masses and to confirm operative clearance of lymph nodes in cancer surgery.

Normal lymph nodes are oval or reniform, within which the oily medium has a diffuse granular distribution. Central translucencies are frequently due to nodules of fat. When invaded by tumour a node is enlarged and has central and round or peripheral crescent-shaped discrete filling defects. Lymphoma and seminoma may cause a foamy soap-bubble appearance due to diffuse

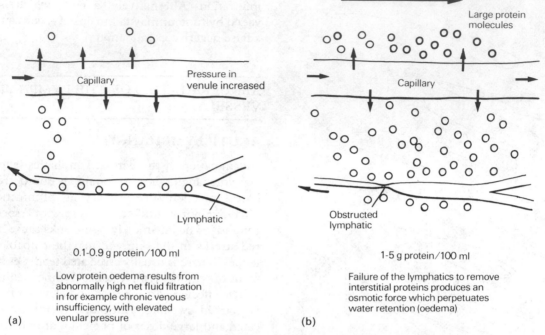

**Fig. 38.3** Types of oedema. (a) Low protein content. (b) High protein content.

from those forms of oedema in which the protein content of the fluid is only 1–9 g/l. Examples of such 'low protein' or 'filtration' oedema are the oedema of hypoproteinaemia, and that which accompanies the raised venous pressure of congestive cardiac failure or venous obstruction.

Lymphoedema is usually subdivided into primary and secondary forms.

## Primary lymphoedema

This is a familial condition caused by developmental abnormalities of the lymphatics. The vessels are hypoplastic and reduced in number, but may show varicose dilatation or even fail to appear. Lymphoedema may be present at birth (congenital lymphoedema or Milroy's disease) but more commonly develops during adolescence and early adult life (lymphoedema praecox). A few cases develop after the age of 35 years (lymphoedema tarda).

*Lymphoedema praecox* predominantly affects females and is unilateral or bilateral. The condition affects upper or lower limbs and begins insidiously as a painless swelling which progresses slowly up the limb. It is often more noticeable after exercise or exposure to warmth, and in the premenstrual period. The swelling is initially soft and pitting, but the high protein content of the retained fluid leads to fibrosis. The limb then becomes permanently enlarged and woody. As with all forms of lymphoedema there is a constant threat of cellulitis and lymphangitis, and a long-term risk of lymphangiosarcoma of the skin.

Lymphoedema is easily distinguished from the soft pitting oedema of congestive heart failure and systemic diseases causing hypoproteinaemia. These are bilateral conditions and as the oedema fluid has a low protein content, fibrosis is rare.

Chronic venous insufficiency gives rise to soft pitting oedema at first. Later this may become firm, rubbery and non-pitting; secondary pigmentation, dermatitis and ulceration may then occur.

*Lymphangiography* is the key to diagnosis (Fig. 38.4). In primary lymphoedema three appearances are described:

1. complete absence of lymphatics (15%)
2. widespread hypoplasia of lymphatics with small and infrequent channels below the knee or in the whole leg (55%) and

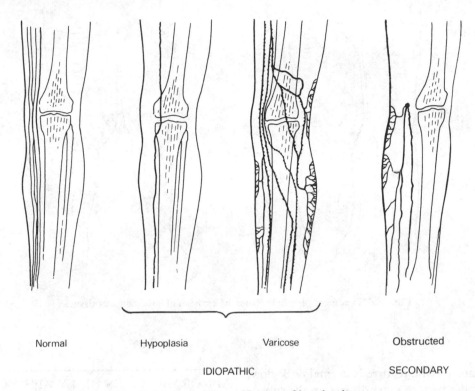

Normal         Hypoplasia         Varicose         Obstructed

IDIOPATHIC                        SECONDARY

**Fig. 38.4** Lymphangiographic types of lymphoedema

3. varicose, dilated and tortuous lymph trunks (30%).

*Treatment.* In the early stages, primary lymphoedema responds to treatment by elevation of the leg at night or to intermittent compression by an inflated cuff to drive fluid out from the swollen limb. A tailored elastic stocking should be worn during the day. Diuretics given in regular cycles have been recommended by some.

It is important to guard against infection by adequate hygiene, prevention of trauma, and prompt treatment of minor infections, e.g. athlete's foot. In some patients who have repeated bouts of streptococcal infection, long-term prophylactic penicillin may be required.

The painless nature of primary lymphoedema means that many patients delay seeking medical aid until faced with the cosmetic problem of a permanently enlarged limb. At this stage the lymphoedema no longer pits and is usually subject to repeated infection. Elevation and mechanical compression are no longer of value. As the failure of lymphatic development is widespread,

there is little point in attempting to construct a 'lymphatic bridge' between limb and trunk. Relief demands the complete excision of skin, subcutaneous tissue and deep fascia from the affected limb. Split-skin grafts of skin removed from the excised tissue are placed directly on the exposed muscle. The limb has a grotesque appearance after this procedure and it is practised only when the swollen limb prevents ambulation, is subject to recurrent infection, or when proliferative nodular changes occur in the skin (Fig. 38.5).

### Secondary lymphoedema

This condition results when the lymph trunks and nodes are obstructed (by tumour, recurrent infection, or infestation with filariasis) or obliterated (by surgery or radiotherapy) (Fig. 38.4). Swelling develops more rapidly than in primary lymphoedema, and is accompanied by dragging discomfort, erythema, and a high risk of recurrent lymphangitis. Lymphangiography demonstrates dilated lymphatics up to the point of the obstruc-

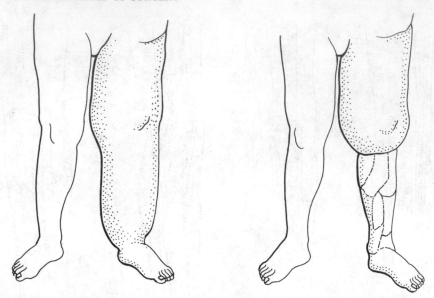

**Fig. 38.5** Treatment of lymphoedema by excision of subcutaneous tissues

tion. A characteristic feature is dermal back-flow, a fine reticular pattern extending from the subcutaneous tissue to the dermis.

Conservative measures such as elevation and compression are of value in the majority of patients. Surgery is seldom indicated and then only if a distinct local lesion has been demonstrated by lymphangiography.

A number of procedures have been used to bypass the lymphatic obstruction. These include burying longitudinal strips of dermis within the muscles to promote access to the deep lymphatics, pedicled omental transplants, and direct anastomosis between dilated lymphatics or transected lymph nodes and the venous system. None of these methods are wholly reliable, although the development of micro-techniques of anastomoses has been a definite advance. Lymphatico-venous anastomoses at several sites in the limb, performed immediately secondary lymphoedema is diagnosed, are reported to give good results. With all other cases, continued elastic support for the limb is an essential part of treatment.

As the upper limb is frequently affected the patient must be warned to avoid minor injuries to the hands. For gardening or any similar occupation gloves must be worn.

## ABNORMALITIES OF LYMPH NODES

The superficial lymph nodes lie subcutaneously and are readily palpable. The skin moves freely over the nodes which normally are oval or kidney-shaped and have a smooth outline. Enlarged nodes retain their shape when involved by infection or lympho reticular neoplasia, but become large, lobulated or nodular and matted when involved by metastatic cancer.

Deep-seated nodes cannot be palpated readily. Enlargement is detected by soft tissue X-rays (mediastinal nodes), lymphangiography (retroperitoneal nodes) and CT scans. With the exception of lymphangiography, these methods indicate only if a node is normal in size and shape. None define the cause of pathological enlargement.

### ACUTE LYMPHADENITIS

Pyogenic infection of lymph nodes is most often due to streptococcal or staphylococcal infection. A typical example is the cervical lymph node enlargement (lymphadenopathy) which accompanies acute tonsillitis. The primary infection may be so trivial as to go unnoticed. For example it may consist only of a tiny puncture wound of the hand or foot, sustained by gardening or walking without shoes. The intervening lymphadenitis may also escape detection.

The affected node or nodes are enlarged, painful and tender, restricting movement of the limb. Fever and leucocytosis are common.

Untreated infection may resolve spontaneously, progress to suppuration and abscess formation, or become chronic.

*Spontaneous resolution* is common. Although the nodes diminish in size, they may never completely return to normal and may remain palpably enlarged for the remainder of the patient's life. There are few normal individuals who do not have palpable nodes in some site or other. The superficial inguinal nodes of the groin are almost invariably enlarged and palpable.

*Suppuration* often leads to neighbouring nodes forming an adherent mass, and breaking down to form a large abscess cavity. The abscess may rupture through the overlying fascia and spread in the subcutaneous tissues to form the superficial loculus of a collarstud abscess (Fig. 38.6). The overlying skin becomes red, hot and shiny, and fluctuation can be elicited. Unless the skin is incised, it will rupture with discharge of the contained pus.

*Chronic infection* is heralded by the nodes becoming smaller and less tender, but they still remain larger and firmer than normal. Systemic signs gradually abate, but it is common for chronic lymphadenitis to run a 'grumbling' course with intermittent episodes of tenderness, node enlargement, and leucocytosis.

*Management.* If lymphadenitis is suspected, a careful search should be made for a primary site of infection within the catchment area of the affected nodes. The largest and most involved

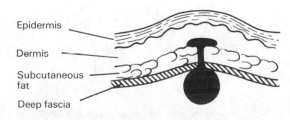

**Fig. 38.6** Collar-stud abscess

Epidermis

Dermis

Subcutaneous fat

Deep fascia

node is usually the first to have been infected. In many cases, the primary site cannot be found or is so trivial that it need not be treated.

In the acute phase, antibiotics are prescribed. Penicillin is usually appropriate as most infections occur outwith hospital. If systemic upset is not marked, oral phenoxymethyl penicillin is given; otherwise parenteral benzylpenicillin is preferred.

If improvement has not occurred within 48 hours, a broad-spectrum antibiotic should be given. In children with acute cervical lymphadenitis this should not be ampicillin. Abnormal reactions to this antibiotic occur regularly in infective mononucleosis which frequently presents with acute lymphadenitis.

Dry heat is sometimes of value to relieve pain over the inflamed nodes. Fluctuation or other local signs of abscess formation indicate incision and drainage of pus. This is best performed under general anaesthesia so that the opening in the fascia can be dilated, the deep loculus evacuated and necrotic material curetted from the node. The incision should be placed to allow dependent drainage and a small corrugated drain inserted to maintain it.

A sample of pus should be sent for culture and determination of sensitivity to antibiotics. A biopsy from the wall of the abscess cavity is performed if there is any doubt as to the nature of the condition.

## CHRONIC LYMPHADENITIS

### Tuberculous lymphadenitis

At one time this was an extremely common cause of neck swelling in children. The deep cervical nodes were painlessly enlarged, and the distribution of node involvement pointed to the likely primary focus of infection. Infection entering through the teeth, tonsils or adenoids involved the upper cervical (jugulo-digastric) nodes, whereas involvement of the lower cervical (supraclavicular) nodes indicated infection coming from the apex of the lung. Generalised lymphadenopathy suggested miliary tuberculosis.

Tuberculous lymphadenitis is now rare in children but occasionally is seen in adults. The nodes enlarge painlessly, become matted together and fixed to adjacent structures. Caseation leads to the formation of a 'cold abscess' which lacks the local and systemic signs of acute inflammation. When a cold abscess ruptures through the deep fascia, the skin reddens, thins, takes on a blue tinge and then gives way to establish an indolent tuberculous sinus.

Not all nodes involved by tuberculosis undergo caseation. In some cases the capsule remains unbroken and the nodes remain discrete. With healing, tuberculous lymph nodes become calcified and are visible radiologically.

Confirmation of tuberculous infection depends on culture of the organism from aspirated material (if the nodes have softened) or from an excised node.

Anti-tuberculous therapy will lead to resolution in the majority of cases. If the nodes remain grossly enlarged after a few weeks of treatment, or if there has been cold abscess formation, surgery is indicated. Then either the enlarged nodes may be excised or more commonly caseous material evacuated. A tuberculous abscess must never be simply drained or secondary infection is inevitable. Primary skin closure is the rule for all surgery performed for tuberculous lesions.

### Virus infections

Both acute and chronic lymphadenitis result frequently from virus infections, e.g. infectious mononucleosis. Occasionally lymph node biopsy may be requested if the diagnosis is in doubt.

### Granulomatous lymphadenitis

This includes a number of forms of chronic non-tuberculous lymphadenitis. Occipital and posterior cervical lymphadenopathy are common in the early stages of rubella; enlargement of the epitrochlear, suboccipital and posterior cervical nodes is a feature of secondary syphilis; lymphadenitis simulating caseating tuberculosis occurs in cat-scratch fever.

## THE LYMPHOMAS

The lymphomas are a group of neoplasms which originate in the primitive reticular cells of the reticulo-endothelial system or their histiocytic or lymphocytic derivatives. The commonest and most important is Hodgkin's disease which is characterised by progressive painless enlargement of lymphoid tissue throughout the body.

## HODGKIN'S LYMPHOMA

This disease is most frequently encountered by the surgeon when patients are referred for diagnosis or for surgical staging of the extent of the disease.

Most patients present with enlarged nodes in the anterior or posterior triangle of the neck or the axilla. The nodes are painless, rubbery and discrete (Fig. 38.7). Rarely the patient presents with an abdominal emergency due to deposits of Hodgkin's tissue causing adhesions or intestinal obstruction. The diagnosis of Hodgkin's disease is confirmed by excision biopsy of an involved node. A full haematological examination and chest X-ray are essential pre-operative investigations. Lymph node dissections in the neck and axilla are more difficult than might be imagined, and good exposure and unhurried dissection are essential. For this reason, general anaesthesia is usually preferred.

*Staging*. The staging of Hodgkin's disease has undergone considerable revision in the past few years. The classification now used most com-

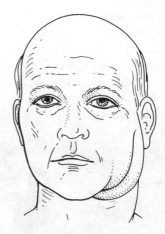

**Fig. 38.7** One type of presentation of nodes in Hodgkin's lymphoma

**Table 38.1** Staging of Hodgkin's disease

| | |
|---|---|
| I | Single lymph node group involved (or one extranodal primary site) |
| II | Two or more lymph node groups involved, on one side of the diaphragm |
| III | Involvement on both sides of the diaphragm ± splenic involvement |
| IV | Extralymphatic spread (including liver involvement) |
| A | No systemic symptoms |
| B | Systemic symptoms (Wt loss > 10% in 6 months Fever Night sweats) |

monly is given in Table 38.1. It is the surgeon's role to provide information from staging laparotomy to supplement clinical and radiological determination of the extent of the disease.

Laparotomy is carried out and splenectomy, wedge needle biopsy of the right and left lobes of the liver, biopsy of the para-aortic nodes at the level of the coeliac axis and duodeno-jejunal flexure, and removal of those nodes which appear abnormal on lymphangiography performed. Radio-opaque clips are placed at the site of node biopsy and at the vascular pedicle of the spleen so that these regions can subsequently be localised on X-ray. In the female, the ovaries and ovarian tubes may be sutured together in the midline behind the uterus to protect them from abdominal radiotherapy. A bone biopsy is performed.

All of the removed material is examined by the pathologist for the presence of Hodgkin's lymphoma tissue. As is the case with all lymph node biopsies, the pathologist should be forewarned in case he wishes fresh samples of tissue for electron microscopy or for corticosteroid receptor assay.

Improved methods of diagnostic imaging are altering the indications for staging laparotomy, which is now less commonly performed.

*Treatment.* The treatment of Hodgkin's disease depends on its stage, and now consists of radiotherapy and chemotherapy, usually with multiple cytotoxic agents given cyclically. Surgery has no place in therapy other than removal of the spleen to reduce the field of radiation required in patients with abdominal involvement. As a result, radiation damage to the left lung and kidney is avoided.

## NON-HODGKIN'S LYMPHOMAS

These are lymphomas other than Hodgkin's disease which were classified previously as lymphosarcoma, reticulosarcoma and follicular lymphoma. All are now grouped as non-Hodgkin's lymphomas but classified according to cell type. Predominantly lymphocytic, predominantly reticulocytic, and mixed types are recognised.

All forms of lymphoma (including Hodgkin's disease) can also be classified according to whether the changes are diffuse or nodular; the former has a more benign course. Extra-nodal disease is more common in non-Hodgkin's than in Hodgkin's lymphoma. The intestine and bone are most commonly involved in young children, the skin and adenoids in young adults.

Certain types of lymphoma are now known to be more common in patients with immune deficiency, lupus erythematosus and Sjogren's disease. Reticulocytic lymphoma of the brain is a long-term hazard in patients on immunosuppressive therapy after renal transplantation. The surgeon is seldom required to establish the diagnosis of non-Hodgkin's lymphoma. Barium studies, lymphangiography and bone marrow examination usually suffice, although lymph node biopsy is sometimes required for confirmation.

Involvement of the stomach and intestine by tumour deposits can give rise to abdominal pain, a mass, fever, anorexia, malabsorption and weight loss. Some patients develop multiple 'punched-out' perforations of the gut at the site of tumour deposits, and present as an acute abdominal emergency. In this event laparotomy is performed and the perforations excised with a rim of surrounding bowel wall to allow histopathological diagnosis. Excision of a length of bowel may be required.

Tissue must always be removed for histology when a surgeon is confronted with an inoperable tumour of the stomach or intestine. Lymphoma can simulate adenocarcinoma in appearance, but is very much more amenable to treatment by radiotherapy and chemotherapy.

The majority of lymphomas of the non-Hodgkin's type are treated by combinations of chemotherapy and radiotherapy. The MOPP regime of nitrogen mustard, vincristine (Oncovin), procarbazine and prednisone, is one of several frequently used. The prognosis of this condition is poorer than that of Hodgkin's disease.

## BURKITT'S LYMPHOMA

This is a poorly differentiated lymphocytic lymphoma first described in East African children. The disease occurs in the tropics and has a similar distribution to malaria. The disease is spread by an insect vector and thought to be virus-induced.

Males are predominantly affected. The area surrounding the jaw is most commonly involved and gives rise to enormous unsightly facial swelling. Most patients have multiple tumour deposits in the kidney, retroperitoneal tissues, ovaries, long bones and central nervous system.

Initially it was believed that one or two injections of cyclophosphamide induced long-term if not permanent remission. A high relapse rate has now been reported and current therapy demands full clinical and pathological staging, and combination chemotherapy with cytosine arabinoside and cyclophosphamide. An immediate remission is induced in the majority of patients, and can be maintained by further courses of combination chemotherapy.

## METASTATIC TUMOUR

All forms of cancer can disseminate by lymphatics and by the bloodstream. The concept that lymphatic invasion takes place first and that entrapment of tumour cells by the regional nodes can delay systemic involvement is no longer acceptable. Although some cells are retained by the regional nodes and give rise to lymph node metastases, others pass through the nodes without being retained, bypass the nodes through more distal lymphatico-venous communications, or enter the bloodstream at the site of the primary disease.

Lymph node deposits are now taken as an indication that the tumour has invaded both lymphatic and blood channels and that there are likely to be systemic deposits elsewhere. Cancer associated with lymph node involvement is incurable by local means alone. Nevertheless, surgical removal of regional lymph nodes may be practised as part of the local control of the disease. This is discussed on page 164.

## MYELOMATOSIS

This disease is a proliferation of plasma cells in the spleen and bone marrow. These cells secrete an abnormal gammaglobulin. The patient is usually over 60 years of age and may present at a surgical clinic because of intermittent bone pain, fractures or nerve pain. Anaemia and an abnormal bleeding tendency may be present and proteinuria (Bence-Jones protein) may be detected.

The most striking feature of the disease is the radiological appearance of punched-out areas in all bones due to the deposits of myelomatous tissue (Fig. 38.8). Occasionally there are obvious swellings along the ribs.

It is important to differentiate these changes from those caused by multiple osteolytic metastases. X-ray of the skull is helpful as this is invariably affected by myelomatosis. The diagnosis is confirmed by demonstration of myeloma cells in the bone marrow and the typical paraproteinaemia.

The treatment of myelomatosis consists of combination chemotherapy. Surgical treatment is required only for stabilisation of pathological fractures.

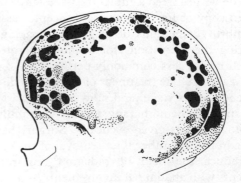

**Fig. 38.8** Radiological appearance of myelomatosis — lytic lesions in the skull

# 39. Endocrine Surgery

## THYROID AND PARATHYROID GLANDS

### THE NORMAL THYROID

#### Anatomy

The thyroid gland lies low in the front of the neck. The right and left lobes overlap the antero-lateral aspect of the trachea and the sides of the larynx and are united by a narrow isthmus which lies across the second and third tracheal rings (Fig. 39.1). The gland weighs 15–20 g. The thyroid and the trachea and oesophagus are freely mobile within a fascial compartment formed by

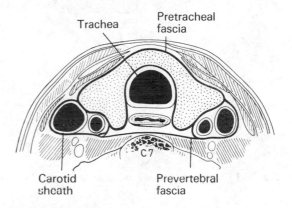

**Fig. 39.2** Anatomy of pre-vertebral fascia

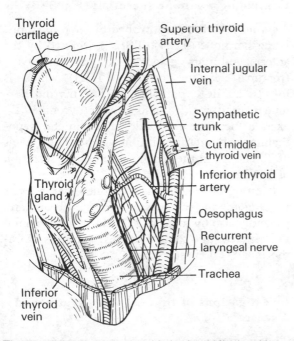

**Fig. 39.1** Anatomy of the thyroid gland (middle thyroid veins are divided)

the pre-tracheal fascia anteriorly, the pre-vertebral fascia posteriorly and the carotid sheath laterally (Fig. 39.2). Anteriorly it is covered by the sternothyroid and sternohyoid muscles, the lower part of the sternomastoid, the investing layer of the deep cervical fascia, the platysma, subcutaneous fat and skin.

The arterial supply is from the superior thyroid artery which branches onto the gland at the superior pole and from the inferior thyroid artery which passes from behind the carotid sheath onto the posterior aspect of the lower third of the gland. The venous drainage is by the superior thyroid veins and variable middle thyroid veins to the internal jugular vein, and by inferior thyroid veins to the innominate veins. Lymphatic drainage passes laterally to the deep cervical chain and inferiorly to the mediastinal glands.

The most important structures related to the thyroid gland are the recurrent laryngeal nerves and the parathyroid glands. The recurrent laryn-

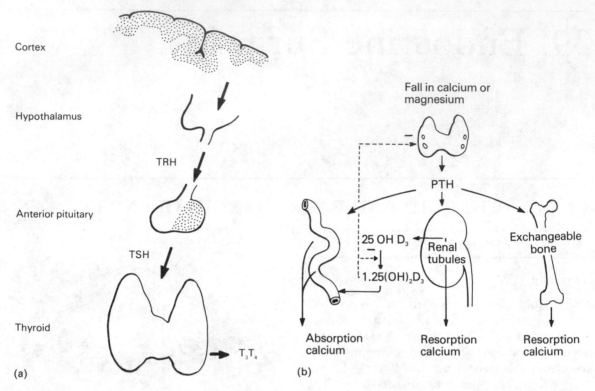

**Fig. 39.3** Control of hormone secretion. (a) Thyroid hormones. (b) Control of parathormone and 1,25 $(OH)_2D_3$ secretion.

geal nerves lie close to the posterior surface of the lower and middle thirds of the thyroid lobes, and pass upwards to enter the larynx. Most parathyroid glands are closely related to the posterior surface of the thyroid lobes, although there are some important variations (p. 564).

## Surgical exposure of the thyroid gland

The thyroid gland is exposed through a transverse skin crease incision placed about midway between the suprasternal notch and the notch of the thyroid cartilage. Laterally it extends almost to the external jugular vein. The incision is deepened through the subcutaneous fat and platysma muscle. Superior and inferior flaps are elevated immediately deep to the platysma, to the level of the notch of the thyroid cartilage and the suprasternal notch respectively. The deep cervical fascia is then incised longitudinally between these two notches and the pre-tracheal fascia is similarly incised to expose the thyroid gland.

## Control of hormone secretion (Fig. 39.3)

Thyroid function is controlled by thyroid stimulating hormone (TSH). TSH is secreted by the anterior pituitary gland in response to thyrotrophin releasing hormone (TRH) which is formed in the hypothalamus. The thyroid hormones thyroxine ($T_4$) and tri-iodothyronine ($T_3$) exert a 'negative feedback' effect on the hypothalmus and anterior pituitary gland. High levels of $T_4$ and $T_3$ in the serum suppress the secretion of TRH and TSH.

Parathyroid function is controlled by the levels of calcium and magnesium in the serum and probably also by those of 1,25-dihydroxy vitamin $D_3$. Increasing concentrations suppress parathormone (PTH) secretion.

## Investigations of thyroid and parathyroid disease

Thyroid function is assessed by measurements of the serum $T_4$ and $T_3$. In pregnancy and during treatment with oestrogens (including oestrogen-containing oral contraceptives) there is an increase in the globulin which binds thyroid hormones. Total $T_3$ and $T_4$ levels are increased. The free thyroxine index in these circumstances provides a measure of the free $T_4$ concentration.

The TSH response to an injection of TRH is measured in suspected thyrotoxicosis and the basal TSH is measured in suspected hypothyroidism. These investigations have replaced radioactive iodine ($^{131}$I) uptake studies in the investigation of thyroid function.

Radioactive isotope scans, ultrasonic scans, aspiration biopsy cytology, or Tru-cut needle biopsy are used in the diagnosis and management of patients with thyroid nodules.

Parathyroid function is assessed by serum calcium and serum PTH levels.

# THYROTOXICOSIS

Thyrotoxicosis is the clinical condition characterised by overproduction of $T_3$ and $T_4$ which are responsible for most of the clinical features. Biochemically the diagnosis rests on the demonstration of increased circulating levels of these hormones.

Three well-defined pathological conditions of the thyroid gland cause thyrotoxicosis. As the hypothalamic-pituitary mechanism is normal, the level of TSH in the serum is reduced or undetectable.

## TYPES

### Graves' disease (diffuse hyperplasia) (75–80%)

This condition is caused by abnormal stimulation of the thyroid by circulating antibodies. The thyroid gland is uniformly hyperactive, very vascular, and on section has a firm meaty appearance. The common clinical features are a diffuse smooth soft symmetrical goitre and exophthalmos. However either or both may be absent even in the presence of severe biochemical disturbance.

If untreated 20% of patients die in acute thyroid crisis; 40% have a chronic course of exacerbations and remissions ending in thyro-toxic cardiac failure. Spontaneous improvement occurs in 30–40% and may lead to hypothyroidism. This natural history explains the high relapse rate after drug treatment is discontinued, and the hypothyroidism rate after surgery.

Repeated episodes of hyperplasia and involution, whether spontaneous or induced by drug treatment, may cause the goitre to become rather nodular in character. This appearance should not be confused with toxic multinodular goitre.

## Toxic multinodular goitre (20–25%)

This condition may develop in a non-toxic multinodular goitre of long standing. Several or multiple nodules become hyperactive and function independent of TSH stimulation. The remainder of the gland is inactive and areas of colloid storage, haemorrhage, fibrosis and calcification are interspersed between the areas of hyperplastic thyroid.

## Solitary toxic adenoma (1–2%)

This is a benign follicular tumour which functions independent of TSH stimulation. The normal 'negative feedback' mechanism totally suppresses the remainder of the thyroid gland.

## CLINICAL FEATURES

Thyrotoxicosis affects females 7–8 times more often than males. It may occur in any of its forms at any age, but typically Graves' disease occurs in younger and toxic multinodular goitre in older patients. Excess $T_3$ and $T_4$ increase the basal metabolic rate and potentiate the actions of the sympathetic nervous system. These effects cause many of the features of thyrotoxicosis.

### Features of increased metabolism

The patient feels hot at rest and is intolerant of a warm environment. Peripheral vasodilatation and increased sweating help to disperse excess body heat. Weight loss is typical, despite increased appetite, but a few patients over-compensate and gain weight. Cardiac output rises to meet the increased metabolic demand. Increased blood flow through the thyroid gland in Graves' disease usually causes a bruit. A palpable thrill or frank pulsation are unusual.

## Features of increased sympathetic activity

Tachycardia is invariably present and persists during sleep. The patient may be aware of palpitations. Atrial fibrillation and cardiac failure are common in older patients in whom there are sometimes few additional features of thyrotoxicosis. Other typical features include a fine tremor of the outstretched fingers, retraction of the upper eyelids, increased gastro-intestinal motility, general hyperkinesia with increased tendon reflexes, and anxiety and emotional instability.

## Features not explained by $T_3$ and $T_4$ excess

Menstrual irregularity and relative infertility are common in thyrotoxicosis. Exophthalmos, ophthalmoplegia, proximal myopathy, pretibial myxoedema, and finger clubbing are variable features in Graves' disease, rare in toxic multinodular goitre, and absent in solitary toxic adenoma.

## DIAGNOSIS

In many patients the diagnosis is evident from the clinical features, but the distinction of mild thyrotoxicosis from anxiety neurosis can be difficult. The diagnosis is confirmed by elevated serum $T_3$ and $T_4$ levels with low or absent TSH. The TSH response to an intravenous injection of 200 $\mu$g TRH is absent owing to atrophy of the anterior pituitary thyrotroph cells. Pure $T_3$ thyrotoxicosis occurs in about 2% of patients. Radioactive isotope scans are only used to confirm that an apparent toxic adenoma is indeed 'hot' and the remainder of the gland is suppressed.

## TREATMENT

Thyrotoxicosis is treated either with anti-thyroid drugs, with radioactive iodine ($^{131}$I) or by surgery.

### Anti-thyroid drug treatment

Carbimazole is the drug of choice. It blocks iodine binding to tyrosine. Symptomatic improvement occurs in about 2 weeks and euthyroidism is achieved in about 6 weeks. When the patient is euthyroid, the dose is either reduced to the minimum necessary to maintain this state or a full blocking dose is continued and thyroxine 0.1–0.15 mg administered daily to maintain euthyroidism. Theoretically, all patients may be treated on a long-term basis provided adverse reactions, particularly skin rash and agranulocytosis, do not occur. In practice, however, long-term anti-thyroid drug treatment implies an enormous load of patients attending follow-up clinics. A trial of anti-thyroid drug treatment for 12–18 months is often advised, but 60–70% of patients will relapse within 2 years of stopping therapy. Early definitive treatment with $^{131}$I or by surgery has many attractions.

### Radioactive iodine

The uncertain risk of mutation of the ovarian or testicular gametes has restricted the use of therapeutic doses of $^{131}$I in Britain in patients less than 40 years of age, except those previously sterilised or unsuitable for other forms of treatment. $^{131}$I is the treatment of choice for patients over 40 years of age whether thyrotoxicosis is caused by Graves' disease, toxic multinodular goitre or solitary toxic adenoma, except when the size of the goitre is sufficient to merit surgery for cosmetic reasons or on account of tracheal deviation and compression. About 60% of patients with Graves' disease, 80% of patients with toxic multinodular goitre, and 50% of patients with solitary toxic adenoma are treated with $^{131}$I. $^{131}$I is also the treatment of choice for the few patients with recurrent thyrotoxicosis after surgical treatment.

The disadvantage of $^{131}$I is the progressive development of hypothyroidism. About 80% of patients are hypothyroid after 15 years and the remainder are at risk indefinitely. Follow-up is essential as thyroxine replacement should be started as soon as hypothyroidism occurs.

There is no evidence that $^{131}$I increases the incidence of leukaemia. It is believed to increase the incidence of thyroid nodules, but not of thyroid cancer.

## Surgery

Surgery is the definitive treatment of choice for patients under 40 years of age whether thyrotoxicosis is caused by Graves' disease, toxic multinodular goitre or solitary toxic adenoma, and for those older patients whose goitre is sufficiently large to require operation. About 40% of patients with Graves' disease, 20% of patients with toxic multinodular goitre and 50% of patients with solitary toxic adenoma are treated surgically. The decline of anti-thyroid drug treatment has resulted in a reduction in the number of significant goitres in those patients with Graves' disease referred for surgery. This facilitates the operation.

Patients are prepared for surgery with anti-thyroid or beta-adrenergic blocking drugs.

## Anti-thyroid drugs

Anti-thyroid drugs are used to achieve clinical and biochemical euthyroidism which is then maintained either by reducing the dose or by adding thyroxine. Treatment is continued until the evening before operation. The claim that potassium iodide 60 mg 8–12 hourly, substituted for anti-thyroid drugs in the last 2 weeks of preparation, reduces the vascularity of the gland and makes it firmer and easier to handle has little substance.

## Beta-adrenergic blocking drugs

Propranolol and sotalol abolish the features of increased sympathetic activity and reduce the $T_3$ and $T_4$ levels slightly. They have little effect on the features of increased metabolism and no effect on the features not explained by $T_3$ and $T_4$ excess. Provided they are used by physicians and surgeons familiar with their actions, they are a safe and effective alternative preparation for surgery although many surgeons still prefer to use anti-thyroid drugs. They are contra-indicated in patients with obstructive airways disease or cardiac failure, and best avoided in diabetic patients as they abolish palpitations as a warning symptom of hypoglycaemia, and impair gluconeogenesis in response to it.

Propranolol 40–80 mg 6-hourly is the usual dose. Symptomatic improvement is achieved rapidly, visits to the out-patient clinic are reduced, and operation may be planned after treatment for a few weeks. The essential criterion of adequate beta blockade is a pulse rate of 80 per minute or less. It is prudent to admit the patient to hospital about 3 days pre-operatively to establish whether minor adjustments in the dose of propranolol are required. The usual dose of propranolol is given on the morning of operation and it is continued for 7 days thereafter. It is important to be vigilant for breakthrough of features of increased sympathetic activity, unexplained pyrexia or excessive sweating in the early post-operative period, and to increase the dose of propranolol as necessary. The addition of potassium iodide 60 mg 8-hourly to beta blockade in the last 2 weeks of preparation reduces $T_3$ and $T_4$ levels by its direct anti-thyroid effect and eliminates this potential complication.

## Bilateral subtotal thyroidectomy

Bilateral subtotal thyroidectomy is performed for Graves' disease and for toxic multinodular goitre. The thyroid gland is exposed and its blood vessels are divided and ligated. The isthmus is divided and each lobe is cut back to leave a postero-medial remnant of about 3 g. The remnants receive their blood supply from branches of small tracheal vessels. As their size is sufficient to protect the recurrent laryngeal nerves and parathyroid glands, formal exposure of these structures is not essential. However most surgeons wisely define the position of both before resecting the gland.

## Total lobectomy

Total lobectomy is performed for solitary toxic adenoma. The recurrent laryngeal nerve must be fully displayed or injury may occur. It is usually possible to conserve the parathyroid glands on their vascular pedicles. If not, the parathyroid tissue on the undisturbed opposite side is sufficient to prevent hypoparathyroidism.

## Results of surgery

Bilateral subtotal thyroidectomy cures thyrotoxicosis in 95% of patients. Recurrent thyrotoxicosis is usually attributed to an inadequate resection, but it may rarely occur even after a near total resection.

Post-operative hypothyroidism occurs in 20–25% of patients. Low $T_4$ and elevated TSH levels are the rule in all patients in the first few months after operation. If they persist for more than 6 months, (or when there are clinical signs of frank hypothyroidism), thyroxine replacement is started. The importance of life-long drug compliance is stressed and these patients are discharged from follow-up after biochemical review has confirmed adequate replacement. Few patients with normal thyroid function 1 year after operation subsequently become hypothyroid and annual biochemical review is sufficient follow-up. Total lobectomy for solitary toxic adenoma always cures thyrotoxicosis and post-operative hypothyroidism is rare.

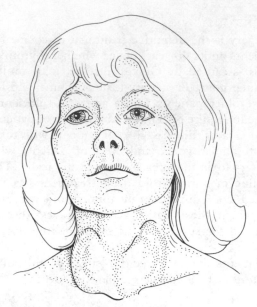

**Fig. 39.4** Goitre

## EUTHYROID MULTINODULAR GOITRE

This is a non-neoplastic enlargement of the thyroid gland. The condition is endemic in areas where dietary iodine is deficient. It also occurs sporadically, with no clearly established cause, and as a reaction to certain drugs. Multinodular goitres vary greatly in size from little more than that of the normal thyroid gland to 150–250 g or occasionally more. Usually the whole gland is involved, but the changes may be confined to one lobe. Section reveals multiple nodules of varied appearance, interspersed with areas of normal thyroid tissue. Some nodules contain abundant gelatinous colloid. Others show degenerative changes with cyst formation, recent or old haemorrhage and calcification.

### Clinical features (Fig. 39.4)

Most multinodular goitres are asymptomatic. Often the goitre causes only minor disfigurement but it may be sufficiently large to cause tracheal compression and dyspnoea, or rarely oesophageal compression and dysphagia. These effects are most likely when retrosternal extension of the gland reduces the size of the thoracic inlet. Haem-

orrhage into a cyst may cause acute pain and a rapid increase in the size of the goitre. When this complication occurs in a retrosternal extension, there may be acute respiratory distress. Rapid painless enlargement is unusual and suggests anaplastic carcinoma or lymphoma.

### Diagnosis

There is seldom difficulty in distinguishing euthyroid multinodular goitre from other goitres. X-rays of the thoracic inlet and chest demonstrate the extent of tracheal deviation or compression and retrosternal extension of the gland. Radioactive isotope scans are often performed but are of little value as 'cold' areas are usually degenerate thyroid tissue and not malignant. In the few patients who present with dysphagia, barium swallow and oesophagoscopy are essential to exclude co-existing intrinsic oesophageal pathology.

### Treatment

Further enlargement of a small multinodular goitre may be prevented by thyroxine replacement, but significant regression of the goitre is unusual. Larger multinodular goitres and those causing symptoms of compression are treated surgically usually by bilateral subtotal thyroidectomy. Retrosternal extensions are accessible through the usual cervical incision. The incidence of post-operative hypothyroidism is much greater than after resections for thyrotoxicosis. It is usual to start thyroxine replacement post-operatively to suppress TSH stimulation and prevent enlargement of the remnants.

## HASHIMOTO'S DISEASE (LYMPHADENOID GOITRE)

Hashimoto's disease is an autoimmune chronic thyroiditis. Autoantibodies to thyroglobulin, colloid, thyroid-cell cytoplasm and microsomes are present in the serum. In most patients the thyroid gland is diffusely enlarged, firm in consistency and pale on section. In some cases the disease is focal and nodular in character. Lymphoid tissue disrupts and replaces the thyroid acini and there is an increase in the fibrous tissue stroma.

### Clinical features

The disease affects females 10 times more often than males and has its maximum incidence at 50 years of age. Most patients are euthyroid but about 20% are thyrotoxic and 5% are hypothyroid when first seen. In time, the disease progresses to hypothyroidism. In most patients there is a diffuse enlargement of the gland, which includes the isthmus and pyramidal lobe to give the characteristic 'butterfly' appearance. In the nodular type there may be confusion with multinodular goitre or carcinoma.

### Diagnosis

The diagnosis is confirmed by the presence of high titres of antithyroid antibodies in the serum. When the goitre is asymmetric or nodular, biopsy is indicated to exclude carcinoma.

### Treatment

Small lymphadenoid goitres are treated with thyroxine replacement and usually regress. Larger goitres and those which cause compression are treated by bilateral subtotal thyroidectomy. Post-operative hypothyroidism is inevitable and thyroxine replacement is required.

## SOLITARY THYROID NODULES

Slow-growing, painless, clinically solitary nodules are a common finding in the thyroid gland. About 50% are adenomas of various histological types. Many others are not neoplasms but simple or blood-filled cysts, or a particularly prominent nodule in an otherwise inconspicuous multinodular goitre. The majority of differentiated thyroid carcinomas also present as clinically solitary nodules, and in most series account for 10% of these.

The incidence of carcinoma is about 30% in 'cold' nodules and only about 6% in 'hot/warm' nodules. However cysts and benign lesions can not be distinguished by radioactive isotope scans. A cyst can be defined by ultrasonic scans although intracystic carcinomas occur occasionally.

Exploration and frozen section histology of all clinically solitary thyroid nodules is standard practice for many surgeons. However an initial fine needle aspiration to distinguish a cyst from a solid tumour has gained in favour. If cystic, the fluid is aspirated completely. Exploration is indicated only if the cytology of the aspirate is suspicious or if the cyst refills.

For solid nodules the aspirate is examined cytologically. Alternatively Tru-cut needle biopsy can be performed. Neither are fully satisfactory as it is not possible to exclude the diagnosis of follicular carcinoma when the biopsy is taken from a follicular adenoma. However, all other thyroid lesions may be diagnosed with confidence by an experienced pathologist. Operation is then performed for diagnosed carcinomas and for all follicular lesions. The treatment of follicular lesions is by total lobectomy.

There is no evidence that direct sampling of carcinomatous thyroid by fine needle aspiration cytology (or by Tru-cut needle biopsy) is associated with an undue risk of tumour implantation in the biopsy tract.

## MALIGNANT THYROID TUMOURS

Malignant thyroid tumours are comparatively rare accounting for less than 1% of all tumours. Females are affected three times more often than males.

The major types of thyroid cancer and their frequency are: papillary adenocarcinoma (45–55%), follicular adenocarcinoma (10–25%), medullary carcinoma with amyloid stroma (0–10%), anaplastic carcinoma (25–40%) and malignant lymphoma (0–10%). Medullary carcinoma arises from the parafollicular 'C-cells' which are derived from the neural crest and secrete calcitonin.

External irradiation of the head and neck in childhood is associated with an increased incidence of thyroid cancer. Some medullary carcinomas are familial and are inherited as an autosomal dominant trait.

### CLINICAL FEATURES

About 70% of papillary carcinomas and 50% of follicular carcinomas present with a solitary thyroid nodule or with diffuse enlargment of one lobe. These swellings are seldom hard and recent rapid growth is uncommon. Cervical lymphadenopathy, either alone or in addition to the thyroid lesion, is present in a further 30% of both tumours. Distant metastases are rare in papillary carcinomas but are present in about 15–20% of follicular carcinomas, usually in bone, lung or liver. Papillary carcinoma is an occasional incidental finding on histological examination of thyroid tissue excised for other reasons. The term 'lateral aberrant thyroid' was formerly used to describe thyroid tissue within cervical lymph nodes. Even in the absence of macroscopic abnormality of the thyroid gland this is now recognised as being metastatic from a well-differentiated papillary thyroid carcinoma.

Medullary carcinoma presents with typically hard enlargement of one or both lobes of the thyroid. Cervical lymphadenopathy occurs in over 50% of patients. Despite elevated serum calcitonin levels, the serum calcium level is almost always normal. Whether the tumour is sporadic or familial, it is often associated with a variety of endocrine abnormalities, most frequently phaeochromocytoma and hyperparathyroidism, but also Cushing's syndrome, diabetes mellitus and carcinoid syndrome. It also may be associated with multiple mucosal neuromas. These syndromes of multiple endocrine neoplasia are further described on p. 583.

It is possible to identify pre-clinical medullary carcinomas by elevated serum calcitonin levels, either basal or in response to an injection of pentagastrin, and this test is used to screen relatives of patients with established disease.

Anaplastic carcinomas and malignant lymphomas present with a rapidly enlarging diffuse hard goitre which is usually partially or completely fixed. Cervical lymphadenopathy is also present in 30% of these tumours. Pulmonary metastases are present in 10% of anaplastic carcinomas. Dyspnoea, stridor and dysphagia are common. Hoarseness from invasion of the recurrent laryngeal nerve or Horner's syndrome from invasion of the cervical sympathetic chain may also occur.

### TREATMENT

Papillary and follicular carcinomas are treated either by total lobectomy including the isthmus, or by total thyroidectomy. On balance, total thyroidectomy is preferred, partly because there is a small risk of intrathyroidal lymphatic spread, but also to eliminate the need for initial ablation of residual thyroid tissue should [131]I later be given to treat distant metastatic disease. However, many surgeons prefer to leave a small remnant of the contralateral lobe to protect the parathyroids. Individual enlarged cervical nodes are removed at thyroidectomy and whenever further lymphadenopathy occurs. High dose thyroxine replacement (0.25 mg daily) is given to totally suppress TSH stimulation. Distant metastases can often be controlled for long periods with thyroxine and [131]I.

Medullary carcinoma is treated by total thyroidectomy. A modified neck dissection is performed for cervical lymphadenopathy. The parathyroid glands are carefully examined because of the association with hyperparathyroidism. The tumour does not respond to [131]I or external radiotherapy.

Operable anaplastic carcinoma, which is rare, is

treated by total thyroidectomy, modified neck dissection for cervical lymphadenopathy and post-operative external radiotherapy. However, many anaplastic carcinomas are inoperable and are treated by external radiotherapy alone. Malignant lymphomas are treated by external radiotherapy.

## PROGNOSIS

Papillary carcinoma has a good prognosis; 10-year survival is about 85%. The outlook in follicular carcinoma with minimal invasion is almost as good, but the 10-year survival for the more invasive lesions is only about 45%. The 10-year survival for medullary carcinoma is about 50%. Malignant lymphoma has a much poorer prognosis and the 5-year survival is about 50%. Anaplastic carcinoma is almost invariably a rapidly fatal condition. 70% of patients die within 1 year and the 5 year survival is less than 5%.

## HYPERPARATHYROIDISM

Primary, secondary and tertiary forms of hyperparathyroidism are recognised (Fig. 39.5).

*Primary hyperparathyroidism* is usually caused by a single adenoma but may also be caused by primary hyperplasia of one or more (usually all) parathyroid glands, and very rarely by a parathyroid carcinoma. Parathyroid adenoma occasionally occurs as part of multiple endocrine neoplasia (p. 583). Ectopic parathormone (PTH) secretion occurs in several non-endocrine tumours.

*Secondary hyperparathyroidism* is a diffuse hyperplastic response of all parathyroid glands to lowered serum calcium levels. The most frequent underlying disease is chronic renal failure. Impaired conversion of 25-hydroxy-vitamin $D_3$ to 1,25-dihydroxy-vitamin $D_3$ by the kidney results in diminished calcium absorption from the intestine. 1,25-dihydroxy-vitamin $D_3$ probably also has a 'negative feedback' effect on PTH secretion, the absence of which further contributes to the secondary hyperparathyroidism. Other causes of secondary hyperparathyroidism are malabsorption syndromes and, rarely, deficient dietary intake of vitamin D and calcium.

*Tertiary hyperparathyroidism* occurs when elevated serum calcium levels supervene in patients with secondary hyperparathyroidism. In some patients this change is the result of autonomous function when an adenoma develops in a hyperplastic parathyroid gland. However in the majority of patients, the large hyperplastic parathyroid glands are unable to suppress their secretion of PTH completely despite rising serum calcium levels in response to treatment.

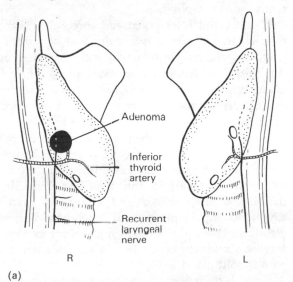

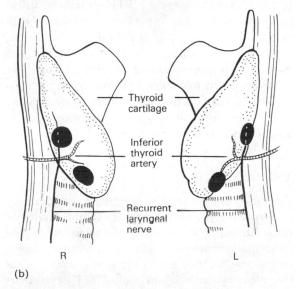

**Fig. 39.5** Types of hyperparathyroidism. (a) Parathyroid adenoma. (b) Parathyroid hyperplasia.

## CLINICAL FEATURES

Primary hyperparathyroidism affects women twice as often as men. The classical presentations include recurrent renal stones, bone disease, peptic ulcer, pancreatitis and a variety of mental symptoms, but an increasing number of cases are now diagnosed biochemically during investigation of other conditions. Irreversible renal damage inevitably occurs in untreated primary hyperparathyroidism. Thus, even mildly elevated serum calcium levels should be fully investigated and the disease treated at the earliest opportunity. Severe bone disease with gross demineralisation, subperiosteal bone resorption (typically seen in the middle and distal phalanges of the fingers), cysts in the long bones, and a 'moth-eaten' skull, is now seldom seen in primary hyperparathyroidism. By contrast, it is a typical feature of secondary and tertiary forms of the disease.

## DIAGNOSIS

The many causes of hypercalcaemia from which primary hyperparathyroidism must be distinguished include metastatic carcinoma in bone, excessive dietary intake of calcium and vitamin D, multiple myeloma, sarcoidosis, and ectopic PTH secretion. The diagnosis is easily made by measuring the serum PTH level. In the presence of hypercalcaemia, elevated PTH levels occur in primary and tertiary hyperparathyroidism and in ectopic PTH secretion. In the latter condition, the primary tumour is usually known, but if it is occult it is impossible to distinguish ectopic PTH secretion from primary hyperparathyroidism. In tertiary hyperparathyroidism there is severe bone disease and the underlying long-standing causative disease is usually evident.

## TREATMENT

Operation is advised for all patients with primary hyperparathyroidism whether symptomatic or not. Attempts to predict the position of the abnormal parathyroid glands by arteriography, radioactive isotope scans, ultrasonic scans, selective venous cannulation with PTH determinations and computerised tomography are unreliable and many surgeons consider them to be unnecessary. Normal and abnormal parathyroid glands are readily identified at a careful exploration.

The thyroid gland is exposed. The middle thyroid veins and superior thyroid artery and vein are divided and ligated and the thyroid lobe is rotated medially. The inferior thyroid artery and the recurrent laryngeal nerve are displayed. The point where they cross is an important landmark and many parathyroid glands are located within 1 cm of it. Almost all superior parathyroids are less than 2 cm above it, and most inferior parathyroids are less than 2 cm below it, although about 20% of inferior parathyroids are below the lower pole of the thyroid gland among the inferior thyroid veins or in the superior cornu of the thymus. Parathyroids sometimes lie within the thyroid gland. Mediastinal parathyroids are rare.

Every effort must be made to locate four parathyroid glands before any tissue is excised. Should only three normal glands be found, thyroid lobectomy and cervical thymectomy are performed on the side of the missing gland and the tissue is submitted for frozen-section histology. In the unusual event that the fourth parathyroid is still not identified, it is necessary to split the sternum to the level of the fourth intercostal space, transect it, and explore the mediastinum. Alternatively, the operation should be discontinued and the patient further investigated by selective venous sampling.

If one gland is enlarged and three glands are normal, the diagnosis is usually that of a parathyroid adenoma. Opinions differ on the extent of the resection. Some excise only the abnormal gland but others also remove two of the remaining normal parathyroids without biopsy of the third normal gland. This allows adequate histological assessment, minimises the possibility of recurrent disease and makes post-operative hypoparathyroidism extremely unlikely. When more than one gland is enlarged, the diagnosis is usually parathyroid hyperplasia and a subtotal parathyroidectomy is performed. The three largest glands and part of the smallest gland are excised, leaving a remnant equivalent in size to a normal parathyroid gland.

Secondary hyperparathyroidism with symptomatic bone disease, metastatic calcification, or both, is an increasing clinical problem in patients on long-term haemodialysis for chronic renal failure. Some patients are managed satisfactorily with 1-hydroxy vitamin $D_3$ (alfacalcidol). This is converted in the liver to 1,25-dihydroxy-vitamin $D_3$ which increases calcium absorption from the intestine and probably also has a 'negative feedback' effect on the parathyroids. Both mechanisms reduce PTH secretion, allowing the bone disease (renal osteodystrophy) to improve.

In some patients, treatment increases metastatic calcification or causes hypercalcaemia. These patients and patients with autonomous tertiary hyperparathyroidism require total parathyroidectomy and autotransplantation of parathyroid fragments equivalent in size to a normal parathyroid gland into the brachioradialis muscle. Post-operatively, treatment is continued with alfacalcidol and calcium to heal the bone disease and minimise the risk of recurrent hyperparathyroidism. If this occurs, revisional surgery may be performed under local anaesthesia and is much easier than re-exploration of a cervical parathyroid remnant.

# COMPLICATIONS OF THYROID AND PARATHYROID SURGERY

## Haemorrhage

Haemorrhage in the confined space deep to the deep cervical fascia causes acute respiratory obstruction. It may be necessary to re-open the wound immediately in the recovery area or ward before returning the patient to theatre for formal exploration and ligation of the bleeding vessel.

## Sputum retention and chest infection

These complications are frequent but generally minor. Physiotherapy should be commenced a few hours after operation to clear tracheal secretion. Otherwise this is retained because of discomfort in the neck and variable degrees of subglottic oedema caused by pressure by the endotracheal tube during operation.

## Nerve injuries

The recurrent laryngeal nerve is the most important nerve at risk. Injuries are more likely during surgery for retrosternal goitres and carcinomas. Traction during dissection causes temporary paralysis in 5% of nerves at risk. Function recovers within 3 months. Accidental division or ligation causes permanent paralysis. Visualisation of the nerves at operation is the best preventative. If transection is noted at operation it is repaired with a single fine suture.

*Unilateral injury* initially causes a non-explosive 'bovine' cough and hoarse voice. Even when paralysis is permanent these features improve as the opposite vocal cord compensates by increased adduction, and atrophy of the paralysed muscles draws the paralysed cord nearer to the midline. Then the final result is a normal voice which tires easily.

*Bilateral injury* usually causes early post operative stridor and ineffective coughing. The patient may require re-intubation and the endotracheal tube is left in place for 7–10 days. If there is no improvement by this time, a tracheostomy is performed. When bilateral paralysis is permanent, both cords are eventually drawn towards the midline causing dyspnoea on exertion and requiring revision of the glottic aperture. This results in a weak voice. It may be necessary to maintain a permanent tracheostomy with a speaking tube for those who do heavy work.

The vocal cords should always be examined before and after thyroid surgery so that recurrent nerve damage can be detected.

The external branch of the superior laryngeal nerve is at risk when the superior pole vessels are divided and ligated. It supplies the crico-thyroid muscle which tenses the vocal cord. Injury causes minor voice changes. Prevention is by avoiding mass ligature of the superior pole vessels.

The cervical sympathetic chain is at risk during exposure and ligation of the inferior thyroid artery. Injury causes Horner's syndrome.

## Hypothyroidism

This is discussed under the diseases for which thyroidectomy is performed. Hypothyroidism may also occur after parathyroid exploration as a consequence of division and ligation of thyroid vessels to display the parathyroid glands.

## Hypoparathyroidism

This condition is manifest by paraesthesia, a positive Chvostek's sign and hypocalcaemia. It is most likely after total thyroidectomy for carcinoma, bilateral subtotal thyroidectomy for Graves' disease with a large goitre, or parathyroid surgery. In such cases monitoring of serum calcium post-operatively is normal. Intravenous calcium supplements are often sufficient to tide the patient over, but oral calcium with or without alfacalcidol may be required for days, weeks or rarely months. Some patients require correction of magnesium deficits before hypocalcaemia will respond to treatment.

## Thyrotoxic crisis

This complication reflects inadequate preparation of a thyrotoxic patient for surgery and should never occur. It is manifest by hyperpyrexia and an acute thyrotoxic and sympathomimetic state. Management is by sedation, intravenous sodium iodide, oral carbimazole and oral propranolol to reduce $T_3$ and $T_4$ levels and block their effects. Intravenous fluids, steroids and oxygen are used as general supportive measures. Salicylates are used to lower fever, and digoxin and diuretics are indicated if cardiac failure occurs.

## Wound infection

This is very uncommon. A frank wound abscess requires drainage.

## Keloid scar

This occurs in a small number of patients, usually when the incision is placed too low on the extended neck and overlies the clavicles when the neck is returned to the normal position. Re-excision and re-suture of the scar is seldom helpful. Local steroid injections may help, but spontaneous resolution usually occurs in 18–24 months, leaving a rather wide but flat scar.

# PITUITARY GLAND

The pituitary gland is small, weighing only 500 mg. It is enclosed within a bony shell, the sella turcica, which is sealed superiorly by a fold of dura mater, the diaphragma sella. Through this passes the pituitary stalk which connects the pituitary to the hypothalamus (Fig. 39.6).

The pituitary consists of two main parts: the adenohypophysis (anterior pituitary) and the neurohypophysis (posterior pituitary). These two parts have different functions and different connections with the hypothalamus.

## ANTERIOR PITUITARY

The anterior pituitary secretes hormones which act on distant targets (Fig. 39.7). It contains solid cords of secreting cells, which by conventional staining with haematoxylin and eosin are of three main types: acidophil, basophil and chromophobe. Using immunofluorescence and other sophisticated stains these cells can be further divided specifically according to the nature of

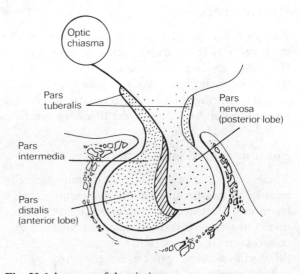

**Fig. 39.6** Anatomy of the pituitary

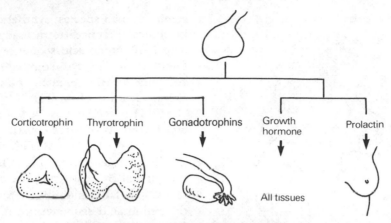

**Fig. 39.7** The anterior pituitary hormones

their secretion. Thus individual cells secrete growth hormone, prolactin, gonadotrophins, ACTH and TSH.

The anterior pituitary develops embryologically from the epithelium of Rathke's pouch, an outgrowth from the pharynx. Some cells are believed to be of neural crest origin and to belong to the APUD system (see p. 583).

The anterior pituitary is connected to the hypothalamus by the hypophyseal portal venous system (Fig. 39.8). A group of veins run down the pituitary stalk to connect capillaries in the median eminence of the hypothalamus with capillaries and sinusoids of the anterior pituitary. This portal system transfers a series of peptide neurosecretory hormones (messengers) from the hypothalamus to stimulate or inhibit the endocrine cells of the pituitary. The most important messengers are growth hormone releasing and inhibiting factors, corticotrophin releasing factor, LH-FSH-releasing hormone, TSH-releasing hormone and prolactin-inhibiting factor (PIF). If the hypophyseal-portal tract is divided disconnecting the anterior pituitary from these hypothalamic influences, the secretion of all hormones but prolactin is suppressed. Prolactin-secreting cells, being released from the inhibitory effect of PIF become overactive and there is uncontrolled prolactin hypersecretion. A complex system of long, short and ultrashort loops form a delicate feedback system by which the secretion of pituitary hormones can be adjusted according to need (Fig. 39.9).

## FUNCTIONS OF PITUITARY HORMONES

### Growth hormone

Containing 191 amino acids (mol.wt. 22 000) growth hormone has a wide variety of functions which include regulation of growth. Inadequate secretion in childhood leads to dwarfism Its metabolic effects include increased uptake of amino acids and protein synthesis with increase in the size of muscles, viscera and glands. Lipolysis is increased and there is increased utilisation of fatty acids causing ketosis. Growth hormone has

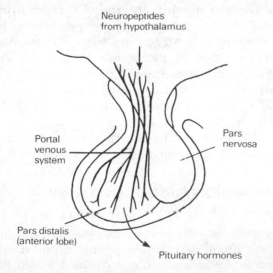

**Fig. 39.8** The hypophyseal-hypothalamic system

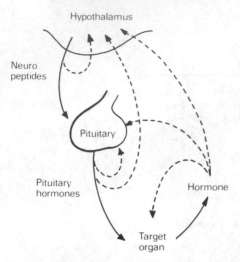

**Fig. 39.9** Feedback systems for control of pituitary hormones

an anti-insulin effect: it increases gluconeogenesis and decreases peripheral utilisation of glucose. In large amounts it augments milk secretion.

Release of growth hormone is stimulated by stress, fasting and hypoglycaemia. It can be inhibited by bromocriptine or chlorpromazine. It stimulates the secretion of somatomedin from liver and kidney, this being responsible for some of its growth-promoting effects. Growth hormone excess causes gigantism in children and acromegaly in adults.

## Prolactin

This hormone is similar in size to growth hormone (mol.wt. 21 500). Normally only small amounts are secreted, but these increase markedly during the night. During pregnancy there is a great increase in the secretion of prolactin which is one of the essential hormones for lobulo-alveolar development of the breast and the initiation of lactation.

Prolactin release is increased by oestradiol, phenothiazines (chlorpromazine) and metoclopramide. Its release is inhibited by L-dopa and bromocriptine.

## Corticotrophin

Human corticotrophin (ACTH) is a 39-amino acid polypeptide. The first 23 amino acids are common to all species: synthetic ACTH, as used in clinical practice (tetracosactrin) contains 24. The 4–10 amino acid sequence is similar to that found in melanocyte-stimulating hormone and accounts for the pigmentation associated with excess secretion of ACTH.

ACTH is secreted as part of a larger molecule which consists of three constituent polypeptides: pro-gamma ACTH, ACTH and β-lipoprotein (LPH). Pro-gamma ACTH is believed to act on the adrenal by sensitising the cells to the action of ACTH. LPH mobilises fat, but also contains the amino acid sequences of metencephalin and β-endorphin which bind to opiate receptors and have analgesic properties.

ACTH itself stimulates the inner zones of the adrenal cortex to secrete cortisol and adrenal androgens. Its secretion is in turn stimulated by corticotrophin-releasing hormone (CRH) which is secreted in response to all forms of stress.

## Glycoprotein hormones

Three glycoprotein hormones are secreted by the pituitary; luteinising hormone (LH), follicle-stimulating hormone (FSH) and thyroid-stimulating hormone (TSH). Each has α and β subunits. The α subunit is common and is shared with human chorionic gonadotrophin, but each has a specific β subunit which endows them with their appropriate actions. FSH stimulates follicle development towards the end of the menstrual cycle and the secretion of oestrogen from the thecal cells. LH triggers ovulation and promotes the formation of the corpus luteum and the secretion of oestrogens and progesterone. In the male FSH stimulates spermatogenesis and LH the secretion of testosterone by the Leydig cells (Fig. 39.10).

TSH promotes the growth of the thyroid and regulates the secretion of thyroid hormones.

## DISORDERS OF THE ANTERIOR PITUITARY

Functioning adenomas of the pituitary probably result from overstimulation by hypothalamic factors. Initially small, and confined within the gland (microadenomas) they slowly increase in

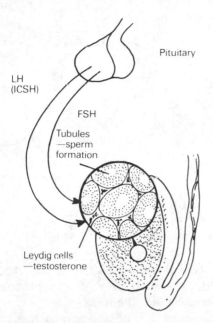

**Fig. 39.10** Control of sexual functions

size and may ultimately expand the sella turcia. Eccentric enlargement is common and produces asymmetry of the pituitary fossa. This can be detected radiologically by lateral tomograms.

Upward extension of an adenoma may stretch the diaphragm or herniate through it as a suprasellar extension. The optic chiasma is compressed and visual defects occur. Air encephalography or CT-scan with contrast enhancement will reveal its size.

It is important that pituitary adenomas are recognised before they enlarge the fossa or extend above it. Haemorrhage may occur into a pituitary adenoma and lead to hypopituitarism.

Three endocrine syndromes are of most surgical relevance.

## Acromegaly

This syndrome, characterised by 'large extremities' is due to excess secretion of growth hormone, usually starting in early adult life. Overgrowth of soft tissue affecting the hands, feet and face gives the patient a characteristic grotesque appearance with a massive coarse face, bulging supraorbital ridges and protruding jaw. Endochondral ossification and periosteal new bone formation accounts for some of these changes. All viscera are enlarged and there is muscle hypertrophy. How-

ever, muscle weakness and cardiac failure develop later. The skin is coarse and greasy and there is acne. Headache, sweating and the carpal tunnel syndrome are common. Glucose tolerance is impaired and galactorrhoea may occur in females.

Growth hormone levels are increased and secretion is not suppressed by glucose or a meal. Increased levels of circulating somatomedin are also described.

Treatment is aimed at restoring growth hormone levels to normal. External radiation will achieve this in 70% of patients but only after several years. Radioactive implants give quicker relief. For small adenomas, transphenoidal surgical removal is now the treatment of choice.

Bromocriptine has also been used but normal levels of growth hormone are achieved in only 20% of patients.

## Hyperprolactinaemia

Prolactin is the commonest hormone to be secreted by pituitary tumours of all types. It causes galactorrhoea; and amenorrhoea, which results from suppression of gonadotrophin secretion. Young women are predominantly affected.

Basal levels of serum prolactin are high, there is absence of the normal nocturnal increase and the response to TRH and metoclopramide is diminished.

Other causes of hyperprolactinaemia, e.g., from drugs, must be excluded.

In view of the importance of preserving pituitary function in this age group, small adenomas are treated by enucleation. Larger tumours are treated by bromocriptine, which inhibits prolactin release and also has been reported to reduce the size of the tumour.

Particular care must be taken during pregnancy as tumour expansion may threaten visual integrity.

## Cushing's disease

This is due to an adenoma affecting ACTH secreting cells. Only 15% are associated with expansion of the pituitary fossa. Removal of the microadenoma or its irradiation relieves the syndrome.

## PITUITARY SURGERY AND RADIATION

Tumours of the pituitary may be removed surgically or destroyed by radiation. The normal pituitary may be removed or destroyed to treat advanced cancer of the breast. Suppression of ACTH secretion causes adrenal atrophy reducing the secretion of DHA-sulphate so that it is no longer available for peripheral conversion to oestrogens.

### Surgical hypophysectomy

The pituitary can be approached surgically from above through the cranium (Fig. 39.11). This operation is undertaken by a neurosurgeon, and involves removing a bony flap and retracting or resecting one or both or resecting one frontal lobe. Alternatively one can dissect down to the fossa between them. This is a major procedure, suitable only for removing the whole pituitary or a large tumour. Loss of smell is a constant complication, and if the pituitary stalk is divided high up diabetes insipidus is permanent and severe. The trans-cranial approach is now reserved for large tumours with suprasellar extensions.

The preferred approach for removing a normal gland, or for enucleating a small adenoma is transphenoidal. The route to the gland is through the ethmoidal or sphenoidal sinuses using an operating microscope (Fig. 39.12). As the pituitary stalk is divided low down within the fossa

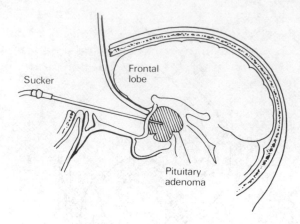

**Fig. 39.11** Transfrontal hypophysectomy

diabetes insipidus is rare. CSF rhinorrhoea may occur, but is usually prevented by placing a free flap of muscle into the fossa.

Occasionally a combined approach is required for large tumours, the gland being exposed both from above (transcranially) and by the anterior transphenoidal route.

### External radiation

The pituitary gland is radio-resistant and at least 10 000 rad is required to affect the function of the normal gland. Smaller doses (4–5000 rad) are used to treat acromegaly and Cushing's disease. A rotational technique is used to protect surrounding nervous tissue.

Larger doses of radiation can be delivered by beams of heavy particles (protons, alpha particles

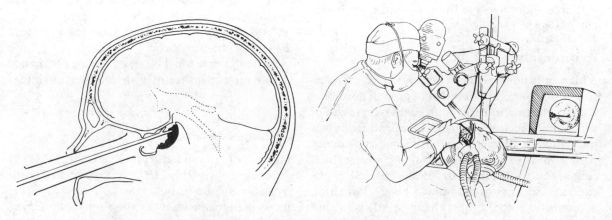

**Fig. 39.12** Transphenoidal hypophysectomy

or neutrons) generated by a cyclotron. These beams are narrow with little scatter and high doses of radiation can be focused on small areas. This form of therapy is available only in a few centres.

### Internal irradiation

The implantation of radioactive sources by trans-ethmoidal or transphenoidal cannulation can readily be accomplished under radiological control (Fig. 39.13). The isotope most commonly used is $^{90}$Yttrium, a beta-particle emitter of high energy but short half-life (64 hours). The activity of the source can be adjusted so as to achieve a complete or partial hypophysectomy.

Diabetes insipidus follows internal radiation only if the dose to the hypothalamic nuclei is significant. The introduction of radioactive implants by the transnasal route may occasionally be complicated by CSF rhinorrhoea. This can be controlled by the transphenoidal exposure of the fossa and the insertion of a muscle patch.

### Maintenance therapy

Following total hypophysectomy cortisol or cortisone therapy is required in a dose of 37.5 mg daily. As aldosterone secretion is unaffected there is no need to administer a mineralocorticoid.

On the other hand, TSH secretion is sup-pressed and hypothyroidism will develop over a period of some months. This requires l-thyroxine 0.1–0.2 mg daily for its control.

As indicated above diabetes insipidus is a common immediate complication of hypophysectomy or insertion of radioactive implants. The complication is transient unless the pituitary stalk or hypothalamus has been damaged. It can be controlled with DDAVP (desmopressin) given either by intra-nasal instillation or by intramuscular injection.

Immediately following hypophysectomy additional cortisol or cortisone therapy is given to cover the normal metabolic response to surgery. When undergoing further stress or trauma a patient who has had a hypophysectomy should be protected by increasing the dose of cortisone

### Posterior pituitary

The neurohypophysis is a secretory and storage unit which includes the nerve cells of the supra-optic and paraventricular hypothalamic nuclei (Fig. 39.14). Fibres pass from these nuclei by the hypothalamo-hypophyseal tract to the median eminence of the hypothalamus and the posterior lobe of the pituitary. The nerve cells secrete arginine vasopressin (antidiuretic hormone) and

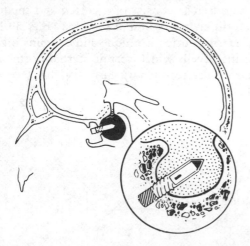

**Fig. 39.13** Implantation of radioactive $^{90}$Y into the pituitary fossa

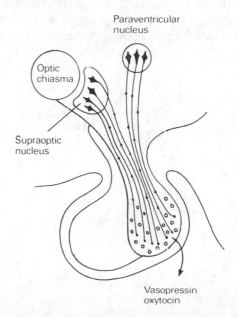

**Fig. 39.14** Neurohypophyseal system

oxytocin, both octapeptides of mol.wt. 1000 which in complexed form pass down the nerve fibres to be stored in vesicles within the pituitary.

Only vasopressin is of surgical import. It increases the permeability of the distal tubule, facilitating the reabsorption of water and so reducing plasma osmolality. Release of vasopressin is governed by osmoreceptors in the hypothalamus related to the internal carotid circulation (sensitive to 2% changes in osmolality) and by the baroreceptors (both high and low-pressure) in the heart and great vessels which monitor arterial and venous pressure.

Failure of secretion of vasopressin results in diabetes insipidus. This may be due to trauma, to inflammatory lesions or to primary or metastatic tumours. Following surgical hypophysectomy permanent diabetes insipidus occurs only if the hypothalamic nuclei are irreparably damaged, e.g. by pulling upon the pituitary stalk, or by its high division. Irradiation, particularly from internal sources, may cause severe diabetes insipidus.

The symptoms of diabetes insipidus are thirst and polyuria. The volume of urine is usually from 5–12 l/day. The urine is dilute with an sp.gr. of 1001–1005 and osmolality of 50–200 mmol/l. The osmolality of the plasma is normal (270–290 mmol/l) or slightly increased.

Inappropriate excess secretion of vasopressin occurs in some patients from a bronchial carcinoma and other paraendocrine tumours. There is hyponatremia, increased extracellular volume and renal loss of sodium. Inappropriate secretion is also associated with positive pressure ventilation following surgery.

# ADRENAL GLANDS

The adrenal glands are small, weighing approximately 4 g each. 90% of normal glands weigh less than 6 g. They are situated above and medial to the kidneys. The right adrenal lies in close contact with the inferior vena cava into which the short wide adrenal vein drains. On the left, the adrenal vein is joined by the inferior phrenic vein before running downwards to enter the renal vein (Fig. 39.15).

The anatomy of the venous drainage of the adrenals is of importance to the surgeon and also to the radiologist. In patients with suspected adrenal disorders, the radiologist may cannulate the adrenal veins to collect blood for hormone assays. The arterial supply arises from the aorta, the renal and phrenic arteries. A leash of small vessels run in the peri-adrenal fat to reach the capsule of the gland.

The adrenals consist of a cortex and medulla which differ in origin and function (Fig. 39.16). The adrenal cortex is unique and contains highly specialised cells which secrete steroid hormones. Some are also secreted by the ovary, the testis and

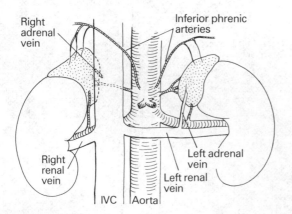

Fig. 39.15 Anatomy and venous drainage of the adrenals

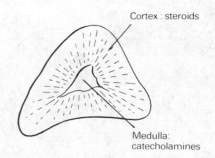

Fig. 39.16 Adrenal gland showing cortex and medulla

the placenta, but only those synthesised in the adrenal cortex are termed corticosteroids. The medulla is part of the sympathetic system. It contains chromaffin cells which secrete the catecholamines adrenaline and noradrenaline.

## ADRENAL CORTEX

Microscopically, three zones can be recognised in the human adrenal cortex (Fig. 39.17). From within out, these are 1. the *zona glomerulosa*, containing small cells arranged in whorls and hoops, 2. the *zona fasciculata*, with radial cords and bundles of clear fat-laden cells and 3. the *zona reticularis*, containing small compact cells arranged indiscriminately. These three zones form two functional layers: an outer, of zona glomerulosa secreting the mineralo-corticoid *aldosterone*; and an inner, the fasciculata-reticularis which secretes the glucocorticoids cortisol and corticosterone, the androgenic steroids androstenedione (A), 11-hydroxy-A and testosterone and their inactive precursor dehydroepiandrosterone sulphate (DHA-S). Precursor steroids for the synthesis of aldosterone are also synthesised and small amounts of progesterone and oestrogens may be formed.

## CONTROL OF ADRENAL CORTICAL SECRETION

The adrenal cortex stores only a fraction of the daily requirements of hormones. They are secreted 'to order' and circulate either bound to an $\alpha$ globulin (95%), or as free steroids (5%).

### Cortisol

15–20 mg of cortisol are secreted daily under the control of pituitary ACTH which is in turn governed by the negative feedback effect of circulating cortisol (Fig. 39.18).

ACTH also stimulates the secretion of androgenic steroids. If excessive, this can cause virilisation. The output of androstenedione and

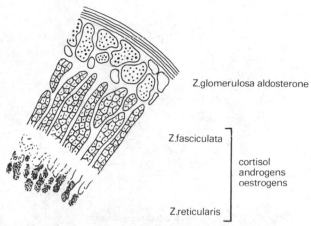

**Fig. 39.17** Zones of adrenal cortex showing functional zones and hormones secreted

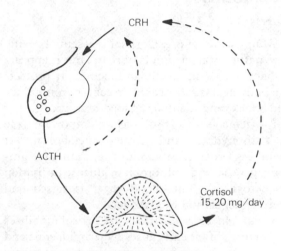

**Fig. 39.18** Control of cortisol secretion

testosterone is normally small: that of DHA-S is 25 mg daily.

### Aldosterone

The mineralo-corticoid aldosterone is secreted in small amounts of 100–200 $\mu$g daily. Circulating levels are low (5–6 ng per 100 ml). Although the secretion of aldosterone is increased by large amounts of ACTH, it is normally controlled by angiotensin. Angiotensin is formed by the action of renin which is secreted by the juxtaglomerular apparatus of the kidney in response to diminished perfusion. Aldosterone secretion is also sensitive to the concentrations of sodium and potassium in the circulating adrenal blood (Fig. 39.19).

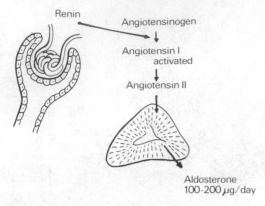

**Fig. 39.19** Control of aldosterone secretion

# FUNCTIONS OF ADRENOCORTICAL HORMONES

## Cortisol

1. *Maintenance of life*. Cortisol is essential to life. The nature of its action is obscure, but it appears to have a vital intracellular function. It protects the body against stress, aids recovery from injury and shock, and maintains blood pressure.

2. *Metabolic*. Cortisol has an important role in carbohydrate and protein metabolism. It mobilises protein (catabolic) and stimulates gluconeogenesis with inhibition of glucose utilisation (diabetogenic). The blood sugar is raised and there is deposition of glycogen.

3. *Fat and water distribution*. Cortisol mobilises body stores of fat and causes hyperlipidaemia and governs the distribution of water and fat. There is a slight mineralo-corticoid effect, with retention of sodium and excretion of potassium but this is of clinical relevance only when circulating cortisol levels are excessive. Renal excretion of water is enhanced.

4. *Other actions*. Excess cortisol causes psychosis and mental instability. It is anti-inflammatory, reducing lymphocyte and eosinophil cell counts in the blood, inhibiting fibroblastic activity and depressing antibody formation.

## Aldosterone

The main action of aldosterone is to facilitate the renal exchange of potassium and hydrogen ions for sodium (Fig. 39.20). It has a similar action on intestinal mucosa, sweat glands and, to a greater

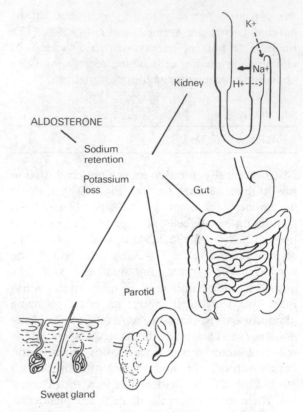

**Fig. 39.20** Actions of aldosterone

or lesser extent, on all cells. Whether potassium or hydrogen is exchanged depends on their availability. In low potassium states, the urine may be acid due to obligatory secretion of hydrogen rather than potassium ion, despite extracellular alkalosis. Sodium retention increases plasma volume but this is limited by an escape mechanism which over-rides the effect of aldosterone and permits sodium excretion.

## Androgens

DHA-sulphate is biologically inactive but is converted in fat, liver and other tissues to testosterone, its 5- reduced products and oestrogen. It is an important source of active hormones in postmenopausal women.

# ADRENALECTOMY

## Indications

Removal of normal adrenal glands is now used rarely in the palliation of metastatic breast cancer.

The operation is restricted to postmenopausal patients and has, as its objective, removal of the source of DHA-sulphate, which is utilised peripherally for conversion to active androgens and oestrogens. Availability of the adrenal suppressing drug aminoglutethimide has offered a method whereby adrenalectomy can be achieved 'medically'.

## Approach

Adrenalectomy is now most commonly indicated for adrenal disorders. These are due to overstimulation inducing hyperplasia or to a tumour. The effect depends on which hormone is excreted to excess. The adrenals may be approached surgically from in front (transabdominally); from the side; or from behind, (through the bed of the 12th rib).

If both glands are to be explored or removed, the lateral approach is less suitable as the patient will have to be turned during operation.

## Maintenance therapy

Following total adrenalectomy, patients must take permanent maintenance steroid therapy. Cortisone acetate 37.5 mg daily or cortisol (hydrocortisone) acetate (30 mg daily) and the synthetic mineralo-corticoid fludrocortisone acetate (100 $\mu$g daily) are given orally. Tests of adequacy of maintenance therapy include estimations of blood pressure in erect and supine positions and serum electrolyte determinations.

During the immediate postoperative period, large doses of steroid must be given to cover the metabolic response to surgery. Cortisol (hydrocortisone) sodium succinate is water soluble and can be given by intravenous infusion during the first 24 hours. Further doses may be given intramuscularly until the patient can take cortisone by mouth. An alternative preparation for intramuscular use is cortisone acetate in a slow release medium.

Oral cortisone is started on day 3–4 and the dose gradually reduced to maintenance levels. A typical dose schedule is given in Table 39.1.

Blood pressure is the best guide to the adequacy of therapy. Should hypotension occur, 100 mg cortisol sodium succinate is immediately given by intravenous injection and an intravenous infusion of saline with added cortisol (200 mg) commenced.

An adrenalectomised patient must be warned to increase the dose of cortisone should stress or infection occur, should carry a card marked with the dose of cortisone and fludrocortisone, and should be able to recognise symptoms of steroid insufficiency (loss of appetite, nausea, cramps, muscle pains and a general feeling of 'floppiness'). If such symptoms develop, the patient should take an extra two tablets of cortisone and report to his or her doctor.

**Table 39.1** Dose schedule for total adrenalectomy (note that cortisone and hydrocortisone [cortisol] are only preparations suitable for use *alone* as replacement steroid therapy). Cotisol acetate has 0.8 potency of hydrocortisone

|  | Parenteral (hydrocortisone sodium succinate or (for IM) cortisone acetate | Oral cortisone acetate (tabs 25 mg) | Total |
|---|---|---|---|
| Day of operation | 100 mg with anaesthetic 100 mg 8-hourly in 500 ml IV (monitor BP) | – | 400 mg |
| D + 1 | 100 mg 8-hourly (by drip or IM) | – | 300 mg |
| + 2 | 50 mg 8-hourly | – | 150 mg |
| + 3 | 50 mg 10 pm | 50 mg 10 am & 4 pm | 150 mg |
| + 4 |  | 50 mg bd | 100 mg |
| + 5 |  | 50 mg am 25 mg pm | 75 mg |
| + 6 |  | 50 mg am 25 mg pm | 75 mg |
| + 7 |  | 25 mg bd | 50 mg |
| + 8 |  | 25 mg bd |  |

Failure to anticipate the need for additional cortisone may precipitate an 'adrenal crisis' with acute hypotension and collapse.

Should this occur, cortisol sodium succinate (100 mg) is administered intravenously and the patient admitted to hospital. An intravenous infusion is set up with 200 mg cortisol sodium succinate in 500 ml saline and a regime similar to that used in the post-adrenalectomy patient is instituted.

## CUSHING'S SYNDROME

The signs and symptoms of Cushing's syndrome are due to prolonged and inappropriate secretion of cortisol. The severity and rate of progression of the disease depends on the amount secreted.

Excess secretion of cortisol may be caused by a functioning tumour of the adrenal cortex (20%) or overstimulation of normal glands by excess ACTH (80%) either of pituitary origin or from an ectopic source (Fig. 39.21).

### Adrenal tumour

A benign adenoma is the commonest adrenal tumour causing Cushing's syndrome. It is almost invariably unilateral and more common in females. Histologically an adenoma contains clear (fasciculata-like) or compact (reticularis-like) cells.

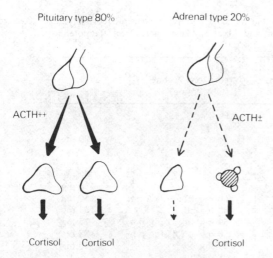

**Fig. 39.21** Types of Cushing's syndrome

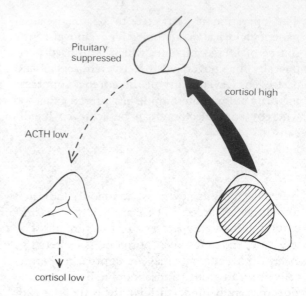

**Fig. 39.22** Effect of adrenal adenoma secreting cortisol on opposite gland

Adrenal carcinoma is a rare cause of Cushing's syndrome. More common in children and young adults, it grows to a large size, is highly malignant and metastasise to liver and lungs.

The autonomous secretion of cortisol from an adrenal tumour inhibits ACTH secretion so that the contralateral gland is atrophic and non-functioning (Fig. 39.22).

### Pituitary disease

This is the commonest cause of Cushing's syndrome accounting for 80% of all cases. There is a basophil or sometimes a chromophobe adenoma of ACTH secreting cells. This may be tiny (microadenoma), large and even invasive. Both adrenals become hyperplastic. This syndrome is called 'Cushing's disease'.

### Ectopic ACTH production

Cushing's syndrome may rarely be caused by the inappropriate secretion of an ACTH-like peptide by a tumour of non-pituitary origin. This may arise in the bronchus, pancreas, thymus and other sites and is usually malignant (Fig. 39.23).

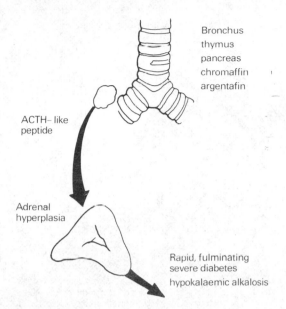

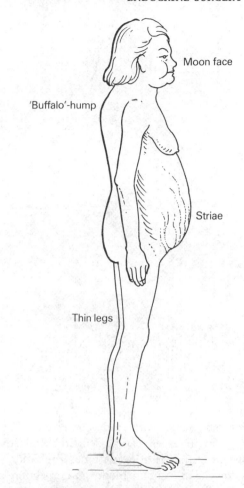

**Fig. 39.23** Ectopic ACTH syndrome

## Clinical features

Cushing's syndrome occurs most frequently in young adult women. The most striking feature is centripetal (truncal) obesity due to redistribution of body water and fat which may produce the classic feature of a buffalo hump (Fig. 39.24). The limbs are spare. 'Mooning' of the face occurs early. In advanced cases the appearances have been likened to a lemon on matchsticks. As a result of protein loss, the skin becomes thin with purple striae, dusky cyanosis and visible dermal vessels; there is muscle weakness, increased capillary fragility, purpura, and osteoporosis. Acne, loss of libido, hirsutism, diabetes and hypertension are common. Amenorrhoea, hypertension and obesity are common early features.

These clinical signs usually develop gradually over several years and can best be recognised by reviewing family photographs. In some cases the course is fulminant, particularly when the patient has an adrenal carcinoma or ectopic secretion of ACTH. Electrolyte disturbance, pigmentation, severe diabetes and psychosis are particularly common in these circumstances. Cachexia is prominent and may overshadow these features.

## Investigation

Before carrying out adrenalectomy on a patient with Cushing's syndrome, the surgeon should

**Fig. 39.24** Typical features of Cushing's syndrome

assure himself:

1. That there is evidence of cortisol hypersecretion outwith normal control. Plasma cortisol will be elevated, its diurnal variation will be lost and it will not be suppressed by *low* dose dexamethasone or increased by insulin hypoglycaemia.

2. That the cortisol excess is considered to be of adrenal origin. If a functioning adrenal tumour is present, ACTH cannot be detected in the plasma and urinary excretion of cortisol is not suppressed by *high*-dose dexamethasone (Fig. 39.25).

3. That the cortisol excess is not of pituitary origin (see below). In Cushing's syndrome due to pituitary causes, plasma ACTH will be inappropriately high and urinary cortisol excretion is suppressed by dexamethasone.

4. That attempts to localise the lesion have been made. The methods used include CT-scans and

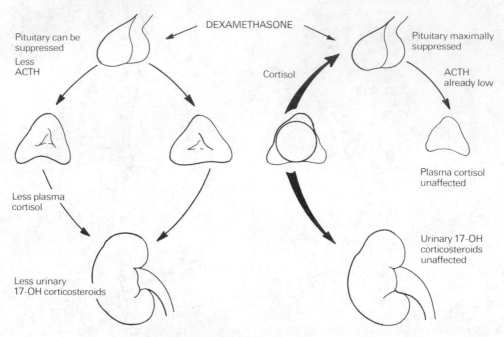

**Fig. 39.25** The dexamethasone suppression test

radioisotopic scans with iodo-cholesterol. The source of cortisol excess can be defined by selective adrenal-vein catheterisation with determination of cortisol levels in venous blood and injection of contrast medium to outline the tumour.

## Treatment

*Adrenal tumour.* The treatment of an adrenal adenoma is removal of the gland with its contained tumour. Only the affected adrenal need be explored. As the other adrenal is atrophic, cortisone therapy is required postoperatively. Once the patient is maintained on small doses, cortisone can gradually be withdrawn when the remaining adrenal will resume normal function.

Carcinomas of the adrenal causing Cushing's syndrome should also be removed if possible, but this may be difficult. Recurrence of tumour, locally and systemically is likely to occur and adjuvant systemic therapy with an adrenal cytotoxin, e.g., opDDD is advised. Unfortunately, this drug has unpleasant gastrointestinal side effects and may not be tolerated.

*Pituitary disease.* The symptoms and signs of bilateral adrenal hyperplasia due to pituitary hyperfunction (Cushing's disease) can be cured permanently by bilateral adrenalectomy, and until recently this was standard treatment. There are disadvantages. The patient must permanently take maintenance therapy and removal of the source of cortisol alters the setting of the feedback mechanism so that the pituitary is no longer suppressed. Large amounts of ACTH are secreted with pigmentation of the skin (Fig. 39.26). In some patients a pituitary adenoma may expand and cause pressure on the optic chiasma.

Irradiation of the pituitary may prevent these effects of adrenalectomy but a direct attack on the pituitary is now preferred treatment, leaving the adrenals undisturbed. Microsurgical removal of the microadenoma is the treatment of choice. Alternatively, the whole gland may be removed or irradiated, either from external or internal sources. Ideally the function of the normal gland should be preserved so that maintenance therapy is not required, and sexual functions and parity are undisturbed.

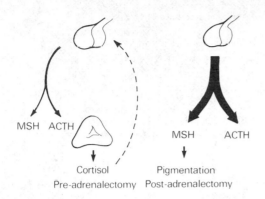

**Fig. 39.26** Mechanisms of postadrenalectomy pigmentation in Cushing's disease

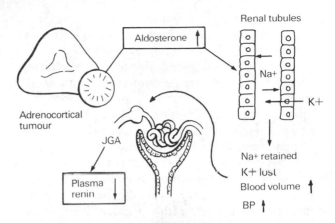

**Fig. 39.28** Effect of primary aldosteronism

In fulminating cases with severe upset, metyrapone, aminoglutethamide or trilostane should be used to prepare the patient for operation. Some surgeons advise such preparation in all cases.

## ALDOSTERONISM

Hyperaldosteronism most commonly occurs as a secondary phenomenon in chronic liver, renal and cardiac disease (Fig. 39.27). Activation of the juxtaglomerular apparatus by diminution in plasma volume, renal ischaemia or excess use of diuretics causes hypersecretion of renin, and increased stimulation of the zona glomerulosa by angiotensin. Primary hyperaldosteronism (Conn's syndrome) is due most commonly to a benign adenoma of the adrenal cortex (Fig. 39.28). The patient is usually a young or middle-aged woman; the lesion is small (1–3 g), single canary yellow in colour and composed of cells of glomerulosa type. Occasionally an adrenal cortical carcinoma causes primary hyper-

aldosteronism; and a number of patients with bilateral adrenal hyperplasia or multiple adrenal microadenomas have been described.

The classical clinical features are due to the metabolic consequences of aldosterone excess, i.e. sodium retention and potassium loss. Now most patients are discovered in the course of investigation at a hypertension clinic.

### Sodium retention

Retention of sodium expands plasma volume and hypertension is the rule. This may be associated with severe headache and visual disturbance but serious retinopathy is uncommon. Oedema is rare.

### Potassium loss

In the early stages of the syndrome the only evidence of potassium loss is a moderate depression of serum potassium. Later there may be episodes of muscle weakness and nocturnal polyuria, the latter due to the effect of hypokalaemia on the kidneys. This is associated with vacuolation and distortion of distal tubular cells.

If unrecognised, the syndrome progresses to a state of severe hypokalaemic alkalosis with attacks of periodic muscle paralysis, tetany and paraesthesia. This full-blown picture is now rare.

### Diagnosis

The finding of a low serum potassium in a hypertensive patient should alert the clinician to the possibility of primary aldosteronism. Investigations are designed to demonstrate:

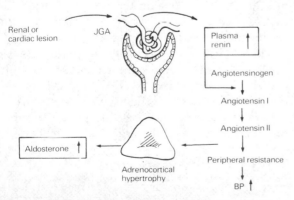

**Fig. 39.27** Mechanism of secondary aldosteronism

1. That there is hypokalaemia. This may require repeated estimations on venous blood samples taken without an occluding cuff.

2. That there is hyperaldosteronism. Estimates of plasma aldosterone are performed by radio-immunoassay at 4-hourly intervals to compensate for diurnal variation. Reduction of blood pressure and reversal of hypokalaemia should follow the administration of spironolactone, an aldosterone antagonist.

3. That aldosterone excess is not secondary

Plasma renin concentration is the critical estimation. In secondary hyperaldosteronism it is increased whereas in the primary form it is undetectable. Spironolactone will raise renin levels in secondary hyperaldosteronism.

If primary hyperaldosteronism is confirmed an attempt should be made to localise the adenoma with a CT or radio-iodo-cholesterol scan. Blood samples are collected from both right and left adrenal and from the inferior vena cava for aldosterone estimations.

Plasma cortisol should always be estimated to exclude the possibility of atypical Cushing's syndrome.

## Treatment

The treatment of primary hyperaldosteronism due to an adenoma is to remove the adrenal and its contained tumour. It is important that the patient first be repleted with potassium by the administration of oral potassium supplements and spironolactone or triamterine.

Primary aldosteronism due to adrenal hyperplasia can be cured by bilateral adrenalectomy but at too great a price. Medical therapy with triamterine and amiloride is preferable to the long-term administration of spironolactone.

## ADRENOGENITAL SYNDROME (ADRENAL VIRILISM)

A genetically-determined enzyme defect leads to deficient secretion of cortisol. The feedback mechanism is activated and there is increased production of ACTH. This causes adrenal hyperplasia and inappropriate secretion of adrenal androgen (Fig. 39.29). The effect depends on the sex and age at which the disease is manifest. Female infants show enlargment of the clitoris and varying degrees of fusion of the genital folds.

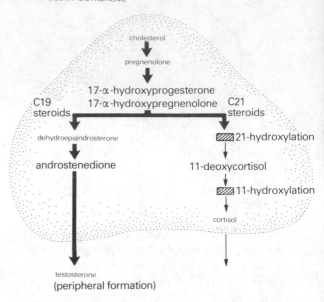

ADRENOGENITAL SYNDROME

**Fig. 39.29** Simplified mechanism of causation of adrenal virilism. 21-hydroxylase deficiency may lead to excessive loss of salt due to aldosterone lack; 11-hydroxylase deficiency to hypertension through accumulation of DOC.

As she develops, other signs of virilism appear leading to precocious heterosexual puberty. Young boys have isosexual precocious puberty.

In both sexes there are striking abnormalities of growth. Bone growth is rapid at first but the epiphyses fuse early so that the final height is stunted. Excess muscle growth produces the 'infant Hercules' appearance. Milder forms of the disease may affect older girls and cause hirsutism and acne. Associated metabolic abnormalities depend on the type of enzyme block. Thus 21-hydroxylase deficiency may lead also to excessive loss of salt due to aldosterone deficiency; 11-hydroxylase deficiency to hypertension through accumulation of 11-deoxycortisol.

The syndrome is effectively treated by glucocorticoid which supplies the patient's needs for cortisol and suppresses ACTH. Surgical correction of the genital abnormality may be required.

Rarely virilism may be due to an adrenal tumour which is usually large and malignant.

## ADRENAL FEMINISATION

Exceptionally, a tumour of the adrenal cortex may secrete oestrogens. Such tumours are usually large and malignant. Endocrine effects are normally recognised only in the male in whom feminisation with gynaecomastia, decreased libido and testicular atrophy occurs. Treatment consists of removal of the tumour but the results are poor. Recurrence and metastatic disease are invariable.

## ADDISON'S DISEASE

Adrenal insufficiency whatever the cause can produce problems in patients undergoing surgery. These have been discussed on page 55. A patient known to have Addison's disease should receive full steroid cover during major surgery as has been detailed on page 575. Awareness that postoperative hypotension may be due to an adrenal cause and treatment with IV hydrocortisone (cortisol) can prove life-saving.

## THE ADRENAL MEDULLA

The adrenal medulla contains chromaffin cells which stain yellow-brown with chromate stains. These are derived from the neural crest and secrete catecholamines into the circulation. The cells belong to the APUD series (see p. 583) and are supplied by preganglionic sympathetic nerves. The adrenal medulla is not essential to life. There are other collections of chromaffin cells in paraganglia in the retroperitoneum, mediastinum and neck.

The normal adrenal medulla produces catecholamines in the ratio 80% adrenaline to 20% noradrenaline. It also secretes dopamine which acts as a precursor to noradrenaline.

## ADRENALINE

This acts on both $\alpha$ and $\beta$ adrenergic receptors to redistribute blood flow by constricting skin and splanchnic vessels and dilating those of the heart, skeletal muscles and brain. It causes tachycardia, induces a sense of panic, and has metabolic effects. These include the conversion of glycogen to glucose in the liver, and an increase in the concentration of free circulating fatty acids.

## NORADRENALINE

This acts on $\alpha$ receptors to constrict all blood vessels and raises the systolic and diastolic pressure. It has little effect on the central nervous system or metabolism.

Small amounts of catecholamines are excreted in the urine in free and conjugated form. Larger amounts are excreted as metabolites, such as 'meta' derivatives (e.g. metnoradrenaline); 4-hydroxy-3-methoxy-mandelic acid (VMA); and 4-hydroxy-3-methoxy-phenylglycol (HMPG).

## PHAEOCHROMOCYTOMA

A phaeochromocytoma is a benign tumour of the adrenal medulla which secretes large amounts of adrenaline and noradrenaline. Phaeochromocytomas also occur in extra-adrenal paraganglionic tissue, most often in the retroperitoneum near the kidneys and occasionally in more distant locations such as the posterior mediastinum, neck, pelvis or urinary bladder. An extra-adrenal phaeochromocytoma secretes only noradrenaline. 99% of all tumours arise within the abdomen, 80% in the adrenals. 20% are multiple and may affect both adrenals.

A phaeochromocytoma averages 5 cm in diameter, is highly vascular and chocolate-brown in colour. Histologically the cells resemble those of the normal adrenal medulla and stain with chromate. Approximately 5% are malignant and metastasise.

Associated conditions are neurofibromatosis, medullary carcinoma of the thyroid (as part of multiple endocrine neoplasia type II), duodenal ulcer and renal artery stenosis.

### Clinical features

Phaeochromocytomas present before the age of 50 years. Their clinical features depend on the proportions of adrenaline and noradrenaline secreted by the tumour. Noradrenaline excess causes hypertension: that of adrenaline metabolic effects (e.g., thyrotoxicosis) and even hypotension.

*Paroxysmal hypertension* is the most characteristic symptom and is due to the sudden release of catecholamines from the tumour. This may be precipitated by abdominal pressure, exercise or postural change. During an attack the blood pressure exceeds 200/100 mmHg and there is headache, palpitations, sweating, extreme anxiety and chest and abdominal pain. Pallor, dilated pupils and tachycardia are features of note.

Alternatively *persistent hypertension* may develop between 30–40 years of age. Then the clinical features are those of severe hypertension associated with moderate or severe retinopathy. Fundal changes include vascular spasm, optic atrophy and blindness. Glycosuria is common. There is mottling of the skin and tingling of the extremities. Extra-adrenal phaeochromocytomas are always associated with persistent hypertension. Micturition may precipitate a syncopal attack if the tumour is in the bladder.

A minority of patients present in other ways. In some metabolic effects predominate and the patient is thyrotoxic. In others there is paroxysmal *hypotension*.

An unsuspected phaeochromocytoma may cause fatal and unexplained collapse after trauma or an operation. For this reason the possibility that a patient has a phaeochromocytoma must never be ignored or the need for further investigations overlooked.

### Investigation

All young hypertensives should be screened for a catecholamine-secreting tumour. The most reliable test is the demonstration of increased urinary excretion of the catecholamine metabolites (VMA) following a paroxysm.

Radiographic localisation of the site of the lesion is performed under full adrenergic blockade. As the tumour is vascular it may be demonstrated by aortography. Selective adrenal venous sampling defines the side of excess catecholamine secretion. Iodine-131-meta-iodobenzylquanidine has recently been shown to be concentrated in chromaffin tissue and is of potential value for radioisotope imaging of phaeochromocytomas.

### Treatment

Surgical removal of the tumour is the treatment of choice. At one time this was hazardous, but the availability of α- and β-adrenergic blocking drugs has reduced the risks. The potential for hypertensive attacks during induction of anaesthesia or handling of the tumour is reduced and tachycardia and arrhythmias are prevented.

The patient should come to operation with both blood pressure and pulse rate controlled. As the blood volume is also restored by preoperative

adrenergic blockade, troublesome hypotension following removal of the tumour does not usually occur. However, maintenance of blood volume during operation is still important.

Long-acting preparations are used. The α-blocker phenoxybenzamine is started 7–10 days preoperatively to control blood pressure. The β-blocker propanolol may then be added to reduce tachycardia. A combined preparation may be used but β-blocking agents should never be given first as cardiac failure may be precipitated.

Atropine should not be used for premedication and thiopentone is best avoided. Enflurane is the preferred anaesthetic. Pulse and blood pressure are monitored; phentolamine and propanolol (short acting α- and β-blocking agents) sodium nitroprusside (which acts directly on vessels independent of adrenergic receptors and gives additional control of hypertension) and blood should be available. Because of the likelihood of multiple tumours both adrenals are explored. While now uncommon (see above), profound hypotension may follow removal of the tumour and must be anticipated.

## NON-ENDOCRINE TUMOURS

### NEUROBLASTOMA

This is a highly malignant tumour of the adrenal medulla arising from primitive sympathetic nervous tissue of neural crest origin. It is one of the commonest malignant tumours of infants and young children and metastasises widely to lymph nodes, liver, bones and lung. Skeletal metastases may be confused with bone sarcoma. 75% of tumours secrete catecholamines.

Treatment by radical surgical excision, radiotherapy and chemotherapy offers the only hope of benefit.

### GANGLIONEUROMA

This is a benign, firm, well encapsulated tumour arising from ganglion cells. It grows slowly, does not metastasise and may reach a large size. Severe diarrhoea may be a feature. Treatment by surgical excision gives excellent results.

# APUDOMAS AND MULTIPLE ENDOCRINE NEOPLASIA

Cells which secrete amines and polypeptide hormones have certain characteristics in common. These are a capacity to store *amines*, e.g. catecholamines (A); the ability to take up amine precursor such as dopamine (PU); and the possession of the decarboxylating enzyme, l-aromatic decarboxylase, which is necessary for amine synthesis (D). The acronym APUD is used to name these cells, which can be defined by specific histochemical and immunofluorescent techniques.

Derived from neural ectoderm, they are believed to migrate from the neural crest to their sites in endocrine tissues where they serve specific functions. For example, APUD cells in the anterior pituitary secrete ACTH; in the adrenal medulla catecholamines; and in the thyroid, calcitonin. APUD cells abound in the intestinal tract, both singly and in conglomerates such as the pancreatic islets. In the gut they are responsible for the secretion of the amines 5-hydroxytryptamine and histamine and a large series of polypeptide hormones (including secretin, cholecystokinin, gastrin, enteroglucagon, somatostatin, vasoactive intestinal peptide) which regulate gastro-intestinal secretions and motor function. Some believe the origin of the gut APUD cells to be endodermal.

Tumours and hyperplasia of APUD cells account for many of the endocrine syndromes described in this chapter and also those which affect the pancreatic islets (see Chapter 36). They are also believed to be responsible for ectopic hormone secretion by tumours at non-endocrine sites such as that of ACTH or serotinin by bronchial carcinomas.

Tumour formation by APUD cells is not limited to single sites. These cells are also implicated in the Multiple Endocrine Neoplasia (MEN) syndromes in which a number of endocrine glands are affected. The commonest syndromes are due to abnormal production of hormones by the anterior pituitary, adrenal medulla, pancreas and the C cells of thyroid. However, parathyroid hyperplasia is also a feature although, as APUD cells do *not* contribute to the formation of parathormone, the mechanism is obscure.

The MEN syndromes are very rare. Inherited as autosomal dominants with varied penetrance, the tumours may be benign or malignant. It is for this reason the preferred term is now Multiple Endocrine Neoplasia (MEN), rather than Multiple Endocrine Adenomas (MEA) as previously used. Two main subgroups are described.

*MEN I* is due to hormone-secreting hyperplasia and/or tumours of the parathyroid, pancreatic islets and anterior pituitary. A variety of non-hormone-secreting tumours may also occur affecting the thyroid, pituitary, adrenal and soft tissues (lipomas). Carcinoid tumours have also been described.

There is a disparity between the clinical presentation and endocrine abnormality. Thus, while most cases present with peptic ulceration or its complications, the most common endocrine abnormality is hyperparathyroidism which is present in 90–95% of cases. Excess secretion of gastrin from pancreatic islet cells occurs in 20–40% and of insulin in 10%. Pituitary syndromes (acromegaly) are rare but chromophobe adenomas of the pituitary are more common.

Treatment is directed at the dominant feature. As hyperplasia of the parathyroid inevitably affects all four glands, these should be removed and a portion of one implanted into an accessible site from which it can be removed if recurrence develops. As the disease is familial, screening of the family is important.

*MEN II*. This inherited syndrome is composed of a triad of medullary carcinoma of the thyroid, phaeochromocytoma and parathyroid hyperplasia. Two main subgroups are described:

*MEN IIa* in which medullary carcinoma of the thyroid is predominant. One-third of cases also have a phaeochromocytoma, parathyroid hyperplasia or both.

*MEN IIb* in which medullary carcinoma of the thyroid and phaeochromocytoma occur without parathyroid abnormality. However, there is overgrowth of nervous tissue to form multiple mucosal neuromas, thickened nerves and ganglioneuromatosis of the gut. There is a typical facies with thick nodular lips Marfan-like habitus with lax ligaments and a tendency to joint subluxation.

Both these syndromes can be diagnosed by the finding of raised plasma calcitonin levels. This reflects excess secretion of calcitonin by the neoplastic parafollicular cells in the thyroid, and this test is used to screen families for occult lesions. A pentagastrin provocation test has also been developed; patients with asymptomatic MEN-II syndrome show a rapid rise of calcitonin following a bolus intravenous injection of pentagastrin.

The surgical treatment of MEN-II is directed primarily at the medullary carcinoma of the thyroid which is treated by total thyroidectomy. In all cases, urinary catecholamine and VMA determinations must be made to exclude phaeochromocytoma so that if one is present it can be treated first. In patients with metastatic carcinoma, doxorubicin is the chemotherapeutic agent of choice and the success of treatment can be monitored by plasma calcitonin levels.

## CARCINOID SYNDROME

This syndrome is due to excessive secretion of 5-hydroxy tryptamine (serotonin) by a tumour affecting APUD cells of argentaffin type (carcinoid tumour) most commonly in the small intestine, the appendix. Rarely, it is caused by inappropriate secretion of serotonin from a tumour.

The syndrome consists of attacks of flushing, which is characteristically patchy in distribution, abdominal colic with diarrhoea and bronchospasm. Heart rate and cardiac output are increased and there may be blood pressure changes. Telangiectases, dependent oedema, tricuspid and pulmonary valvular lesions occur. Excretion of the metabolite of serotonin, 5-hydroxy-indole acetic acid, is increased.

The presence of the syndrome is indicative of large tumour mass. It therefore occurs only in patients with malignant carcinoid and gross metastases.

Carcinoid tumours of the small bowel and appendix are described on pages 406 and 416.

# 40. Urological Surgery

## INVESTIGATIONS

### HISTORY

The majority of patients who present in a urological clinic have either a sign or symptom which suggests an abnormality in the urinary tract. Thus a patient with blood in the urine (haematuria), *irrespective of other symptoms*, requires a full urological investigation.

There are also those patients who present in other clinics complaining of symptoms which may be due to urological problems, e.g. backache from metastatic prostatic carcinoma, fever of unknown origin from renal carcinoma, lethargy and anaemia due to obstructive renal failure or headaches from hypertension of renal origin. Since common things occur commonly, an elderly male complaining of difficulty in passing his urine *probably* has outflow tract obstruction due to benign enlargement of the prostate (benign prostatic hyperplasia, BPH). But, he may also recently have been prescribed a diuretic so causing the change in his urinary habits.

Environmental factors must not be ignored. In some parts of the world, bilharziasis is a common cause of haematuria. In the industrialised world, there may have been contact with certain carcinogenic agents which, years later, cause bladder cancer.

### URINARY TRACT SYMPTOMS

The site of *pain* must be accurately defined. Pain in the 'side' could either originate from the chest, loin or spinal column. Renal pain occurs in the renal angle i.e. that angle between the 12th rib and the sacrospinalis muscles. Ureteric pain (or colic) may start in the renal angle but typically radiates forwards and downwards into the groin and to either the testes or labia. When the bladder is obstructed acutely, there is characteristic severe central lower abdominal pain. Chronic bladder obstruction may produce only a vague lower abdominal ache even although the bladder is grossly distended. Bladder abnormalities and prostatic diseases may also cause ill-defined perineal or penile pains. A prostate which is grossly enlarged can encroach into the rectum and cause rectal symptoms, including *tenesmus*. The recognition of penile and testicular pain is usually easy.

Urinary symptoms have a 'patois' of their own. *Frequency of micturition* is recorded numerically. Thus D/N = 6/3 indicates that the frequency by day is × 6 and that by night × 3. A *poor stream* and *dribbling* are characteristic of a mechanical obstruction in the outflow tract. *Urgency* describes the sudden uncontrollable urge to empty the bladder. *Strangury* is *slow* and painful micturition. This may be associated with *incontinence (urge incontinence)*. *Stress incontinence* indicates an involuntary loss of urine due to stress such as straining to lift, running or even laughter. *Dysuria* is *painful micturition* which is often described as being of a burning or scalding nature.

The patient may use a wide range of phrases to describe alterations in urinary habits. The interrogation must aim to reveal whether the patient is describing obstruction (e.g. poor stream) detrusor contraction (e.g. urgency), infection (e.g. frequency, dysuria) or a more sinister sign of malignancy (e.g. dark, discoloured or brown urine).

## EXAMINATION

Examination should be full, and not confined to the urinary system. Thus, cardiological, neurological and gynaecological problems may be associated with urinary signs and symptoms. Since many urological patients are elderly they must be assessed as to their fitness for further investigations and operative treatment. For example the cardiovascular state of a patient may be relevant to subsequent investigations (e.g. the need for an anaesthetic) or treatment (e.g. the administration of oestrogens for carcinoma of the prostate).

Physical examination of the *kidneys* is difficult. The patient must be able to relax the abdominal muscles so that the kidney can be lifted with a hand behind the loin and palpated by the other hand pressing downwards (Fig. 40.1). The *ureter* cannot be palpated even though it does pass close to the posterior fornix of the vagina. The *bladder*, if enlarged, is central and rises up out of the pelvis; it is dull to percussion and in a patient with chronic retention who is lying flat and relaxed, is visible. Abnormalities of adjacent abdominal organs must be sought. For example a mass in the iliac fossa could be ovarian in origin.

In the male, examination must include the groins, hernia sites, cords, testes and epididymes, which are examined both with the patient standing up and lying down. The penis should always be examined. If it is uncircumcised it must be confirmed that the foreskin retracts and that the glans and meatus are normal.

In the female, the vulva, urethra and vagina must be examined; a speculum examination should be carried out if there is any suspicion of a vaginal or cervical abnormality.

(However, a full pelvic examination for both male and female is best carried out under general anaesthesia with a muscle relaxant).

A rectal examination is mandatory, not only to examine the prostate but to detect abnormalities of the anal margin (e.g. haemorrhoids, fissures) and lower rectum (e.g. carcinoma).

## ROUTINE INVESTIGATION

### Urine

Routine 'side-room' examination of the urine consists of testing for protein and sugar with proprietary test-papers. Testing for protein is a simple guide to glomerular function. Provided that there is no urinary tract infection, normal urine is almost protein-free. A protein leak of more than 150 mg/24 hrs requires further investigation of the kidneys. The detection of sugar in the urine may point to a diagnosis of diabetes and urinary symptoms may be related to this.

In surgical practice the routine *microscopic examination* of a fresh specimen of urine is of limited value. However, the presence of red cells or pus cells may support a diagnosis of stone or infection. Other abnormalities in the urinary sediment are more relevant in renal parenchymal disease.

For *microbiological examination* of the urine, a fresh sample must be collected in a sterile container. In order to avoid contamination by normal urethral flora, the patient is asked to pass some urine into the toilet, then the next part into a special container, then the remainder into the toilet — hence the expression a *mid-stream specimen* of urine (MSU). In the microbiological laboratory, the specimen will usually be examined microscopically for pus cells only. A more detailed microscopic examination of the urine, e.g. for crystals, casts or ova, will need to be carried out on a fresh specimen in the side room of a ward or clinic. To detect organisms the microbiologist will culture the urine on a suitable medium. He will also determine the sensitivity of any organism against antimicrobial agents.

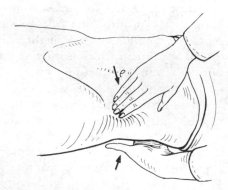

**Fig. 40.1** Palpation of the kidney

## Blood

A guide to overall renal function is provided by measuring blood urea or creatinine. Urea is the major end-product of protein metabolism but the blood level may be influenced by diet and urine flow rate. As the blood urea does not rise unless the glomerular filtration rate is reduced to 50% of normal, considerable renal damage can exist in the presence of a normal blood urea. The measurement of serum creatinine is preferred since it is stable, independent of urine flow and little influenced by diet.

The blood chemistry may also be examined to exclude a metabolic disorder. The haemoglobin should be checked and will be low in a patient with chronic renal disease. The ESR may be markedly raised in idiopathic retroperitoneal fibrosis, a cause of ureteric obstruction.

A search for tumour-secretory products (*tumour markers*) in the blood may help to diagnose and monitor malignant disease. In tumours of the testis, human chorionic gonadotrophin and α feto protein are valuable tumour markers. Serum acid phosphatase is also a useful marker for carcinoma of the prostate.

## Intravenous urography

The basic radiological investigation of the urinary tract is an *intravenous urogram* (IVU). It consists firstly of a plain X-ray of the abdomen and pelvis to show the areas of the kidneys, ureters and bladder. In addition to demonstrating the lumbar spine and pelvis, opacities such as stones in the region of the urinary tract will be shown.

An iodine-containing contrast material is then injected intravenously and serial X-rays taken as the contrast is excreted.

The concentration of contrast is influenced by the urine flow which, in turn, depends on the hydration of the patient. Routine preparation for an IVU should include fluid restriction for 12 hours. As faeces within the large bowel will diminish the radiographic outline of the urinary tract, an aperient may be given on the day before the X-ray.

An IVU demonstrates the renal pelvis and calices and the rate of emptying from the kidneys.

The calibre of the ureters is seen as they pass to the bladder. After the bladder has filled with contrast, the patient empties the bladder and a 'post micturition' X-ray is taken to show the efficiency of bladder emptying and to indicate the amount of residual urine.

When there is an obstruction, there is delayed excretion of the contrast. Then delayed X-rays, up to 24 hours after the contrast injection, may give added detail of the affected kidney and ureter.

## SPECIAL INVESTIGATIONS

### Other radiological tests

To define the ureter, pelvis and calices more clearly a *retrograde uretero-pyelogram* may be necessary (Fig. 40.2). This consists of the retrograde injection of contrast material through a ureteric catheter placed in the lower ureter. With improved techniques of intravenous urography a retrograde injection is now less commonly used.

To demonstrate the renal vessels a *renal angiogram* is performed. A catheter is passed into the aorta via a femoral artery up to the level of the renal arteries where contrast medium is injected and serial films taken. If better definition is required the renal vessels may be selectively catheterised. The main uses of this test are for the detection of stenosis of the main renal artery, the vascularity of a renal mass, or as a preliminary to embolisation to infarct a kidney.

To define the bladder, to detect uretero-vesical reflux or to examine the bladder neck and urethra a *micturating cysto-urethrogram* (MCU) is required. The bladder is filled by catheter with contrast material and its emptying studied by X-ray screening. An *ascending urethrogram* in which contrast medium is injected into the urethra and X-rays taken can be used to define strictures, but is less useful than an MCU.

### Ultrasound

The main use of ultrasound in the urinary tract is to distinguish between solid tumours and cysts of the kidney. Other uses include the detection of peri-renal collections of fluid such as may occur

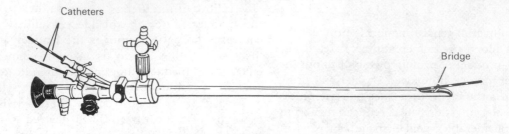

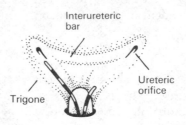

**Fig. 40.2** Cystoscopy and ureteric catheterisation

around a transplanted kidney, and the characterisation of masses in the pelvis. Ultrasound is of limited value in determining the size or spread of tumours.

## Nuclear imaging

Methods using radiolabelled substances are used for two main purposes:

1. To detect *metastases in bones*: $^{99m}$Technetium labelled methylene diphosphonate (MDP) is the most reliable method for detecting metastases in carcinoma of the prostate.

2. To measure *renal function*: $^{99m}$Technetium labelled chelates, DTPA (diethylene tetramine penta-acetic acid) and DMSA (dimercaptosuccinic acid) are used for this purpose. DTPA is rapidly excreted through the glomerulus and can be used to provide a measure of the glomerular filtration rate from each kidney. DMSA is concentrated in the renal tubule. As only 5% is excreted, static imaging can be carried out some 2 to 3 hours after injection. Parenchymal defects, such as tumours, haematoma, lacerations or ischaemia may be demonstrated. Differential renal function can be quantified from the DMSA concentration in each kidney.

## Urodynamics

In their simplest form, urodynamic studies refer to the measurement of the maximum urinary flow rate during micturition by a flow meter. Normally the flow rate exceeds 20 ml/sec. A flow rate of less than 6 ml/sec for a voided volume of 150 ml or more, is abnormal. The urinary stream may be so poor that no such quantification is necessary, but in a proportion of patients with equivocal urinary symptoms, the flow rate can be of help in determining the degree of obstruction.

For additional information on the dynamic activity of the urinary tract, measurements of flow rate are combined with *cystometry*. This provides a measure of the residual urine, the capacity of the bladder, the capacity at the time a desire to void occurs and the detrusor pressures when the bladder is full and at maximum flow rate. Detrusor muscle pressure is recorded continuously and any spontaneous contractions during the filling of the bladder may indicate an unstable bladder (a cause of urgency and urge incontinence). The pressures along the length of the urethra may also be measured (urethral pressure profile).

These measurements are of particular value in distinguishing between bladder and urethral abnormalities in the incontinent patient. They also assist in distinguishing between neurological, pharmacological and mechanical causes of outflow tract symptoms.

## Semen analysis

Microscopic examination of the semen is a basic investigation in an infertile male. The specimen is collected 3 days after the last ejaculation and examined within 2 hours. Normal semen has a volume of 2–6 ml; a sperm concentration 20–120 $\times$ $10^6$/ml. More than 60% of the sperms are motile at 2 hours.

The morphology, biochemistry and viability of the sperm may also be studied. In selected cases, immunological tests may help determine the cause of infertility.

## Biochemical screening for stones

The main metabolic causes of urinary tract stones are hyperparathyroidism, idiopathic hypercalciuria, hyperoxaluria and cystinuria. All patients with urinary tract calculi should be screened for such an underlying metabolic abnormality. Serum calcium, phosphate, oxalate and uric acid are measured. More detailed investigation requires the 24-hour collection of urine for calcium, phosphate, oxalate and uric acid excretion. The composition of passed or removed stones should be analysed to determine their metabolic type.

## URINARY TRACT OBSTRUCTION — OUTFLOW TRACT

The *outflow* tract is that part of the urinary tract which extends from the bladder neck through the urethra to the external urinary meatus. In the older male it is most commonly obstructed by benign hyperplasia of the prostate; in the younger male the obstruction may be due to a stricture. Carcinoma of the prostate is a less frequent cause of obstructive symptoms.

## BENIGN PROSTATIC HYPERPLASIA (BPH)

## Pathology

From about the age of 40 years the prostate undergoes progressive change in size and consistency. Enlargement results from hyperplasia of periurethral glandular tissue forming adenomas in the central zone of the prostate. These characteristically form lateral 'lobes' and, often a 'middle lobe'. The normal prostatic tissue is gradually compressed to form a shell or capsule around these adenomas. There is considerable variation in the growth rates of the adenomas and in the proportion of stromal and epithelial tissue. A prostate that has been previously infected or has a preponderance of stromal tissue will be firm and fibrous; adenomas with epithelial preponderance can grow to large discrete masses of total weight greater than 100 g. These changes are generally referred to as benign prostatic hyperplasia (BPH).

The enlarging adenomas lengthen and obstruct the prostatic urethra, interfere with the sphincter mechanisms of the internal meatus and lead to the signs and symptoms of prostatic obstruction. In order to overcome increasing outflow resistance, the bladder detrusor muscle hypertrophies. The muscle bands form trabeculae between which saccules may form diverticula. Occasionally a diverticulum may become quite large — even larger than the bladder. Bladder diverticula empty poorly and are liable to the three main complications of urinary stasis: infection, stones and tumour.

With progressive inability to empty the bladder completely, the risk of urinary infection and stone formation increases. Bladder stones have become rare in Western countries but are often seen in areas of poor nutrition and especially in children. The stones are typically of the infective type, mixed calcium oxalate and phosphate. Eventually the residual urine may be greater than 1 litre (chronic retention) leading to progressive obstruction and dilatation of the ureters (hydroureter) and pelvi-caliceal system (hydronephrosis) with, ultimately, obstructive renal failure (Fig. 40.3).

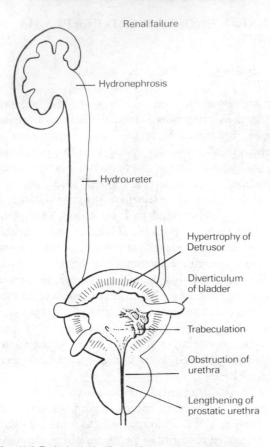

Renal failure

Hydronephrosis

Hydroureter

Hypertrophy of Detrusor

Diverticulum of bladder

Trabeculation

Obstruction of urethra

Lengthening of prostatic urethra

**Fig. 40.3** Pathological effects of prostatic hyperplasia

## Clinical features

The pathological changes at the bladder neck produce variable signs and symptoms which correlate poorly with the size of the prostate. Frequency, urgency and dysuria are common. Nocturia may become increasingly troublesome and inconvenient. The force of the stream will be noticeably weaker and, with straining in an attempt to empty the bladder, bleeding may occur from vessels at the bladder neck. These clinical features may be separated into two main groups. There are those that are due to obstruction — slow stream and hesitancy and those that are due to an unstable detrusor muscle — urgency and urge incontinence. These latter irritative symptoms, alone, are not an indication for prostatectomy.

Increasing frequency may deceive the patient into thinking that he is passing an adequate amount of urine whereas the bladder may be full though painless. Such frequency may progress to dribbling incontinence. It is this patient who is liable to the signs and symptoms of obstructive uraemia, including drowsiness, anorexia and personality changes.

Some patients may suddenly stop passing urine (acute retention). This may be precipitated by a urinary infection, cold weather or excessive alcohol, each of which can cause sufficient congestion of the bladder neck to tip the balance from difficult micturition to acute painful retention. If the obstruction has already led to chronic retention of urine (the patient being unable to empty his bladder completely), acute-on-chronic obstruction may occur. If the patient has a bladder stone he may have obstructive symptoms during micturition and there may also be bladder pain at the end of micturition.

Examination of a patient with symptoms of prostatism will reveal little except enlargement of the gland on rectal examination. The enlargement is symmetrical and smooth with a median groove between the two lateral 'lobes'. The consistency of an adenoma is described as *rubbery*. Asymmetry or a hard consistency should raise a suspicion of malignancy. In a patient with an acute painful retention of urine, the size of the prostate is more difficult to determine. This is partly due to the pelvic discomfort but also to the fullness of the bladder which changes the normal relationship of the prostate to the lower rectum so that the gland appears to be larger than it is. In the patient with chronic retention, the painless enlarged bladder rises up out of the pelvis — almost to the umbilicus. Even if the shape is not visible, the area will be dull on percussion. In addition, the patient with chronic retention may be ill from obstructive uraemia.

## Investigations

All patients must have a basic assessment of renal function, and their haemoglobin and serum electrolytes measured. As symptoms of dysuria and frequency may be principally related to a urinary infection (which will require to be treated) the urine must be cultured in all cases. The serum acid phosphatase is measured if the consistency of the gland raises the suspicion of a neoplasm. Intravenous urography is necessary to detect the extent of any of the secondary effects of obstruction on the bladder (e.g. diverticula, stones) and upper urinary tract, and especially to assess the residual urine after micturition. If the patient is uraemic, urography with a high dose of contrast and delayed X-rays will be required.

In some patients, and especially in the elderly, neurological or pharmacological causes of changes in micturition must be remembered. A urodynamic assessment may be necessary.

## Treatment

The main clinical decision is whether or not the patient requires an operation on the prostate. There is no acceptable alternative treatment which will reduce the size of the gland. There are three clinical groups, each requiring a different approach to management.

*1. Symptomatic only.* The assessment of the severity of symptoms is influenced by the age of the patient, the social inconvenience caused and their rate and progression. Thus, a young man may be greatly inconvenienced by symptoms that are quite acceptable to one who is elderly. If there is difficulty in determining the exact role of the prostate in causing these symptoms, urodynamic measurements may be helpful, especially if the symptoms appear to be irritative rather than obstructive.

Once it is established that the prostate is the principal problem, prostatectomy is recommended. Very few patients are unfit for this and only a history of a myocardial infarction within 3 months should defer it.

*2. Acute retention.* This is an emergency requiring admission to hospital. If there is a history of prostatism, conservative measures to encourage micturition (sedation, a warm bath) only delay inevitable catheterisation. A self-retaining (Foley) catheter (16 F) is passed using strict asepsis, and connected to a closed bladder drainage system. Should it not be possible to pass a urethral catheter, a suprapubic cystostomy should be performed. A specimen of urine is cultured and antibiotics given only if there is microbiological evidence of an infection.

Only if the history of prostatism is short should the urethral catheter be removed after 12 hours and this may be followed by normal voiding. However such a patient should be advised to have a prostatectomy. Otherwise, routine pre-operative investigations are performed with operation on the next available operating day.

*3. Chronic retention.* It is essential to determine whether or not the patient has developed any of the complications of obstruction, especially renal damage. Though the upper urinary tracts may be dilated, renal function is not necessarily impaired.

If the patient is well, with no haematological or biochemical disturbance, there is no indication for preliminary bladder drainage and prostatectomy may be planned in the usual way.

If the patient is uraemic, with associated biochemical abnormalities, his general fitness for operation must be assessed. Uraemia alone is not a contraindication but hyperkalaemia, dehydration or other evidence of fluid and electrolyte disturbance must be corrected by intravenous fluids. The bladder is catheterised, and prostatectomy is carried out as soon as the patient is judged to be fit. It is not necessary to wait unduly long for the blood urea to return to normal as the risk of infection from prolonged catheterisation may be a more serious hazard.

The relief of chronic obstruction is almost always followed by a diuresis due to the combination of an osmotic (urea) diuresis and renal tubular changes resulting from back pressure. These losses will be detected by careful intake/output fluid charts; the blood pressure should be monitored and intravenous fluid replacement may be necessary.

Only exceptionally will a patient be considered unfit for prostatectomy. He will then need a permanent self-retaining catheter.

Prostatectomy may be performed either by open or closed (endoscopic) techniques.

*Open prostatectomy.* Earlier open procedures were by a transvesical approach in which the bladder was opened and the adenomatous obstruction enucleated from the capsule. Later, a retropubic approach was used in which the adenoma was enucleated through a transverse incision in the prostatic capsule (Fig. 40.4a). These open procedures are now reserved for the

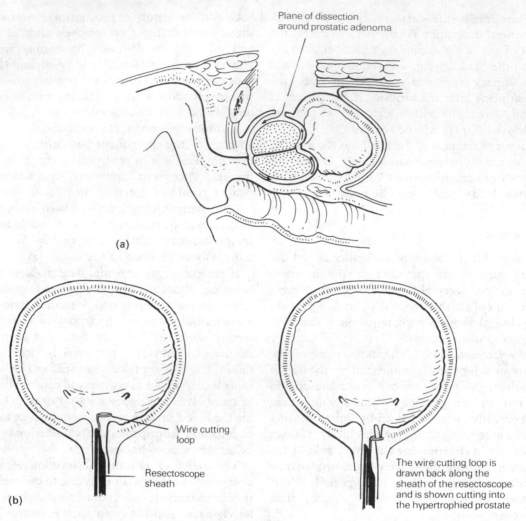

Plane of dissection
around prostatic adenoma

(a)

Wire cutting
loop

Resectoscope
sheath

(b)

The wire cutting loop is
drawn back along the
sheath of the resectoscope
and is shown cutting into
the hypertrophied prostate

**Fig. 40.4** a) Retropubic prostatectomy, b) Transurethral resection of the prostate

removal of very large adenomata or when another procedure, e.g. removal of a bladder diverticulum, is required. Apart from the length of hospitalisation (approx 10–14 days) and the presence of an abdominal wound, enucleation of some of the smaller adenomata may damage the external sphincter mechanism and cause incontinence. This is a particular problem with more fibrous glands and those that contain cancer.

*Closed (endoscopic) prostatectomy* — transurethral resection (TUR). The prostate gland is removed, piecemeal, by electro-resection using an instrument called a resectoscope (Fig. 40.4b). The disadvantage of a lengthy apprenticeship in acquiring the skill to perform this procedure is greatly outweighed by patient acceptance, short hospitalisation (5–7 days) and the precision of removal of the obstructing tissue. It is now universally accepted as the method of choice. Great damage can be inflicted in the prostatic urethra and even the bladder by the inexpert use of a resectoscope, and experience in the technique is essential.

If the patient should have a bladder stone this may be crushed with a lithotrite or removed by a suprapubic lithotomy. If there is a diverticulum with a narrow neck, this should be removed through a suprapubic transvesical approach. If the diverticulum is shallow with a wide neck then only the prostatectomy need be done.

## Post-operative care

After either form of prostatectomy, the bladder must be drained by a urethral catheter to allow free drainage while the prostatic bed begins to heal and bleeding stops. After a TUR, the catheter is removed usually on the 3rd post-operative day; after an open procedure, because of the bladder or prostate incision, the catheter is usually removed on the 7th post-operative day.

The main post-operative hazard is bleeding. In an open procedure, blood vessels at the bladder neck are sutured but bleeding within the capsule is less easy to control. In a TUR, coagulation of the blood vessels is more precise but not always complete. If post-operative bleeding is excessive, a clot may form and lead to obstruction (clot retention). Various techniques are used to minimise this hazard: a good flow of urine can be induced by diuretics or continuous irrigation through a three-way urethral catheter established.

The results from all forms of prostatectomy have continued to improve but transurethral resection is now recognised as the procedure of choice. It has the lowest morbidity and mortality (1.3%) and the hospital stay is 50% less than that following other procedures.

## MALIGNANT PROSTATE OBSTRUCTION

Carcinoma of the prostate is discussed on page 602 *et seq.*

## BLADDER NECK OBSTRUCTION

Occasionally, the obstruction to the outflow tract appears to be at the bladder neck. The prostate is often quite small giving rise to the expression — 'prostatism without a prostate'. The aetiology may be an infective condition such as prostatitis or schistosomiasis or a neurological condition such as with diabetes or a prolapsed intervertebral disc. More commonly, the obstruction is due to dyssynergia which is the failure of the bladder neck to open when the detrusor contracts.

Characteristically, bladder neck dyssynergia is found in the younger middle-aged man — i.e. an age too young to expect BPH. His urinary stream is poor, though he may have thought it normal for him, and there may be frequency and urgency.

The muscular dysfunction that causes dyssynergia may be improved by alpha-blocking drugs. However, endoscopic incision or excision of the bladder neck is preferable to long term drug treatment but surgery is contraindicated if the risk of retrograde ejaculation and therefore infertility should be of concern to the patient.

## URETHRAL OBSTRUCTION

Lesions of the urethra may be congenital, traumatic, infective or malignant. Each may result in outflow tract obstruction (Fig. 40.5). Foreign bodies, including urinary stones, may also cause obstruction. Any of these causes may be complicated by infection, with periurethral abscess, fistulae and stones occurring as late complications.

## Pathology

*Congenital lesions.* Congenital valves in the posterior urethra occur only in boys. These lie at the level of the verumontanum and may cause gross obstructive changes in the bladder and upper tracts at birth. The diagnosis is confirmed by micturating cysto-urethrography and treatment is by endoscopic incision of the valves.

Diverticula of the urethra are rare causes of obstruction. More commonly, diverticula of the urethra occur as a secondary effect of obstruction in women.

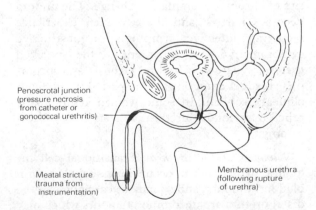

Fig. 40.5 Common sites and causes of urethral stricture

*Urethral trauma.* An important late sequel of urethral trauma is a stricture whose severity is related both to the site and the extent of injury. Thus, a posterior urethral stricture that follows major trauma to the pelvis may be surrounded by dense fibrous tissue, whereas a stricture of the bulb of the urethra may be surrounded by healthy tissues. The former requires major reconstructive surgery, but the latter may be readily managed either by urethral dilatation or incision.

It must be remembered that rough inexpert use of any instrument (including a catheter) in the urethra can be followed by stricture formation.

*Infective lesions.* In the male, the principal organism responsible for inflammatory change, scarring and stricture of the urethra is *Neisseria gonorrhoeae*. The periurethral glands of the bulb of the urethra are the main site of the infection and when treatment is inadequate, stricture formation in this area is likely.

The long-term use of a self-retaining catheter, not necessarily associated with infection, may also cause an inflammatory reaction in the urethra. This may result in a stricture, most commonly at the external meatus.

The foreskin may also cause problems due to infection (balanitis), narrowing of the orifice, or to it becoming retracted and stuck (paraphimosis). These are discussed on page 611.

In the female the paraurethral glands, sometimes called the 'female prostate', may become the site of chronic inflammatory change. The urethra becomes narrow and these women experience recurring infective symptoms or obstructive symptoms without infection — the so-called *urethral syndrome.* Urethral stenosis and incomplete bladder emptying are but part of this difficult clinical problem. In some women symptomatic relief may follow urethral dilatation or urethrotomy.

*Tumours of the urethra.* Transitional cell tumours, which often occur in association with bladder tumours, and squamous carcinoma of the distal urethra are uncommon tumours which may cause obstructive symptoms.

## Clinical features

The change in micturition due to a urethral narrowing may be indistinguishable from that which occurs with BPH. However, a stricture should be considered if there is a previous history of urethral infection, instrumentation or trauma.

The external meatus must always be examined and if present the foreskin retracted for full inspection. The urethra is palpated: it is possible for a stone to lodge in the urethra yet the patient still pass his urine, though with difficulty. In women, the urethra is best examined as part of a cystourethroscopy under general anaesthesia: the urethra can then be palpated against the shaft of the cystoscope.

## Investigations

An intravenous urogram may show only incomplete bladder emptying. An ascending urethrogram may not show the posterior urethra adequately because of spasm; a micturating cysto-urethrogram (MCU) in which the behaviour of the urethra during micturition is studied on the X-ray screen, is preferred. A urodynamic assessment of the urethra *and bladder* may be indicated for more complex problems, especially when neurological and mechanical problems co-exist.

The final investigation to assess a urethral lesion is urethroscopy. This procedure should be considered as a cystourethroscopy since both urethra and bladder are always examined as a routine. The site and character of the lesion is determined and the degree of narrowing is measured.

## Treatment

The precise site and extent of a stricture will have been established by these investigations. Many simple strictures are treated easily by repeated dilatation using either plastic or metal bougies or may be incised under a direct vision using a urethrotome. Most simple short strictures in the region of the bulb respond well to this type of treatment but there is a risk of recurrence which may require some form of operative reconstruction (a urethroplasty). In this procedure a strip of full-thickness skin is used to restore the normal calibre of the urethra.

A long persistent stricture of the anterior urethra will require a two-stage plastic reconstruction. A tight fibrous post-traumatic stricture of the membranous urethra may require transpubic excision of the scar tissue and urethral reconstruction. Stenosis of the meatus is treated by meatoplasty.

Where the foreskin cannot be retracted normally (phimosis) and especially if infections are troublesome, circumcision is recommended.

If paraphimosis is present without gross oedema, it may be possible to reduce it manually, compression of the glans allowing the constricting band to be drawn forwards. Otherwise it is necessary to incise the constricting band. Circumcision may be carried out at a later date (see p. 611).

## URINARY TRACT OBSTRUCTION — UPPER TRACT

The upper urinary tract includes the renal pelvicaliceal system and the ureters. As with any tubular structure, obstruction may be due to extrinsic, intrinsic or intraluminal causes.

In the kidney, stones within the pelvi-caliceal system and congenital abnormality of the pelviureteric junction are the main causes of obstruction: both cause hydronephrosis. In the ureter, the common causes of obstruction are:

1. *Extrinsic* — retroperitoneal fibrosis; external pressure, e.g. carcinoma cervix

2. *Intrinsic* — transitional cell tumours, tuberculosis/bilharziasis, ureterocele, ectopic ureter, vesicoureteric reflux, megaureter

3. *Intraluminal* — calculi

More rarely, a sloughed renal papilla or blood clot (from a tumour) may obstruct either kidney or ureter.

During pregnancy the ureters dilate, probably as a result of external compression by the baby.

## RENAL AND URETERIC CALCULI
### Pathology

Stones which form in the kidney are of two main types — infective and metabolic.

An *infective* stone is whitish, chalky and crumbles or breaks easily. It is composed mainly of calcium, ammonia and magnesium phosphates. Such stones develop wherever drainage in the urinary tract is impaired and are usually associated with an anatomical abnormality such as a diverticulum or with long-term recumbency or paraplegia. Their formation indicates an established infection which cannot be eradicated by antibiotics alone. As the stone enlarges, drainage is further impaired and there is progressive damage to the kidney.

A *metabolic* stone, commonly of calcium oxalate, is usually hard and dark with an irregular sharp surface. It develops as a result of an abnormality of the constituents of the urine. There may be an abnormal concentration of normal constituents e.g. by dehydration, excess excretion of normal constituents (e.g. calcium as in hyperparathyroidism, uric acid as in gout) or there may be abnormal constituents (as in the metabolic disorder of cystinuria). Probably several aetiological factors must occur together or in sequence for a stone to form in the urinary tract. As indicated above, all patients with urinary calculi should be screened for metabolic abnormalities.

### Clinical features

Renal pain and ureteric colic are characteristically unilateral. Renal pain is dull and aching; ureteric colic acute and severe and occuring in waves which pass down along the line of the ureter. A stone may cause bleeding or there may be symptoms of urinary tract infection. However, a stone in the kidney may remain silent, even one large enough to fill the pelvis and calices (staghorn in appearance).

### Investigation

An intravenous urogram will usually provide all the necessary information on the anatomical position of the stone(s). Routine haematological and biochemical tests are needed to assess overall renal function and to exclude metabolic causes of stones. A urine sample is cultured to determine if there is infection. If an obstruction is acute, relief of that obstruction is the prime clinical need; but if the obstruction is chronic and has caused renal damage, the surgical approach will be influenced by the function of that kidney. This is best determined by radioisotope methods.

## Treatment

Symptomatic treatment is necessary as soon as the diagnosis has been confirmed. Large doses of pethidine may be required to relieve pain. The addition of anti-spasmodics may assist the passage of the stone. The likelihood of spontaneous passage depends both on the size of the stone and the smoothness of its surface. A stone of less than 0.5 cm in diameter should pass down the ureter. If it becomes fixed, with increasing hydroureter and hydronephrosis, or if the urine is infected, the stone must be removed.

A stone in the lower ureter, below the pelvic brim, may be coaxed out endoscopically using a stone basket. The instrument must be used with great care — serious damage to the ureter may otherwise result. Other fixed stones will require a direct surgical approach for removal (ureterolithotomy).

Surgical techniques for the removal of fixed stones within the kidney have improved in recent years. Provided the affected kidney contributes more than 10% of the total renal function, attempts to save the kidney should always be made. Removal of a stone from the renal pelvis (pyelolithotomy) should be straightfoward.

Stones that extend into the calices or are multiple and occupy most of the pelvi-caliceal system, may need to be removed through an incision into the cortex of the kidney (nephrolithotomy). Clamping of the renal vessels gives a bloodless field for operation. If this is to be prolonged for more than 30 minutes, cooling of the kidney (to 15°C), is recommended. The inside of a calix may be examined by a nephroscope and small stones removed with forceps or by trapping in a fibrin coagulum. If stones in the lower calices have damaged the lower part of the kidney a partial nephrectomy may be necessary.

Recently, the techniques of percutaneous removal and ultrasonic destruction of small to medium size renal stones have been developed. It seems likely that up to 50% of renal stones will be suitable for treatment by either of these methods.

# PELVI-URETERIC JUNCTION (PUJ) OBSTRUCTION (IDIOPATHIC HYDRONEPHROSIS)

## Pathology

Narrowing at the junction between the renal pelvis and the ureter is a common cause of hydronephrosis. As the cause of the narrowing remains obscure the term *idiopathic hydronephrosis* is appropriate. Electron microscopy of the narrow area shows normal muscle cells with normal innervation but the muscle bundles are separated by an excess of collagen fibres which may prevent relaxation of the segment. This abnormality of the PUJ is likely to be congenital. It is often bilateral and it is seen in very young children. Gross hydronephrosis may, however, present at any age.

## Clinical features

Idiopathic hydronephrosis may be the cause of a large painless mass in the loin; in its grossest form the volume of urine in the hydronephrotic sac may simulate free fluid in the peritoneal cavity. The more usual moderate sized hydronephrosis causes ill-defined renal pain or ache which may be exacerbated by drinking large volumes of tea or beer; the patient may regard these symptoms as 'indigestion'. Rarely, there may be no symptoms and a non-functioning hydronephrotic sac may be found incidentally.

## Investigations

An intravenous urogram, with or without delayed films, will provide sufficient information in most cases. The calibre of the ureter in a PUJ obstruction is normal. There are a few patients in whom there is doubt as to whether the dilatation of the pelvis and calices is truly obstructive in nature. Methods to resolve this include urography and renography during an induced diuresis, and antegrade pressure/flow measurements.

## Treatment

Operations on the pelvi-ureteric junction to relieve an obstruction (pyeloplasty) are designed to remove the obstructing tissue and to refashion the PUJ so that the lower part of the renal pelvis drains freely into the ureter (Fig. 40.6). On occasions, an aberrant vessel to the lower pole of the kidney crosses the PUJ and gives the appearance of having caused the obstruction (though this is unlikely): in this situation, the PUJ is reconstructed in front of these vessels.

It is not possible to predict the degree of recovery of function (if any) of a kidney after relief of the obstruction. A grossly hydronephrotic kidney should be removed; but if the contralateral kidney is also impaired, even a poorly functioning kidney should be preserved.

## RETROPERITONEAL FIBROSIS

### Pathology

Fibrosis of the retroperitoneal connective tissues may encircle and compress the ureter(s) causing hydroureter and hydronephrosis. Fibrosis occurs in three groups of conditions:

*Idiopathic.* In this, the largest group, the fibrosis extends across the pelvic brim to involve the ureters and vena cava. The aetiology is unknown though it may be associated with methysergide or analgesic abuse. Mediastinal fibrosis or palmar fascial fibrosis (Dupuytrens contracture) may co-exist.

*Malignant.* In this group the fibrosis contains malignant cells and represents a metastatic process from primary sites as various as breast, stomach, pancreas and colon; any part of the ureter may be affected.

*Reactive fibrosis.* Radiotherapy to pelvic organs, resolving blood clot after major vascular or other surgical procedures or extravasation of sclerosants (e.g. phenol for a nerve block) can lead of fibrotic change in the retroperitoneum.

Since the gross appearance of all three groups of fibrosis may be similar, biopsy of the tissue is essential for diagnosis.

### Clinical features

Obstruction due to pelvi-ureteric fibrosis may cause symptoms similar to idiopathic hydronephrosis, i.e. ill-defined renal pain or ache. Some patients complain of low backache.

### Investigation

An intravenous urogram will show hydronephrosis and usually, hydroureter down to the level of the obstruction. The anatomy of the ureter is often hard to define and a retrograde ureteropyelogram under X-ray screening may be required. It is rarely necessary to pass a ureteric catheter up to the kidney — although it is characteristic of retroperitoneal fibrosis that a ureteric catheter will pass easily through what appears to be a severe obstruction.

A markedly raised erythrocyte sedimentation rate (ESR) is commonly found in patients with idiopathic retroperitoneal fibrosis.

### Treatment

The relief of obstruction may be difficult. The ureter is dissected out of the fibrous sheet of tissue (ureterolysis) and wrapped in omentum to prevent further involvement in the fibrous process. Although obstruction due to idiopathic retroperitoneal fibrosis may regress with steroid treatment, ureterolysis and biopsy should be the

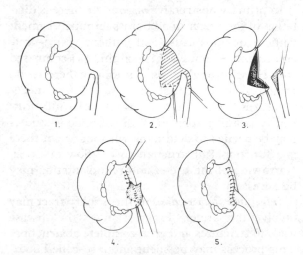

Fig. 40.6 Anderson-Hynes pyeloplasty

primary treatment and steroids reserved for any recurrence of obstruction.

## TRANSITIONAL CELL TUMOURS (See also Urothelial Tumours, p. 601.)

Though most commonly arising in the bladder, transitional cell tumours may occur in any part of the urothelium. During endoscopy, a tumour of the lower ureter may be seen protruding through the ureteric orifice. Tumours higher up the ureter may not be detected until late: a change in the intravenous urogram may not be obvious until there is a significant degree of obstruction. The tumour may bleed and the clot may cause colic and obstruction.

Although a transitional cell tumour in the upper urinary tract may appear suitable for local excision, radical excision (nephro-ureterectomy) is recommended because of the difficulties in follow-up examination of this area. Conservative surgery may be considered in the elderly and *will* be necessary for those with bilateral upper tract tumours.

## MISCELLANEOUS CONDITIONS

A variety of congenital and acquired abnormalities of the ureter and ureteric orifice may result in obstruction.

A *ureterocele* develops behind a pin hole ureteric orifice; the intra-mural part of the ureter dilates, bulges into the bladder and can become very large. Incision of the pin hole opening will relieve the obstruction.

An *ectopic ureter* occurs with a congenital duplication of one or both kidneys (duplex kidneys). Developmentally, the ureter has two main branches and if this arrangement persists the two ureters of the duplex kidneys may drain separately into the bladder (Fig. 40.7). One of the ureters will enter normally on the trigone, the ectopic ureter (from the upper renal moiety) may enter either the bladder or, more rarely, the vagina or seminal vesicle.

A ureter that is ectopic within the bladder is liable to have an ineffective valve mechanism so that urine passes *up* the ureter on voiding (vesicoureteric reflux). Reflux can occur in normally sited ureters if the normal intra-mural ureter fails to act as a valve. The pressure of refluxing urine

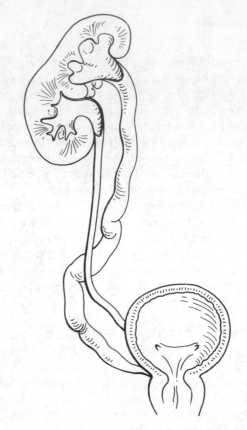

**Fig. 40.7** Duplex kidney

behaves as an intermittent obstruction which in children may lead to serious renal damage. Vesicoureteric reflux is treated by reimplantation of the ureter with the formation of an effective valve.

In primary obstructive *megaureter* there is dilatation of the ureter in all but its terminal segment without obvious cause and without vesico-ureteric reflux. Although this condition is compared with Hirschprung's disease, normally there are no ganglionic cells in the ureter so that the megaureter cannot be due to neuromuscular incoordination. Radiographic and pressure/flow studies may be needed to determine whether or not there is a functional obstruction to the flow of urine. Narrowing of the ureter and reimplantation may be necessary.

*Infections. Tuberculosis* of the urinary tract may involve the ureter. Progression of the disease leads to strictures and even complete obstruction. This process may be silent and a so-called autonephrectomy may be detected at a later date. This is now rare. *Bilharziasis* affecting the urinary tract is common in parts of Africa and in the Middle East. Ureteric fibrosis and obstruction are part of the process that can affect the whole of the urinary tract if untreated. Many patients present in such an advanced state of the disease that surgical treatment is not feasible.

Both these infections require specific drug treatment. When the ureters are involved and obstructed a variety of reconstructive surgical procedures may have to be considered to conserve renal function and to correct obstruction and/or reflux.

## RENAL CYSTS

Simple cysts of the kidney are usually single. They are almost always asymptomatic and of interest only because they are often found incidentally on an IVU. The differential diagnosis between a cyst and a renal carcinoma must then be made. Ideally, both the diagnosis and treatment of a cyst are accomplished at the same session in the Radiology Department (Table 40.1). Fluid from the cyst is examined cytologically; if there is a suspicion of tumour cells, then the cyst must be explored. Malignant change in a cyst can occur but is very rare.

Polycystic kidney disease is a congenital anomaly (dominant) that affects *both* kidneys and often leads to chronic renal failure in middle life. Despite their very large size the kidneys cause few symptoms. Infection or bleeding into a cyst can occur and may require exploration to relieve the symptoms. These kidneys may be a cause of haematuria.

## TUMOURS OF THE URINARY SYSTEM

Benign adenomas are small and usually incidental findings. Haemangiomata are rare but may cause dramatic haematuria.

Primary malignant tumours are nephroblastoma (or Wilms' tumour) in children and renal carcinoma in adults. Metastases from other tumour sites may occasionally be found in the kidney.

**Table 40.1**

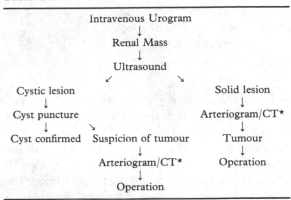

*More precise tumour staging may be obtained from computed tomography (CT); an arteriogram will give more information about renal vessels and tumour vascularity.

## NEPHROBLASTOMA

These usually occur in children under 4 years and account for 10% of all childhood malignancies.

### Pathology

The tumour is probably derived from embryonic mesodermal tissue and microscopically has a mixed appearance of spindle cells, epithelial cells and muscle fibres. The growth is rapid and there is early local spread including invasion of the renal vein. Invasion of the renal pelvis is late so that haematuria is not common. Tumours presenting in the first year of life have a better prognosis than those diagnosed later. Distant metastases most commonly appear in the lungs, liver and bones.

### Clinical features

The cardinal sign is a large abdominal mass which is often first noted when bathing the baby. Some of the unusual clinical features associated with a renal carcinoma in adults, e.g. fever or hypertension, may also be present.

### Investigations

An intravenous urogram is carried out. The main differential diagnosis is from a neuroblastoma affecting the adrenal (see p. 582) but other causes of a large kidney such as hydronephrosis and cystic disease must be considered. The tumour is bilateral in 5 to 10% of cases.

The chest is X-rayed.

### Treatment

A transabdominal nephrectomy with wide excision of the mass is carried out after preliminary ligation of the renal pedicle. This is followed by radiotherapy and chemotherapy using a combination of actinomycin-D and vincristine. As a result of this treatment, the prognosis of this tumour has improved greatly. Five-year survival rates (previously 10%) are now 80%.

## RENAL CARCINOMA

This is the most common malignant tumour of the kidney. The incidence in males is three times greater than in females, and most patients are over 40 years of age.

### Pathology

The tumour arises from renal tubules. Haemorrhage and necrosis within the tumour gives a characteristic mixed golden yellow and red appearance to the cut surface. Microscopically there are the clear and granular cell types, the former more common. There is early spread of the tumour into the renal pelvis, causing haematuria. Invasion of the renal vein often extending into the inferior vena cava also occurs early. Direct spread into perinephric tissues is common. Lymphatic spread occurs to para-aortic nodes, while blood borne metastases (which may be solitary) may develop almost anywhere in the body.

### Clinical features

The triad of pain, haematuria and a mass are important but late features. A remarkable range of systemic effects may occur early. These include fever, a raised ESR, polycythaemia, disorders of coagulation, and abnormalities of plasma proteins and liver function tests. The patient may present as a pyrexia of unknown origin (PUO) or rarely with a neuromyopathy.

Systemic effects may also be due to secretion by the tumour of such products as renin, erythro-poietin, parathormone and gonadotrophins. These abnormalities disappear when the tumour is removed but may reappear when metastases develop.

### Investigations

The investigation of a renal carcinoma is that of a 'space occupying lesion' or 'mass' in the renal parenchyma. The main differential diagnosis of such a mass is between a simple cyst and carcinoma. The sequence of investigations used is that which gives the maximum information with the least number of tests and which facilitates the diagnosis and treatment of simple renal cysts. These include ultrasonography, needle aspiration CT scan and arteriography (Table 40.1).

Additional information about the extent to which a tumour has spread into the renal vein is obtained from an inferior vena cavagram. A chest X-ray including tomograms and an isotope bone scan are performed to detect metastases.

### Treatment

A radical nephrectomy that includes the perirenal fascial envelope and ipsilateral para-aortic lymph nodes is standard treatment. Preoperative radiotherapy is of no benefit but post-operative radiotherapy may be given if the surgical excision is incomplete. Infarction of the kidney by renal artery embolisation at the time of the arteriogram can be used to reduce the vascularity of the tumour mass and assist the removal of larger tumours. There is no effective chemotherapy for this tumour, although some are believed to be hormonally sensitive.

Because of the unusual features associated with renal carcinomas, a nephrectomy should always be considered. Not only may systemic effects disappear, but there may even be regression of a solitary metastasis. Solitary metastasis tend to remain single for long periods of time and excision or radiotherapy is often worthwhile.

## UROTHELIAL TUMOURS

The urothelium is the transitional cell lining of the urinary tract that extends from the renal papilla to the external urinary meatus. Approximately 8000 new cases of tumours arise from this source each year in the United Kingdom. The incidence of these tumours is increasing, possibly due to environmental carcinogens.

There is a high incidence of urothelial cancer in workers in certain chemical, dyestuff and rubber moulding industries. This has led to the identification of carcinogens (naphthylamines and benzidine) which are now banned from industrial use. Carcinogens associated with hairdressing and leather work have also been suspected. Smoking and analgesic abuse are also associated with a higher incidence of urothelial cancer.

The vast majority of urothelial tumours occur in the bladder.

## Pathology

Almost all tumours are transitional cell carcinoma. A squamous carcinoma may occur in urothelium that has undergone metaplasia, usually due to chronic inflammation or irritation following a stone or bilharziasis. An adenocarcinoma is a rarity which occurs in a urachal remnant in the dome of the bladder.

The appearance of a transitional cell tumour ranges from a delicate papillary structure to a solid ulcerating mass. The appearance correlates well with their subsequent behaviour — papillary tumours are relatively benign while those which ulcerate are more malignant. A *biopsy* is essential:

1. To confirm the diagnosis.
2. To determine the cell differentiation (grade).
3. To determine the depth to which the tumour has penetrated the bladder wall (stage).

The TNM system of tumour classification is applied to bladder tumours. Two problems lead to difficulties in their assessment:

1. The T category, the clinical assessment of the tumour, requires a bi-manual examination under anaesthesia to judge the penetration through the bladder wall (especially for T2 and T3 tumours, see Fig. 40.8).

2. The P category, the pathological description of the precise depth of penetration by the tumour, may be impossible to determine on a specimen

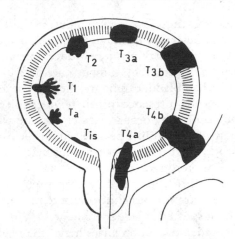

**Fig. 40.8** T categories of bladder tumour

that does not include the full thickness of the bladder wall.

In practice, the combined information on T and P categories will enable a decision on the best form of treatment.

## Clinical features

More than 80% of patients will have noted haematuria which is usually painless. It should be assumed that such bleeding is from a tumour until proved otherwise. In women, symptoms of cystitis are so common that occasional bleeding may be thought to be part of an infective problem. In men symptoms of prostatism are common and may include bleeding.

Bleeding at the end of micturition, and especially if the colour is pink/red, suggests that the site of bleeding is in the bladder; uniformly dark-coloured urine suggests that the source is in the upper tract.

A tumour at the lower end of a ureter or a bladder tumour involving the ureteric orifice may cause obstructive symptoms but usually there are few other complaints apart from discolouration of the urine. Examination is usually unhelpful. A rectal examination will detect only the far-advanced tumour.

## Investigations

The urine may show obvious blood. Cytology of the urine is not helpful in the initial assessment but can be used in the follow-up of certain patients, e.g. those exposed to industrial carcinogens. The detection of mutagens in the urine by microbiological testing is a new development.

Because upper tract tumours are much less common than bladder tumours, they can be overlooked in the presence of an obvious bladder tumour. Both may occur together and the whole of the urothelium must be assessed on the excretion urogram. If there is a suspicious defect in the ureter, a ureteropyelogram is necessary.

Cystourethroscopy and examination under anaesthesia are the basic investigative procedures for all suspected bladder tumours. With the patient under relaxation anaesthesia, the bladder and tumour are then examined bimanually to determine the depth of spread. The physical features of the tumour(s) are noted, the normal bladder mucosa is inspected and biopsies taken from the tumour and any suspicious area. For some tumours the definitive treatment may then be carried out.

### Treatment

*Upper tract tumours.* The management of these tumours is mentioned on page 598.

*Superficial bladder tumours.* Small superficial tumours (T0 and T1) are treated by endoscopic diathermy, or if larger than 2–3 mm, by transurethral resection. Provided the base is small, bulky tumours may also be resected but the urologist may prefer to open the bladder and excise the base together with at least a 1 cm margin of healthy bladder wall (partial cystectomy). A partial cystectomy is especially suitable for a tumour of this type in the upper half of the bladder. In that site transurethral resection is awkward and even unsafe.

Histological examination may show that an apparently superficial tumour has invaded superficial bladder muscle (T2). Provided the resection was complete and the tumour was well or moderately well-differentiated no further treatment is indicated. If, however, the tumour was poorly differentiated and the exact depth of invasion could not be determined, treatment should be as for an invasive tumour (see below).

Intravesical chemotherapy using Epodyl or Thiotepa is useful to treat multiple low-grade transitional cell carcinoma and to reduce the recurrence rate of low-grade superficial tumours. The drug is instilled weekly for 3 months and then the bladder is re-examined. If there has been a response, regular treatment is recommended. If there are further new tumours, they will require to be treated by extensive diathermy or even cystectomy.

*Invasive bladder tumours.* The management of an invasive (T3) tumour is much debated. The combination of a short pre-operative course of radiotherapy followed by total cystectomy is recommended for the younger (under 65 years) patient. The morbidity and mortality of such a radical procedure increases with age and some surgeons believe that a radical course of radiotherapy is a better option. Unfortunately this may not always cure the tumour and a 'salvage' cystectomy may be needed for tumour recurrence or for such symptoms as intractable bleeding.

A cystectomy will always necessitate diversion of the urine. In an ileal conduit (or ureteroileostomy) the ureters are implanted into a short segment of ileum which then opens on the abdominal wall as an ileostomy (Fig. 40.9). Alternatively, the ureters may be implanted into the sigmoid colon — ureterosigmoidostomy — but complications of renal infection and metabolic disturbances make this procedure less popular (Fig. 40.10).

An invasive T4 tumour, fixed to the pelvis or surrounding organs, is inoperable and only symptomatic palliative primary treatment can be given.

The role of chemotherapy in combination with any of these treatments is not yet known. Response rates for palliation with chemotherapy are poor.

The prognosis of bladder tumours depends on the stage and grade of the tumour. The 5-year survival rate varies from 20–30% in those with deep muscle invasion to 50–60% in mucosal tumours. Overall the 5-year survival rate is about 35%.

Invasive tumours may sometimes develop in the posterior (prostatic) urethra. These tend to be aggressive in behaviour and require aggressive combination treatment.

## CARCINOMA OF THE PROSTATE

In the UK this is the 6th most common malignancy in males, arising in 6000 new patients per

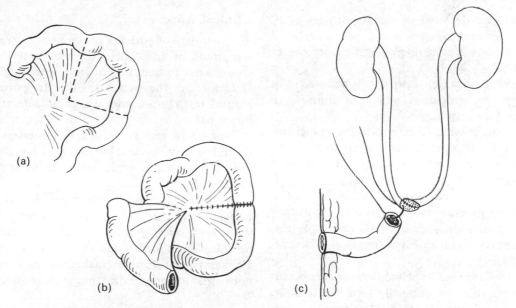

**Fig. 40.9** Ileal conduit urinary diversion. (a) & (b) Isolation of segment of ileum. (c) Uretero-ileal anastomosis.

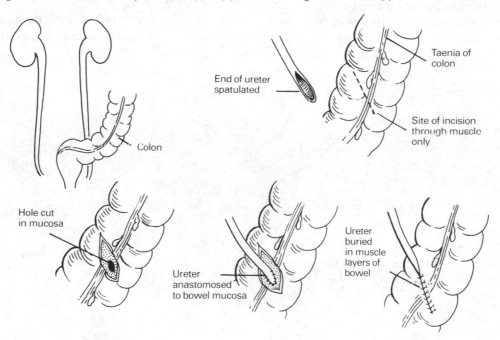

**Fig. 40.10** Ureterosigmoidostomy

annum and increasing in frequency. The tumour is common in North Europe and US (particularly in negroes) but rare in China and Japan. Rare under 50, uncommon under 60, the mean age at presentation is approximately 70 years. The aetiology is unknown but endocrine-related and possibly viral factors are implicated.

## Pathology

Almost all malignant tumours of the prostate are carcinomas. Microscopically, carcinoma of the prostate is not always easy to diagnose. This is especially true of small foci; if a prostate is examined by serial sections such a malignant focus will be detected in almost all men of 80 years of age and over.

Three degrees of biological malignancy can be recognised:

1. Clinical, in which a prostate is believed to be malignant on palpation and this diagnosis is confirmed by histology.

2. Latent, in which a tumour is found incidentally, usually in a prostatectomy specimen.

3. Occult, in which the tumour presents with metastases.

The TNM system of classification for carcinoma of the prostate is T0: a latent, incidentally diagnosed tumour; and T1–4 showing progressive degrees of involvement of the gland. These are shown in Fig. 40.11.

Metastatic spread to pelvic lymph nodes occurs early. One third of clinically localised tumours will have node involvement. Metastases to bone, principally the lumbar spine and pelvis are common; more than half of all new cases have such metastases.

## Clinical features

The majority of patients present with 'prostatic' symptoms of frequency, urgency and dysuria. One quarter present with acute retention of urine. Occasionally the tumour extends posteriorly around the rectum and causes an alteration in bowel habit.

Symptoms and signs due to metastases are much less common and include back pain, weight loss, anaemia and obstruction to the lower ends of the ureters.

On rectal examination the prostate feels nodular and stony hard. The diagnosis must never be made on clinical grounds alone; many irregular prostates even with nodules are not malignant. Conversely 10–15% of malignant prostates are not palpably abnormal on rectal examination.

## Investigation

Since most patients present with outflow tract obstruction, an intravenous urogram and serum

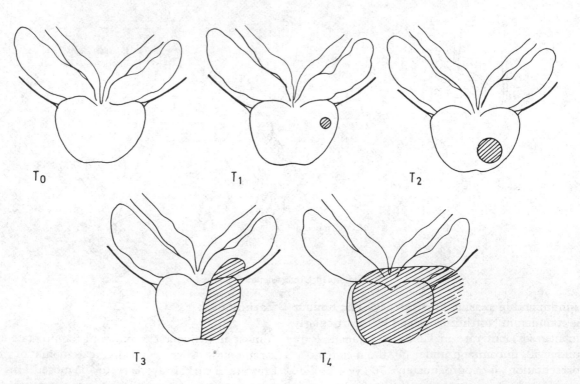

**Fig. 40.11** T categories of prostatic carcinoma ($T_0$ — microscopic; $T_1$ — intracapsular and impalpable; $T_2$ — palpable nodule within gland; $T_3$ — extending beyond capsule; $T_4$ — fixed)

creatinine are used to assess the urinary tract. An X-ray of the pelvis or lumbar spine, to investigate backache, may show ostcosclerotic metastases as the first evidence of a prostatic malignancy.

Whenever possible, the diagnosis should be confirmed either by a needle biopsy of a suspicious part of the prostate or by histological examination of tissue removed by endoscopic resection should this be necessary to relieve outflow tract obstruction.

The patient is assessed for metastases (M category) by measuring the serum acid phosphatase and by a skeletal survey by X-ray or radioisotope bone scan. Serum acid phosphatase is a useful marker of tumour metastases though normal values do not rule out spread of the tumour. Its main use is as a monitor of response to treatment and progress of the disease. A bone scan is more sensitive in detecting metastases than X-rays or acid phosphatase and is a useful monitor of the progress of this disease.

Lymphography is practised by some, but is inaccurate and therefore unnecessary. A staging pelvic lymph node dissection is also unnecessary because the usual treatment recommended in the United Kingdom would not be influenced by the information gained.

## Treatment

Prostatic cancer, like that of the breast, is sensitive to endocrine influences. In 1941 Charles Huggins, Professor of Urology in the University of Chicago, concluded from a series of experimental studies that since the growth of all types of prostatic cells could be inhibited by oestrogens or castration and stimulated by androgens, then the malignant prostate might also respond to endocrine manipulation. This concept led to the first successful treatment of this tumour.

The management is best considered in four clinical groups:

*1. Incidental or focal cancer.* Such a patient will have had a prostatectomy. The diagnosis will have been made incidentally on histological examination of the prostatic tissue. A patient with a focus of well differentiated carcinoma who has no evidence of bone metastases, has a normal life expectancy. Since these men have no other symptoms and no other evidence of tumour, they should only be watched. If the focus was undifferentiated, treatment by radiotherapy should be considered. Such tumours can recur and progress to a more advanced stage of clinical cancer.

*2. Localised prostatic cancer; no evidence of bone metastases.* Radiotherapy is recommended; endocrine treatment should be kept in reserve until there is evidence of progression of the tumour. A radical excision of the prostate is practised in some parts of the world but not in the United Kingdom.

*3. Metastatic prostatic cancer.* These form the largest number of patients. They should be treated either by orchiectomy or by oestrogens (stilboestrol 1 mg tds). Oestrogens should not be given to a patient with cardiovascular disease since salt-retention may precipitate further cardiovascular problems including hypertension and cerebro-vascular bleeding.

*4. Secondary treatment.* A small proportion of patients fail to respond to endocrine treatment. A larger number of patients respond for a year or two, but then the disease progresses. Other oestrogens, or progesterones, are of limited value but chemotherapy with 5-fluorouracil, cyclophosphamide or nitrogen mustard may be effective. Radiotherapy will relieve localised bone pain. For severe generalised bone pain, a hypophysectomy can be effective palliative treatment.

## Prognosis

The prognosis of a patient with an incidental finding of carcinoma of the prostate (focal) is that of the normal population. With tumours localised to the prostate a 10 year survival rate of 40–50% can be expected but if metastases are present this falls to 10%. Only 50% of such patients will survive 3 years. The overall 5 year survival rate of all patients with carcinoma of the prostate approximates 25%.

## TESTICULAR TUMOURS

Tumours of the testis, although uncommon, occur mainly in younger men between the age of 20 and 40 years. In the United Kingdom there are about 500 new cases per annum. These tumours have two particular features: 1. They secrete 'tumour markers' which provide good indices for both diagnosis and prognosis. 2. The prognosis in the non-seminomatous tumours has been dramatically improved by recent advances in chemotherapy.

## Pathology

There are two main cell types — seminoma and teratoma. These account for 85% of all tumours of the testis. Malignant lymphoma, yolk-sac tumours, interstitial cell tumours and Sertoli cell/mesenchyme tumours comprise the remainder.

*Seminoma.* This tumour arises from seminiferous tubules and is of relatively low grade malignancy. The cut surface has a uniformly grey appearance. Microscopically, the cell type varies from well differentiated spermatocytes to undifferentiated round cells. Metastases occur mainly via the lymphatics and may spread to the lungs.

*Teratoma (Non-seminomatous tumours).* This tumour arises from primitive germinal cells. The tumour may contain cartilage, bone, muscle, fat and a variety of other tissues and is classified according to the degree of differentiation. Well differentiated tumours are the least aggressive. A trophoblastic teratoma represents the other extreme and is highly malignant. Most teratomas have an in-between pattern. Occasionally, both teratoma and seminoma occur in the same testis.

## Clinical features

The history is often vague. The patient may blame an injury or there may be pain and swelling suggestive of inflammation. In this event the patient may wrongly have received treatment for 'acute epididymitis'. Very rarely, a patient may complain of gynaecomastia (usually associated with a teratoma).

Irrespective of the history, any new, painless testicular lump in a young man (20–40 years) must always be regarded with suspicion. A hydrocele in a young man demands early exploration. A testicular tumour may be accompanied by a blood-stained effusion in the tunica vaginalis.

The peak age for a teratoma is 20–30 years and

for a seminoma 30–40 years: however, either may occur at any time from childhood to old age.

## Investigations

Immediately a tumour is suspected, and before orchiectomy, blood should be examined for $\alpha$-feto protein and the $\beta$-subunit of HCG. The levels of these classic 'tumour markers' are increased should the disease be extensive.

Accurate staging of the tumour requires detailed investigations that include lymphography and intravenous urography, CT scans of lungs, liver and retroperitoneal area, and an assessment of the renal function and pulmonary function.

Staging classification (Royal Marsden Hospital):

  I Lymphogram negative, no evidence of metastases
 II Lymphogram positive, metastases confined to abdominal nodes
III Involvement of supra and infra diaphragmatic lymph nodes. No extra lymphatic involvement.
IV Extra lymphatic involvement

## Treatment

Through an inguinal incision the cord is ligated and divided at the internal ring and the testis removed. Subsequent treatment depends on the histological report. Radiation to regional nodes (paravertebral) remains the treatment of choice for a seminoma since this tumour is very radiosensitive.

The management of a teratoma is more debatable because of the wide histological variations. Traditionally X-ray therapy was advised but the use of combination chemotherapy (vincristine, actinomycin-D, bleomycin plus cisplatinum) has now greatly improved the prognosis and has indicated the need to evaluate the exact place of radiotherapy and also of retroperitoneal lymph node dissection as part of management.

The tumour markers, $\alpha$ feto protein and beta HCG are most valuable in monitoring the response to treatment and in detecting recurrent disease. Both markers should be measured at regular intervals in all patients with testicular tumours for at least 2 years after they are considered to be tumour free.

Computerised tomography, in addition to being useful for staging the tumour, can be used to follow the response of enlarged lymph nodes to treatment.

### Prognosis

The 5-year survival rate for seminoma is 90–95%. That for teratomas is more variable and depends on tumour type, stage and volume. More favourable tumours may have a 95% 5-year survival rate but in more advanced cases 60–70% is more usual.

## CARCINOMA OF THE PENIS

This unusual tumour is generally attributed to poor hygiene associated with a non-retractible foreskin; it is very rarely recorded in a circumcised man. It occurs only in the elderly.

### Pathology

The tumour may be either a papillary or an ulcerating squamous cell carcinoma. Local spread is early and it may ulcerate and fungate. Lymphatic spread to inguinal lymph nodes is common but infection of the tumour may also lead to inguinal node enlargement.

### Clinical features

The patient may present with either a purulent or blood-stained discharge. Unfortunately a more advanced ulcerating lesion is common and some may present only when much of the penis is destroyed and the inguinal lymph nodes are involved.

### Investigations

The diagnosis must be confirmed by biopsy.

### Treatment

Early tumours respond dramatically to bleomycin. An initial circumcision is required to keep the tumour area clean and treat any infection. Advanced tumours require partial amputation and bilateral bloc dissection of the inguinal lymph nodes. Inoperable tumours are treated by palliative radiotherapy.

---

## TRAUMA

---

### KIDNEY AND RENAL PEDICLE

#### Aetiology and pathology

*Open injuries*. The kidney and renal pedicle may be injured by either a gun-shot wound or by stabbing. A percutaneous needle biopsy of the renal parenchyma can, inadvertently, cause severe bleeding and rarely an arteriovenous fistula. Open lacerations of the parenchyma, collecting system or pedicle are usually associated with other injuries within the abdomen.

*Closed injuries*. These are of two types:

1. *Direct blunt injury* as when a child slips and falls against the edge of the bath or, as in sports injuries, where there is a blow or kick in the loin. These injuries are commonly associated with fractured ribs and, on the right side, an injury to the liver.

2. *Major trauma* such as in aircraft or road accidents in which there is deceleration. The pedicle is injured rather than the kidney. Deceleration injuries to the pedicle may cause intimal tears, spasm or thrombosis of the vessels.

The late effects of renal trauma include a perirenal collection of urine (urinoma), scarring of the kidney or renal artery stenosis (hypertension). Hydronephrosis may be an early or late complication.

#### Clinical features

While a gunshot wound is obvious, a penetrating wound from a knife may appear trivial even should it involve several important deep structures.

Commonly, a child or young person presents with a history of injury (sometimes trivial) to the loin, followed by haematuria. Usually, the worse the haematuria, the worse the renal damage.

Thus, a bruise or contusion of the kidney causes mild haematuria, a laceration causes moderate haematuria, while a fragmented kidney causes gross haematuria. A mass in the loin which is increasing in size is characteristic of severe injuries.

In severe injuries there will also be signs of shock (tachycardia, low blood pressure, pallor and sweating). These patients may have injuries to other organs.

Damage to the renal pedicle may cause few signs or the patient may be severely shocked.

## Investigations

An intravenous urogram is urgently performed to determine the extent of renal damage. A shocked patient must be resuscitated but urographic information about the other kidney must always precede emergency surgery.

In a mild contusion the urogram may be normal. With increasing damage there is distortion of the renal outline, calices and extravasation of contrast. Non-visualisation of the kidney implies serious damage, especially to the pedicle, and is an indication for angiography.

Angiography is also helpful in assessing parenchymal/vascular damage in those cases where surgical exploration is considered; it is not necessary in a patient who needs urgent exploration.

A DMSA renal scan and ultrasound are of more help in the follow-up of an injured kidney than in its immediate care.

## Treatment

A contusion of the kidney is managed conservatively by bed rest and observation.

A laceration, if part of an open injury, needs exploring to determine the overall extent of the damage. Lacerations from a closed injury may be treated conservatively at first, but should the haematuria persist or the loin swelling increase, exploration is carried out. Severe lacerations with fragmentation of the kidney should be explored.

The extent of the operation depends on the severity of the laceration. Whenever possible a partial nephrectomy is preferable.

## URETER

### Aetiology and pathology

*Open injuries.* Rarely, a ureter may be damaged by a knife or a bullet. This is always associated with other injuries.

The principal cause of injury to a ureter is an operation involving the colon, rectum, bladder, major abdominal blood vessels and, most commonly of all, the uterus. The anatomical relationship of the ureter to these organs makes it inevitable that it can be affected by direct spread of a variety of pathological conditions. Surgical damage may lead to complete or partial obstruction with subsequent hydronephrosis, or to a urinary fistula. A fistula may occur either immediately, if damage to continuity is not recognised at operation, or later, if the injury to the ureter is one which causes later necrosis. The urine may leak to the skin (cutaneous fistula), form a 'urinoma' or after a gynaecological operation leak through the vagina (uretero-vaginal fistula).

*Closed injuries.* The ureter is occasionally involved in major accidents of 'run-over' type.

### Clinical features

The patient may complain of renal pain after an operation. However, even a completely obstructed kidney may cause few symptoms. If there is infection in the obstructed kidney then the patient may be extremely ill with pain, fever and rigors.

Any excessive 'watery' discharge from a wound is suspicious. A urinary fistula may cause little or no symptomatic upset but if infection is added the patient may become extremely ill.

### Investigations

A rapid way to determine whether a watery discharge is urine or serum is to measure the concentration of urea in the fluid. Alternatively, intravenous methylene blue will quickly appear in a urinary leak. An intravenous urogram will show the side of the damage. Whether the ureter is cut or injured, there is always some hold-up in the contrast on the affected side. This differs from the urogram in a patient with a *vesico-vaginal* fistula where the upper tract is usually normal.

If there is still uncertainty as to whether a vaginal leak is from ureter or bladder discolouration of a vaginal swab after the intravesical instillation of methylene blue will confirm that the leak is from the bladder.

Occasionally, cystoscopy and ureteric catheterisation are indicated.

## Treatment

Early exploration of the wound is advised to avoid the risks of infection. Provided it is of sufficient length, a damaged lower ureter may be reimplanted directly into the bladder. If the ureter is short, then the gap may be bridged by a tube of bladder (Boari flap) (Fig. 40.12) or simply by drawing up the bladder and fixing it to the psoas muscle (psoas hitch).

If the ureter is too short for these procedures, it may be joined to the other ureter (uretero-ureterostomy). However, if there is infection, or the patient has a limited prognosis from the primary disease, it may be best to remove the kidney or to embolise the renal artery.

## BLADDER

### Aetiology and pathology

*Open injuries*. Penetrating injuries to the bladder can occur when a person falls and is impaled on a fence. Then, bladder, urethra and rectum are all likely to be damaged. The bladder may be injured in the course of extensive cancer operations in the pelvis. Occasionally a large inguinal or femoral hernia may include bladder in the medial wall of the sac, and this may be damaged during repair of the hernia. Unrecognised injuries during surgical procedures may lead to a wound fistula, a vesico-vaginal fistula or a vesico-colic fistula.

Fistulae may also occur as a result of inflammatory or neoplastic bowel disease.

*Closed injuries*. Two types of closed bladder injury may occur. Two different mechanisms are involved.

1. *Intraperitoneal*: Typically, the person has been drinking alcohol, has a full bladder and is assaulted and kicked in the abdomen. The dome of the bladder ruptures and urine extravasates into the peritoneum (Fig. 40.13a). There is intestinal ileus and abdominal distension.

2. *Extraperitoneal*: Usually, this rupture is due to a major road traffic accident in which the pelvis is fractured (Fig. 40.13b).

An extraperitoneal leak in the bladder may also occur in the course of resecting the prostate or a bladder tumour. Should this occur the urine creates a local inflammatory reaction such that the small bowel may become adherent to the pelvic peritoneum. This is dangerous should the patient later require pelvic irradiation.

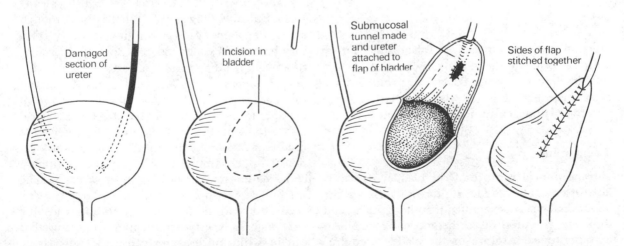

**Fig. 40.12** Boari flap

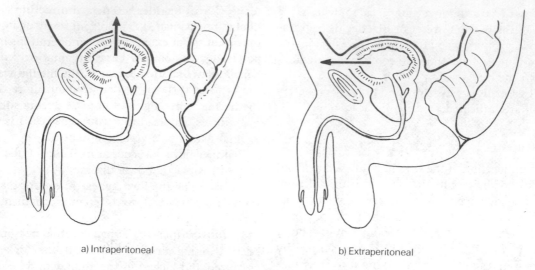

a) Intraperitoneal  b) Extraperitoneal

**Fig. 40.13** Rupture of the bladder

## Clinical features

The ileus and distension that occur with intraperitoneal rupture of the bladder are often detected late because of the circumstances surrounding the injury. However, the patient will soon note that he is anuric and seek advice.

Extraperitoneal extravasation of urine, if part of a major accident, will only add to what already are severe pelvic symptoms. When the leak occurs during an endoscopic procedure the patient will later complain of suprapubic pain with varying degrees of lower abdominal tenderness.

## Investigations

Generally, the circumstances of the bladder injury will establish the diagnosis. If confirmation of a bladder injury is required, a water soluble contrast material is injected via a urethral catheter and the bladder examined on the X-ray screen.

## Treatment

Intraperitoneal rupture of the bladder demands laparotomy. The bladder rupture is oversewn, the abdominal viscera examined for other injuries and drainage by urethral catheter established. An extraperitoneal rupture of the bladder requires surgical exploration to remove blood and serum, to correct bony injuries, to close the tear in the bladder and to establish bladder drainage.

If urine has extravasated during any pelvic operation, a urethral catheter to keep the bladder empty is usually all that is necessary. Very rarely a suprapubic drain may be required.

## URETHRA

### Aetiology and pathology

*Open injuries.* A penetrating injury may rarely involve either the anterior or posterior urethra.

*Closed injuries.* 1. *Anterior urethra*: Typically this is due to 'falling astride' a hard object though a well aimed boot can cause a similar injury. This may be either a contusion or laceration. A laceration may be either partial or complete.

2. *Posterior urethra*: The mechanism of injury to this part of the urethra is similar to that for an extraperitoneal rupture of the bladder, e.g. road traffic accident. For such an injury to damage the urethra, a fracture of the pubis or fracture-dislocation of the pelvis must occur. Both posterior urethra and bladder are damaged in 10% of cases. The urethral rupture may be either partial or complete.

An injury to the posterior urethra may also be iatrogenic. Inexpert instrumentation of the urethra can tear the mucosa and cause a false passage and subsequent stricture formation.

## Clinical features

Anterior urethral injuries are usually located at the bulb of the urethra so that the patient presents with a haematoma of the perineum. Should this haematoma become infected, there may be sloughing of the skin, urethra and even scrotal tissues.

Because of the mechanism of injury, the patients with posterior urethral tears are usually shocked and require resuscitation before a detailed assessment of the pelvic injuries can be made. If the patient has passed clear urine the bladder and urethra are probably intact. If there is blood at the external meatus a urethral injury must be suspected. A distended bladder can occur either because of spasm of the urethral sphincter or because of a torn posterior urethra.

## Investigations

If the physical signs suggest an *anterior urethral* injury and the patient has passed clear urine, no further steps need be taken. If there is blood at the external meatus or the urine is blood-stained, a urethrogram using a water soluble contrast material may demonstrate the extravasation.

There is a strongly held view that any investigative procedure of the posterior urethra is dangerous and may worsen the urethral injury. A catheter should never be passed in the Emergency Room — 'just to see'.

If the patient should pass clear urine then nothing further should be done. If however the urine is blood stained, a retrograde urethrogram may be carried out. The radiological distinction between an extraperitoneal bladder rupture and a rupture of the membranous urethra may be difficult. Catheterisation for these injuries is best carried out at the time of other surgical procedures with full aseptic precautions.

## Treatment

The patient with an injury to the bulb of the urethra will have a perineal haematoma. This will resolve if the urethral injury is only a contusion. As there is always the risk of infection prophylactic antibiotics are indicated.

A large haematoma may need to be drained. If this is necessary, the urethra is likely to be lacerated. The extent of injury should be examined and the urethra repaired if possible. The bladder is drained either by a urethral or by suprapubic catheter.

The treatment of a posterior urethral injury will depend on the expertise available. It is quite acceptable to perform a suprapubic cystostomy and deal with the injury to the urethra at a later date. If, however, a laparotomy is necessary for other reasons, this may also give an opportunity to pass a catheter. If the rupture is incomplete, the catheter will act as a splint. If the rupture is complete, the ends of the urethra can be approximated and splinted by the catheter.

The late complication of these injuries is stricture.

# SURGERY FOR OTHER ASPECTS OF EXTERNAL GENITALIA

## PENIS

### Circumcision

The foreskin is normally non-retractile in the first few months of life. By the end of the first year 50% will retract; but it may be 3–4 years before all will do so. Provided that the parents are reassured of these facts, there is no reason, *apart from religious grounds*, to remove the foreskin within the first few years of life.

In some children the foreskin remains non-retractile beyond these limits and this should be treated by circumcision. Otherwise, secretions may collect under the foreskin, leading to infection (balanitis) and narrowing of the orifice (phimosis). In those whose foreskin may retract, but not easily, pain during intercourse may be a problem in later years. If there are difficulties in keeping the glans and coronal sulcus clean, accumulated secretions may predispose to carcinoma of the penis.

Urologists are familiar with the problem of a non-retractile foreskin should the patient later need a cystoscopy or urethral catheterisation.

If a poorly retracting foreskin should remain

retracted it can act as a tight band and cause engorgement and oedema of the glans (paraphimosis. Management is urgent: it may be possible to compress the glans and draw the foreskin forwards but, should this fail, the tight band must be incised under general anaesthesia. Later elective circumcision is advocated.

## Congenital abnormalities

*Hypospadias.* Failure of fusion of embryonic folds results in abnormal placing of the external urinary meatus along the ventral surface of the penis. The opening may be coronal, penile, scrotal or even perineal. With these latter sites the corpus spongiosum is scarred and fibrosed leading to a ventral curvature or *chordee* of the penis.

Treatment is to correct the chordee by excising the fibrosis and then to perform one of several available plastic surgical techniques to make a new urethral opening in the normal position on the glans. These procedures should be completed before the boy goes to school.

*Epispadias.* In this condition, the external urinary meatus opens on the dorsal surface of the penis. The extent of the abnormality varies from a penile abnormality to a gross failure in development of the bladder and urethra. Severe deformity is due to extension of the cloacal membrane onto the lower abdominal wall preventing the two halves of the wall from closing over the developing bladder. As a result, the mucosa of the whole bladder and the ureteric orifices are exposed and form the infra-umbilical part of the abdominal wall (exstrophy). The urethra lies opened out and the testes are undescended; additional abnormalities include separation of the symphysis pubis and rectal prolapse.

Reconstruction of these deformities is not always successful and urinary incontinence may remain a major problem and require treatment by a urinary diversion.

## Disorders of erection

*Priapism.* In this uncommon condition there is a maintained erection, unassociated with sexual desire. It occurs in association with leukaemia, disorders of coagulation, renal dialysis and sickle-cell trait and is believed due to sludging of venous blood in the sinuses of the corpora cavernosa. Thus the painful erection affects the corpora cavernosa but not the corpus spongiosum or glans.

A variety of non-operative methods to relieve the congestion, e.g. spinal anaesthesia or heparinisation have been tried but all fail. Aspiration of the thickened blood is also ineffective.

Operative treatment by a venous shunt (e.g. saphenous vein to corpus cavernosum or corpora cavernosa to corpus spongiosum), when carried out within 6–12 hours, gives satisfactory results and the patient can achieve normal erections subsequently.

If treatment is delayed or incomplete, the erectile tissue is damaged and the patient will be impotent.

*Peyronie's disease.* This is the occurrence of a hard fibrous plaque (or plaques) in the wall of a corpus cavernosum causing a lateral curvature of the penis. The cause is obscure but is probably related to trauma leading to hard scar tissue formation in a corpus cavernosum. In addition to the deformity the patient complains of pain during intercourse.

Various treatments including cortisone injections, vitamins and radiotherapy have been tried for this condition, but without much success. Excision of the plaque with replacement by a dermal patch graft or excision of a wedge of tissue on the convex (opposite) border of the penis may prove effective. It is suggested that the condition will eventually improve without treatment but reliable data are scarce.

## Impotence

Impotence may be psychogenic, organic or drug-induced. Although *loss of libido* may be due to a generalised illness or endocrine disease, the majority of patients who complain of *impotence* have a psychosexual disturbance which may require psychosexual therapy.

1. *Psychogenic* causes can be established from a careful history that includes details of sexual habits. However, it is always important to exclude organic causes so that the correct advice may be given to the patient.

2. *Organic* impotence may occur with diabetes

mellitus, neurogenic disorders, after major pelvic injury or operations (e.g. total cystectomy), vascular disease of the pelvic vessels (e.g. Leriche syndrome), priapism and Peyronie's disease. Most of these conditions cause irreversible impotence, but angiography may help to define a treatable abnormality of the arterial supply to the penis.

There is no drug treatment, and the only treatment in selected cases is to implant a pair of inflatable silicone rods into the corpora cavernosa to allow successful intercourse.

3. *Drug induced* impotence occurs in patients receiving oestrogen treatment for prostatic cancer. In addition, a range of anti-hypertensive drugs may cause loss of erection or inability to ejaculate. Drugs such as barbiturates, benzodiazepams, corticosteroids, phenothiazines and spironolactone may all affect libido.

## SCROTUM

Examination of the scrotal contents should follow a simple routine. With the patient supine, the configuration of the scrotum and the scrotal wall is first observed. The contents of the scrotum are then palpated between the thumb and index and middle fingers. In sequence the testes, head, body and tail of the epididymis, the cord and the external inguinal ring are checked. With the patient standing and the doctor seated, examination of the contents is repeated, specifically excluding an inguinal hernia and a varicocele (see below).

### Undescended testes (cryptorchidism)

Normally both testes should be in the scrotum within 6 months of birth. However, the testes may be excessively mobile and readily retract towards the external inguinal ring or into the inguinal canal, especially when the patient is examined in a cold room. Such *retractile* testes may easily be misdiagnosed as being incompletely descended. Care must be taken to examine the baby in a warm room or after a bath.

Undescended testes are of two types: incompletely descended and ectopic.

1. *Incomplete descent of the testis.* Such a testis is arrested in its *normal* pathway to the scrotum. Usually this is within the inguinal canal, more rarely within the abdomen. The testis is smaller than normal and cannot be palpated. Its ability to produce sperms is doubtful.

As the spermatic cord is short, such testes are difficult to bring down into the scrotum by operation (orchiopexy). If this can be carried out before the age of 6 years the testis may be of some use; otherwise it should be removed.

On occasions an incompletely descended testis is situated just inside the external inguinal ring through which it can be coaxed (*emergent testis*). If the child is approaching puberty when this diagnosis is made, a 5-day course of human chorionic gonadotrophin may encourage enlargement and descent.

Testes that remain incompletely descended have a one in 40 chance of becoming malignant; the risk is doubled if the testis is retained in the abdomen.

2. *Ectopic testis.* It is important to distinguish an ectopic from an incompletely descended testis. An ectopic testis has developed normally but after passing through the external inguinal ring its further descent is impeded. Either it remains in the superficial inguinal pouch (common) or is transposed to perineal, femoral or pre-pubic sites (rare).

Because an ectopic testis is normal in size, it is palpable and its cord is normal. Operative placement in the scrotum (orchiopexy) is achieved without difficulty.

Provided orchiopexy is done at an early age, preferably before 6 years, spermatogenesis is believed to occur normally. However, even if the diagnosis is not made until later (frequently this is just before puberty), orchiopexy should still be performed. The use of gonadotrophins to treat ectopic testes is illogical.

*Orchiopexy.* The operation of orchiopexy consists of mobilising the testis and its cord and placing the testis in the scrotum. Various methods are used to stop the testis from retracting back towards the inguinal canal. The simplest is to place the testis in a pouch between the dartos muscle and scrotal skin (Fig. 40.14).

As indicated above, mobilisation of an ectopic testis and placement in a dartos pouch is easy.

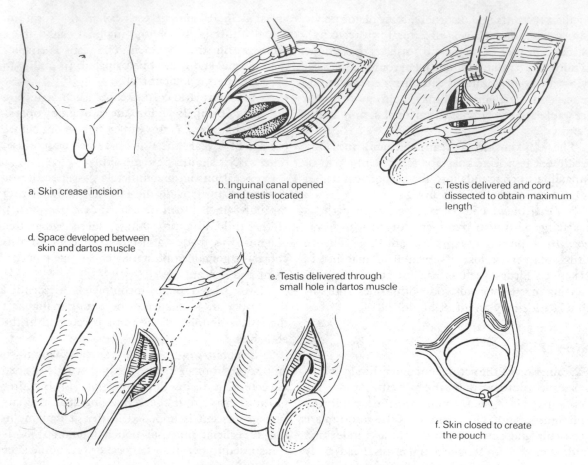

a. Skin crease incision

b. Inguinal canal opened and testis located

c. Testis delivered and cord dissected to obtain maximum length

d. Space developed between skin and dartos muscle

e. Testis delivered through small hole in dartos muscle

f. Skin closed to create the pouch

**Fig. 40.14** Dartos pouch fixation of testis

Because of the shorter cord, an incompletely descended testis can be brought into the scrotum only with difficulty and various manoeuvres may be necessary to gain length.

### Torsion of the testis

Torsion of the testis is due to an abnormality of the visceral layer of the tunica vaginalis which completely covers the testis so that it is suspended within the parietal layer and can twist the cord. Torsion is a surgical emergency. Delay in diagnosis or treatment may lead to loss of the testis.

The characteristic history is of a teenager who suddenly develops an acutely tender, swollen testis. There may be a history of minor trauma or of previous episodes of pain in the testis due to partial torsion. On examination there is a red, swollen hemiscrotum which is usually too tender to palpate. Misdiagnosis of the swelling as an epididymo-orchitis, which is rare in teenagers, is a serious error.

The scrotum must be explored as soon as possible so that the twist can be reversed and the blood supply restored. If this is not done within 12–18 hours, the testis infarcts and must be excised. If the testis is viable it is fixed, e.g. by creating a dartos pouch. Since the underlying abnormality of the tunica is bilateral, the other testis must be fixed to its parietal tunica vaginalis *at the same time*. Otherwise, torsion may occur later on that side. This could be disastrous for the fertility of the patient.

### Hydrocele

The collection of fluid in the tunica vaginalis resulting in an enlarged but painless scrotum is a common condition, especially in older men. The inconvenience of its size usually leads the patient to seek advice.

The cause of most hydroceles is unknown (idiopathic). The fluid is straw-coloured and rich in protein. In some it develops as a reaction to epididymo-orchitis and rarely, but more sinister, it may develop with a malignant testis (secondary hydrocele). Then the fluid may be blood-stained.

On examination of the scrotum there is a smooth oval swelling above which a normal spermatic cord can be palpated. The fluid around the testis transilluminates when a torch is held against the scrotum but in long-standing hydroceles this may be difficult to elicit owing to fibrosis and thickening of its wall. It is important always to seek this physical sign and also to examine carefully the neck of the scrotum to exclude an inguinal hernia as the cause of the swelling.

It may be possible to palpate the testis and confirm that it is normal, but this is unusual as it lies behind and is enveloped by the hydrocele. If there is doubt about an associated pathology, the fluid should be aspirated by needle and syringe and the testis re-examined. If there is still doubt, immediate exploration is indicated to exclude a testicular tumour.

Injury to the scrotum may result in a swelling that resembles a hydrocele but does not transilluminate because the tunica has filled with blood (*haematocele*).

Aspiration alone does not cure an idiopathic hydrocele and the tunica soon refills with fluid. It is possible to obliterate the sac by injecting a sclerosant after aspiration but, preferably, it should be excised, or everted so that recurrence is prevented.

Should the hydrocele fluid become infected, incision and drainage of the pus are necessary. Similarly, a haematocele may require treatment by incision and drainage.

## Cyst of the epididymis

Cysts in the epididymis arise from diverticula of the vasa efferentia. The distinction between a cyst(s) of the epididymis and hydrocele is easy. Epididymal cysts are almost always multiple and therefore nodular on palpation; they are located above and behind the testis which is palpably separate from the cysts and they always transilluminate brightly.

A solitary epididymal cyst may even resemble a testis, so giving rise to fables of three testes.

Sometimes the fluid within an epididymal cyst is opalescent and contains sperms — a *spermatocele*. Usually the fluid is clear.

It is better to leave these cysts alone unless increasing size warrants excision. This operation requires careful dissection to remove the cyst completely. Often several other little cysts are present which, if not removed, will eventually increase in size and produce a so-called recurrence. If all the cysts are removed, the pathway for sperms will almost certainly be damaged. A bilateral operation could result in sterility.

## Varicocele

The veins of the pampiniform plexus are dilated and tortuous producing a swelling in the line of the spermatic cord resembling a 'bag of worms'. It is more common on the left side because of the right-angled drainage of the testicular vein into the renal vein, which renders it more liable to stasis. In some men, varicocele is associated with infertility. A dragging sensation in the scrotum may cause concern.

Treatment by scrotal support is now not advised. The spermatic vein can be ligated at the internal inguinal ring or embolised through a venous cannula inserted by femoral or jugular routes.

## Epididymo-orchitis

Acute epididymo-orchitis is the preferred term to describe either acute orchitis or acute epididymitis, for both testis and epididymis are involved in an acute inflammatory reaction. Further, the spermatic cord is often thickened (funiculitis). After an infection has subsided, the epididymis alone may remain thickened and irregular, so that chronic epididymitis may be diagnosed. Thus a late effect of tuberculosis is an irregularly hard (craggy) epididymis.

Apparent involvement of the testis alone may be a feature of viral infections such as mumps orchitis. Late syphilis results in a gumma of the testis, but this is now seen only in museum specimens.

The usual cause of epididymo-orchitis is bacterial, either from an infected urine or gonococcal urethritis. The affected side of the scrotum is swollen, inflamed and very tender. In all cases the urine or urethral discharge must be cultured. Sometimes there is no evidence of an infective cause and a viral aetiology may be suspected.

Treatment is by an antibiotic selected by the result of culture of the organism, bed rest and a scrotal support. If there is any doubt about the diagnosis, the testis should be explored.

Abscess formation is now rare but should signs of localisation or fluctuation develop, the pus should be drained. An important late complication of epididymo-orchitis is infertility.

## INFERTILITY

The investigation and management of an infertile marriage requires the assessment of both partners, but only aspects of male infertility will be discussed here. While more patients are now being referred for investigation, the management of infertility is still very limited in its success. Often it consists only of clarifying the diagnosis and appropriate counselling.

A detailed history is essential, particularly enquiring into factors that may contribute to an abnormal sperm count. These include previous operations (e.g. hernia), illness (e.g. mumps, tuberculosis), bacterial infection (e.g. gonococcal), certain drugs (nitrofurazone, cyclophosphamides and possibly some tranquillisers). Excessive smoking, alcohol intake, obesity and working in a hot environment may all suppress spermatogenesis. Enquiry of psychosexual problems including impotence or premature ejaculation, should also be made.

Physical examination may be entirely normal. Body build and hair distribution are noted. Testicular size is a crude but useful guide to spermatogenic potential. Thus a tall male with female hair distribution and pea-sized testes almost certainly has Klinefelter's syndrome. Examination of the scrotum may reveal dilated spermatic veins (varicocele).

The principal investigation in the male is an analysis of the seminal fluid. The values given as 'normal' are only a guide, for undoubtedly pregnancy can occur with low sperm concentrations (oligozoospermia). However, the lower the concentration of sperms the less the chance of pregnancy.

If a patient has no sperm (azoospermia) it is necessary to distinguish between obstruction and primary spermatogenic failure. This may be possible by measuring plasma FSH. A normal value indicates obstruction which is usually in the epididymis. In these patients the testes are also normal in size. More detailed tests such as immunological compatibility and chromosome analysis may be necessary but these require special facilities.

## Management

There is no treatment for a patient with azoospermia due to primary spermatogenic failure. A testicular biopsy to confirm the diagnosis is all that can be done.

Azoospermia due to obstruction may be treated by a bypass anastomosis (epididymovasostomy). This may be successful if the obstruction is in the tail of the epididymis but if it is elsewhere in the epididymis or in the vasa efferentia, the results are very poor.

The initial treatment of a patient with oligozoospermia is to reduce weight, improve dietary and smoking habits and adjust occupation. It is always helpful to ensure that the patient has an understanding of the basis of reproductive biology and especially the timing of intercourse in relation to the menstrual cycle. These measures alone often lead to a successful pregnancy.

The role of a varicocele as a cause of infertility is debatable. There is evidence that some varicoceles affect testicular temperature and therefore spermatogenesis and ligation of these veins is widely practised to avoid this effect. Most series have shown overall improvement in semen analysis following the ligation, but such studies are uncontrolled.

Drug treatment for oligozoospermia is disappointing: clinical trials are in progress but no one treatment can at present be recommended. As a result various worthless drugs continue to be prescribed.

## VASECTOMY AND VASECTOMY REVERSAL

Bilateral ligation of the vasa deferentia, in the neck of the scrotum, is now widely practised as a form of permanent contraception. The procedure is usually done as an out-patient, using local anaesthesia. Each vas is ligated, divided and the ends separated in order to avoid recanalisation.

It is essential that the post-operative semen analysis be checked at 6–8 weeks to confirm azoospermia. Three negative tests are required for assurance that fertilization cannot occur.

Reversal of vasectomy may be requested, usually because of remarriage. Reported pregnancy rates vary from 50–80% following this microsurgical procedure.

---

## SURGERY FOR DISORDERS OF CONTROL OF MICTURITION

### ANATOMY OF THE OUTFLOW TRACT

The *fundus* of the bladder consists of interlacing bundles of smooth muscle, the detrusor, which do not lie in defined layers. They are attached to the deep muscle layer of the trigone. During the storage phase of micturition the detrusor stretches to accommodate the increased volume of urine but without an increase in intravesical pressure (compliance).

The *trigone* forms the base to the bladder and includes both ureteric orifices and the internal urethral orifice. It has two muscle layers: 1. the superficial trigonal muscle which merges with the ureteric muscle and extends down into the proximal urethra and 2. the deep trigonal muscle to which is attached the detrusor muscle.

The *proximal urethral mechanism* (internal meatus) consists of a loop of the detrusor, the superficial trigonal muscle and, in the male, a circular smooth muscle — the pre-prostatic sphincter. This sphincter is richly supplied with sympathetic nerves and closes tightly with ejaculation.

The *distal urethral mechanism* (external sphincter) consists of the intrinsic urethral (striated) muscle which surrounds the urethra distal to the verumontanum and forms the external urethral sphincter. It is supplied by parasympathetic nerves. The periurethral skeletal muscle of the pelvic floor surrounds this sphincter and is supplied by the pudendal nerve.

In the *female*, the external urethral sphincter extends over the whole length of the urethra but is most prominent in the mid-third of the urethra which it surrounds. Proximally, there is no equivalent of the pre-prostatic sphincter in the male and distally the periurethral muscles of the pelvic floor provide the main support.

## NEUROLOGICAL CONTROL OF MICTURITION

### Parasympathetic

Parasympathetic nerves arise from S2, 3 and 4 as pre-ganglionic axons, then relay through the pelvic ganglia and, as post-ganglionic nerves, supply the detrusor muscle, the smooth muscle of the urethra and intramural striated muscle of the external sphincter. These nerves (cholinergic) stimulate detrusor contraction and maintain urethral closure.

### Sympathetic

Sympathetic nerves arise from D11–L1. The exact role of the sympathetic nerves in the control of micturition has not been fully clarified. It is now known that alpha-adrenergic receptors at their nerve terminals are mainly in the smooth muscle of the proximal urethra, whereas beta receptors are in the fundus of the bladder. The alpha receptors respond to noradrenaline by stimulating contraction, while the beta receptors relax smooth muscle.

### Somatic

The pudendal nerves arise from S2, 3 and 4 and supply the striated muscles of the pelvic floor. Afferent nerves are carried in both the parasympathetic and pudendal pathways and transmit sensory impulses from the bladder, urethra and pelvic floor. These sensory impulses not only pass to the cerebral cortex and the micturition centre but also to the cord as part of the spinal cord reflexes. Thus bladder filling stimulates afferent impulses which then stimulate pelvic floor contraction, so adding to urethral compression.

### Cortex

Cortical control is a basic part of the micturition cycle described below. The higher centres suppress detrusor contractions and their main influence is to inhibit micturition until such times that it is appropriate to micturate. Afferent impulses pass to the brain via the posterior columns and lateral spinothalamic tracts. Thus bladder sensation is transmitted bilaterally and is lost only when both tracts are divided. The cortical centres are situated in the anteromedial aspect of the frontal lobe, the cingulate gyrus and the paracentral lobule.

## MICTURITION CYCLE

The series of events that occur continuously within the bladder are known as the micturition cycle, which has three phases:

1. *Storage (or filling) phase.* Because of the high compliance of the detrusor muscle the bladder fills steadily without either bladder sensation or change in intravesical pressure. Eventually the volume is sufficient to induce the desire to void, which marks the end of this phase.

2. *Postponement (or inhibitory) phase.* Voluntary control is now exerted over the desire to void, which then disappears, temporarily. Compliance of the detrusor allows further increase in capacity until the next desire to void. Just how often this desire need be inhibited depends upon many circumstances, not the least of which is finding a suitable place in which to void.

3. *Emptying (or micturition) phase.* The act of micturition is initiated first by voluntary and then by reflex relaxation of the pelvic floor, followed by reflex detrusor contraction. Intravesical pressure remains greater than the urethral pressure until the bladder is empty.

The normal control of micturition requires the co-ordinated reflex activity of autonomic and somatic nerves as described in the preceding paragraphs. These responses require normal anatomical structures and normal innervation. Thus a patient with an extensive carcinoma of the prostate that has damaged the sphincter mechanisms and a patient with a spinal cord injury that has damaged the innervation are examples which illustrate the two main groups of patients with disorders of micturition. These are 1. those with a structural disorder and 2. those with a neurogenic disorder.

## 1. STRUCTURAL DISORDERS

### Investigation of structural disorders

In the assessment of all abnormalities of function affecting the lower urinary tract there may be difficulty in interpretation of the findings because of dual pathology. For example, incontinence in an elderly man may be due to cortical deficiency resulting from cerebral degeneration but could also be due to chronic outflow tract obstruction resulting from prostatic hypertrophy.

The history is important but it may be deceptive, mainly because different abnormalities can produce similar symptoms. The exact character of the urinary abnormality must be determined so that, if possible, structural causes can be separated from neurological causes. Details of drug treatment are noted. Diuretics and drugs with anticholinergic side effects may tip the balance when there is already dysfunction. Urine is tested for glycosuria and infection.

In addition to the intravenous urogram there is now a range of more specific methods for assessing micturition but they are not all absolute requirements for a diagnosis. Their value lies in resolving specific clinical questions that will influence management. These methods include radiology (cystourethrography), urodynamics (cystometrogram and urethral pressures) and direct inspection (cystourethroscopy and pelvic examination under anaesthesia).

In summary, a full clinical history and physical examination, with cystourethroscopy and bimanual examination of the pelvic contents, remain the basic initial methods for investigation of structural disorders.

## STRUCTURAL CHANGES CAUSING INCONTINENCE IN THE MALE

### 1. After operations

The male is vulnerable to disorders of control of micturition because removal of the prostate gland is a common operation. In this operation the internal urethral mechanism is deliberately excised posteriorly but the distal mechanism is left strictly alone; any damage to this sphincter will affect continence. Episodes of incontinence commonly follow removal of the urethral catheter but stop within several days. More persistent incontinence can be classified as follows.

*Dribbling incontinence.* This is due to structural damage to the external urethral mechanism. It is uncommon and recovery is unlikely. Treatment is by an appliance or an operative procedure that narrows the urethra.

*Stress incontinence.* This occurs with any sudden increase in abdominal pressure, as with coughing. Since the damage to the sphincter is mild it usually responds to physiotherapy.

*Urge incontinence.* This is not due to sphincter weakness but to involuntary bladder contractions in an uninhibited or unstable bladder. Removal of the prostatic obstruction alone is usually sufficient to correct the symptoms of urgency and urge incontinence but antispasmodic drug treatment may be necessary.

*Enuresis.* Bed-wetting that occurs after prostatectomy is due to either urge incontinence or poor tone in the pelvic floor or both. Physiotherapy and drug treatment may help.

Other operative procedures on the urethra, such as repeated dilatations for urethral stricture or urethroplasty, may be followed by incontinence as classified above.

## 2. With disease

*Carcinoma of the prostate* may grow locally to involve the adjacent urethral structures; repeated transurethral resections for recurring obstruction may be necessary. The net effect of these is to change the posterior urethra into a rigid tube so that dribbling incontinence occurs, i.e. urine leaks during the storage phase. Either an indwelling catheter or condom incontinence appliance may be necessary.

*Benign prostatic enlargement* may induce urgency of micturition either alone or with other obstructive symptoms. An early sign of benign enlargement, a 'post-micturition dribble', is probably due to a small amount of urine that is trapped between the proximal and distal mechanisms. A similar complaint may occur with prostatitis and early outflow changes of bilharziasis (the development of chronic retention with overflow or dribbling incontinence is referred to on p. 591).

Chronic illness and debility, especially in an elderly patient, may lead to incontinence because of poor tone in the periurethral striated muscle of the pelvic floor; this may be worsened by some loss of the cortical inhibition of micturition.

## STRUCTURAL CHANGES CAUSING INCONTINENCE IN THE FEMALE

Incontinence of urine in women is more prevalent than generally suspected. As many as 50% of nulliparous young women may have some degree of stress incontinence and in approximately 20% this may be a daily occurrence. Overall, approximately 10% of women aged 15–64 are incontinent twice or more per month; this figure rises rapidly in older patients and in geriatric units. Only a fraction of the younger women seek advice, either because of embarrassment or stoical acceptance of some incontinence as a normal event.

### 1. After childbirth operations

Multiparous women commonly lose some of the tone in the muscles of the pelvic floor with each pregnancy. Symptoms may range from occasional stress incontinence to dribbling incontinence. Examination shows weakening of the pelvic floor muscles and anterior vaginal wall (*cystocele*). It is important to distinguish stress incontinence from urge incontinence, for the former responds to surgical procedures designed to support the bladder neck and strengthen the anterior vaginal wall, while the latter should be treated by drug therapy. Stress incontinence is characterised by an involuntary loss of urine that occurs with coughing, laughing, sneezing or any activity that raises the intra-abdominal pressure suddenly. A cough, however, may stimulate involuntary detrusor contractions, which causes motor urge incontinence. This differential diagnosis can be made only by a urodynamic assessment. Urge incontinence may thus be motor, due to unstable detrusor contractions, or sensory, in which infection or stones produce excessive sensory stimulation.

In parts of the world where obstetric services

are poor, prolonged labour may lead to a *vesico-vaginal fistula* which presents as continuous dribbling incontinence. The association with delivery is usually clear, but a small fistula may be missed. Investigation of dribbling incontinence must distinguish between urethral damage and a fistula. Treatment consists of either closing the fistula *per vaginam* or a procedure to support the bladder neck.

The operation of hysterectomy may be followed by urinary incontinence, suggesting damage to the ureter(s) at the time of operation. Again, the association of an operation and incontinence should indicate a diagnosis of uretero-vaginal fistula and investigations are directed to establishing which ureter has been damaged. Treatment consists of reimplanting the ureter into the bladder.

## 2. With diseases

*Cystitis.* In addition to the symptoms of frequency, urgency and dysuria, this common condition in women sometimes causes sensory urge incontinence. Treatment of both the infection and bladder spasm is required.

*Chronic interstitial cystitis (Hunner's ulcer)* This chronic inflammatory condition, in addition to causing frequency and dysuria, may also cause urgency and urge incontinence. Treatment of this condition is often unsatisfactory. Hydrostatic dilatation may be effective or the patient may respond to treatment with steroids.

*Urethral syndrome.* This condition is characterised by symptoms of cystitis but there is no infection. There may be some incontinence. These patients often have a degree of urethral stenosis and treatment by urethral dilatation or incision may be successful. However, the urethral syndrome usually responds to treatment by regulating micturition habits and by careful perineal hygiene.

*Ectopic ureter.* Dribbling incontinence in a child should raise the suspicion of an ectopic ureter in which the lower of the two ureters from a kidney opens outside the control of the urethral mechanism. The abnormal ureter must be relocated in the bladder.

*Carcinoma of the cervix* or its treatment by radiotherapy may cause vesico-vaginal fistula and hence incontinence.

## 2. NEUROGENIC DISORDERS

### Investigation of neurogenic disorders

As with the investigation of structural disorders a full history, including an interview with relatives, is required. Examination must include the plantar reflexes and the sensation and tone of the anal canal. Once again, glycosuria and urinary infection should be sought.

Urodynamic, radiological and electromyographic studies may all be required to determine the appropriate management.

## AETIOLOGY OF ABNORMAL MICTURITION

### 1. In the cortex

*Diseases* affecting the frontal lobe can alter the pattern of micturition, increasing or decreasing the frequency or affecting the social awareness of incontinence. Lesions such as cerebral thrombosis or cerebral degeneration may produce incontinence by failing to inhibit the postponement phase of micturition. The paracentral lobule controls the activity of skeletal muscle, so that lesions in this area may cause sustained pelvic and perineal muscular contraction. It must be remembered that a disorder of micturition may be accentuated by or even be due to the physical inability to prepare for micturition.

*Emotional states* may affect the postponement of micturition, giving rise to 'giggle' incontinence and possibly to enuresis in some patients. Incontinence with epilepsy is also due to a loss of inhibitory control. Hysteria can lead to acute retention in women. *Sensory stimuli* may be excessive, as with the pain of cystourethritis in women, and the patient may develop 'sensory urge incontinence'.

*Drugs* including alcohol, may alter the cortical control of micturition. Sedatives may affect the postponement phase and precipitate incontinence, especially at night. The intoxicated patient may lack the mental alertness to maintain continence or may continually suppress the desire to void, leading to prostatic congestion and retention.

## 2. In the spinal cord

Two aspects of disease or injury to the spinal cord will influence the nature and prognosis of the disordered micturition: the level of the disease and the completeness or incompleteness of the damage.

*Injury to the spinal reflex centre ( S2, 3, 4 ).* The injury is usually a fracture of the spine at the level of T12, L1 which damages the conus medullaris. The bladder distends without sensation and the external sphincter is flaccid. Thus the cystometrogram is flat. The patient develops retention with overflow but emptying is possible with abdominal straining or hand pressure.

*Injury above the sacral segments (upper motor neurone lesions).* Trauma such as fractures of the cervical spine, whiplash injuries or gunshot wounds are the most common injuries to the spinal cord. *Tumours* such as angiomata may compress the cord or the cord may be injured during surgical removal of the tumour. *Diseases* affecting the spinal cord include multiple sclerosis and transverse myelitis.

If the central connections are disrupted, the patient develops a reflex bladder which, because of the uncoordinated action of the detrusor and sphincter, leads to a thick-walled, trabeculated, overactive bladder. Usually the central connections are not completely disrupted and there may be some sensation and some cortical inhibition.

## 3. In the pelvic nerves

*Operative procedures* may interrupt the autonomic pathways, especially when the dissection involves the side walls of the pelvis as in a radical dissection of the rectum or the uterus. Similarly, a lumbar sympathectomy or surgery for aortic aneurysm may disrupt the neural pathways in the pelvis.

Diseases affecting the autonomic system, principally diabetes mellitus, affect the control of micturition.

With the loss of sensation and contraction, the bladder becomes an atonic sac, prone to the main complication of stasis infection. The external sphincter remains closed by uninhibited tonic contractions, but the internal sphincter is partly open since it partly depends upon detrusor activity.

## 4. In the bladder

*Primary failure of the detrusor* has been described but usually it is a sequel to chronic overdistension.

*Atonic bladder* following overdistension. The atonic myogenic bladder is caused by prolonged outlet obstruction and is found in the late stages of bladder decompensation. The commonest cause is silent prostatic obstruction, where progressive loss of the desire to void results in overflow incontinence. In women, conscious prolonging of the postponement phase can lead to a large, atonic bladder.

## GENERAL PRINCIPLES OF MANAGEMENT OF DISORDERS OF MICTURITION:

1. The diagnosis must be as complete as possible. More than one mechanism may account for the disordered micturition.

2. Infection is the single most sinister complication; every effort is made to avoid this.

3. Renal damage (from vesicoureteric reflux) and infection account for most of the morbidity and mortality.

4. Early management of a spinal injury consists of continuous bladder drainage with a fine urethral catheter. Avoid infection.

5. If there is evidence that the spinal reflex is intact, reflex activity may return to the bladder.

6. Reflex activity leads to uncoordinated micturition; the bladder becomes thick-walled and sacculated and there is vesicoureteric reflux.

7. If there is no reflex activity, manual expression of the large atonic bladder is necessary.

8. If manual expression is unsatisfactory, incision of the distal urethral mechanism is necessary. Resection of the proximal urethral mechanism may also be needed.

9. If the complications of reflux and recurrent urinary infection are severe, urinary diversion is indicated.

10. Since there are no effective devices to keep an incontinent female dry, a urinary diversion may need to be done early.

# 41. Appendices

## PRACTICAL PROCEDURES

### VENEPUNCTURE

The ante-cubital fossa is the most convenient site for venepuncture. Here the median cubital vein, median vein of forearm and the cephalic vein are easily accessible but the median nerve and the brachial artery must be avoided. A 21-gauge needle is used for adults and a 23-gauge needle for children. A venous tourniquet is placed around the upper arm. Small veins become more engorged if the fist is clenched several times or if the veins are tapped briskly. The skin is cleaned with isopropyl alcohol and the elbow is fully extended. The needle is inserted obliquely through the skin overlying the vein in a 'two step' fashion: first through the skin, then through the vein wall. A distinct reduction of resistance to the passage of the needle is appreciated as the lumen of the vein is entered. The needle is advanced 2 or 3 mm within the vein and then stabilised with the left thumb (Fig. 41.1). The plunger of the syringe is gently withdrawn until the volume of blood required is obtained. The tourniquet is released and the needle is withdrawn. Pressure over the

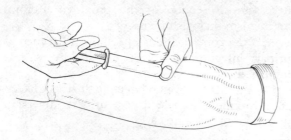

**Fig. 41.1** Venepuncture

puncture site for 1 minute prevents haematoma formation. The needle is removed from the syringe and the blood is gently injected into appropriate tubes. Tubes which contain anticoagulants must be gently inverted several times to allow sufficient mixing to prevent clot formation. The tubes are now labelled with the patient's name and hospital number, and the time and date of sampling. Preliminary or delayed labelling introduces an unacceptable risk of error.

### VENEPUNCTURE FOR BLOOD CULTURE

This requires more stringent preparations than routine venepuncture. The hands are washed and dried on a sterile towel. An assistant applies the venous tourniquet. The patient's skin is prepared with isopropyl alcohol applied with a sterile cotton wool ball carried on sterile forceps. Venepuncture is performed with strict 'no touch' technique and blood is withdrawn. The needle is withdrawn from the vein, removed from the syringe and a second needle is substituted to inject 5 ml aliquots of blood into paired blood culture bottles — two aerobic, two anaerobic and two containing penicillinase if the patient is already being treated with penicillin. All bottles are immediately sent to the laboratory and/or placed in an incubator at 37°C.

### PERIPHERAL VENOUS CANNULATION

Most intravenous infusions are given into the cephalic vein in the forearm or into a vein on the flexor or extensor aspect of the forearm. In these situations the cannula does not cross joints.

Splints are unnecessary and the patient may use the arm freely. Cannula units comprise an outer polythene or teflon sheath — the cannula proper — and an inner metal needle. 'Venflon', 'Intraflon', 'Abbocath', 'Quick-Cath' and 'Medicut' are convenient. A 16 or 18-gauge cannula is used for most purposes in adults but a 14-gauge cannula is required for rapid blood transfusion. The preliminary preparation for venepuncture is repeated. A small bleb of local anaesthetic is raised intradermally at the proposed site of skin puncture. The vein is steadied by the left thumb which applies gentle pressure and traction distally. Venepuncture is made with the cannula unit and is confirmed by 'flashback' of blood into the observation chamber at the top of the metal needle. The cannula unit is advanced 2–3 mm within the vein (Fig. 41.2). The left hand is now used to advance the cannula proper up the vein while the right hand withdraws the inner metal needle simultaneously. The venous tourniquet is released, the infusion tubing set previously primed with isotonic saline solution is connected to the cannula and the infusion is commenced. The cannula is fixed securely to the skin with adhesive tape and the infusion tubing is folded in a U-loop and also secured with adhesive tape (Fig. 41.3).

Peripheral intravenous cannulation requires no more than clean hands, antiseptic skin preparation and a strict 'no touch' technique for the part of the cannula which lodges within the vein and its end to which the infusion tubing is connected. Cannula sites are inspected daily and the cannula is removed at the first sign of swelling or local tenderness over the vein.

## CENTRAL VENOUS CANNULATION

A central venous cannula is used to measure the central venous pressure or for parenteral nutrition. Long cannulas (60 cm) are inserted via the basilic vein at the elbow and short cannulas (20–30 cm) are inserted directly into the subclavian or internal jugular veins. Cannula units vary considerably but a 16-gauge cannula is generally used. 'Surcath' and 'Intramedicut' are preferred because the teflon cannula is introduced through and retained by a short outer cannula. This avoids the risks of accidental division of the cannula and possible embolisation inherent in the 'Bardicath' and 'Drum-Cartridge' systems in which the cannula is introduced through and retained by a metal needle. 'Nutricath' is a silastic cannula specially designed for long term intravenous nutrition.

Central venous cannulas are always inserted under sterile conditions, ideally in the operating theatre. The operator scrubs up and wears a gown and gloves. The patient's skin is prepared with antiseptic solution and draped with sterile towels. The precise method for insertion of each cannula unit is clearly described in the manufacturer's instructions which must always be consulted.

Local anaesthesia is used. Cannulation of the basilic vein is performed above the elbow skin crease to permit free use of the arm. In other respects the procedure is similar to peripheral venous cannulation. Cannulation of the internal jugular vein and subclavian vein is performed with the patient tipped 20°-head down to achieve adequate venous congestion. Preliminary test venepuncture with a 21 or 19-gauge needle identifies the vein without risk of trauma to adjacent structures. The cannula is then inserted with confidence.

The *internal jugular vein* is best entered in the triangle between the sternal and clavicular heads of the sterno-mastoid muscle. The operator stands behind the patient's head which is rotated

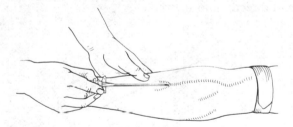

**Fig. 41.2** Peripheral venous cannulation

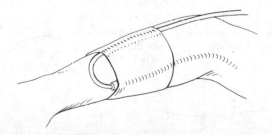

**Fig. 41.3** Cannulation and infusion tubing secured

a few degrees towards the opposite side. The cannula is introduced at the apex of the triangle at an angle of 45° to the skin. It is directed downwards parallel to the sagittal plane or up to 15° medially (Fig. 41.4).

The *subclavian vein* is best entered by the infraclavicular approach. The infra-clavicular pulsation of the subclavian artery is defined with the left index finger. The cannula is introduced 5 mm medial to this point, just below the clavicle, and directed upwards at an angle of 45° to the sagittal plane, passing immediately below the clavicle and in front of the first rib to enter the subclavian vein at a depth of some 4–5 cm (Fig. 41.5).

Other approaches to the internal jugular vein and the subclavian vein are also available. All approaches have the potential hazard of entering the pleural cavity. It is therefore essential to check the correct placement of the cannula in the venous system by a 'flowback' test. The infusion tubing set previously primed with isotonic saline solution is connected to the cannula. The infusion fluid bag is then lowered below the level of the patient and the clip on the tubing released. Blood flows retrogradely up the tubing. If this does not occur the cannula is not in the venous system. The head-down position is now changed to horizontal and the fluid bag is raised above the patient. Free flow now occurs into the superior

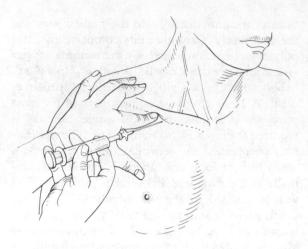

Fig. 41.5 Cannulation of subclavian vein

vena cava. A penetrated chest X-ray is taken to visualise the tip of the cannula. It may need to be advanced or withdrawn. When a satisfactory position is obtained in the superior vena cava the cannula is sutured to the skin to prevent accidental dislodgement. The skin puncture site is dabbed with antiseptic solution and covered with a sterile dressing.

Cannulas inserted for intravenous nutrition are tunnelled in the subcutaneous tissue to emerge on the chest at a distance from the site of the initial cannula skin-venepuncture (Fig. 41.6). This minimises the risk of sepsis spreading down the tract and directly into the vein.

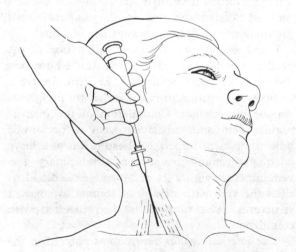

Fig. 41.4 Cannulation of the internal jugular vein. Note the triangle between the sternal and clavicular heads of sternomastoid.

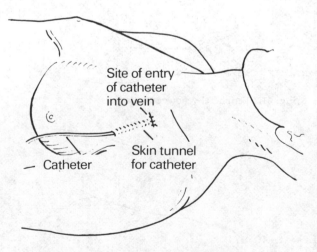

Site of entry of catheter into vein

Skin tunnel for catheter

Catheter

Fig. 41.6 Skin tunnel for central venous catheter

## CENTRAL VENOUS PRESSURE MANOMETRY

A T-piece with a three way tap at the junction of its limbs is connected between the central venous cannula and the infusion set. The bottom of the vertical limb of the T-piece is secured against the zero mark on a centimetre scale. The infusion flows through the horizontal limb and the cannula.

The patient is placed horizontal, the mid thoracic point (the point at which the mid-axillary line is intersected by a vertical plane from the sternal angle) is marked and the zero level on the centimetre scale is adjusted with the aid of a spirit level to lie in the same horizontal plane as the mid-thoracic point (Fig. 41.7). Alternatively, the sternal angle can be used as a reference point for +5 cm on the scale.

The three-way tap is turned first to allow fluid to fill the vertical limb of the T-piece to about 20–25 cm, and then to allow the vertical limb to drain into the central venous cannula. The level of fluid in the vertical limb drops rapidly and then stabilises, falling and rising between 0.5–1.0 cm with inspiration and expiration. The lowest point of the meniscus on inspiration measures the central venous pressure in centimetres of water above the mid-thoracic point. The normal range is 5–12 cm. As soon as the measurement is made, the three way tap is turned to restore flow from the infusion set through the cannula. Sequential measure-

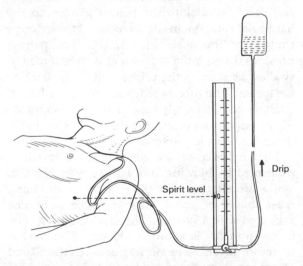

**Fig. 41.7** CVP Manometry. Note the mid thoracic point marked with a black dot — the zero reference point.

ments must be made with the patient lying horizontal.

Low central venous pressure is corrected by rapid infusion of crystalloid, colloid or blood as appropriate and in sufficient volumes to restore the central venous pressure to the normal range. High central venous pressure indicates fluid overload and further intravenous infusions are strictly limited.

## VENOUS CUTDOWN CANNULATION

This procedure is rarely required. Even when it is impossible to cannulate a peripheral vein, it is seldom difficult for an experienced operator to cannulate the internal jugular vein or the subclavian vein. However, profound hypovolaemic shock is the occasional exception. In this condition delays are unacceptable and a cutdown cannulation of the basilic vein at the elbow, the cephalic vein in the delto-pectoral groove or the long saphenous vein at the ankle or groin may be life-saving. The latter site has the singular advantage that the end of the sterile infusion set may be inserted directly into the vein but this is only a temporary expedient in a grave emergency as it is associated with the risk of ilio-femoral venous thrombosis.

Venous cutdown cannulation is performed under local anaesthesia and with sterile conditions. The skin is incised transversely over the chosen vein. The subcutaneous fat is opened with the points of dissection scissors. The vein is exposed and cleared all round over a length of 1 cm. The distal end of this segment is ligated with an absorbable ligature. The proximal end is elevated on a second absorbable ligature to prevent venous backflow and a transverse venotomy is made with a scalpel. The largest cannula that will fit the vein is introduced through the skin 2 cm below the incision and passed up the vein (Fig. 41.8). The proximal ligature is tied securely but without undue compression of the cannula. The infusion set is then connected to the cannula and the infusion commenced rapidly. The skin is closed with non-absorbable sutures and the cannula is sutured to the skin to prevent accidental dislodgement. Finally the wound and the skin puncture site are dabbed with antiseptic solution and covered with a sterile dressing.

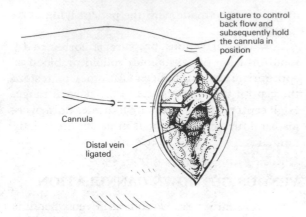

Fig. 41.8 Venous cutdown cannulation

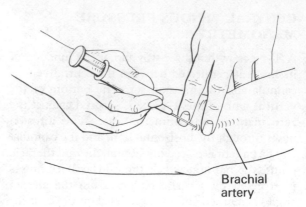

Fig. 41.9 Brachial artery puncture

## ARTERIAL PUNCTURE

Arterial puncture is performed to measure the $Pa_{O_2}$, $Pa_{CO_2}$, pH and bicarbonate concentration or to monitor arterial pressure. The brachial artery at the elbow or the radial artery at the wrist are the sites of choice for arterial puncture. A 21-gauge needle and preferably a glass syringe, containing a metal agitator, are used. Five thousand units of heparin in 1 ml solution are drawn into the syringe. The plunger of the syringe is fully withdrawn and the air in the barrel and excess heparin are expelled. The residual heparin not only anticoagulates the blood but also lubricates the syringe. A second needle is substituted to avoid local anticoagulation of the needle tract with heparin.

The course of the artery is defined by palpation of its pulse between two fingers placed longitudinally 1 cm apart. The skin is cleaned with isopropyl alcohol. The needle is inserted at an angle of 45° to the skin, bevel upwards, and advanced directly into the artery (Fig. 41.9). Blood pulsates into the syringe under its own pressure; 4–5 ml is sufficient. The needle is withdrawn and an assistant applies firm pressure over the puncture site for 3 minutes to prevent haematoma formation. The needle is removed from the syringe, any small air bubbles are expelled through the nozzle and a cap is then applied. The syringe is gently inverted several times to heparinise the blood. The sample is sent immediately for analysis. If any delay is anticipated the syringe must be placed in ice.

To monitor arterial pressure, an indwelling cannula is inserted and connected to a manometer.

## INTUBATION

### NASOGASTRIC INTUBATION

The patient is asked to sit up for this procedure. If the patient is particularly apprehensive, the nostril may be anaesthetised with local anaesthetic spray. A size 14F or 16F radio-opaque tube is used for most adults but a size 18F or 20F tube is preferred for patients with intestinal obstruction. The tube is thoroughly lubricated with KY jelly and then passed into the nostril parallel to the hard palate and not in the direction of the external contour of the nose (Fig. 41.10). The patient breathes through the mouth and is encouraged to swallow as soon as the tube is felt at the back of the throat. The tube is gently advanced with each swallow and is readily passed into the stomach. Sips from a glass of water help those who find it difficult to swallow spontaneously.

The presence of the tube in the stomach is confirmed by blowing 20 ml air rapidly down it, while auscultating over the stomach; a bubbling noise should be heard. Gastric contents are now aspirated with a syringe. The ideal length of tube in the stomach is about 10–15 cm. The tube is therefore advanced to midway between the 50 and 60 cm marks and then secured firmly to the nose and cheek with adhesive tape.

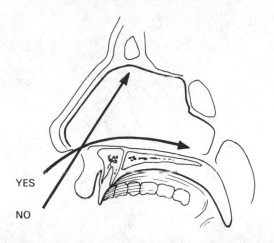

**Fig. 41.10** Nasogastric intubation. Note the correct direction to insert the tube

## OESOPHAGEAL TAMPONADE

The Sengstaken tube is a gastric aspiration tube with inflatable gastric and oesophageal balloons, distension of which compress the overlying oesophageal and high gastric veins. It is used for the emergency treatment of bleeding oesophageal varices.

A modification, the Minnesota tube (Fig. 41.11), has an additional channel to allow the aspiration of saliva from the oesophagus above the level of the oesophageal balloon.

Before passing the tube, the oesophageal and gastric balloons are checked. It is also important that efficient suction apparatus is available. The nose is anaesthetised with local anaesthetic spray and the tube is thoroughly lubricated with local anaesthetic jelly. The tube is passed through the nose or mouth and into the back of the throat. As with routine nasogastric intubation, the patient is encouraged to swallow and the tube is gently advanced with each swallow. The procedure is, however, much more uncomfortable and few patients with bleeding varices are able to cooperate well with the operator. Coughing and spluttering is usually a sign that the tube is in the larynx and it must be withdrawn before further attempts are made to advance it.

The tube is passed so that the junction between the oesophageal and gastric balloon is 50 cm from the incisor teeth and the gastric balloon is inflated with 30 ml gastrografin. An X-ray is taken to confirm that the balloon is inflated in the stomach. The balloon is now filled with water to a total volume of 150 ml and then drawn back to impact at the cardia. An assistant holds the tube in this position with slight tension. The oesophageal balloon is inflated with air to a pressure between 30 and 40 mmHg, checked by attachment

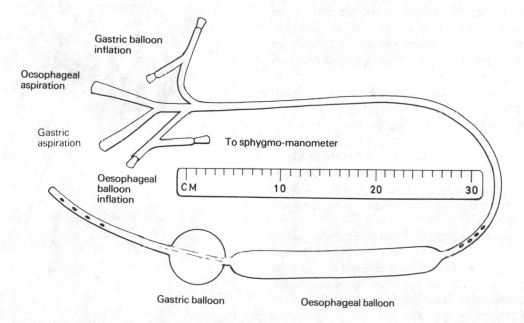

**Fig. 41.11** Minnesota tube

to a sphygmomanometer. A 5 cm cube of sponge rubber is secured around the tube as close to the nose as possible. The assistant now releases the tube and the sponge pulls back snuggly against the nose. This ensures continuous 'fixed traction' on the tube with reliable compression of varices in the gastric fundus in addition to those in the oesophagus.

The stomach is aspirated regularly through the main lumen of the tube. The oesophagus cannot be aspirated with the Sengstaken tube and saliva starts to pool as soon as the oesophageal balloon is inflated. The patient is therefore nursed semi-prone so that saliva may be spat out of the mouth. With the Minnesota tube these secretions can be aspirated.

It is essential to deflate the oesophageal balloon for 5–10 minutes every 6 hours to avoid the risk of ischaemic necrosis of the oesophageal mucosa. If possible, the pressure in the oesophageal balloon should be reduced to 25 mmHg after 12 hours. Normally the tube is not kept in position for more than 24 hours.

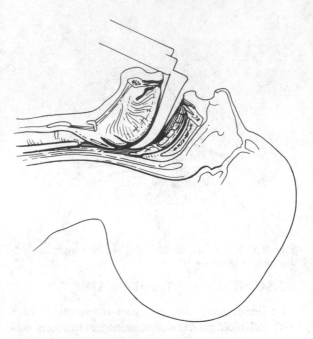

**Fig. 41.12** Laryngoscope in position

## ENDOTRACHEAL INTUBATION

The operator stands behind the patient's head. The neck is slightly flexed and the head is extended. Dentures are removed. Secretions or vomit are cleared from the mouth and pharynx with suction. An assistant presses on the cricoid cartilage to prevent reflux of oesophageal contents into the pharynx.

The Mackintosh laryngoscope is held in the left hand. The curved blade is passed down the right side of the tongue to engage the tip in the vallecula anterior to the epiglottis (Fig. 41.12). The assistant hooks a finger in the right angle of the mouth to improve the view while the laryngoscope is lifted vertically and the blade pulls the tongue and epiglottis forwards to expose the vocal cords (Fig. 41.13).

A lubricated, cuffed endotracheal tube is passed under direct vision between the vocal cords and into the trachea. The average external diameter of suitable tubes is 9 mm for adult males and 8 mm for adult females. The cuff of the tube is inflated with a few ml of air. The assistant discontinues cricoid pressure and the laryngoscope is removed.

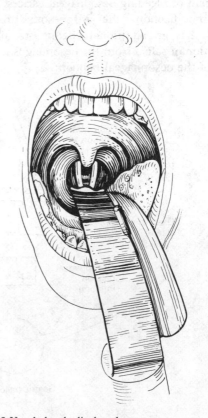

**Fig. 41.13** Vocal chords displayed

"By holding Penis ventically

S Shape converted to J.

The endotracheal tube is connected to a re-breathing bag or a self inflating 'Ambu-bag' and ventilation is started. The chest is observed and auscultated to confirm inflation of both lungs.

## URETHRAL CATHETERISATION

Urethral catheters are inserted under sterile conditions. The operator scrubs up and wears a gown and gloves. The patient's skin is prepared with antiseptic solution and draped with sterile towels. All items that will be required are laid out on the sterile catheter tray.

For *males* a 14 or 16F self-retaining Foley balloon catheter is used (Fig. 41.14). If the operator is right-handed, the penis is grasped with the left hand. Traction is applied down the shaft to retract the prepuce. All further manoeuvres are performed with the right hand.

The glans and the inner aspect of the prepuce is prepared with antiseptic solution applied by a swab carried in forceps. The catheter is lubricated by drawing it across a large drop of sterile KY jelly on a gauze swab. The catheter is then placed in a kidney dish which is transferred to rest over the patient's thighs close to the penis. The penis is held vertically and the catheter is introduced using forceps (Fig. 41.15). When the catheter is in the bulbar urethra, the penis is directed towards the feet and the remainder of the catheter is inserted. Urine flows into the kidney dish. The left hand is released from the penis and used to steady the inflation limb for the catheter balloon while 10–20 ml water is injected. The catheter is gently withdrawn until the balloon engages at the bladder neck. The prepuce is drawn down over the glans to prevent paraphimosis.

The sterile drainage tube is fitted to the cath-

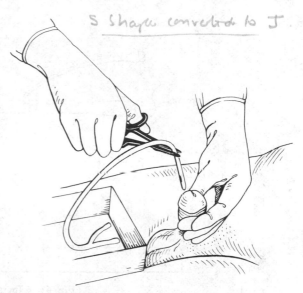

**Fig. 41.15** Catheterisation (alternatively the catheter can be 'milked out' of its plastic container)

eter and secured to the pyjama trousers to avoid traction directly on the catheter.

For *females* an 18 or 20F self-retaining Foley balloon catheter is used. The labia minora are separated with the thumb and fingers of the left hand to expose the urethral meatus immediately anterior to the vagina. The pudenda is now swabbed with antiseptic solution. Two swabs are used, each being swept once across the pudenda from anterior to posterior and then discarded. The remainder of the procedure is performed in a similar fashion to catheterisation in the male, although the catheter need only be inserted to half its length before the drainage tube is connected and the balloon is inflated.

## SUPRAPUBIC CATHETERISATION

Suprapubic catheterisation is indicated when urethral catheterisation cannot be performed or is contraindicated. The bladder must be distended to at least midway between the pubic symphysis and the umbilicus. The 16F 'Ingram Trocar Catheter' (Fig. 41.16) of the Foley type is inserted under sterile conditions.

The operator scrubs up and wears a gown and gloves. The patient's skin is prepared with antiseptic solution and draped with sterile towels. Local anaesthetic is infiltrated at an angle of 70°

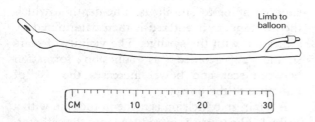

Limb to balloon

CM    10    20    30

**Fig. 41.14** Foley balloon catheter

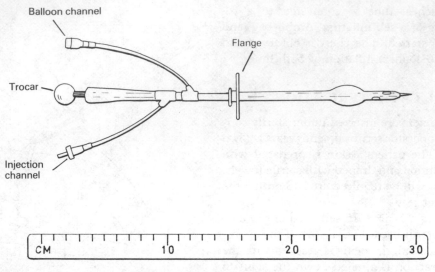

Fig. 41.16 Ingram trocar catheter

through all layers of the mid line of the abdominal wall two finger breadths above the pubic symphysis. The depth at which the bladder lumen is entered is then determined by aspiration with the syringe.

A 6 mm stab incision is made in the skin with a scalpel. The shaft of the catheter is held firmly between left thumb and index finger some 4–5 cm higher than the estimated depth of the bladder lumen. This prevents 'overshoot' as the right hand thrusts the trocar and catheter through the abdominal wall (Fig. 41.17). The catheter is advanced fully with the left hand while the trocar is withdrawn simultaneously with the right hand. An assistant engages the sterile drainage tube to the catheter. The catheter balloon is inflated with 5 ml water. The length of catheter within the

bladder is adjusted so that the balloon is 2–3 cm away from the bladder wall. The snug fitting flange is slid down the catheter to make contact with the skin and then sutured to it to prevent accidental displacement of the catheter.

## ABDOMINAL PARACENTESIS

Abominal paracentesis is performed to relieve the discomfort caused by abdominal distention with ascitic fluid or to obtain a specimen of ascitic fluid for cytological examination. The bladder must be empty. A 'Trocath' peritoneal dialysis catheter with multiple side perforations over a length of 8 cm is inserted under sterile conditions (Fig. 41.18). The operator scrubs up and wears a gown and gloves. Local anaesthetic is infiltrated at an angle of 70° through all layers of the abdominal wall either in the midline one-third of the way between the umbilicus and the pubic symphysis or in the right or left iliac fossa at the junction of the outer to middle thirds of a line from anterior superior spine to umbilicus. The depth at which the peritoneum is entered is then determined by aspiration with the syringe. The vicinity of scars should be avoided, as adhesion formation between scar and bowel increases the risk of puncture of the bowel.

A 3 mm stab incision is made in the skin with a scalpel. The trocar is introduced into the catheter. The shaft of the catheter is held firmly between

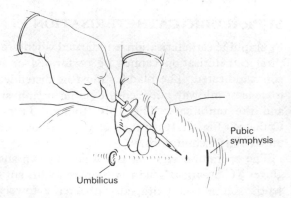

Fig. 41.17 Suprapubic catheterisation

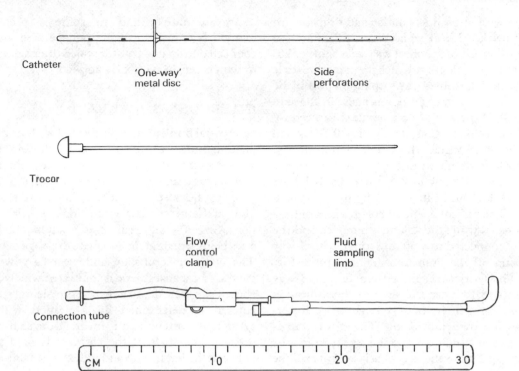

Fig. 41.18 'Trocath' peritoneal dialysis catheter

left thumb and index finger some 4–5 cm higher than the estimated depth of the peritoneum. This prevents 'overshoot' as the right hand thrusts the trocar and catheter through the abdominal wall into the peritoneum (Fig. 41.19).

The catheter is advanced further with the left hand while the trocar is withdrawn simultaneously with the right hand. If resistance is noted, the catheter is withdrawn 2–3 cm, rotated 180°

and then advanced again. The minimum final length of catheter within the peritoneal cavity must be 10 cm. If this position is not obtained, the side perforations of the catheter may lie within the abdominal wall and allow troublesome extravasation of ascitic fluid in the subcutaneous tissues. The 'one-way' metal disc is slid down the catheter to make contact with the skin and secured to it with adhesive tape. The catheter is cut across some 4 cm above the metal disc and attached by the connection tube with flow control clamp to a sterile drainage tube.

## PLEURAL ASPIRATION

Pleural aspiration is performed to drain a large pleural effusion. The patient sits upright and rests his elbows and forearms on a table. The 7th or 8th intercostal space is identified and marked in the plane of the inferior angle of the scapula. Lower spaces are not suitable as the diaphragm lies too close to the chest wall. The procedure is performed under sterile conditions. The operator scrubs up and wears a gown and gloves. The patient's skin is

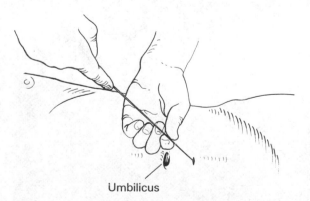

Fig. 41.19 Insertion of peritoneal dialysis catheter

prepared with antiseptic solution and draped with sterile towels. Local anaesthetic is infiltrated through all layers of the chest wall at an angle of 70° downwards. The depth at which the pleural space is entered is determined by aspiration with the syringe. A 2 mm stab incision is made in the skin with a scalpel and a wide bore needle with a central stilette inserted so that its tip lies 0.5–1.0 cm obliquely downwards within the pleural cavity. The needle is stabilised in this position by an old artery forceps, a screw-lock or alternatively by the left thumb and index finger resting firmly against the skin. The patient is told to hold his breath for a few moments while the stilette is removed and the needle is connected to a 50 ml syringe with 3-way tap closing off the limb to a drainage tube (Fig. 41.20). The syringe is aspirated until full, the 3-way tap is turned to close the limb to the aspiration needle and the contents of the syringe are ejected via the drainage tube into a jug. The 3-way tap is turned to close the limb to the drainage tube and the cycle of aspiration and ejection is repeated. The procedure is stopped when the patient starts to cough — often the case after 1.0–1.5 litres has been removed — or when the aspiration is complete. The patient is told to hold his breath again for a few moments while the needle is withdrawn and the skin puncture site is covered with a sterile dressing.

An alternative, and to some a preferable method, is to insert a small drainage tube which is connected to an underwater sealed drainage system to which gentle suction is applied.

## INTERCOSTAL INTUBATION

Intercostal intubation is performed to drain a large pneumothorax or haemothorax. For the former, the second intercostal space in the mid clavicular line is most suitable and for the latter the ninth intercostal space in the posterior axillary line is preferred. A 'Trocar Catheter' is inserted under sterile conditions. Size 20–26F is suitable for adults, the larger sizes being essential for adequate drainage of blood. The operator scrubs up and wears a gown and gloves. Local anaesthetic is infiltrated widely at the chosen site. The depth at which the pleural space is entered is determined by aspiration with the syringe. A stab incision is made in the skin with a scalpel. The shaft of the catheter is held firmly between the left thumb and index finger some 3 cm higher than the estimated depth of the pleura. This prevents 'overshoot' as the right hand thrusts the trocar and catheter through the chest wall in the chosen interspace into the pleural cavity (Fig. 41.21).

The point of the trocar is directed towards the apex of the pleural cavity. The catheter is then advanced with the left hand while the trocar is

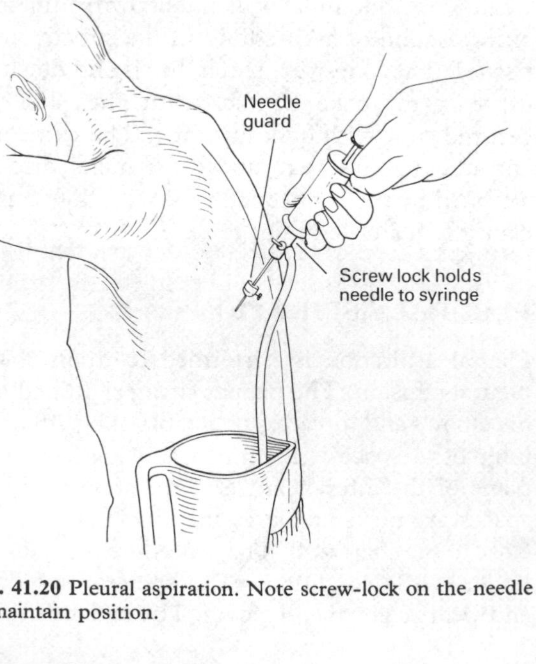

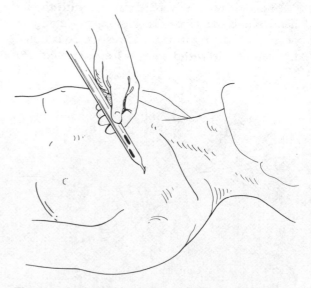

**Fig. 41.20** Pleural aspiration. Note screw-lock on the needle to maintain position.

Needle guard

Screw lock holds needle to syringe

**Fig. 41.21** Intercostal intubation with 'Trocar Catheter'

withdrawn simultaneously with the right hand. The catheter is clamped with a heavy artery forceps. The catheter is then sutured to the skin with a heavy suture to prevent accidental dislodgement. A 'Z' suture is placed loosely in the skin around the emerging catheter. The catheter is connected to a sterile drainage tube which emerges under a waterseal in a drainage bottle (Fig. 41.22). The artery forceps is removed from the catheter and the patient is asked to cough gently to expel much of the air or blood within the chest. The drainage bottle may then be connected to a suction apparatus to maintain a negative pressure of 30–40 mmHg and prevent loculation of air or fluid.

The catheter may be removed 12–24 hours after drainage has ceased, and chest X-ray confirms a well expanded lung. The patient is told to hold his breath for a few moments. An assistant presses the margins of the skin wound against the catheter. The 'Z' suture is held taut, the catheter is removed and the suture is tied firmly. A sterile dressing pad is applied over the sutured wound. A repeat chest X-ray is performed to confirm that air has not entered the pleural cvaity during removal of the catheter.

## LUMBAR PUNCTURE

Lumbar puncture is performed to obtain samples of cerebro-spinal fluid or to insert therapeutic substances or spinal anaesthetic agents. The patient lies on the left side on a firm couch with the spine flexed and the knees drawn up to the abdomen. This position opens up the interspinous spaces. The right shoulder and right hip must lie vertically above the left shoulder and left hip. Lumbar puncture is performed under sterile conditions. The operator scrubs up and wears a gown and gloves.

The patient's skin is prepared with antiseptic solution and draped with sterile towels. The space between the spinous processes of the 3rd and 4th lumbar vertebrae is identified at the point where the vertical line joining the highest points of the iliac crests crosses the spine. Local anaesthetic is infiltrated in this space to a depth of 2–3 cm. A lumbar puncture needle with a central stilette is inserted in the mid line and aimed towards the umbilicus. At a depth of 3–4 cm the dura is pierced. A distinct drop in resistance to the further passage of the needle confirms that it is in the subarachnoid space. The stilette is removed and cerebro-spinal fluid drips out of the needle.

The needle is removed when the procedure is completed and the puncture site is covered with a sterile dressing. The patient must lie flat in bed for the next 24 hours. Severe headache is an indication that cerebro-spinal fluid is leaking through the dura into the epidural space. This is managed by an epidural 'blood patch' — a procedure best performed by an anaesthetist familiar with epidural anaesthetic techniques.

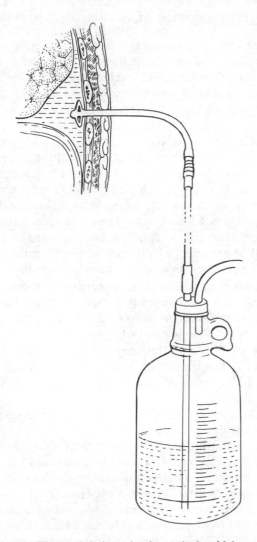

**Fig. 41.22** Waterseal drainage bottle attached to Malecot catheter

## WOUND SUTURE

The operator must practise the techniques of surgical knot tying first with heavy cord and then on patients undergoing elective surgery under general anaesthesia. Thereafter he may consider suturing minor superficial incised lacerations and only later progress to deeper or ragged lacerations. All wounds are thoroughly cleaned with antiseptic solution and a generous volume of local anaesthetic is then infiltrated into the surrounding tissues. Lignocaine 1% is usually used. The maximum dose for adults is 200 mg, so the volume is limited to 20 ml. Lignocaine with adrenaline (1:200 000) may be preferred but must never be used on fingers, toes or penis, as vasoconstriction may cause ischaemic necrosis.

Wounds are sutured under as near sterile conditions as possible, although, in busy casualty departments, it is accepted that gowns are unnecessarily cumbersome and gloves alone will generally suffice. Once the local anaesthetic has become effective, the entire wound is inspected. Incised lacerations present few problems. The layers are usually easily defined and foreign body fragments are uncommon. Ragged lacerations are more difficult. The layers are sometimes difficult to define and foreign body fragments including grit, glass, clothing and hair are common. These are removed and the wound is irrigated with antiseptic solution or with hydrogen peroxide. The irregular margins of all damaged tissue layers are excised leaving healthy regular tissue defects to be sutured.

In the face, excision must be restricted to an absolute minimum.

In suturing wounds, several principles should be followed:

1. Tissues should be handled gently. Rubbing wounds with swabs to remove blood should be avoided — swabs should be *pressed* on to the wound and blood allowed to soak into the swab, which is then removed.

2. Haemostasis should be meticulous.

3. Foreign material or devitalised tissue should be removed. Heavily contaminated wounds are best not sutured primarily but treated by delayed primary or secondary suture.

4. 'Dead' spaces in the wound should be closed using absorbable sutures (catgut or Dexon). If this is not possible, a drain or drains should be led from the dead space prior to closing more superficial layers or, alternatively, the wound left open and subsequently treated by secondary suture or by skin grafting.

5. Sutures should be tied just tight enough to approximate tissues without tension. Excessively tight sutures, or the use of tension to approximate skin or deeper tissues, causes ischaemia of the wound edges, with delay in healing, and an increased risk of wound infection.

## SUTURING THE SKIN

Non-absorbable sutures are generally preferred for skin, and require removal subsequently. Interrupted sutures are preferred, and have the advantage over continuous sutures that, should the wound become infected, removal of one or two appropriately sited stitches may allow adequate drainage of the wound.

The sutures should be placed equidistant from one another, and with equal 'bites' on either side of the wound. A sufficient number of sutures should be inserted to maintain apposition of the skin edges without any gaping between sutures. More than this is unnecessary. The size of bite will be determined by the amount of subcutaneous fat present, and by whether or not the subcutaneous fat has been separately sutured. In the abdomen, the bite is approximately 5 mm on either side of the wound whereas, on the face, a 1 or 2 mm bite is usual. The wound edge is picked up using *toothed* dissecting forceps and the needle introduced through the skin as close to vertical as possible, and brought out on the other side at a similar angle.

Similar principles apply when using a continuous suture.

A subcuticular stitch, inserted as a continuous suture, is preferred by some surgeons, and has the advantage of avoiding the small pinpoint scars at the site of entry and exit of the traditional suture, or the ugly cross hatching that results if sutures are tied too tightly or left in too long.

The following times are normally recommended for removal of sutures:

face and neck — 4 days
scalp — 7 days
abdomen and chest — 7-10 days
limbs — 7 days
feet — 10-14 days

However, cosmetic results as good as those achieved by subcuticular suturing can be obtained by removing sutures in half the above times, and replacing them by adhesive strips (Steristrip, Clearol, etc).

## SUTURE MATERIALS

### Non-absorbable

Non-absorbable sutures fall into three basic categories:

*Natural braided* e.g. silk. This has good 'handling' qualities, and knots easily and securely. It has the disadvantage of causing significant tissue reaction, and is possibly associated with a higher rate of wound infection than synthetic materials.

*Synthetic monofilament* e.g. nylon, prolene. These sutures pass easily through tissues, and cause little tissue reaction. They are, however, rather more difficult to handle than silk, and the knot is rather insecure, so that multiple 'threads' are required to ensure security.

*Braided synthetic* e.g. Mersiline, Ethibond, braided nylon. These sutures attempt to combine the virtues of both the above types, without their disadvantage, and are now the preferred materials for skin suture.

### Absorbable sutures

Absorbable sutures (catgut [plain or chromic], Dexon, Vicryl and PDS are rarely used in skin, apart from in circumcision, where removal of sutures may be uncomfortable for both patient and nurse. They have been recommended for children, who may view the removal of sutures with apprehension, and fail to cooperate, but catgut tends to cause too much tissue reaction and synthetics take too long to be absorbed and fall off. Absorbable sutures are also being used for subcuticular skin closure, although hypertrophic scarring has been reported with this technique.

## SUTURE GUAGE

Very fine sutures (4/0 or 5/0) are recommended for the face, neck, hand and digits. Elsewhere, sutures of 3/0 or 2/0 gauge are used. Sutures of larger than 2/0 gauge are not necessary for skin.

## OTHER TECHNIQUES

### Adhesive strips

Provided that the skin surface around the wound is flat, adhesive strips (Steristrip, Clearol) may be used instead of sutures. The cosmetic effect is good. Such strips may be used to replace sutures after early removal.

### Metal clips or staples

Metal clips (e.g. Michel clips), or staples are used by some surgeons, particularly on thyroid incisions, and are favoured by many gynaecologists. They give a good cosmetic result, but have the disadvantage that they catch easily on clothing, producing discomfort.

### Needles

Needles used in skin suture are cutting needles. Near the point they are triangular in cross section, with one side of the triangle being longer than the other two. When inserting the needle, this longer side should be parallel to the wound edge.

The needles may be hand held, or used with a needle holder. Hand held needles may be straight or curved, while holder designed needles, which are generally smaller, are always curved in varying degrees.

---

## ANTIBIOTICS IN SURGICAL PRACTICE

## PRINCIPLES IN THE USE OF ANTIBIOTICS

Antibiotics reduce mortality and morbidity in surgical practice when used correctly. Their casual or unplanned use, however, may result in the emergence of resistant strains of bacteria in a ward or hospital population. A policy for the use of antibiotics is therefore desirable. It must be kept under regular review because of continuing changes in the patterns of bacterial resistance to antibiotics. In conjunction with a bacteriologist, the resistance patterns of all pathogens isolated from sputum, urine, bile, pus and blood should be recorded over a 6-month period. A policy may then be devised which 'rests' those antibiotics to which resistance is developing. Knowledge of resistance permits more appropriate use of antibiotics in circumstances where it is necessary to give 'blind' treatment, for example, in life threatening infections where antibiotics must be prescribed before the results of culture and sensitivity tests are known. In these circumstances a Gram-stained film of the appropriate specimen may give some idea of the likely infecting organism. In other circumstances the most likely infecting organism must be surmised and therapy started according to the antibiotic policy. The principles behind an antibiotic policy may be summarised as follows:

1. Selection of an antibiotic for an organism which has been shown to be fully sensitive to it.

2. Restriction of the use of antibiotics to which resistance has been demonstrated.

3. Rotation of antibiotics so that exposure of a particular organism to a particular antibiotic is limited.

The following are guidelines when prescribing antibiotics:

1. The spectrum of an antibiotic should be known accurately — a broad spectrum antibiotic is avoided if a narrow spectrum antibiotic is suitable.

2. The most potent antibiotics are reserved for life-threatening infections.

3. Antibiotics which may be used systemically are not used topically.

4. Antibiotics are given in full dose and at the correct intervals.

5. Bacteriological proof of the eradication of pathogenic organisms is obtained at the end of treatment.

6. Except in one or two rate sites (e.g. lung abscesses) antibiotics are not used to treat abscesses as an alternative to surgical drainage.

7. The side effects of antibiotics should be known and monitored.

8. Expensive antibiotics are not used where equally effective cheaper alternatives are suitable.

## EMERGENCY USE OF ANTIBIOTICS

### Chest infection

In chest infection the most common pathogens are *Streptococcus pneumoniae* and *Haemophilus influenzae*. Both are sensitive to ampicillin, erythromycin, cotrimoxazole and cephalosporins. Other chest pathogens are *Staphylococcus aureus*, *E. coli*, *Klebsiella pneumoniae* and *Pseudomonas*. Generally, these should be treated only when they have been grown from sputum and are considered to be truly pathogenic. In many instances they simply represent a 'replacement' flora after antibiotic treatment of other conditions. If time does not permit sensitivity testing and these organisms are causing life-threatening chest infection, *Staphylococcus* should be treated with flucloxacillin, *E. coli* and *Klebsiella* with gentamicin and *Pseudomonas* with tobramycin or mezlocillin.

### Acute urinary tract infection

In acute urinary tract infection, *E. coli* or other coliforms are the causative organisms in about 80% of cases. Cotrimoxazole is the drug of choice. For severe pyelonephritis or septicaemia caused by urinary infection, gentamicin is preferred.

### Wound infection

Wound infections normally do not require antibiotic treatment but spreading cellulitis around a wound is the exception. After clean operations, cellulitis is normally caused by streptococci and benzyl penicillin is the antibiotic of choice. After operations on the gastro-intestinal tract, cellulitis may be caused by anaerobic streptococci or bacteroides and metronidazole with penicillin is preferred. Frank wound abscesses require surgical drainage.

## Peritonitis

In peritonitis the infecting flora initially depends on the level of the alimentary tract from which the condition originates. Coliforms, streptococci and staphylococci predominate when the source of peritonitis is in the upper alimentary tract and anaerobic streptococci and bacteroides predominate when the source of peritonitis is in the lower alimentary tract. As time elapses the whole spectrum of bacteria is involved in the peritoneal infection. In early cases it may be acceptable to choose a relatively limited antibiotic cover but in most instances 'complete spectrum' cover with gentamicin and clindamycin or with gentamicin, metronidazole and penicillin is the best treatment.

## Septicaemia

In septicaemia 'complete spectrum' cover is indicated (as in peritonitis above) until the causative organism and its sensitivity have been defined from blood cultures.

# PROPHYLACTIC USE OF ANTIBIOTICS

The prophylactic use of antibiotics is established in the following situations:

## Chronic bronchitis

Patients with chronic bronchitis subject to intermittent exacerbations are given prophylactic antibiotics. Ampicillin, cotrimoxazole or tetracycline are suitable. They are commenced shortly before operation and continued for several days afterwards.

## Tetanus

Patients with accidental wounds which have the potential risk of infection with *Clostridium tetani* are given prophylaxis described on page 65. The wounds are treated by meticulous debridement or, if delayed, by excision.

## Gas gangrene

Patients with ischaemic limbs which require amputation are at considerable risk of developing gas gangrene. Benzyl penicillin is given one hour pre-operatively and continued 6-hourly for 3–5 days.

## Meningitis

Patients with compound skull fractures and technically compound basal skull fractures involving the paranasal sinuses, the mastoid air cells or the middle ear are at risk of developing meningitis. Ampicillin and flucloxacillin is given for several days, or for basal fractures, until cerebro-spinal fluid rhinorrhoea or otorrhoea ceases.

## Prevention of endocarditis

Patients with congenital, rheumatic and degenerative valve disease, septal defects, or prosthetic heart valves are at risk of bacterial colonisation during bacteraemia and are given prophylactic antibiotics. For dental treatment outside hospital, amoxycillin 3 g orally one hour before treatment is more convenient than intra-muscular penicillin. For dental treatment in hospital, benzyl penicillin 1 g and gentamicin 80 mg intra-muscularly are suggested. For minor surgery involving the gastro-intestinal or genito-urinary tract, ampicillin 1 g and gentamicin 80 mg are given intra-muscularly one hour before operation. For cardiac surgery, flucloxacillin 500 mg and gentamicin 80 mg are given intravenously just before skin incision, 8-hourly for 24 hours, and one hour before removal of chest drains.

## Gastrointestinal and genito-urinary surgery

Patients undergoing gastro-intestinal and genito-urinary surgery, whether elective or emergency, are at risk of wound infection, intra-abdominal infection and septicaemia. Many methods have been advocated in the past decade to reduce this. A single large dose of antibiotic appropriate for the predicted bacterial flora, administered intravenously on induction of anaesthesia is probably the most convenient and effective method. In particularly contaminated surgery and in emergency surgery, three additional doses 8-hourly post-operatively may confer further benefit. Antibiotic lavage of the operative field and the incision is another rational approach to prophylaxis though not as yet widely practised.

### Prosthetic implants

Prophylactic antibiotics are obligatory when any prosthetic material is inserted. Staphylococcal infection is the most serious problem if prophylaxis is omitted in, for example, heart valve replacement, cardiac pacemaker insertion, ventriculo-venous shunts, aortic graft, joint prostheses, mammary prostheses or polypropylene mesh repairs of massive abdominal wall defects. However, other bacteria may also be involved and a more 'complete spectrum' cover immediately pre-operatively and 8-hourly post-operatively for 24 hours is usually given.

### Immune suppressed patients

Patients who have suppression of their immune mechanisms, either as a result of disease, or as a result of therapy (e.g. transplant patients) should receive antibiotic prophylaxis when undergoing surgery. The choice of antibiotic will be dictated by the type of operation as outlined in the preceding paragraph.

## MEDICO-LEGAL PROBLEMS

Surgeons, more than any other medical practitioners, are confronted in every day practice by medico-legal problems.

## CONSENT TO TREATMENT

A doctor may not force his recommendations onto a patient. Treatment performed without consent may amount to assault and result in litigation. In every instance, the patient should be given as much information about proposed treatment as the doctor considers to be in his best interest. For minor procedures, verbal consent is adequate but, for operative procedures, written consent must be obtained. The nature and purpose of the proposed operation are explained to the patient by a doctor. The patient is then asked to sign a consent form which the doctor countersigns. For patients under the age of 16 years, written informed consent of the parent or guardian is obtained.

If immediate treatment is necessary to save the patient's life, verbal consent is acceptable. When the patient's condition does not allow even this, the proposed treatment should be discussed with a near relative but if no-one is readily available, the patient should be given whatever treatment is immediately necessary.

If a patient is compulsorily detained under the Mental Health Act, treatment immediately necessary to preserve life and health may be given without consent. For all other procedures, the informed written consent of the patient should be obtained before an operation is performed. If the patient is unable or unwilling to give his consent to a non-urgent operation, it should not be performed. If this prohibition jeopardises the patient's health, the surgeon and psychiatrist should act in good faith and in the best interests of the patient.

Patients with mental illness who are not compulsorily detained under the Mental Health Act have exactly the same rights as the ordinary patient.

Jehovah's Witnesses who consent to operation but refuse to consent to transfusion of blood or blood products place the surgeon in a dilemma. If the surgeon agrees to the limitations set by the patient, a conditional consent form which is prepared by the Defence Societies, should be signed by the patient and countersigned by the surgeon and a witness. In an acute life-threatening situation he must take such action as he believes necessary to preserve life.

## THE OPERATION

### Pre-operative examination

Every patient about to have an operation under general anaesthesia must be examined pre-operatively. The responsibility for this may rest with either the surgical staff or the anaesthetic staff. The declared policy of the individual surgical unit should be known to all staff working in it. The history should include a list of previous operations and previous anaesthetics (noting any untoward reactions to either), past history and a systematic enquiry including current drugs and known allergies. In addition to full physical examination, urinalysis must always be performed. Full blood count, chest X-ray and ECG are prudent for all but the shortest examinations under anaesthetic and supplementary respiratory function tests and arterial blood gas analysis may be relevant in patients about to undergo major surgery. The decision whether or not a patient is fit for anaesthetic and the proposed operation rests with the anaesthetist and the surgeon in consultation.

### Pre-medication

Ideally the pre-medication should be ordered directly by the anaesthetist. In many instances, however, local policy dictates that the surgical staff prescribe the pre-medication. The anaesthetist should be consulted if there is any doubt about the drug or the dose to be given.

### Safeguards against wrong operations

Performing a wrong operation or operating on the wrong patient is both avoidable and indefensible. A series of safeguards to prevent these disasters has been recommended by the Defence Societies. In summary they are:

1. All patients wear identity bracelets including forenames, surname and hospital number. This is checked when the patients is sent to theatre. In a paediatric ward the identity bracelet is of the type which cannot be removed by the child.

2. The operation list shows the patient's full name, hospital number and the nature of the operation.

3. Patients are sent for by name and number by the senior nurse in the operating theatre.

4. The anaesthetist checks that the correct patient has been brought to the anaesthetic room.

5. The surgeon sees the patient and reviews the case notes before the anaesthetic is commenced.

The following safeguards are recommended to prevent an operation on the wrong side, limb or digit:

1. The side to be operated on is marked by the surgeon with an indelible ink before the patient comes to theatre.

2. The words right and left are written in full in the patient's notes and on the operation list.

3. To avoid ambiguity in describing digits, the fingers are described as thumb, index, middle, ring and little finger and the toes are described as great, 2nd, 3rd, 4th and little toe.

### DISCHARGE AGAINST MEDICAL ADVICE

When a patient decides to discharge himself from hospital and the doctor feels that discharge is not in the best interests of the patient, the reasons for this advice are clearly explained. The patient is asked to sign a form which indicates that he is voluntarily taking his own discharge from hospital against the advice of his doctor. His signature on this form is witnessed by two persons. The general practitioner is informed about the patient's discharge from hospital, his condition and any further treatment which is considered advisable.

When the patient has a mental illness, the doctor may feel that there are grounds for compulsory detention under the Mental Health Act. The mental welfare officer is contacted. If he agrees that detention under the Act is in the best interests of the patient or society, he will make application to the Court for formal admission to a Mental Hospital and compulsory detention.

### CONFIRMATION OF DEATH

It is the statutory duty of the doctor who has attended the deceased during his last illness to supply a death certificate to the Registrar of Deaths. Although a certificate may be issued if the body has not been seen after death, it is desirable that identification and examination are performed. The pupils are tested for reaction to light. The precordium is auscultated for heart sounds, and the optic fundus is inspected with an ophthalmoscope for fragmentation of blood in the retinal vessels.

There are circumstances in which a death certificate should not be issued until the death has been reported to the coroner in England and

Wales or the procurator fiscal in Scotland. These include sudden death when the doctor has not seen the patient before, or in England and Wales when a doctor has not attended the deceased within 14 days of death; death after trauma or neglect or in suspicious, unnatural or violent circumstances; death during an operation or before recovery from an anaesthetic; death within 24 hours of admission to hospital; deaths about which complaints or litigation may be expected.

If the doctor is in any doubt about issuing a death certificate, he should discuss the matter first with the coroner or procurator fiscal.

## CREMATION

Before a cremation may take place, two medical certificates are required — forms B and C. Form B is completed by the usual medical attendant of the deceased or the doctor signing the death certificate. Form C is completed by a medical practitioner of at least 5 years standing who is neither a relative of the deceased, nor a partner of the doctor completing Form B. A fee is payable for each certificate.

## REMOVAL OF TISSUES FOR TRANSPLANTATION

Under the Human Tissues Act of 1961, a registered doctor who is satisfied that life is extinct, may remove the required organ for transplantation provided either the deceased had requested in writing or orally in front of two witnesses that his body be used for therapeutic purposes, medical education or research *or* the person in possession of the body is satisfied that the deceased expressed no objection and the next of kin have no objection to removal of tissues for transplantation.

The increasing use of life support systems which maintain respiratory function for patients suffering very severe head injury or spontaneous intra-cerebral catastrophe has resulted in the definition of stringent criteria of 'brain death'. When these criteria have been confirmed independently by two senior doctors, withdrawal of the life support system may be considered after discussion with the patient's next of kin.

Members of transplant teams should not be involved in these decisions. If the relatives are favourably disposed towards tissue transplantation, organs may be removed before the life support system is disconnected.

## CLINICAL RESEARCH

Clinical research presents moral and ethical problems rather than legal ones. Proposed research projects should be presented in detail to the Hospital Ethics Committee. Approval may be expected when the research project has a direct bearing on the illness for which the patient is being treated and does not involve additional invasive or painful investigations. Ethical criteria are stricter when the research project may contribute to the advancement of knowledge but is of no immediate benefit to the patient. Nevertheless, approval is usually given provided there is no unnecessary pain and no risk to the patient's health or well-being. If ethical doubt persists, the matter is referred to a Defence Society.

Informed verbal consent is always obtained from the patient and written consent is prudent in all but the simplest projects.

## LABORATORY REQUESTS AND REPORTS

Great care must be taken in labelling and completing all laboratory request forms and in labelling specimen containers. Inappropriate advice may result from incorrect information on the request forms, incorrect or insufficient samples, or by sending the request form for one patient with the specimen from another patient. The greatest potential hazard is in blood transfusion where labelling errors may result in a fatal incompatible blood transfusion. Before blood transfusion is commenced, the patient's name, hospital number, date of birth, blood group and number on each unit of blood are checked at the patient's bedside to ensure that they correspond on the laboratory form and on the blood bag label. This is confirmed by a second observer.

Laboratory reports must be scrutinised and acted upon without undue delay and individual surgical units must define policies to ensure that important information is not overlooked. Important outstanding reports may be available by telephone from laboratories at certain times and so permit earlier treatment of critically ill patients than is achieved by awaiting the 'routine' arrival of the written report. Such communications should be made directly to the ward doctor or alternatively written in a book specially identified for this purpose.

## CONFIDENTIALITY

The professional relationship between a doctor and his patient is based on the understanding that information given to the doctor in his professional capacity is confidential. There are, however, instances in which breach of professional secrecy is justified. In Court, a doctor may be directed to divulge information. He may request that this information is disclosed in writing but if this is overruled, failure to comply risks prosecution for contempt of court. Professional secrecy may also be breached when a doctor feels he has a duty to protect the patient or an innocent third party from avoidable harm. There are three common situations in which this problem arises.

The first is fitness to drive a motor vehicle. If, for example, a patient is subject to fainting or fits or to a lack of motor coordination which will impair his ability to drive safely, efforts should be made to persuade him to notify the licencing authority. The introduction of the driving licence valid until the 70th birthday placed a great burden of responsibility on the driver to report any disability and an equal burden of responsibility on the doctor to persuade him to do so. If the patient does not agree to divulge the information himself, it is considered ethical for the doctor to disclose it to the licencing authority.

The second is non-accidental injury to children. When a doctor suspects he is dealing with non-accidental injury to a child, it is considered ethical to disclose confidential information. Health authorities should be able to investigate actual or possible cases of non-accidental injury to children. If this service is not available, the childrens officer of the local authority, or the officers of the National Society for the Prevention of Cruelty to Children, are appropriate persons to inform. The doctor should advise the parents that it is in the interests of the child to disclose clinical information to the appropriate authority and that it is preferable to do so with their agreement.

The third is police investigation of a crime. A doctor may be asked to divulge information given in confidence. Only if it clearly appears to be in the interests of public safety to do so should the information be given. In doubtful cases, the prudent doctor will consult his Defence Society.

In all other circumstances, requests for confidential information should be denied unless the patient has given informed written consent.

## NOTIFIABLE DISEASES

All doctors must remember that certain diseases are by statute notifiable to health authorities. In surgical wards anthrax, dysentery, erysipilas, food poisoning and tuberculosis are most likely to be suspected.

All cases of diarrhoea of undetermined cause; of gas gangrene and clostridial wound infections; and patients with suspected serum hepatitis should be reported to the hospital infection officer without delay. So also should any unusual 'runs' of wound or other infections in the ward.

## THE POLICE

There are frequent occasions in surgical practice when the doctor comes into contact with the police. Even when the police are acting in the interests of the patient, information should only be disclosed with the consent of the patient. As has been stated previously, the doctor may be faced with difficult decisions when the police are investigating a crime by the patient. The duty of the doctor in possession of information which might assist the police in their pursuit of a criminal is not clear in law and must be left to individual conscience and judgement. In most circumstances the doctor will seek guidance from his defence society before divulging to the police information received in professional confidence. However, when the nature of the crime is extreme or the potential dangers to society are great, the doctor may feel that these factors take precedence over the rules of professional secrecy.

When an in-patient is in police custody, it is usual for a police officer to remain with him during his stay in hospital. When there is not an accompanying police officer, the police may request information about time of discharge of the patient from hospital and this should be given. When a patient is brought to hospital after a road traffic accident, the question of driving under the influence of alcohol frequently arises. The police may request a blood sample for blood alcohol analysis. The doctor in charge should satisfy himself that neither the request for the sample nor the actual taking of it will be prejudicial to the patient's condition. The sample should not be taken by the hospital staff but by the police surgeon. Blood taken by a hospital doctor from an unconscious patient as part of the routine admission investigations should not be made available to the police. If requested, it may be preserved in the hospital and released later if the patient or his legal representative consent.

## COURT APPEARANCE

Most doctors will at some time be required to appear in court. For the junior doctor it will usually be as a witness to fact, having been involved in the care of the patient in the case. For the senior doctor it will usually be as an expert witness whose specialised knowledge is such that he is called solely to express his opinion.

Legible and comprehensive notes must be made when treating any patient whose case is likely to result in legal proceedings. They must be referred to before appearance so that a clear knowledge of the facts is available.

Divulgence of professional confidence in court evidence is considered under 'confidentiality'.

## CLINICAL RECORDS

The importance of accurate and legible clinical records in hospital practice cannot be over-emphasised. Complaints against hospital doctors frequently allege that clinical examinations have been omitted or have been cursory or claim that wrong treatment has been given. Oral evidence to refute this is more likely to impress the court if it is backed up by a contemporary entry in the clinical notes. It should be remembered that in the event of a complaint against a doctor, a court may require the case records to be examined by the medical advisors of the complainant. Thus facetious or rude entries should never be made in case notes.

Case notes remain the property of the Secretary of State, but as indicated above there are occasions in which a court may order compulsory disclosure of clinical notes. In such instances the applicant issues a summons to the doctor or hospital accompanied by written evidence to justify the application. The doctor or hospital may then request a hearing at which the arguments for and against the production of case notes are heard. If the court orders the production of the case notes they are disclosed to the applicant's medical advisors only and not to his legal advisors or to the applicant himself. Whenever such applications are made, the doctor should seek advice from his defence society immediately.

## PROFESSIONAL NEGLIGENCE

Negligence may be defined as a failure to display the competence and to exercise the care which might reasonably be expected of the doctor and which results in damage to the patient. Two common examples which affect junior hospital doctors are prescribing an antibiotic for a patient who is known to be hypersensitive to it and failing to X-ray a patient in whom there is clinical doubt about bone injury. More obvious examples of negligence are operation on the wrong patient, limb or digit.

When a letter of complaint is received from a patient or his lawyer, the case notes are carefully perused and a factual report about the case is made. Copies are sent first to the doctor's defence society and to the hospital legal advisor. A further copy is retained by the doctor. All correspondence including the letters of complaint, threats of proceedings or claims for compensation are forwarded to the defence society. If the incident involved an instrument, needle, swab or foreign body, this should not be discarded.

# Index